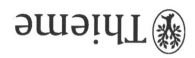

Experimental Research Methods in Orthopedics and Trauma

Hamish Simpson, DM (Oxon), MA (Cantab), FRCS (Edinburgh & England)
Professor of Orthopedic Surgery
Department of Orthopaedics and Trauma
University of Edinburgh
Edinburgh, United Kingdom

Peter Augat, PhD
Professor of Biomechanics
Paracelsus Medical University
Salzburg, Austria

Director
Institute of Biomechanics
Trauma Center Murnau
Murnau am Staffelsee, Germany

257 illustrations

Thieme
Stuttgart • New York • Delhi • Rio de Janeiro

Library of Congress Cataloging-in-Publication Data

Simpson, A. Hamish R. W., author.
Experimental research methods in orthopedics and
   trauma / Hamish Simpson, Peter Augat.
      p. ; cm.
Includes bibliographica references and index.
ISBN 978-3-13-173111-1 (alk. paper) – ISBN 978-3-13-
173121-0 (eISBN)
I. Augat, Peter, author. II. Title.
[DNLM: 1. Biomedical Research. 2. Orthopedics–methods.
3. Biomechanical Phenomena. 4. Musculoskeletal Diseases.
5. Orthopedic Procedures–methods. WE 20]
   RD732
   616.7'027–dc23

                                        2014019935

© 2015 by Georg Thieme Verlag KG

Thieme Publishers Stuttgart
Rüdigerstrasse 14, 70469 Stuttgart, Germany
+49 [0]711 8931 421, customerservice@thieme.de

Thieme Publishers New York
333 Seventh Avenue, New York, NY 10001 USA
+1 800 782 3488, customerservice@thieme.com

Thieme Publishers Delhi
A-12, Second Floor, Sector-2, Noida-201301
Uttar Pradesh, India
+91 120 45 566 00, customerservice@thieme.in

Thieme Publishers Rio de Janeiro, Thieme Publicações Ltda.
Edifício Rodolpho de Paoli, 25° andar
Av. Nilo Peçanha, 50 – Sala 2508,
Rio de Janeiro 20020-906 Brasil
Tel: +55 21 3172-2297 / +55 21 3172-1896

Cover design: Thieme Publishing Group
Typesetting by DiTech

Printed in Germany by Aprinta   5 4 3 2 1

ISBN 978-3-13-173111-1

Also available as an e-book:
eISBN 978-3-13-173121-0

Important note: Medicine is an ever-changing science undergoing continual development. Research and clinical experience are continually expanding our knowledge, in particular our knowledge of proper treatment and drug therapy. Insofar as this book mentions any dosage or application, readers may rest assured that the authors, editors, and publishers have made every effort to ensure that such references are in accordance with **the state of knowledge at the time of production of the book.**

Nevertheless, this does not involve, imply, or express any guarantee or responsibility on the part of the publishers in respect to any dosage instructions and forms of applications stated in the book. **Every user is requested to examine carefully** the manufacturers' leaflets accompanying each drug and to check, if necessary in consultation with a physician or specialist, whether the dosage schedules mentioned therein or the contraindications stated by the manufacturers differ from the statements made in the present book. Such examination is particularly important with drugs that are either rarely used or have been newly released on the market. Every dosage schedule or every form of application used is entirely at the user's own risk and responsibility. The authors and publishers request every user to report to the publishers any discrepancies or inaccuracies noticed. If errors in this work are found after publication, errata will be posted at www.thieme.com on the product description page.

Some of the product names, patents, and registered designs referred to in this book are in fact registered trademarks or proprietary names even though specific reference to this fact is not always made in the text. Therefore, the appearance of a name without designation as proprietary is not to be construed as a representation by the publisher that it is in the public domain.

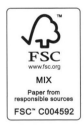

Contents

Contents

Foreword

Advances in basic research ultimately drive advancements in clinical care. When we as orthopedic surgeons contemplate the treatments available to us today in comparison to those a generation ago we readily appreciate that the effectiveness of our diagnostic and therapeutic armamentarium greatly exceeds that of our predecessors. This is driven in large part by technological advances in imaging, biomechanics, molecular biology, nanotechnology, and bioinformatics. While progress has been real, it can be argued that orthopedic surgery is somewhat behind the curve in translating these basic advances to improvements in clinical practice. Thus, the publication of this book on experimental research methods is particularly timely. The editors have compiled a series of contributions from a group of interdisciplinary scientists with expertise in a broad array of scientific disciplines. This expertise has been brought to bear in developing a comprehensive volume on state-of-the-art research methodologies that can be applied to improvement in the care of patients with musculoskeletal injuries. This volume will be of value not only to basic researchers, but also to clinician scientists who are on the front lines of musculoskeletal research. In addition, this volume will be an important resource for orthopedic surgical trainees who need to learn the basics of experimental methodology so that they have the tools to interpret the orthopedic literature in their professional lives. *Experimental Research Methods in Orthopedics and Trauma* is a valuable contribution to our specialty.

Joshua J. Jacobs, MD
Professor and Chairman
Department of Orthopaedic Surgery
Rush University Medical Center
Chicago, Illinois, United States

Endorsement by the International Combined Orthopaedic Research Societies (I-CORS) Member Organizations

We are delighted that a book covering the spectrum of research methodologies in trauma and orthopaedics has been produced. The diverse specialties of the contributors and their wide geographical spread will ensure that the reader is presented with a comprehensive analysis of the available techniques. We consider that researchers commencing a musculoskeletal research project will find this book a very useful starting point.

Constituent Members

Jiake Xu, MD, PhD
Australia & New Zealand Orthopaedic Research
    Society

Andrew McCaskie, MB, ChB, MMus, MD, FRCS, FRCS
    (T&O)
British Orthopaedic Research Society

John Antoniou, MD, PhD, FRCSC
Canadian Orthopaedic Research Society

Steven Boyd, PhD
Canadian Orthopaedic Research Society

Ling Qin, PhD
Chinese Orthopaedic Research Society

Gang Li, PhD
Chinese Orthopaedic Research Society

Ting ting Tang, MD, PhD
Chinese Orthopaedic Research Society

Nicola Baldini, MD, PhD
European Orthopaedic Research Society

Nobuo Adachi, MD
Chairperson of Committee on International Affairs
Japanese Orthopaedic Association

Gun-Il Im, MD
Korean Orthopaedic Research Society

Theodore Miclau, MD, Chair, ICORS
Orthopaedic Research Society

Je-Ken Chang, MD
Taiwanese Orthopaedic Research Society

Oscar Kuang Sheng Lee, MD
Taiwanese Orthopaedic Research Society

Associate Scientific Members

R. Geoff Richards, PhD, FBSE
AO Foundation

X. Ed Guo, PhD
International Chinese Musculoskeletal Research
    Society (ICMRS)

Candidate Members

Suresh Sivananthan, MD
Asean Pacific Orthopaedic Research Society

Feza Korkusuz, MD,
Turkish Orthopaedic Research Council

Gautum Shetty, MS
Indian Orthopaedic Research Society

Preface

Medical science flourishes when it is carried out as a multi-disciplinary endeavour. To achieve this, medical scientists apply research methods from numerous scientific disciplines to unravel clinical problems. With the rapid development of science, the available research methods have become more varied, intricate and often more difficult to understand. Therefore, the medical scientist faces the challenge of choosing from a range of highly ingenious research tools and understanding their application for their own research endeavour. In addition, the interested reader of medical research papers is sometimes faced with mystifying descriptions of continuously developing research methodologies and need to have these elucidated.

This book on experimental research methodologies is compiled by scientists from numerous disciplines, but all of whom have a common interest in musculoskeletal science. Orthopaedic surgeons, musculoskeletal physicians, biologists, engineers, physicists and mathematicians have composed a total of 54 chapters on research methodologies in musculoskeletal science. The general strategy for translational research involves defining a research question from a clinical problem, carrying out experiments to answer this question and then applying the findings back to the patient. The research question may be best answered with a patient investigation, an in vivo model, a cell culture experiment, a biomechanical measurement study, or a mathematical in silico model. This book provides a comprehensive summary of up-to-date research methodologies across this spectrum of types of study and is dedicated to the medical scientist interested in interdisciplinary research. While each chapter has been written by a specialist in the respective field, the aim has been to educate and teach the medical scientist who needs a comprehensive introduction. Thus, reading a chapter from this book will introduce you to the respective field and enable you to understand the research methodology and the findings obtained with its application, but will not necessarily enable you to accomplish a very specialized research task. Our book will also provide you with abundant practical advice and explanations of key terminology. This will familiarize you with each research area and will facilitate your participation in research activities.

Hamish Simpson
Peter Augat

Acknowledgments

The OTC Foundation would like to thank sincerely all contributors to this book: the OTC Research Committee who conceptualized its scope and content, the chapter authors who made available their knowledge and donated their time, and the editors and section editors who accompanied the shaping of the book from its beginnings to its final presentation. Volker Alt, Taco Blokhuis, Kurt Hankenson, Gabby Joseph, Thomas Link, Chuanyong Lu, and Esther van Lieshout are specially thanked for section editing of the book.

The editors are greatly indebted to Vivien Gourlay and Sandra Augat who assisted them in managing the preparatory process with diligence, dedication, and patience.

The OTC Foundation is also grateful to Stryker for a research grant, which made this book possible.

Richard Helmer
Managing Editor
OTC Foundation

Contributors

Rana Abou-Khalil
Senior Research Fellow
INSERM UMR1163
Université Paris Descartes-Sorbonne Paris Cité
Institut Imagine
Hôpital Necker-Enfants Malades
Paris, France

Kishan Victoria Aldridge, BSc(Hons), MBChB(Hons), MRCS(Ed), MSc
ECAT Clinical Lecturer University of Edinburgh
MRC Human Genetics Unit
The MRC Institute of Genetics and Molecular Medicine
The University of Edinburgh
Western General Hospital
Edinburgh, Scotland, United Kingdom

Roland Aldridge, PhD
Clinical Lecturer and Honorary Special Registrar in General Surgery
Department of Clinical Surgery
The University of Edinburgh
Edinburgh, Scotland, United Kingdom

Volker Alt, MD, PhD
Deputy Clinic Director
Department of Orthopaedic Trauma Surgery
University Hospital Giessen-Marburg GmbH, Campus Giessen
Justus-Liebig-University Giessen
Giessen, Germany

Andrew A. Amis, Prof. FREng, DSc(Eng)
Professor of Orthopaedic Biomechanics
Department of Mechanical Engineering
Imperial College London
London, United Kingdom

Richard van Arkel, MEng
Imperial College London
Department of Mechanical Engineering
London, United Kingdom

Peter Augat, PhD
Professor of Biomechanics
Paracelsus Medical University
Salzburg, Austria
Director
Institute of Biomechanics
Trauma Center Murnau
Murnau am Staffelsee, Germany

Astrid D. Bakker, PhD
Associate Professor
Department of Oral Cell Biology
Academic Centre for Dentistry Amsterdam (ACTA)
University of Amsterdam and VU University Amsterdam
MOVE Research Institute Amsterdam
Amsterdam, The Netherlands

Spencer Behr, MD, PhD
Assistant Professor
Department of Radiology and Biomedical Imaging
University of California San Francisco (UCSF)
San Francisco, California, United States

Pinaki Bhattacharya, PhD
KU Leuven - University of Leuven
Department of Mechanical Engineering
Leuven, Belgium

Taco Johan Blokhuis, PhD
Department of Surgery/Traumatology
Utrecht University Medical Center
Utrecht, The Netherlands

Torsten Blunk, PhD
Department of Trauma, Hand, Plastic and Reconstructive Surgery
University of Würzburg
Würzburg, Germany

Gordon William Blunn, PhD
John Scales Centre for Biomedical Engineering
Institute of Orthopaedics and Musculoskeletal Science
Division of Surgery and Interventional Science
University College London
Royal National Orthopaedic Hospital
Middlesex, United Kingdom

Joseph Borrelli, Jr, MD
Orthopedic Surgeon
Texas Health Physicians Group
Texas Health Arlington Memorial Hospital
Arlington, Texas, United States

Nathalie Bravenboer
Senior Researcher
Department of Clinical Chemistry
MOVE Research Institute Amsterdam
VU University Medical Center
Amsterdam, The Netherlands

Wing-Hoi Cheung, PhD
Associate Professor
Department of Orthopaedics and Traumatology
The Chinese University of Hong Kong
Shatin, Hong Kong, China

Simon Kwoon Ho Chow, BSc, MSc, PhD
Department of Orthopaedics and Traumatology
The Chinese University of Hong Kong
Shaitin, Hong Kong, China

Nicholas Clement
Department of Orthopaedics and Trauma
Edinburgh University
Edinburgh, Scotland, United Kingdom

Melanie Jean Coathup
Senior Lecturer in Orthopaedics
John Scales Centre for Biomedical Engineering
Institute of Orthopaedics and Musculoskeletal Science
Division of Surgery and Interventional Science
University College London
Royal National Orthopaedic Hospital
Middlesex, United Kingdom

Céline Colnot, PhD
INSERM UMR1163
Université Paris Descartes-Sorbonne Paris Cité
Institut Imagine
Hôpital Necker-Enfants Malades
Paris, France

Luca Cristofolini, PhD
Professor of Biomechanics
Department of Industrial Engineering
School of Engineering and Architecture
University of Bologna
Bologna, Italy

Dieter R. Dannhorn, PhD
Owner and General Manager
Dr Dannhorn Consulting and More
Erolzheim, Germany

Hannah Darton
PhD Student
Imperial College London
Department of Mechanical Engineering
South Kensington Campus
London, United Kingdom

Marcel Dijkgraaf, PhD
Consultant in Clinical Research Methodology and
  Statistics
Clinical Research Unit
Academic Medical Center Amsterdam
Amsterdam, The Netherlands

Lutz Dürselen, PhD
Professor of Biomechanics
Head of Joint Biomechanics Research Group
Institute of Orthopaedic Research and Biomechanics
Centre of Musculoskeletal Research Ulm
Ulm University
Ulm, Germany

Sebastian Eberle, PhD
Computational Engineer
KRP-Mechatec Engineering GbR
Munich, Germany

Regina Ebert, PD PhD
Orthopedic Center for Musculoskeletal Research
University of Würzburg
Würzburg, Germany

Nan van Geloven, PhD
Biostatistician
Clinical Research Unit
Academic Medical Center Amsterdam
Amsterdam, The Netherlands

Allen Edward Goodship, BVSc, PhD, MRCVS
Emeritus Professor of Orthopaedics
John Scales Centre for Biomedical Engineering
Institute of Orthopaedics and Musculoskeletal Science
Division of Surgery and Interventional Science
University College London
Royal National Orthopaedic Hospital
Middlesex, United Kingdom

Rob de Haan, PhD
Professor of Clinical Epidemiology
Clinical Research Unit
Academic Medical Center Amsterdam
Amsterdam, The Netherlands

Camilla Halewood, MEng, MBiomedE
Biomechanical Engineer
Department of Mechanical Engineering
Imperial College London
London, United Kingdom

David Hamilton, PhD
Department of Orthopaedics
University of Edinburgh
Edinburgh, Scotland, United Kingdom

Kurt D. Hankenson, DVM, PhD
Associate Professor
Department of Physiology
Associate Director
Laboratory for Comparative Orthopedic Research
Michigan State University
East Lansing, Michigan, United States

Markus O. Heller, PhD
Professor of Biomechanics
University of Southampton
Bioengineering Science Research Group
Faculty of Engineering and the Environment
Southampton, United Kingdom

Christoph Henkenberens
Department of Trauma Surgery
University Hospital Giessen-Marburg GmbH,
Campus Giessen, Germany
Laboratory of Experimental Trauma Surgery,
Justus-Liebig-University
Giessen, Germany

Safa Herfat, PhD
Orthopaedic Trauma Institute
Department of Orthopaedic Surgery
University of California at San Francisco
San Francisco General Hospital
San Francisco, California, United States

Paul Hindle, MBChB, MRCS (Eng), RAF
Trauma and Orthopaedic Registrar
The Royal Infirmary of Edinburgh
Edinburgh, Scotland, United Kingdom

Timothy M. Jackman
Department of Biomedical Engineering
Boston University
Boson, Massachusetts, United States

Franz Jakob, Prof. Dr.
Orthopedic Center for Musculoskeletal Research
Orthopedic Department
University of Würzburg
Würzburg, Germany

Ineke D.C. Jansen, PhD
Department of Periodontology
Academic Centre for Dentistry Amsterdam (ACTA)
University of Amsterdam and VU University Amsterdam
MOVE Research Institute Amsterdam
Amsterdam, The Netherlands

Richard T. Jaspers, PhD
Assistant Professor
Laboratory for Myology
MOVE Research Institute Amsterdam
Faculty of Human Movement Sciences
VU University Amsterdam
Amsterdam, The Netherlands

Paul J. Jenkins, MBChB, MRCS(Ed)
Consultant Orthopaedic Surgeon
Glasgow Royal Infirmary
Glasgow, Scotland, United Kingdom

Gabby B. Joseph, PhD
Musculoskeletal and Quantitative Imaging Research Group
Department of Radiology and Biomedical Imaging
University of California San Francisco
San Francisco, California, United States

Petra Juffer, PhD
Department of Oral Cell Biology
Academic Centre for Dentistry Amsterdam (ACTA)
University of Amsterdam and VU University Amsterdam
MOVE Research Institute Amsterdam
Amsterdam, The Netherlands

Christian Kaddick, PhD
EndoLab
Mechanical Engineering GmbH
Rosenheim, Germany

Grace Kim, PhD
Sibley School of Mechanical & Aerospace Engineering
Cornell University
Ithaca, New York, United States

Jenneke Klein-Nulend, PhD
Professor
Department of Oral Cell Biology
Academic Centre for Dentistry Amsterdam (ACTA)
University of Amsterdam and VU University Amsterdam
MOVE Research Institute Amsterdam
Amsterdam, The Netherlands

Barbara Klotz
Orthopedic Center for Musculoskeletal Research
University of Würzburg
Würzburg, Germany

Kwong-Man Lee, PHD
Scientific Office
Lee Hysan Clinical Research Laboratories
Chinese University of Hong Kong
Shatin, Hong Kong, China

G. Harry van Lenthe, PhD
KU Leuven - University of Leuven
Department of Mechanical Engineering
Leuven, Belgium

Xiaojuan Li
Musculoskeletal and Quantitative Imaging Research
    Group
Department of Radiology and Biomedical Imaging
University of California San Francisco
San Francisco, California, United States

Esther M.M. Van Lieshout, MSc PhD
Associate Professor
Erasmus MC, University Medical Center Rotterdam
Trauma Research Unit, Department of Surgery
Rotterdam, The Netherlands

Thomas M. Link, MD, PhD
Professor of Radiology
Chief, Musculoskeletal Imaging
Clinical Director
Musculoskeletal and Quantitative Imaging Research
Department of Radiology and Biomedical Imaging
University of California San Francisco
San Francisco, Califorrnia, United States

Chuanyong Lu, MD
Orthopaedic Trauma Institute
Department of Orthopaedic Surgery
University of California at San Francisco
San Francisco General Hospital
San Francisco, California
Department of Pathology
SUNY Downstate Medical Center
Brooklyn, New York, United States

Punyawang Lumpaopong, PhD
Imperial College London
Department of Mechanical Engineering
London, United Kingdom

Thomas J. MacGillivray
Senior Research Fellow
Clinical Research Imaging Centre
Queen's Medical Research Institute
University of Edinburgh
Edinburgh, Scotland, United Kingdom

Ralph Marcucio, PhD
Orthopaedic Trauma Institute
Department of Orthopaedic Surgery
University of California at San Francisco
San Francisco General Hospital
San Francisco, California, United States

Gabriel McDonald
Engineer
Saint-Gobain
Boston, Massachusetts, United States

Jeffrey Meier, MD
Department of Radiology
University of Colorado, Denver
Aurora, Colorado, United States

Birgit Mentrup
Orthopedic Center for Musculoskeletal Research
University of Würzburg
Würzburg, Germany

Marjolein C. H. van der Meulen, PhD
Sibley School of Mechanical & Aerospace Engineering
Cornell University
Ithaca, New York
Hospital for Special Surgery
New York, New York, United States

Theodore Miclau, MD
Orthopaedic Trauma Institute
Department of Orthopaedic Surgery
University of California at San Francisco
San Francisco General Hospital
San Francisco, California, United States

Leanora Anne Mills, FRCS Orth&Tr
Consultant Orthopaedic Surgeon
Royal Aberdeen Childrens Hospital
Aberdeen, Scotland

Elise F. Morgan, PhD
Orthopaedic & Developmental Biomechanics Lab
Departments of Mechanical and Biomedical
  Engineering
Boston University
Boston, Massachusetts, United States

Iain R. Murray, BMedSci, MRCSEd, Dip SEM, PhD
ECAT Clinical Lecturer, Scottish Centre for Regenera-
  tive Medicine
The University of Edinburgh
Edinburgh, Scotland, United Kingdom

Frank Niemeyer, PhD
Scientific Computing Centre Ulm (UZWR)
University of Ulm
Ulm, Germany

Geert von Oldenburg
Director Research and Development
Biomechanics & Systems Integration
Stryker Trauma & Extremities
Schönkirchen, Germany

Thomas R. Oxland, PhD
Director
ICORD
Blusson Spinal Cord Centre
Vancouver, BC, Canada

Bidyut Pal, PhD
Research Associate
Department of Mechanical Engineering
Imperial College London
London, United Kingdom

Pankaj Pankaj, PhD
Reader
Institute for Bioengineering
School of Engineering
The University of Edinburgh
King's Buildings
Edinburgh, Scotland, United Kingdom

Janak L. Pathak
Department of Oral Cell Biology
Academic Centre for Dentistry Amsterdam
University of Amsterdam and VU University
  Amsterdam
MOVE Research Institute Amsterdam
Amsterdam, The Netherlands

Catherine Jane Pendegrass
John Scales Centre for Biomedical Engineering
Institute of Orthopaedics and Musculoskeletal
  Science
Division of Surgery and Interventional Science
University College London
Royal National Orthopaedic Hospital
Middlesex, United Kingdom

John Rasmussen, Prof. PhD
Department of Mechanical and Manufacturing
  Engineering
Aalborg University
Aalborg, Denmark

Ines L.H. Reichert, FRCS (Tr & Orth), MD, PhD
Consultant Orthopaedic and Trauma Surgeon
Hon Sen Lecturer
King's College
London, United Kingdom

Johannes B. Reitsma, MD, PhD
Associate Professor
Julius Center for Health Sciences and Primary Care
University Medical Center Utrecht
Utrecht, The Netherlands

Jim Richards, Prof. of Biomechanics, PhD, MSc, BEng
Allied Health Research Unit
University of Central Lancashire
Preston, Lancashire, United Kingdom

Dieter Rosenbaum, Prof. PhD
Institut für Experimentelle Muskuloskelettale
  Medizin
Universitätsklinikum Münster
Westfälische Wilhelms-Universität Münster
Münster, Germany

Erin Ross
Edinburgh Orthopaedic Engineering Centre
The University of Edinburgh
Edinburgh, Scotland, United Kingdom

Reinhard Schnettler
Department of Trauma Surgery
University Hospital Giessen-Marburg GmbH Campus
Giessen, Germany
Laboratory of Experimental Trauma Surgery
Justus-Liebig-University
Giessen, Germany

Andreas Martin Seitz, PhD
Institute of Orthopaedic Research and Biomechanics
Centre of Musculoskeletal Research Ulm
Ulm University
Ulm, Germany

James Selfe, Prof. of Physiotherapy, PhD, MA, GDPhys, FCSP
Allied Health Research Unit
University of Central Lancashire
Preston, Lancashire, United Kingdom

Scott Ian Kay Semple, PhD SRCS
Reader
Clinical Research Imaging Centre
Queen's Medical Research Institute
Edinburgh, Scotland, United Kingdom

Ulrich Simon, PhD
Scientific Computing Centre Ulm (UZWR)
University of Ulm
Ulm, Germany

Hamish Simpson, DM (Oxon) MA (Cantab), FRCS (Edinburgh & England)
Professor of Orthopedic Surgery
Department of Orthopaedics and Trauma
University of Edinburgh
Edinburgh, United Kingdom

Innes D M Smith
Orthopaedic Research UK Clinical Research Fellow
Musculoskeletal Research Unit
Department of Orthopaedic and Trauma Surgery
The University of Edinburgh
Edinburgh, Scotland, United Kingdom

Andre F. Steinert, Prof., Dr. med.
Department of Orthopaedic Surgery
Orthopedic Center for Musculoskeletal Research
Julius-Maximilians-University Würzburg
Würzburg, Germany

J.M. Stephen, PhD
Imperial College London
Department of Mechanical Engineering
London, United Kingdom

Michael Tanck, PhD
Assistant Professor
Department of Clinical Epidemiology, Biostatistics and Bioinformatics
Academic Medical Center, University of Amsterdam
Amsterdam, The Netherlands

David Volkheimer
Institute of Orthopaedic Research and Biomechanics
University of Ulm
Ulm, Germany

Robert James Wallace, PhD
Department of Orthopaedics
University of Edinburgh
Edinburgh, Scotland, United Kingdom

Christopher C. West, MBChB, BMedSci (Hons), MRCS (Eng)
Clinical Research Fellow and
Honorary Registrar in Plastic Surgery
The Centre for Regenerative Medicine
The University of Edinburgh
Edinburgh, Scotland, United Kingdom

Hans-Joachim Wilke
Institute of Orthopaedic Research and Biomechanics
University of Ulm
Ulm, Germany

Zohar Yosibash, DSc
Hans Fischer Senior Fellow
Institute for Advanced Study
Technical University of Munich
Munich, Germany
Professor of Mechanical Engineering
Computational Mechanics Laboratory
Department of Mechanical Engineering
Ben-Gurion University of the Negev
Beer-Sheva, Israel

Yan-Yiu Yu, PhD
Research Scientist
Orthopaedic Trauma Institute
Department of Orthopaedic Surgery
University of California at San Francisco
San Francisco General Hospital
San Francisco, California, United States

Part 1

Why Do We Need Experimental Research?

1 Evidence-Based Research

Hamish Simpson

Poor quality research has little or no value; therefore, it is essential that we ensure that any research we carry out is to a high standard. Guidelines have been published by several bodies, such as the Wellcome Trust and the UK Medical Research Council for Good Research Practice; these cover the ethical and data protection aspects of good research. For clinical research, several frameworks have been suggested in order to ensure a high standard of research. These include the CONSORT statement for the reporting of clinical trials and the principles of evidence-based medicine. Many of the requirements in these clinical frameworks can be considered in a preclinical research setting and if followed will ensure that the preclinical research is carried out to the highest standards.

1.1 Lessons to Be Learned from Evidence-based Medicine for Preclinical Research

In 1996, David Sackett wrote that "Evidence-based medicine is the conscientious, explicit and judicious use of current best evidence in making decisions about the care of individual patients."[1]

Evidence-based medicine is the integration of best research evidence with clinical expertise and patient values. Evidence-based medicine asks questions, finds and appraises the relevant data, and harnesses that information for everyday clinical practice. Evidence-based medicine follows five steps encompassed within the five "A"s:
1. Ask as answerable question
2. Find the relevant Articles (the evidence)
3. Critically Appraise the evidence (validity, impact, applicability)
4. Apply
5. Assess

The same steps can be applied to translational research. In particular, it is very important to formulate a clear clinical question from a patient's problem.

Asking the right question can be difficult, yet it is fundamental to carrying out relevant translational research. One framework that has been suggested to help formulate the question for evidence-based medicine is "PICO." This framework states that a "well-built" question should include four parts, referred to as PICO, that identify the patient problem or population (P), intervention (I), comparison (C), and outcome(s) (O). Not all translational research can be fitted into this framework, but it does stress the importance of starting with the right question and the necessity of having appropriate control groups.

The next two steps of evidence-based medicine are also entirely relevant to preclinical research, namely finding the relevant previous publications and critically appraising this literature to ensure that the experimental design is optimized. In addition, it is important that the model, whether it is biomechanical, in vitro, in silico, or in vivo, is valid for the question being addressed. For instance, although muscle structure is similar in different mammals, the structure of bone and its propensity for remodeling vary in different mammals, and it is essential this is taken into account in ensuring the model is valid (see Chapter 42).

1.2 Lessons to Be Learned from Clinical Trial Design for Preclinical Experiments

The second framework described for the reporting of clinical trials but also of relevance to preclinical research is the CONSORT statement outlined in ► Table 1.1. The items of particular relevance to preclinical research are outlined in ► Table 1.2.

Of particular note are the statements about minimizing bias (see also Chapter 54). Frequently, this is not done in preclinical research,[2,3] even when it adds little to the complexity of the design. For example, (1) randomization: Ideally the allocation of specimens (for biomechanical or in vitro work) or animals (for in vivo studies) should be randomized in a similar manner to patient randomization for clinical trials. (2) The assessments should be carried out in a blinded manner. For instance, if the number of positive cells on a histological section are being counted, the assessor should be unaware of which group the histological section has come from. (3) Multiple observers should be used if possible.

If the steps outlined for clinical research, which are relevant to preclinical research, are applied, the standard of the preclinical research will rise and with this the degree to which the preclinical studies can be applied clinically will increase.

For in vivo preclinical studies, an excellent fuller reporting guideline has been produced by Kilkenny and co-authors[4]: The ARRIVE guidelines (► Table 1.3).

1.3 Levels of Evidence

For clinical research, studies should be graded for quality and weight according to five levels of evidence, the hierarchy of clinical evidence:

Table 1.1 The CONSORT Framework

Title and abstract		
	1a	Identification as a randomized trial in the title
	1b	Structured summary of trial design, methods, results, and conclusions (for specific guidance, see CONSORT for abstracts)
Introduction		
Background and objectives	2a	Scientific background and explanation of rationale
	2b	Specific objectives or hypotheses
Methods		
Trial design	3a	Description of trial design (such as parallel, factorial) including allocation ratio
	3b	Important changes to methods after trial commencement (such as eligibility criteria), with reasons
Participants	4a	Eligibility criteria for participants
	4b	Settings and locations where the data were collected
Interventions	5	The interventions for each group with sufficient details to allow replication, including how and when they were actually administered
Outcomes	6a	Completely defined prespecified primary and secondary outcome measures, including how and when they were assessed
	6b	Any changes to trial outcomes after the trial commenced, with reasons
Sample size	7a	How sample size was determined
	7b	When applicable, explanation of any interim analyses and stopping guidelines
Randomization		
Sequence generation	8a	Method used to generate the random allocation sequence
	8b	Type of randomization; details of any restriction (such as blocking and block size)
Allocation concealment mechanism	9	Mechanism used to implement the random allocation sequence (such as sequentially numbered containers), describing any steps taken to conceal the sequence until interventions were assigned
Implementation	10	Who generated the random allocation sequence, who enrolled participants, and who assigned participants to interventions
Blinding	11a	If done, who was blinded after assignment to interventions (e.g., participants, care providers, those assessing outcomes) and how
	11b	If relevant, description of the similarity of interventions
Statistical methods	12a	Statistical methods used to compare groups for primary and secondary outcomes
	12b	Methods for additional analyses, such as subgroup analyses and adjusted analyses
Results		
Participant flow (a diagram is strongly recommended)	13a	For each group, the numbers of participants who were randomly assigned, received intended treatment, and were analyzed for the primary outcome
	13b	For each group, losses and exclusions after randomization, together with reasons
Recruitment	14a	Dates defining the periods of recruitment and follow-up
	14b	Why the trial ended or was stopped
Baseline data	15	A table showing baseline demographic and clinical characteristics for each group
Numbers analyzed	16	For each group, number of participants (denominator) included in each analysis and whether the analysis was by original assigned groups

Table 1.1 (*continued*)

Title and abstract		
Outcomes and estimation	17a	For each primary and secondary outcome, results for each group, and the estimated effect size and its precision (such as 95% confidence interval)
	17b	For binary outcomes, presentation of both absolute and relative effect sizes is recommended
Ancillary analyses	18	Results of any other analyses performed, including subgroup analyses and adjusted analyses, distinguishing prespecified from exploratory
Harms	19	All important harms or unintended effects in each group (for specific guidance, see CONSORT for harms)
Discussion		
Limitations	20	Trial limitations, addressing sources of potential bias, imprecision, and, if relevant, multiplicity of analyses
Generalizability	21	Generalizability (external validity, applicability) of the trial findings
Interpretation	22	Interpretation consistent with results, balancing benefits and harms, and considering other relevant evidence
Other information		
Registration	23	Registration number and name of trial registry
Protocol	24	Where the full trial protocol can be accessed, if available
Funding	25	Sources of funding and other support (such as supply of drugs), role of funders

Table 1.2 Components of the CONSORT Framework of Particular Relevance to Preclinical Research

Abstract	1	Structured summary of trial design, methods, results, and conclusions
Background and objectives	2	Specific objectives or hypotheses
Methods	3	The interventions for each group with sufficient details to allow replication, including how and when they were actually administered
Outcomes	4	Completely defined prespecified primary and secondary outcome measures, including how and when they were assessed
Sample size	5	How sample size was determined
Randomization	6	Type of randomization; details of any restriction (such as blocking and block size)
	7	Mechanism used to implement the random allocation sequence (such as sequentially numbered containers), describing any steps taken to conceal the sequence until interventions were assigned
Blinding	8	If done, who was blinded after assignment to interventions (e.g., researchers or those assessing outcomes) and how
Statistical methods	9	Statistical methods used to compare groups for primary and secondary outcomes
Results	10	For each group, losses and exclusions after randomization, together with reasons (an experimental flow diagram should be considered)
Harms	11	All important harms or unintended effects in each group
Discussion	12	Interpretation consistent with results, balancing benefits and harms, and considering other relevant evidence
Funding	13	Sources of funding and other support (such as supply of drugs), role of funders

Table 1.3 Animal Research: Reporting in Vivo Experiments: The ARRIVE Guidelines

Item		Recommendation
Title	1	Provide as accurate and concise a description of the content of the article as possible.
Abstract	2	Provide an accurate summary of the background, research objectives including details of the species or strain of animal used, key methods, principal findings, and conclusions of the study.
Introduction		
Background	3	a. Include sufficient scientific background (including relevant references to previous work) to understand the motivation and context for the study, and explain the experimental approach and rationale. b. Explain how and why the animal species and model being used can address the scientific objectives and, where appropriate, the study's relevance to human biology.
Objectives	4	Clearly describe the primary and any secondary objectives of the study, or specific hypotheses being tested.
Methods		
Ethical statement	5	Indicate the nature of the ethical review permissions, relevant licenses (e.g., Animal [Scientific Procedures] Act 1986), and national or institutional guidelines for the care and use of animals, that cover the research.
Study design	6	For each experiment, give brief details of the study design, including: a. The number of experimental and control groups. b. Any steps taken to minimize the effects of subjective bias when allocating animals to treatment (e.g., randomization procedure) and when assessing results (e.g., if done, describe who was blinded and when). c. The experimental unit (e.g. a single animal, group, or cage of animals).
		A timeline diagram or flow chart can be useful to illustrate how complex study designs were carried out.
Experimental procedures	7	For each experiment and each experimental group, including controls, provide precise details of all procedures carried out. For example: a. How (e.g., drug formulation and dose, site and route of administration, anesthesia and analgesia used [including monitoring], surgical procedure, method of euthanasia). Provide details of any specialist equipment used, including supplier(s). b. When (e.g., time of day). c. Where (e.g., home cage, laboratory, water maze). d. Why (e.g., rationale for choice of specific anesthetic, route of administration, drug dose used).
Experimental animals	8	a. Provide details of the animals used, including species, strain, sex, developmental stage (e.g., mean or median age plus age range), and weight (e.g., mean or median weight plus weight range). b. Provide further relevant information such as the source of animals, international strain nomenclature, genetic modification status (e.g., knockout or transgenic), genotype, health/immune status, drug- or test-naïve, previous procedures, etc.
Housing and husbandry	9	Provide details of: a. Housing (e.g., type of facility, specific pathogen free; type of cage or housing; bedding material; number of cage companions; tank shape and material, etc., for fish). b. Husbandry conditions (e.g., breeding program, light/dark cycle, temperature, quality of water, etc., for fish, type of food, access to food and water, environmental enrichment). c. Welfare-related assessments and interventions that were carried out before, during, or after the experiment.
Sample size	10	a. Specify the total number or animals used in each experiment and the number of animals in each experimental group. b. Explain how the number of animals was decided. Provide details of any sample size calculation used. c. Indicate the number of independent replications of each experiment, if relevant.

Table 1.3 (continued)

Item		Recommendation
Allocating animals to experimental groups	11	a. Give full details of how animals were allocated to experimental groups, including randomization or matching if done. b. Describe the order in which the animals in the different experimental groups were treated and assessed.
Experimental outcomes	12	Clearly define the primary and secondary experimental outcomes assessed (e.g., cell death, molecular markers, behavioral changes).
Statistical methods	13	a. Provide details of the statistical methods used for each analysis. b. Specify the unit of analysis for each dataset (e.g., single animal, group of animals, single neuron). c. Describe any methods used to assess whether the data met the assumptions of the statistical approach.
Results		
Baseline data	14	For each experimental group, report relevant characteristics and health status of animals (e.g., weight, microbiological status, and drug- or test-naïve) before treatment or testing (this information can often be tabulated).
Numbers analyzed	15	a. Report the number of animals in each group included in each analysis. Report absolute numbers (e.g., 10/20, not 50%). b. If any animals or data were not included in the analysis, explain why.
Outcomes and estimation	16	Report the results for each analysis carried out, with a measure of precision (e.g., standard error or confidence interval).
Adverse events	17	a. Give details of all important adverse events in each experimental group. b. Describe any modifications to the experimental protocols made to reduce adverse events.
Discussion		
Interpretation/scientific implications	18	a. Interpret the results, taking into account the study objectives and hypotheses, current theory, and other relevant studies in the literature. b. Comment on the study limitations including any potential sources of bias, any limitations of the animal model, and the imprecision associated with the results. c. Describe any implications of your experimental methods or findings for the replacement, refinement, or reduction (the 3Rs) of the use of animals in research.
Generalizability/translation	19	Comment on whether, and how, the findings of this study are likely to translate to other species or systems, including any relevance to human biology.
Funding	20	List all funding sources (including grant number) and the role of the funder(s) in the study.

1. Level 1
   a) Systematic reviews of randomized control trials
   b) Randomized control trials
2. Level 2 Cohort studies
3. Level 3
   a) Case-controlled trials (comparisons made but not randomized)
   b) Observational studies (including surveys and questionnaires)
4. Level 4
   a) Case series
   b) Case reports
5. Level 5 Editorials, expert opinion

In a similar way, preclinical research can be graded into different levels depending on the quality of the experimental design and the number of "dropouts" (▶ Fig. 1.1).

The higher the level of evidence of a piece of research, the more notice is taken of the conclusions in applying them to the patient. Preclinical research has been considered by some to come at the bottom of this pyramid of evidence; however, if the preclinical research is carefully designed so that it represents the clinical scenario accurately and performed to a high standard with steps taken to avoid bias, then it should be placed higher up the pyramid and potentially above the level of case series (▶ Fig. 1.2). In some clinical

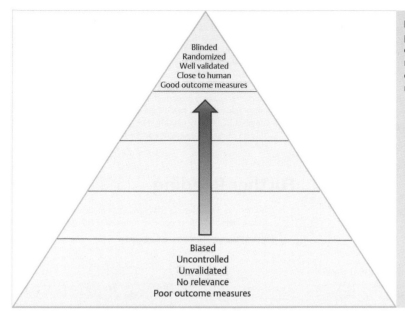

Fig. 1.1 There is a spectrum of quality of preclinical studies, ranging from poorly conducted studies in models that do not resemble the human situation to well-designed experiments in clinically relevant models of the disease.

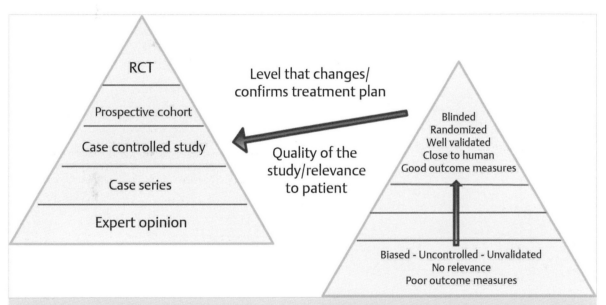

Fig. 1.2 Well-conducted research in relevant clinical models can have a greater impact on guiding the treatment for a patient than low-level clinical research. Therefore, top-level preclinical studies can slot in the hierarchy of evidence toward the middle of the pyramid rather than at the bottom of it.

areas, this may mean that it is the highest level of evidence available and as such should have a major influence on patient management.

In addition to informing patient care directly, preclinical studies also have a role in the design of clinical trials for complex interventions. According to Campbell et al,[5] complex interventions are "built up from a number of components, which may act both independently and interdependently." Evaluating complex interventions can pose a considerable challenge. Preclinical studies inform the preliminary phase of the design of studies for the evaluation of complex interventions (see following box) and as such they have a crucial role in ensuring that clinical trials address the right question with the right design.

<table>
<tr><td>

Medical Research Council Framework for Design and Evaluation of Complex Interventions

Stepwise approach (on paper)

Phase 0—Preclinical or theoretical (why should this intervention work?)

Phase 1—Modelling (how does it work?)

Phase 2—Exploratory or pilot trial (optimizing trial measures)

Phase 3—Definitive randomized controlled trial

Phase 4—Implementation

</td></tr>
</table>

References

[1] Sackett DL, Rosenberg WM, Gray JA, Haynes RB, Richardson WS. Evidence based medicine: what it is and what it isn't. BMJ 1996; 312: 71–72

[2] Kilkenny C, Parsons N, Kadyszewski E et al. Survey of the quality of experimental design, statistical analysis and reporting of research using animals. PLoS ONE 2009; 4: e7824

[3] Landis SC, Amara SG, Asadullah K et al. A call for transparent reporting to optimize the predictive value of preclinical research. Nature 2012; 490: 187–191

[4] Kilkenny C, Browne WJ, Cuthill IC, Emerson M, Altman DG. Improving bioscience research reporting: The ARRIVE guidelines for reporting animal research. J Pharmacol Pharmacother 2010; 1: 94–99

[5] Campbell NC, Murray E, Darbyshire J et al. Designing and evaluating complex interventions to improve health care. BMJ 2007; 334: 455–459

Further Reading

van der Worp HB, Howells DW, Sena ES et al. Can animal models of disease reliably inform human atudies? PLoS Med 2010;7(3): e1000245

2 Establishing a Basic Research Facility in Orthopedic Surgery

Chuanyong Lu, Safa Herfat, Céline Colnot, Ralph Marcucio, and Theodore Miclau

The initiation of research programs requires complex decision-making as directional, logistical, and financial considerations must be evaluated. The greatest barriers to the development of new basic research facilities include available technical expertise, space, and finances. The establishment of an orthopedic laboratory should be based on research interest, expertise, funding, and the surrounding research environment. Collaboration between multiple disciplines and centers is key to the success of a research program. Here, we outline some of the major research directions in orthopedics and list the basic equipment to set up a laboratory for cellular and molecular biology, biomechanics, and tissue engineering of musculoskeletal tissues.

Because our population is aging and the rate of automobile accidents worldwide is increasing, musculoskeletal problems continue to represent a significant source of death and disability, with growing societal and economic burdens. Although our knowledge about musculoskeletal diseases has been greatly improved in the last decades, we are still facing challenges and have limited options to treat fracture nonunions, large segmental bone/joint defects, degenerative joint diseases, failed implants, and ligament injuries. Research into the normal biology of musculoskeletal tissues, the diseases and injuries associated with these tissues, and the underlying mechanisms of musculoskeletal tissue regeneration continue to gain importance. These investigations often require a multidisciplinary approach including basic cellular and molecular biology, bioengineering, biomechanics, and clinical research. Collaboration between disciplines and centers with different expertise is essential to continue to advance the field. A team of self-motivated scientists and experienced technicians is key to the success of a laboratory. The purpose of this chapter is to address issues that may be of interest to the development of new basic science research programs and initiatives. A brief review of the current and developing areas of orthopedic research is included, and the resources required for establishing a new biology, tissue engineering, or biomechanics research laboratory are described.

2.1 Development of a Basic Biology Laboratory

2.1.1 Research Directions for a Biology Laboratory

The goal of orthopedic research is to develop better treatments to prevent, cure, or slow down the progress of musculoskeletal disorders. Research into basic cellular and molecular mechanisms of skeletogenesis, skeletal tissue regeneration, and musculoskeletal disorders is critical to the accomplishment of this goal.

Embryonic Skeletal Development

The human skeleton forms through two distinct processes: endochondral ossification and intramembranous ossification. During endochondral ossification, progenitor cells differentiate into chondrocytes and form cartilage first, which is then replaced by bone. All the long bones in our body (except for the clavicle) develop through this process. Intramembranous ossification occurs through direct bone formation; examples are the flat craniofacial bones. Bone development is a highly regulated process that involves multiple transcription factors, such as SOX-9 and cbfa-1, and their downstream molecules. Since bone regeneration in adults largely recapitulates the process that occurs during embryonic skeletal development and shares similar regulating mechanisms, the findings in skeletogenesis frequently lead to novel therapeutic targets for bone repair. For example, molecules such as matrix metalloproteinase-9, matrix extracellular phosphoglycoprotein, and wnt proteins are expressed during both skeletogenesis and adult bone repair. Further research demonstrated that matrix extracellular phosphoglycoprotein and wnt proteins could promote osteogenesis in vitro or in vivo.

Bone Regeneration

Bone repair is initiated by an acute inflammatory response, which is followed by the recruitment of skeletal progenitor cells, differentiation of chondrocytes and osteoblasts, formation of bone and cartilage, and remodeling of the callus. Inflammation plays an important role in fracture healing by modulating angiogenesis, stem cell recruitment, and callus remodeling. Numerous cytokines, growth factors, and molecules are involved in fracture healing. Expression of tumor necrosis factor-α, interleukin (IL)-1, IL-6, IL-10, IL-18, vascular endothelial growth factor, and bone morphogenetic proteins (BMPs) are detected in fracture calluses.[1,2,3] The contribution of these molecules, cytokines, and inflammatory cells to fracture healing is a focus of current orthopedic research. Other important research topics of bone regeneration are determining the sources of repairing cells, improving bone regeneration in patients with diabetic mellitus or peripheral vascular diseases, and treating large bone defects.

Cartilage Repair

Although we have been studying cartilage repairs for decades, it still remains a challenge to regenerate cartilage with the morphology, chemical compositions, biomechanical properties, and long-term functions comparable to native cartilage. Articular cartilage has a poor capacity to repair itself after injury and tends to heal through the formation of fibrocartilage, which has inferior biomechanical characteristics to resist compression stress compared to normal articular hyaline cartilage. Further understanding of the differences between hyaline cartilage and fibrocartilage, as well as the molecular mechanisms that govern chondrocyte differentiation and extracellular matrix production, could provide clues on how to direct cells to produce hyaline cartilage instead of fibrocartilage. In this field, growth factors such as transforming growth factor (TGF)-β, insulinlike growth factor-1, fibroblast growth factor-2, and BMP-7 may be exploited to improve cartilage regeneration.

Fibrocartilaginous tissues, such as meniscus and intervertebral disk, are equally challenging to regenerate because of the lack of adequate blood supply and the high demand for mechanical loading. The intervertebral disk is composed of three tissues: the cartilage endplate, nucleus pulposus, and annulus fibrosus. These three types of tissue create architecture with a greater level of complexity than that of articular cartilage. Successful regeneration of intervertebral disk may require the regeneration of all three tissues in one implant. Tissue engineering will play an important role in cartilage regeneration, and the right scaffolds, cells, and growth factors need to be tested.

Soft Tissue Regeneration

Muscles, tendons, and ligaments along with blood vessels and nerves are closely associated with bone. The basic biology of muscle and muscle repair is relatively well understood compared to other soft tissues. However, further advances are needed to treat devastating diseases such as Duchenne muscular dystrophy and to improve muscle repair. The biology of tendons and ligaments is now being better understood with the identification of key molecular pathways and cells involved in these tissues. Like muscle and bone healing, tendon and ligament healing is initiated by an inflammatory response that may be modulated to stimulate repair. The key issue with current tendon repair strategies is the difficulty in achieving functionality that is equal to that of the preinjured state, which makes it necessary to explore new growth factors and cells to accomplish the task. In addition, we need to optimize the mechanical stimuli and postsurgical rehabilitation. Tissue engineering may provide promising solutions to tendon or ligament repair in difficult cases such as anterior cruciate ligament (ACL) rupture.

Arthritis

Rheumatoid and degenerative arthritis affects a large proportion of the population and are leading causes of disability. The role of inflammation in the pathogenesis of arthritis has been well established, and several groups of drugs have been developed to tackle inflammation and thus modify the progression of disease. One example is the use of tumor necrosis factor-α antagonists in rheumatoid arthritis. Recent studies have also focused on the role of stem cells in the pathogenesis of arthritis and on the therapeutic effects of mesenchymal stem cells (MSCs) on arthritis, taking advantage of the immune-regulatory effects of MSCs.

Mesenchymal Stem Cells

Stem cell biology is a hot topic in the field of orthopedic research. Experimental studies have shown that stem cells that contribute to fracture healing could derive from peripheral circulation and bone marrow. Transplanted MSCs can differentiate into osteoblasts and chondrocytes in fracture calluses. In addition, MSCs have paracrine effects by expressing potent growth factors and cytokines that modulate angiogenesis, inflammation, and stem cell recruitment/differentiation. The paracrine effects of MSCs in fracture healing have not been fully determined. There is evidence showing that MSC-conditioned medium can improve fracture healing.[4] Current research on MSCs is hindered by the lack of specific surface markers and the inefficiency of in vivo cell tracking techniques.

One recent major achievement in stem cell research is the discovery of induced pluripotent stem (iPS) cells. The iPS cells were first established by retrovirus-mediated transduction of four transcription factors (c-Myc, Oct3/4, SOX2, and Klf4) into mouse fibroblasts or human fibroblasts. The current trend is to use fewer transcription factors or small chemical compounds to reprogram somatic cells. iPS cells have the potential to differentiate toward osteoblasts,[5] indicating their value in bone regeneration. However, the risk of tumorogenesis of iPS cells needs to be addressed prior to clinical application.

2.1.2 Infrastructure and Equipment of a Biology Laboratory

The infrastructure required to run an orthopedic basic research laboratory is similar to any other biological laboratory. Fume hoods are required to vent noxious and dangerous chemicals. An animal housing facility is necessary if work will be performed on any in vivo model. If work is to be performed on established or primary cell lines, then a separate cell culture room should be considered. By isolating cell culture facilities, reduced foot traffic around the incubators and hoods will aid in keeping cultures free of bacteria and mold. Another part of the laboratory should be set aside for processing, sectioning, and staining of histological specimens. This area should be located in a "dust-free" area away from drafts that will create difficulty handling ribbons of histology sections. Work with radioactive materials can be made safer by defining and restricting use of these materials to dedicated areas of the laboratory. Similarly, a dedicated imaging suite that contains all of the microscopes that will be used for documentation and analysis of data will allow undisturbed specimen viewing, will allow the room to be darkened for specialized imaging such as epifluorescence, and will reduce the amount of dust that accumulates on working parts of the microscope. Basic equipment for a biology laboratory is listed in ▶ Table 2.1.

2.2 Development of a Tissue Engineering Laboratory

2.2.1 Research Directions of a Tissue Engineering Laboratory

Tissue engineering is a science of tissue regeneration using combinations of scaffolds, cells, and growth factors. A tissue engineering research team should have expertise in biomaterials, cell biology, molecular biology, and animal surgeries. Advances in the research of novel biomaterials, scaffold fabrication, and growth factors, in combination with improved understanding of the cellular and molecular mechanisms of musculoskeletal tissue regeneration, will further progress this field.

Biomaterials and Scaffolds

The most commonly used biomaterials for bone and cartilage regeneration include (1) natural materials such as collagen, gelatin, fibrin gel, silk, chitosan, and demineralized bone matrix; (2) synthetic materials such as poly(L-lactic acid), poly(glycolic acid), and polycaprolactone; and (3) mineral components such as hydroxyapatite, tricalciumphosphate, and bioglass. Scaffolds can be fabricated synthetic materials by electrospinning, thermally induced phase separation, or three-dimensional (3D) computer-assisted printing. To facilitate mineralization, mineral components can be mixed with other materials before fabrication or deposited on the surface of scaffold. Scaffolds should have the right compositions and 3D structure to facilitate cell adhesion, stem cell recruitment, proliferation, and differentiation. Optimization of the porosity and components has been extensively explored. Recent advances in 3D printing technique allow the fabrication of scaffold with multiple layers that recapitulate the biomechanical property and environment for bone, cartilage, or ligament regeneration in the same construct.

For example, scaffolds for articular cartilage are made with two layers, one desirable for cartilage regeneration

Table 2.1 Infrastructure and Equipment of a Biology Laboratory

Infrastructure and equipment	
Personnel	Cell biologist, molecular biologist, developmental biologist
Space	Dedicated space for tissue processing and sectioning, RNA extraction, cell culture, and radioactive materials
Chemicals	Fume hoods, inflammable cabinet
Cell culture	Dissecting microscope, cell culture hood, incubators, water bath, low-speed centrifuge, revert microscope with fluorescence capability, liquid nitrogen tank, access to fluorescence-activated cell sorting equipment
Molecular biology	Reverse transcription–polymerase chain reaction, polymerase chain reaction, electrophoresis, nano drop spectrophotometer, spectrometer, western blotting equipment, setup for in situ hybridization, centrifuges, access to microarray equipment
Histology	Tissue processing equipment; microtomes for paraffin sectioning, frozen sectioning, and undecalcified tissue sectioning; microscopes; histomorphometry equipment (stereology or BioQuant system; BioQuant Inc., San Diego, CA); equipment for immunostaining
Surgery	Surgery room, surgery table, fracture apparatus, drill, saw, general surgical instruments, anesthesia machine (isoflurane), dissecting microscope, animal facility
Bone analysis	X-ray machine, microcomputed tomography, dual-energy X-ray absorptiometry, biomechanical equipment, Fourier transform infrared spectrometer

and another for subchondral bone formation. To facilitate the attachment of ligament to bone, a stratified or multiphasic scaffold is designed for interface tissue engineering.[6] Stem cells or growth factors can be added to the scaffolds to achieve better results.

Stem Cells

Research on stem cells is a major component for tissue engineering. Currently, most studies are using stem cell transplantation to improve tissue regeneration, in which stem cells are collected, cultured, and expanded in vitro with or without differentiation before being transplanted in vivo. Cell transplantation provides repairing cells to the site and may employ the paracrine effects of transplanted cells. However, cell transplantation is limited by several disadvantages including an additional surgery to collect cells for culture, expensive cell culture procedures, and risk of contamination. Recently, scientists have explored the efficiency of cell homing, which uses growth factors to recruit host cells into the scaffolds, to improve tissue regeneration. As a proof of concept, anatomically correct scaffolds for rabbit humeral condyle were fabricated, incorporated with TGF-β3, and implanted in rabbits. Without delivering exogenous stem cells with the scaffold, this approach of cell homing was able to regenerate a functional humeral condyle in these animals, which exhibited an articular surface of hyaline cartilage.[7] In the direction of cell homing, further research is necessary to find out the most potent growth factors for MSCs recruitment in both in vitro and in vivo settings.

Growth Factors

Numerous growth factors are capable of improving skeletal tissue regeneration, among them are BMPs, TGF-β, platelet-derived growth factor, fibroblast growth factors, vascular endothelial growth factor, and stromal cell–derived factor-1, etc. As our understanding of stem cell biology improves, this list will get longer. To regenerate different types of tissue, specific growth factors should be chosen. For examples, BMPs are potent for bone regeneration, whereas TGF-β3 is useful for cartilage repair.[7] The safety of these growth factors in humans has not been fully established. Controlled release may lower the dose of growth factors, thus decreasing their side effects and cost.

Large Tissue Regeneration and Vascularization

One of the goals and challenges of tissue engineering is to repair large tissue defects. Large skeletal defects have a limited healing capability due to multiple factors. One factor is the lack of repairing cells or growth factors, which can be corrected by transplanting or homing MSCs. Another important factor is inadequate blood supply or inefficient revascularization. Adding proangiogenic factors to scaffolds facilitates tissue regeneration. Bioreactors allow the regeneration of large anatomically shaped tissues in vitro with scaffold and seeded cells; however, currently there is no available technique to build a working vascular system into these regenerates. The viability of a large regenerate produced in a bioreactor would therefore be significantly compromised, which hinders the clinical application of in vitro organ regeneration.

2.2.2 Infrastructure and Equipment of a Tissue Engineering Laboratory

A laboratory focusing on skeletal tissue engineering shares similar equipment as a biology laboratory for cell culture, histological, cellular, and molecular analyses. In addition, a tissue engineering laboratory should have special equipment for scaffold fabrication, as well as those

Table 2.2 Infrastructure and Equipment of a Tissue Engineering Laboratory

Infrastructure and Equipment	
Personnel	Stem cell biologist, chemist, molecular biologist, collaboration with veterinarians for large animal models
Space	Dedicated space for cell culture and scaffold fabrication
Chemicals	Fume hoods, inflammable cabinet
Scaffold fabrication	Electrospinning setup (a spinneret, a high-voltage direct current power supply, a syringe pump, and a grounded collector), freeze drying machine, 3D-Bioplotter (EnvisionTEC, Dearborn, MI), computers, bioreactors
Cell culture	Dissecting microscope, cell culture hood, incubators, water bath, low-speed centrifuge, revert microscope with fluorescence capability, access to fluorescence-activated cell sorting equipment, access to in vivo fluorescence imaging system
Histology	Tissue processing equipment; microtomes for paraffin sectioning, frozen sectioning, and undecalcified tissue sectioning; microscopes; histomorphometry equipment (stereology or BioQuant systems; BioQuant Inc., San Diego, CA)
Molecular biology	Reverse transcription–polymerase chain reaction, polymerase chain reaction, electrophoresis, nano drop spectrophontometer, spectrometer, western blotting equipment, setup for in situ hybridization, centrifuges, access to microarray equipment
Surgery	Surgical room, surgical table, general surgical instruments, fracture apparatus, drill, saw
Bone analysis	X-ray machine, microcomputed tomography, dual-energy X-ray absorptiometry, biomechanical equipment, Fourier transform infrared spectroscopy

for in vitro and in vivo tissue regeneration. ▶ Table 2.2 lists some of the basic equipment for tissue engineering.

2.3 Development of an Orthopedic Biomechanics Laboratory

2.3.1 Research Directions of a Biomechanics Laboratory

Orthopedic biomechanics is an area of orthopedic research that focusses on applying theoretical and experimental mechanics to study the musculoskeletal system. The role of biomechanics is critical in establishing design parameters and evaluation criteria for orthopedic treatments, surgical techniques, devices, and implants. Orthopedic biomechanics researchers are currently studying the musculoskeletal system using a variety of approaches that include experimental biomechanical analysis (in vivo and in vitro) and computational analysis (modeling and simulation).

Together, experimental and computational approaches continue to increase our knowledge of normal biomechanics, as well as having implications for orthopedic injuries, conditions, and treatments. Although most laboratories may focus on either experimental or computational approaches, some employ both. For example, a sports biomechanics laboratory may acquire kinematic measurements for an athlete and then use these measurements to build musculoskeletal models for further biomechanical analysis. Both computational and experimental approaches are currently being used for sports medicine research investigating the biomechanical effects of ACL injuries, evaluating ACL reconstruction techniques and grafts types, determining how ACL injuries lead to long-term complications such as osteoarthritis, and establishing functional tissue engineering parameters for artificial ACL replacements.

Orthopedic biomechanics researchers are expanding the technical applications of imaging, modeling and simulation, material testing, robotics, and measurement instrumentation. Recent advances in technology now allow a level of accuracy in motion measurement that was previously not attainable. These new technologies have made it possible to measure in vivo motion more accurately and reproduce the in vivo condition more accurately when conducting in vitro biomechanical testing. Advanced modeling software (e.g., Mimics; Materialise, Leuven, Belgium) now allows investigators to build accurate 3D models from data acquired from various imaging modalities. These 3D models can then be imported into finite element software to perform computational biomechanics analysis of musculoskeletal tissues, surgical techniques, and devices. Sensors needed for in vivo and in vitro measurement of joint and tissue deformations and loads also continue to evolve.

Functional tissue engineering is an example of a cutting-edge research topic in orthopedic biomechanics research, which involves different approaches to orthopedic research. Tissue engineering parameters are needed to design and manufacture effective repairs and replacements for load-bearing structures. Parameters such as the in vivo stresses and strains in native and repair tissues during different activities of daily living will serve as important design criteria for tissue-engineered constructs. Determining how engineered constructs and repair tissues interact with mechanical forces, both in vivo and in vitro, is also important. This will require investigators to determine the effects of biomechanical factors on tissue repair in vivo and the optimal mechanical stimuli needed to enhance tissue regeneration in vitro.

In Vivo Biomechanical Analysis

This includes sports medicine and human performance laboratories where researchers perform analysis of activities of daily living (e.g., gait) and athletic motions (e.g., jumping/landing, cutting). Using motion measurement systems and force plates, researchers can perform inverse dynamics analysis to estimate muscle and joint forces, and determine the effects of injury/deficiency, injury preventative training regimens, and treatments (operative and nonoperative) on joint function.

Advances in technology have provided increasingly accurate methods for quantifying the effects of injury and repair. Knee kinematics can now be measured very accurately using a dynamic stereo X-ray system for acquiring high-speed stereoradiographic images during an in vivo, functional activity. Conventional kinematics, contact paths, and deformations of soft tissues can be determined using the dynamic stereo X-ray system and computed tomography (CT) or magnetic resonance imaging (MRI) scans. Although the system is too expensive for most laboratories to set up and maintain, this system can achieve a level of joint motion measurement accuracy needed for ligament and cartilage research. Optical systems, which measure joint motions from reflective skin markers, are more affordable and widely used. Although these systems offer less accurate joint motion measurements due to skin markers not being rigidly attached to the bones, the measurement accuracy is acceptable to identify differences in joint kinematics between healthy, injured, and repaired joints, as well as to identify predictors of injuries in athletes and evaluate the effect of interventions.[8]

In Vitro Biomechanical Testing

Using material testing systems or robotics, researchers can determine normal joint and tissue biomechanics, investigate the biomechanical effects of pathological conditions (e.g., osteoarthritis) and injuries, as well as evaluate (operative and nonoperative) treatments, devices, and implants. Many biomechanics laboratories focus their efforts on evaluating medical devices or biomechanically evaluating various surgical methods (e.g., single versus double bundle ACL reconstructions). These devices are usually implanted into cadaveric samples or surgical methods are performed on cadaveric samples and biomechanically evaluated by integrating technologies such as a material testing system, radiography, and custom-designed jigs to reproduce physiological loading of the cadaveric sample (▶ Fig. 2.1 and ▶ Fig. 2.2). Advances in technologies such as 6-degree-of-freedom robotic

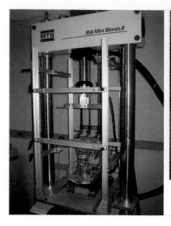

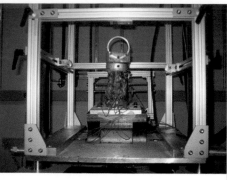

Fig. 2.1 Pure moment testing system for spine laxity measurements.

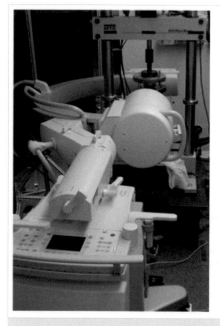

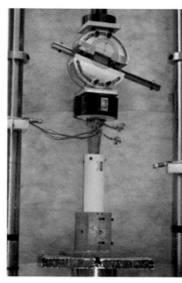

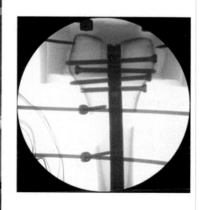

Fig. 2.2 Implant subsidence can be monitored throughout a fatigue test by integrating fluoroscopy and material testing systems.

manipulators now allow investigators greater flexibility in reproducing physiological loading conditions by offering the capabilities to reproduce the 6-degree-of-freedom joint kinematics to measure joint loads (stiffness-based testing),[9] apply joint loads to measure joint laxity, or simultaneously apply joint motions and loads to reproduce physiological loading conditions (hybrid control).

Computational Analysis Using Modeling and Simulation

Computational techniques are very useful for biomechanical analysis, which would be difficult to perform experimentally, such as determining the biomechanical contributions of bone microstructure or performing biomechanical analysis of a device-tissue interface. Computational methods can also serve as a cost-effective alternative to experimental testing. However, experimental biomechanical testing is usually required to determine properties needed for computational models or to validate these models.

Accurate anatomical morphologies for computational models can be acquired using actual data from imaging modalities (e.g., MRI). The finite element method is a computational technique that is widely used by both academic research and industry research and development laboratories to evaluate medical devices. Some of the recent applications for finite element analysis include the design optimization of devices and implants using finite element analysis models, determining the biomechanical role of tissue microstructure and the mechanisms of initial failure, and determining the risk of bone damage and implant subsidence due to implant malalignment.

Computational methods are also used to simulate the biomechanics of the musculoskeletal system using simulation software. Musculoskeletal models are currently being developed to investigate the normal biomechanics of musculoskeletal tissues and joints, as well as to understand how musculoskeletal conditions alter joint and tissue biomechanics. These models can also be used to evaluate surgical techniques and nonoperative treatments, as well to determine injury predictors. Advances in modeling software now allow investigators to create patient-specific 3D anatomical models from CT or MR images, and use these models to design patient-specific surgical techniques and predict surgical outcome, thereby serving as valuable surgical planning tools.

2.3.2 Infrastructure and Equipment of a Biomechanics Laboratory

An orthopedic biomechanics laboratory can be established with an experimental or computational focus. In vitro experimental methods usually require expensive high load capacity mechanical testing systems or high payload industrial robots costing over $100,000 with installation costs, as well as access to cadaveric specimen. However, biomechanical testing of weaker soft tissues can be conducted using less costly lower capacity testing systems (e.g., TestResources [Shakopee, MN] Tabletop Test Machines). In vivo experimental research usually requires expensive motion capture systems and access to human or animal subjects that must be approved by an institutional review board or committee (e.g., Institutional Review Board, Institutional Animal Care and Use Committee). Computational biomechanics research can be conducted with minimal equipment, but it does require access to modeling and simulation software, some of which require costly licenses. ▶ Table 2.3 lists some of the recommended equipment and staffing needs to consider acquiring or gaining access to when establishing an orthopedic biomechanics laboratory. All biomechanical research approaches will require mathematical and statistical software for data and statistical analysis.

In addition to the equipment listed in ▶ Table 2.3, other items that are helpful in an experimental testing laboratory include:
- Sufficient laboratory space for equipment, specimen storage (freezers), specimen dissection and preparation (e.g., potting for specimen fixation).
- Basic surgical tools and standard tools (e.g., a drill).
- Access to machining equipment to reduce time and costs when designing fixtures, jigs, and testing rigs for biomechanical testing.
- When conducting biomechanical testing involving bone tissue, a dual-energy X-ray absorptiometry scanner can be used as a helpful tool for screening bone quality.

- Six-degree-of-freedom robot with high payload allows for greater flexibility in applying physiological loads or displacements to complex joints such as the knee.
- Commercially available joint simulators (e.g., ADL Knee Simulator [AMTI, Watertown, MA]).

Other items that are helpful for in vivo biomechanics analysis include:
- Implantable sensors (e.g., strain gauges) or instrumented implants
- Electromyography
- Imaging systems (e.g., dynamic stereo radiography and open upright MRI)

Other software and equipment considerations for a computational research laboratory include:
- Three-dimensional modeling software (e.g., Mimics) is helpful for acquiring anatomical morphologies for computational models or fitting devices to patient-specific anatomical contours for more accurate simulations and analysis.
- Access to a material testing system to validate computational biomechanical analysis with experimental testing.
- Access to scanning electron microscopes and micro-CT for modeling tissue microstructure.

For conducting research on devices and implants, it is important to develop partnerships with companies and collaborations with clinicians. Many orthopedic medical device companies fund research projects conducted by academic biomechanical laboratories.

Although some of these companies may have the staff and testing systems required to conduct biomechanical tests in-house, working with an academic laboratory offers an unbiased evaluation and access to experienced clinical and engineering faculty on a per project basis. Through industry partnerships, an orthopedic biomechanics laboratory that focuses on testing medical devices and implants can minimize the high cost of attaining orthopedic hardware. It is also ideal that the biomechanics laboratory has access to clinical collaborators (i.e., orthopedic surgeons). Their clinical perspective can help define the clinically focused research problems and clinically relevant research questions that should guide the orthopedic biomechanics research. Ideally, trained orthopedic surgeons should perform all surgical procedures and device implantations for research specimens.

Lastly, access to equipment, technical expertise, and resources can be attained through collaboration with other departments within an academic institution or outside collaboration with other institutions. This may offer a better approach to orthopedic biomechanics research as it allows each laboratory to focus efforts on a specific area or niche. It is difficult for a single laboratory to master the knowledge and acquire all of the equipment needed for a broad field of research such as orthopedic biomechanics.

Table 2.3 Infrastructure and Equipment of a Biomechanics Laboratory.

In Vitro Experimental Orthopedic Biomechanics Research	
Equipment (Commercially Available Examples)	• Accurate motion measurement system (Optotrack; NDI, Waterloo, Ontario, Canada)
	• Axial/torsional tester high-capacity loading frame (Mini Bionix; MTS, Eden Prairie, MN)
	• High- and low-load capacity 6-degree-of-freedom load cells (MC5 and MC3; AMTI, Watertown, MA)
	• High-accuracy, low-load testing system for smaller specimens (Electroforce System; Bose, Eden Prairie, MN)
	• Radiography (e.g., C-arm; Philips, Amsterdam, The Netherlands)
Staffing	• Mechanical engineer(s) for testing jig and rig design and fabrication
	• Biomedical engineers(s) for tissue dissection and preparation
	• Access to an electrical engineer to design, install, and troubleshoot electrical sensors and systems
In Vivo Experimental Orthopedic Biomechanics Research	
Equipment (Commercially Available Examples)	• Motion capture system (Vicon, Centennial, CO)
	• Force platforms (Kistler, Amherst, NY)
	• High performance computer(s) with motion and force analysis software (Visual3D Software; C-Motion, Germantown, MD)
Staffing	• Kinesiologist or biomedical/biomechanical engineer for motion analysis
Computational Orthopedic Biomechanics Research	
Equipment (Commercially Available Examples)	• High performance computer(s) with finite element or other modeling software (Abaqus; Dassault Systèmes Simulia Corp., Providence, RI)
Staffing	• Mechanical, biomechanical, biomedical, or computer engineers with modeling and simulation experience

References

[1] Lange J, Sapozhnikova A, Lu C et al. Action of IL-1beta during fracture healing. J Orthop Res 2010; 28: 778–784

[2] Yu YY, Lieu S, Lu C, Miclau T, Marcucio RS, Colnot C. Immunolocalization of BMPs, BMP antagonists, receptors, and effectors during fracture repair. Bone 2010; 46: 841–851

[3] Einhorn TA, Majeska RJ, Rush EB, Levine PM, Horowitz MC. The expression of cytokine activity by fracture callus. J Bone Miner Res 1995; 10: 1272–1281

[4] Wang CY, Yang HB, Hsu HS et al. Mesenchymal stem cell-conditioned medium facilitates angiogenesis and fracture healing in diabetic rats. J Tissue Eng Regen Med 2011; 6: 559–569

[5] Li F, Bronson S, Niyibizi C. Derivation of murine induced pluripotent stem cells (iPS) and assessment of their differentiation toward osteogenic lineage. J Cell Biochem 2010; 109: 643–652

[6] Lu HH, Subramony SD, Boushell MK, Zhang X. Tissue engineering strategies for the regeneration of orthopedic interfaces. Ann Biomed Eng 2010; 38: 2142–2154

[7] Lee CH, Shah B, Moioli EK, Mao JJ. CTGF directs fibroblast differentiation from human mesenchymal stem/stromal cells and defines connective tissue healing in a rodent injury model. J Clin Invest 2010; 120: 3340–3349

[8] Hewett TE, Myer GD, Ford KR et al. Biomechanical measures of neuromuscular control and valgus loading of the knee predict anterior cruciate ligament injury risk in female athletes: a prospective study. Am J Sports Med 2005; 33: 492–501

[9] Herfat ST, Boguszewski DV, Shearn JT. Applying simulated in vivo motions to measure human knee and ACL kinetics. Ann Biomed Eng 2012; 40: 1545–1553

Further Reading

Caplan AI. Why are MSCs therapeutic? New data: new insight. J Pathol 2009; 217: 318–324

Mao JJ, Stosich MS, Moioli EK et al. Facial reconstruction by biosurgery: cell transplantation versus cell homing. Tissue Eng Part B Rev 2010; 16: 257–262

Takahashi K, Tanabe K, Ohnuki M et al. Induction of pluripotent stem cells from adult human fibroblasts by defined factors. Cell 2007; 131: 861–872

3 Good Laboratory Practice and Quality Control

Geert von Oldenburg

The need to follow good laboratory practice (GLP) when conducting preclinical safety and efficacy tests and studies was fostered in recent years by those authorities guiding and deciding upon medical device release for human use. To fulfill this requirement, medical device industry strongly adopted GLP procedures when conducting such safety and efficacy tests and studies.

Having experienced the benefits of GLP, industry now occasionally feels a quality awareness discrepancy when cooperating in basic or applied research with outside institutions, which have not yet installed the main pillars of GLP.

It has become evident that even when performing research studies or testing outside the direct scope of preclinical safety and efficacy tests and studies, following certain GLP rules is a prerequisite for high-quality output. It is thus the purpose of this chapter to introduce the key elements of GLP and quality control as based on international standards and guidance documents. Using the experience from a mechanically profiled testing laboratory in medical device industry (trauma implants), it gives examples of how the normative requirements may be translated in organizational and procedural terms.

3.1 Definitions

GLP is a quality system concerned with the organizational process and the conditions under which nonclinical health and environmental safety studies are planned, performed, monitored, recorded, archived, and reported.[1,2]

3.2 Scope of Good Laboratory Practice

GLP shall be applied for nonclinical safety and efficacy studies that support or are intended to support marketing permits and claims for medical devices for human use.[1]

However, it has to be emphasized that even in those cases where GLP is not mandatory, at least following its main guidelines is suggested: Neglecting them puts quality of work and results at risk; conclusions drawn on incorrect results may be wrong and thus subsequent work steps (like design optimization of a newly developed product based on non-GLP prototype testing) may waste valuable resources. GLP thus also helps to do it right the first time.

3.3 Key Elements of Good Laboratory Practice

There are two main groups of requirements to be addressed when implementing GLP[3]:
- Management requirements
- Technical requirements

This section will define and explain those requirements in detail.

3.3.1 Management Requirements

Organization

The laboratory shall be or refer to a legal entity that can be held responsible and accountable for its work. A legal entity may be an association, corporation, partnership, proprietorship, trust, or individual that has legal standing in the eyes of law.

The laboratory has to have managerial, technical, and quality personnel, which needs the authority and resources necessary to properly carry out their duties. The laboratory needs to have a technical management installed that has overall responsibility for technical operations and provision of resources. In addition, a quality manager needs to be established who has direct access to the leadership level. All personnel must be held free of any influences that may adversely affect the quality of their work.

The organization including responsibilities, authorities, and interrelation of all personnel needs to be properly defined and described. The management needs to provide and enable adequate supervision of all staff, including trainees, by persons familiar and trained in methods and procedures. ▶ Fig. 3.1 shows a sample of an organizational chart that fulfills the requirements set forth per ISO 17025.[3]

Management System

The laboratory leadership shall establish a management system that is appropriate for the work scope of the laboratory. The management system may be documented in policies, programs, procedures, instructions, and charts that are necessary to operate the laboratory in a controlled and effective manner and to assure the quality of test results.

A core element of the management system is the quality management handbook, which includes the commitment to good professional practice and quality testing, the statement of the laboratory's standard work scope, and the quality-related purpose of the management

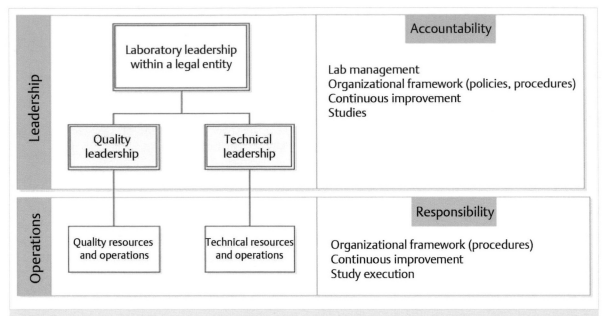

Fig. 3.1 Sample of an organizational chart for a good laboratory practices–guided laboratory facility. Fulfills requirements per ISO 17025.[3]

system. The quality management handbook shall be available and communicated and trained to all laboratory personnel.

Management Reviews

The management system along with the technical and quality activities shall be periodically reviewed by the leadership team to ensure continuing suitability and effectiveness of policies and procedures, and to introduce necessary changes and improvements.

Input sources for the management review may be policies, procedures, quarterly or monthly business reports prepared from laboratory personnel, audit reports, corrective action and preventive action (CAPA) summary reports, any external bodies' assessments, results of interlaboratory comparisons, and customer feedback and complaints.

Review outcome should result in a clear action list for improvement including objectives, action planning, and timelines for completion.

The management review is a key component of the continuous improvement process the laboratory shall constantly strive for. This applies to its whole body of policies, procedures, and activities on management and quality as well as the technical side. The typical cycle for improvement is shown in ► Fig. 3.2.[4]

Document Control

The laboratory management needs to establish procedures to control all documents that form part of its

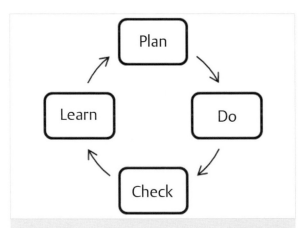

Fig. 3.2 Cycle of continuous improvement to be applied in a good laboratory practices facility.[4]

management system: Besides the aforementioned policies, programs, and procedures, these may be standards, drawings, software, equipment manuals, etc. The document control should include guidelines for filing, archiving, approval, and issue control.

Control of Records

It is recommended that procedures be established for identification, indexing, collection, archiving, maintenance, and disposal of quality and technical records. This also applies to any electronically stored data. The system must ensure that all information on a test or study potentially influencing quality of results is easily accessible and retrievable (e.g., when the need to repeat a study arises or questions on the validity and correct data analysis are raised in, for example, statistics).

Complaints, Control of Nonconforming Testing Work

The laboratory must have policies and procedures for how to deal with nonconformances. Those must ensure responsibilities, authorities, and regulated steps to take in order to implement containment measures, evaluate the significance of any nonconforming work, execute corrections, take corrective actions, verify their efficacy, decide on and execute customer notification, and work recall if needed.

In order to address this requirement, it is recommended a CAPA system be installed under quality management. Such a system focuses on the investigation of root causes of nonconformities in order to prevent their recurrence (corrective action) or to prevent occurrence (preventive action).

Internal Audits

The laboratory shall periodically perform internal audits to check compliance of any management and technical activities versus policies, procedures, standards, and regulations.

It is the responsibility of the laboratory quality manager to plan and organize those audits as required. Major deviations shall be treated per the laboratory CAPA system and audit reports should be a major input to the management reviews periodically performed.

Customer Relations

A key for successful and efficient cooperation with high-quality study and testing outcome is proactive communication to the customer. This spans from exact definition of the study request and requirements via an agreement on the study protocol and methods including involved subcontractors, followed by regular updates on the progress of the study execution and on to final discussion of the study report and outcome.

It is obvious that each necessary deviation from an originally agreed protocol has to be communicated and agreed with the customer as well.

Review of Study or Test Requests

The laboratory management needs to ensure that the requirements to conduct a study including the methods to be used are adequately defined and that the capabilities and resources are available. In this regard, any deficits have to be resolved before any work commences.

Subcontracting of Work

The same requirements as listed previously and in the following do apply in case the laboratory subcontracts its work or parts of its work to a subsupplying laboratory. As far as the quality of the work results is concerned, this also applies to any equipment or auxiliaries purchased from subcontractors.

3.3.2 Technical Requirements

General

Several factors determine the correctness and reliability of the tests performed by a laboratory. The main ones are human factors; accommodation and environmental conditions; the sampling and handling of test items; test, calibration, and validation methods; the equipment used; the measurement traceability; and correctness of statistical methods applied.

Personnel

The technical laboratory management shall ensure adequate competence of all those personnel planning and performing tests as well as documenting those including sign-offs.

Adequate supervision of all personnel still in training must be ensured. All work tasks performed have to be based on appropriate education, training, experience, and/or demonstrated skills as required. The laboratory management shall formulate goals with respect to education, training, and skills of its personnel. A policy and procedures for identifying training needs and training provision guidelines should be set up. Effective and relevant training programs should be conducted with care, with effectiveness checks implemented.

Job descriptions must be available for all positions for clear orientation. They should at least contain responsibilities and duties (managerial, technical, quality), expertise and experience required, qualification and training programs required, managerial duties, and reporting lines.

The Accommodation and Environmental Conditions

The accommodation and environmental conditions shall facilitate correct and repeatable performance of the tests. All conditions that may influence the quality of work results need to be controlled and recorded.

Depending on test subject, this may be electromagnetic disturbances, radiation, illumination environment, humidity, temperature, or vibration levels. Accommodation has to ensure that no cross-contamination of samples occurs. Good housekeeping must be ensured by appropriate means and measures.

It is highly recommended that a line clearance program be installed that guarantees that only those sample, auxiliaries, and equipment currently needed in progressing an ongoing test or study be openly available and present in the operation facility. All other items should be safely stored away in dedicated areas.

Equipment

The laboratory needs to be furnished with all items of sampling, measurement, and test equipment required for correct preparation, performance, and analysis of test results. The equipment shall be capable of achieving the accuracy needed and comply to standards required to be fulfilled for the test subject. All equipment must have appropriate instructions for use and be operated by authorized personnel only. Equipment that may have influence on results quality must be labeled with calibration data.

Calibration

The laboratory shall have an established program and procedures for the regular calibration of its equipment. This should include information on equipment items to be calibrated, purpose and scope of calibration per equipment item, calibration method and auxiliaries needed, output, and acceptance criteria. The personnel (internal/external) in charge of calibration should be defined.

Handling of Test Items

The laboratory shall have procedures for the receipt, handling, transportation, storage (e.g., environmental conditions), retention, and/or disposal of test items. This includes all provisions to protect them from any damage or alteration. This should be flanked by a procedure that guarantees that samples may be clearly identified throughout their laboratory life from initial receipt to final retention or disposal.

Test Methods and Their Validation

General

The laboratory shall use appropriate methods for testing. The method includes sampling (sample size, preparation, handling, transport, storage), test process operation, determination of accuracy, estimation of measurement uncertainty, statistical techniques, and calibration data. If any equipment is used, the method is flanked by needed instructions on the use and operation of all relevant equipment.

Method choice

Select methods that are appropriate for the test purpose. Standardized, published methods are preferred (e.g., international standards, national standards, guidelines from reputable technical organizations, relevant scientific texts or journals).

Obviously, laboratory-developed methods or methods adopted from published ones but tailored to the test requirements may also be used, if appropriate and validated. Development and implementation of a new and advanced testing method require highly qualified personnel equipped with appropriate means. Such development requires sufficient scientific, technical, and regulatory degrees of freedom, leaving a fruitful playground for theoretic and experimental research to develop, mature, and standardize the new method.

As soon as this is accomplished, a new method should be properly described, before implementing and operating it. This should include the following information: test identification, scope, test items to be tested, parameters to be determined, apparatus and equipment needed, reference to standards and materials needed, environmental condition requirements, description of the procedure, criteria for approval/rejection, data to be recorded, method of analysis, statistics to be applied, method of results presentation, and measurement uncertainty.

Validation of methods

Validation is the confirmation by examination and provision of objective evidence that particular requirements for a specific intended use are fulfilled.

All nonstandardized methods or standardized but modified methods shall be validated. Validation techniques may include calibration using reference standards and materials, comparison of results achieved with other methods, interlaboratory comparisons (round robin), systematic assessments of factors influencing results, and assessment or evaluation of measurement uncertainty.

The method capabilities determined within the validation have to be compared to the methods specification of the requirements. The method can be claimed valid only if those requirements are proven to be fulfilled.

Validation is always a balance between costs, risks, and technical possibilities. For instance, there are cases in which the range of uncertainty of the values can only be given in a simplified way due to lack of information. However, there must be procedures in place for estimating uncertainty of measurement. Guidelines may be found in DIN (Deutsches Institut für Normung) 1319.[5] It has to be considered that not only physical test systems must be validated but also any software that is part of a test system or forming an autonomous one (e.g., finite element analysis models).

To assure the continued validity of test methods, it is recommended to periodically perform tests on certified reference materials or to replicate tests on retained items.

Example from medical device industry: method validation

As an example from the medical device industry, ► Fig. 3.3 shows a standard form for the justification

and validation of a new biomechanical test method (e.g., dedicated to mechanical testing of bone plates or intramedullary nails). All requirements as given per ISO (International Organization for Standardization) 17025 are addressed when filling this form properly.

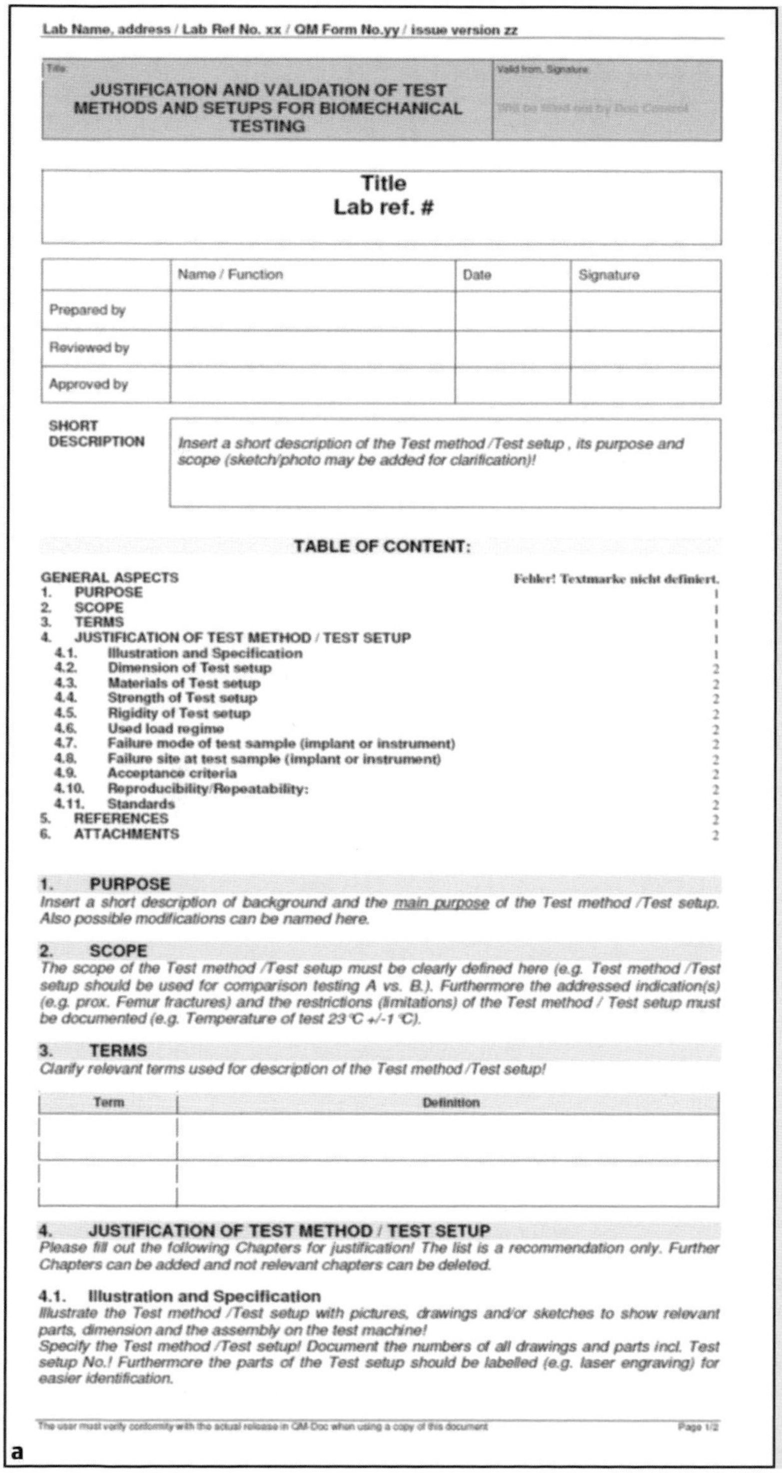

Lab Name, address / Lab Ref No. xx / QM Form No.yy / issue version zz

Title:	Valid from, Signature:
JUSTIFICATION AND VALIDATION OF TEST METHODS AND SETUPS FOR BIOMECHANICAL TESTING	Will be filled out by Doc Control

Title
Lab ref. #

	Name / Function	Date	Signature
Prepared by			
Reviewed by			
Approved by			

SHORT DESCRIPTION — *Insert a short description of the Test method /Test setup , its purpose and scope (sketch/photo may be added for clarification)!*

TABLE OF CONTENT:

GENERAL ASPECTS

1.   PURPOSE
Insert a short description of background and the main purpose of the Test method /Test setup. Also possible modifications can be named here.

2.   SCOPE
The scope of the Test method /Test setup must be clearly defined here (e.g. Test method /Test setup should be used for comparison testing A vs. B.). Furthermore the addressed indication(s) (e.g. prox. Femur fractures) and the restrictions (limitations) of the Test method / Test setup must be documented (e.g. Temperature of test 23 ℃ +/-1 ℃).

3.   TERMS
Clarify relevant terms used for description of the Test method /Test setup!

Term	Definition

4.   JUSTIFICATION OF TEST METHOD / TEST SETUP
Please fill out the following Chapters for justification! The list is a recommendation only. Further Chapters can be added and not relevant chapters can be deleted.

4.1.   Illustration and Specification
Illustrate the Test method /Test setup with pictures, drawings and/or sketches to show relevant parts, dimension and the assembly on the test machine!
Specify the Test method /Test setup! Document the numbers of all drawings and parts incl. Test setup No.! Furthermore the parts of the Test setup should be labelled (e.g. laser engraving) for easier identification.

The user must verify conformity with the actual release in QM-Doc when using a copy of this document   Page 1/2

a

Fig. 3.3 (a,b) Slim process and form to determine and document method justification and validation. Example from the medical device industry.[5,6]

4.2. Dimensions of Test setup
The key dimensions of Test setup must be documented, see Chapter 4.1. and justified. The used dimensions (e.g. CCD-angle, offset, lever arms etc.) may be derived from and justified by human anatomy and taken from e.g. Stryker Osteosynthesis Bone Database or subject related literature.

4.3. Materials of Test setup
The used materials (Renshape BM5166, PU-foams, Steel, etc) for test sample fixation must be listed. The choice of the material should be explained.

4.4. Strength of Test setup
The strength of the Test setup must be sufficient. Calculation and assessments should be documented here. Keep in mind that the purpose is not to measure the setup but the sample.

4.5. Rigidity of Test setup
If applicable, the rigidity of the Test setup should be assessed and documented here. The setup rigidity should not influence the test result. To reach that, the rigidity of the Test setup can be determined separately and afterwards the setup rigidity can be subtracted from the test result to determine the real sample rigidity.
In other cases an adaptation of the setup rigidity to the real condition (human anatomy) may be useful.

4.6. Used load regime
The reasons for using the applied load regime should be explained and justified here, e.g. by literature (bending load, torsional load, etc.) or other sources (e.g. Calculations using Anybody software). Furthermore the load regime can be chosen according to and justified by assessment of clinical failure mechanisms (e.g. Complaints show nail cracks generated by bending forces - Bending forces can be used for the Test setup up).

4.7. Failure mode of test sample (implant or instrument)
The failure mode generated by the Test setup should be confirmed by clinical experience, by literature or other sources (e.g. fatigue failure or static failure; nail failure, screw failure, screw pull out or cut out) and documented in this section.

4.8. Failure site at test sample (implant or instrument)
The location of failure generated by the Test setup should be documented here and if possible confirmed by clinical experience reports, literature or complaint data.

4.9. Acceptance criteria
General acceptance criteria for validity of the Test setup can be listed here (e.g. Test setup must produce a fatigue failure of nail). Product test related acceptance criteria may vary from one test to another depending on the tested product. These special acceptance criteria have to be listed in the Test Plan and Test Protocol. If an acceptance criterion is defined, please include an adequate rationale!

4.10. Reproducibility/Repeatability:
Reproducibility/Repeatability shall be given and documented. Consideration and calculation regarding measurement uncertainty (see DIN 1319-3) shall be documented in this section.

4.11. Standards
Document if at all and which parts of the Test method /Test setup are based on a Standard (ASTM, ISO, etc.). Parameters based on standards do not need further justification.

5. REFERENCES
List all references used for the justification in chapter 4. Suitable references are for instance:
- Current standards
- Test Reports
- Literature articles
- Complaints reported to Stryker (incl. PER-number)
- Monographs and White Papers
- Clinical experience of surgeons (meeting minutes)
- Calculations

6. ATTACHMENTS AND FILING
Attach useful data to this document (e.g. drawings, sketches, calculations, meeting minutes etc.)! The signed document as well as all belonging attachments shall be filed in separate folder (hardcopy) at the lab site where the Test method /Test setup was developed and usually located.

b

Fig. 3.3 (*continued*) Slim process and form to determine and document method justification and validation. Example from the medical device industry.[5,6]

Reporting Results

Generally, results have to be reported accurately, clearly, unambiguously, and objectively. The laboratory should have a procedure for the correct preparation of a study or test report accompanied by a standard form to be used. The report should contain a title, name and address of the laboratory, issue date and number, the location where tests were carried out, a unique identification of the test report, an identification and description of the methods used (including all deviations from originally agreed method), description and condition of items tested or studied, sampling plan, and procedures used by the laboratory.

The report should further contain all relevant results, correct units of measurement (using the International System of Units, if possible), statistical analysis, and statement on uncertainties of measurements. Interpretations of results are allowed but have to be clearly marked as such. Those interpretations may include statements on compliance/noncompliance of the results with previously set acceptance criteria and recommendations on how to use the results or suggestions for test item improvement.

3.4 Test or Study Flow

Based on ISO 17025 requirements along with our own experience with a test laboratory in the medical device industry, a study flow chart is suggested and shown in

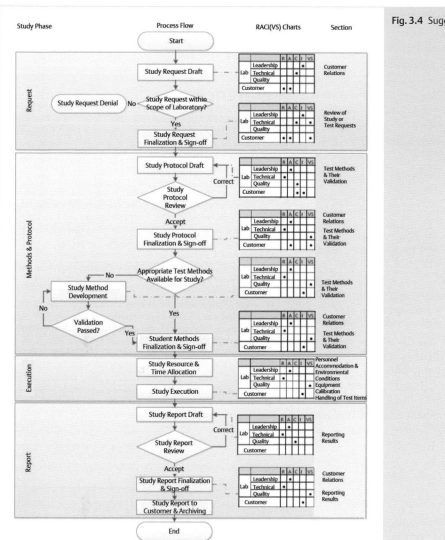

Fig. 3.4 Suggested test or study flow chart.

▶ Fig. 3.4. Along with the sequential steps of a study, the chart lists the personnel involved in each step in a RACI (VS) structure, as defined per ▶ Table 3.1. It makes reference to several sections of this chapter, where more details/requirements may be found for each study step, respectively.

3.5 Formal Aspects: Accreditation and Certification

Laboratories may apply for accreditation to comply to GLP guidelines. The accreditation is dedicated to a specific spectrum of tests and analyses, and based on periodic site audits from legal authorities like Deutsche Akkreditierungsstelle in Germany, UKGLP monitoring program in the United Kingdom, or the American Association for Laboratory Accreditation in the United States. Accreditation attests an institution to follow specific GLP guidelines and to have the technical competence to perform a specific test spectrum. The audit requirements may be based on different standards outlining GLP requirements nationally or internationally.

Alternatively, institutions may be certified that they implemented and follow certain GLP guidelines—like ISO 17025 requirements—within their work scope. The certificate is not dedicated to a specific spectrum of tests or analyses.

3.6 Conclusion

GLP describes a methodology to be followed in order to obtain reliable, repeatable, reproducible, and consistent study and testing results. This can be achieved by installing and continuously strengthening the two key pillars of GLP: a quality-oriented management system along with adequate and qualified technical resources.

Table 3.1 Definition of RACI(VS), tailored to a good laboratory practices–regulated study flow.[7,8]

R	Responsible	In charge of executing a task in a defined and correct manner
A	Accountable	Being held (legally) accountable that a task has been executed in a correct manner.
C	Consulted	Consulted for test item–specific/technical/scientific/subject matter expertise.
I	Informed	Informed about status, results, deviations, etc.
VS	Verify and sign	Verify by review conformance to laboratory and study-specific procedures, protocols, and requirements. Sign off, if this verification is passed.

On the one hand, the enhanced application of GLP in the medical device industry throughout recent years revealed clear advantages, fostering the "do it right the first time" approach. On the other hand, the regulatory and documentary requirements associated with GLP may sometimes be felt as an innovation hindrance and ballast. Thus, where experimental and thought process freedom is needed, this playground must always be ensured to guarantee continuous improvement and vital innovation in any methods development.

However, as soon as a method is established and used for purposes like publishing on biomechanical characteristics with clinical relevance, the key pillars of GLP shall be followed.

References

[1] U.S. Food and Drug Administration. CFR - Code of Federal Regulations Title 21-Food and Drugs Chapter I-Food and Drug Administration. Department of Health and Human Services. Part 58 Good laboratory Practice for Nonclinical Laboratory Studies. Silver Spring, MD: U.S. Food and Drug Administration; 2012

[2] Organisation for Economic Cooperation and Development. OECD series on principles of good laboratory practice and compliance monitoring. Environmental Directorate, Chemicals Group and Management Committee. Number 1. OECD Principles on Good Laboratory Practice (as revised in 1997). Paris, France: Organisation for Economic Cooperation and Development; 1998

[3] European Committee for Standardization. General requirements for the competence of testing and calibration laboratories (ISO/IEC 17025:2005). Brussels, Belgium: European Committee for Standardization; 2005

[4] Wolf G. Irrtümer um den, Deming'schen PDCA-Zyklus. Qulaität und Zuverlässigkeit 54. München, Germany: Hanser Verlag; 2009

[5] DIN Deutsches Institut für Normung e. V. DIN 1319. Grundlagen der Meßtechnik. Berlin, Germany: Beuth Verlag GmbH; 1996

[6] Gerber C, v. Oldenburg G. Divisional quality form DQF30-XXX. Kiel, Germany: Stryker Osteosynthesis; 2011

[7] Jacka M, Keller P. Business process mapping: improving customer satisfaction. New York: John Wiley and Sons; 2009:257

[8] Blokdijk G. The service level agreement SLA guide-SLA book, templates for service level management and service level agreement forms. Fast and easy way to write your SLA. Brisbane, Australia: Emereo Pty Limited; 2008

4 How to Prepare for a Period in Research

Ines L.H. Reichert

Fortune favors the prepared mind. – Louis Pasteur
  One sometimes finds what one is not looking for.
– Alexander Fleming

This chapter aims to provide tips and hints for the clinician in training to prepare effectively for a "time out" in research. The motivation to do so may be driven by interest in a particular field of research and the wish to add "experience in research" to the portfolio. Often, the latter is required to advance to the next position on the career ladder. For nonclinical researchers, the next career step may be to carry out a higher degree and the question "why spend time in research" will be redundant, but other questions concerning the research topic, choice of supervisor, and funding will be just as applicable.

Spending time in research gives one the chance to explore a research question thoroughly and add a completely different aspect to the clinical training path. The "time out" of clinical practice should culminate in completing a project, publishing a paper, and/or submitting a thesis. Furthermore, this time should give the basis for a lifelong understanding, if not continuation, of research.

Frequently, the clinician will not be aware how far he or she steps out of the comfort zone of clinical work by embarking on a full- or part-time research project.

The only way to prevent disappointment is to plan and prepare the proposed period in research—making it a very precious time in every sense. This chapter will address a number of points that are worthwhile considering beforehand.

4.1 Why Spend Time in Research?

A doctor in training contemplating spending time in research must have a good reason to do so, as clinical and research activities demand different frames of mind. The unfamiliarity of the world of research with its distinctive expectations and own ways of measuring success should not be underestimated. It is important to understand the inherent differences in work pattern between clinical and research work.

Also, it cannot be stressed enough that progress may be slow and unpredictable. There may be initial failure, which can put the enthusiastic but inexperienced researcher under a significant amount of strain.

Lastly, a major concern for clinical trainees may be that time in research and thus away from the clinic might result in a loss of practical skills (e.g., in the operating theater). In reality, a preset time away from clinical work of 1 or even 3 years will not make as much of a difference in the long run as often initially feared. However, the timing of the research period needs to be considered carefully. In some countries, such as the United Kingdom, academic training programs have been introduced and the overall period of training may be extended to ensure all training objectives are satisfied.

A final thought may be that spending time in research will make the trainee a better doctor. While in general exposure to research methodology will enhance critical thinking and thus further the practice of evidence-based medicine, the reality of conducting a research project will be largely unconnected to direct clinical practice. Of course, the future results of the conducted research project might contribute to the evidence important for that field of medicine. Furthermore, the clinician spending time in research will gain insight in the research process, leading to new knowledge. This appreciation will be invaluable at a later stage in the clinical career when the exposure to new products and new techniques requires constant critical appraisal.

4.2 What Is Different in Research?

Time at medical school, as the name suggests, is laid out to learn and accumulate facts and combination of facts, usually in descriptive sciences. In clinical attachments, students observe and absorb clinical experience. Basic sciences are touched on in broad terms, but not enough to allow the experience of deductive reasoning.

The medical student usually only gathers glances on how novel facts are being reached. The processes of formulating a hypothesis, designing an experiment, scrutinizing the methods, and collecting and analyzing data are not practiced in medical school.

During the first foundation years in the clinic, the young doctor, still not fully graduated, is challenged to follow the pace of clinical work. This usually demands alertness, good communication, and quick organization. Clinical work follows demands posed from the outside (i.e., the timetable of work on the wards, clinics, and theater sessions)—this starts when one sets foot into the hospital and finishes when leaving. Day to day, the clinician deals with the problems that are presented: patients who require decisions, treatment, and operations. These decisions have their own momentum and urgency, and, particularly in orthopedic surgery, are often solved with an immediately visible and appreciable result (e.g., a radiograph showing the fixation of a fracture). During clinical work, there may be busy times with a number of demands happening at once. An exception is the operating theater, as it provides a relative oasis of calm. This is a place for only one task and allows the required concentration for the surgery to be performed. In general, the clinical world requires quick attention to new patients and new problems. And usually the clinician is able to go home with the sense of having completed a satisfactory "day at the office."

Research demands an entirely different mindset. The researcher starts by formulating the research question. In contrast to clinical life, the problem will not be presented by a patient, but will be actively sought out by the researcher. The research question will go beyond a problem posed by an individual patient and seeks to find a true answer to a given question. Guidance by the research supervisor with academic experience will be vital at this stage. Equally, the researcher will determine how to solve the problem and which methodology would serve best to reach a valid answer. The necessity of funding will be referred to in more detail later on. The researcher with a clinical background will learn to apply research techniques, which are usually unfamiliar, requiring practice (e.g., cell culture, microdissection).

The researcher will perform most of the technical work alone and will interpret the results. The day will be structured around access to the laboratory but in general the working day will be self-motivated. The supervisor will help with the time frame, but much of the organization and daily prioritization will be left to the researcher. Lastly, after a successful time in research, the trainee/investigator will need to present and publish the results.

The relative lack of a structured day will be unfamiliar for anybody coming from a clinical environment. In research, it is definitely not enough just "to show up." While in the clinic each patient sets a mini-problem, the research project consists of facets that come together only at the end of a prolonged period of time and effort. There are days where results or progress are not tangible. As a side effect, each working day has an ill-defined end. For the motivated researcher, there is always more to do, leading to an entirely different stress from the surgical "adrenaline." The day of the clinician resembles a series of sprints, whereas conducting a research project is more akin to running a marathon.

4.3 What Does a Clinician Bring to a Research Laboratory?

It should not be forgotten that the clinician will bring a number of points, views, and attributes to the team that will be very valuable. The clinician will be rigorous in looking for and understanding the clinical relevance of each project, and will help the team with communication of the clinical problem underlying the research question.

Furthermore, the limited time in research and the need to achieve results in this period can help to drive the chosen research project forward. The surgical mindset tends to select the best practical solution to a problem rather than getting lost in a myriad of theoretical considerations.

The discipline instilled in medical school and the long hours required for a clinical day will also benefit the time in research. Lastly, there are a number of projects where clinical experience or operative skills can be of direct use for the project, may it be experimental research with animals or clinical research with patients.

4.4 Spending Time in Research —the Right Decision?

4.4.1 Motivation and Expectations

Before considering a time in research, it will be very useful to be clear about the underlying motivation and expectation (▶ Table 4.1). The motivation for each individual may encompass various aspects ranging from interest in the subject to advancing the career, all of them being valid points. However, it is worthwhile to think of alternatives: Interest in the subject does not necessarily require taking time out for research. Conversely, there are other ways to distinguish the career (e.g., doing a specialist fellowship, adding a master of business administration degree or law course, or spending time in a reputable unit abroad).

There will also be intermediate options of pursuing a research project that may not require taking time out. It may be possible to take part in a clinical research project, such as writing up a case series, in a unit that collects outcome data in a prospective manner.

Occasionally, a laboratory project in a well-set-up unit may only require the commitment of 1 or 2 days per week. However, both of these "intermediate options" will require a similar degree of preparations in order to be certain that these aims will have a good chance of being achieved at the end of the attachment.

Another option is a structured program such as a master of science degree, which will provide a teaching program and require the conclusion of a small project rather than an extensive piece of original work. Enrollment for a master of science degree may be more predictable than spending the time for a self-organized research project.

Motivation of a clinical trainee is often determined by the example set by a leading surgeon, physician, or researcher. The inspiration by an individual might lead to the wish to reach similar skills in the treatment of patients, surgical technique, or conducting research. Furthermore, the exposure to debate might lead to awareness of topical questions in the field and the wish to contribute to the solution. Such exposure to a research question is likely to lead to strong motivation.

Table 4.1 Summary: Key Points to Consider before Deciding on a Period in Research

Is "time out" the best option for me?		
	What would I like to achieve?	
		Research experience, publication, research degree, thesis
	How much time will I need?	
		Discuss a realistic full- or part-time estimate with an academic advisor
	Are there alternatives?	
		Think out of the box. What is my main motivation? • Career enhancement • Interest in the topic • Research experience
How best to organize it?		
	When is the best time?	
		Before or within a specialist training program
	What is the best research topic for me?	
		Broad or specific field of interest
		Basic science or clinical
		Research methodology
	How will I find a supervisor to work with?	
		Academic unit, topic, reputation
		Conferences and debates
		Personal meeting
	What funding is required?	
		Cost of research, basic salary, university fees
	How and when to secure funding	
		In advance • Grant application • Research Fellowship • "Soft money" in agreement with the supervisor and department

Motivation fueled by interest and inspiration will be a good starting point for the endeavor of research. The junior clinician who has not been exposed to a scenario where such motivation can be gleaned from should make this the first point of preparation.

Advice

Attend regional or national meetings, watch debates between senior surgeons/physicians, and read the background of these topics. Does this hold your interest and lead to the wish to find a solution? Would you like seeing yourself contributing to the debate with new facts in a few years?

4.5 How Best to Prepare—Essentials

4.5.1 Timing

The best time for a period in research is usually after completion of a predetermined step in clinical training (i.e., a professional examination) or before starting the next clinical period. The first such opportunity would be as an undergraduate doing an intercalated bachelor of science degree. Following graduation, if there is a break between basic and higher training, this can be a suitable time to carry out a research project (e.g., in the United Kingdom after the MRCS exams). This is the point of time where an additional point on the curriculum vitae is usually most needed, but where also the danger is greatest to be misled to spend a less than worthwhile time out. Therefore, it is preferable to be assured of a clinical training slot in the field that one would wish to practice in. A better time is often a year or two after starting a clinical training program in surgery or medicine. In general, if a trainee is taking time out within the training program, it is best to arrange it to return to clinical work at least 1 year before any clinical exams. There may also be options to carry out higher degrees as a part-time student, while remaining in the clinical post. Another opportunity, the last as trainee, would be after the final specialty exam (e.g., in the United Kingdom, the FRCS [Tr & Orth] exam). This time could constitute a research fellowship, possibly in addition or combination with a clinical fellowship before the end of the fixed years of training. At this final stage of training, the interested candidate would certainly be very aware which specific clinical field is preferred to specialize in and thus be able to tailor the research project to strengthen long-term career prospects.

Conversely, a medical student may choose a research project in a basic science subject such as anatomy or physiology and the skills acquired will be applicable in a range of clinical fields. Moreover, the generic aspects of any research experience are not to be overlooked and are worth taking into account. The deciding factors for the choice of timing will be motivation, opportunity, and career progress, making it counteractive to be too rigid with the perception of a "best" time per se.

Advice

Try to be ahead of the game. If you are thinking of taking time out to conduct a research project, consider and plan it as early as you can. As a rule, the further advanced you are in your clinical training, the more useful will be a research project in a specialized aspect of your chosen field. Motivation will play a considerable role in the choice of the time.

4.5.2 Must It Be a Research Degree?

A period in research may be considered useful when the time spent on a project reveals results worth publishing, ideally as presentation and publication. The extent of a study leading to a publication may be as small as a report on a case series or the description of a novel surgical technique.

Alternatively, the framework of a thesis will allow the researcher to develop a project, apply new techniques, and create novel data. The thesis in itself will be recognition of this structured effort. The results of a thesis are usually worth presenting and publishing. A thesis will need more time and commitment than getting involved in a small aspect of an existing project. A thesis will require an academic supervisor and postgraduate studies for a thesis will also attract registration fees. The time required to complete a thesis varies, usually 2 years are anticipated for a medical doctorate degree and 3 years for a doctorate in philosophy. A clinician often perceives this as too long and anticipates finishing the thesis ahead of schedule, which in reality might be ambitious. If the research project has been very well set up in advance and all of the necessary licenses and facilities are in place, the experimental work may be carried out in a period of 1 to 2 years of full-time research. Under this circumstance, analysis and writing up will need to be accomplished while one has returned to clinical work, and this is a considerable challenge. It is therefore highly recommended to have completed the first draft of the thesis before returning to clinical work.

Advice

Decide clearly on what you would like to achieve in the time you are willing to invest. As soon as you are prepared to spend a year or longer, you should consider registering for a higher degree. A "time out" in research should be planned in an academic unit. Doing a thesis will provide you with a more thorough experience and lead to more recognition, irrespective of a publication.

4.5.3 What Type of Degree?

At an undergraduate stage, a bachelor of science degree may be very useful to gain a first insight into research. Equally, a master of science degree may be very valuable for a predictable research experience at an early stage. A medical doctorate thesis may just be possible with limited time out, provided there has been careful planning. If you are taking time out in the region of a year or two, it will almost certainly be possible to complete a medical doctorate. However, if the research project is generating good results, there may not be a large difference between the effort required to write up a thesis for a medical doctorate and a doctorate in philosophy. Finally from the point of view of being involved in research in the future, it is far preferable to do a doctorate in philosophy.

Advice

Opt for a master of science degree if your aim is a limited but structured insight into research. However, if you would like to be involved in research per se, do a doctorate in philosophy degree if at all possible.

4.5.4 Supervisor and Subject

The choice of supervisor may be the most important point of the preparation. The search for a supervisor will be initially orientated on the research subject, but as outlined in the following the supervisor for the research period will be ideally chosen with more than a purely pragmatic aspect in mind. Most academic professors will have a range of interests and be able to supervise a variety of subjects. There are several scenarios: Firstly, the supervisor may approach the potential researcher/trainee. This is possible in an academic unit where there is an ongoing research program and projects are planned well in advance. This is an excellent scenario as the researcher/trainee may have an opportunity to shape the project and may be included as a named person on a funding proposal. However, a certain degree of caution is advised to be certain that the project has a good chance to get off the ground and to be concluded.

The second, and possibly more common scenario, is that of the researcher/trainee approaching the supervisor. The selection of the supervisor is based on their reputation, the field of interest, previous publications, the institution, and the location. Personal contact will be a deciding factor as both parties will need to work together closely for the duration of this project. Mutual respect and trust will be absolute requirements. The mutual connection and ability to work with each other may be even more important than the subject. The choice of supervisor usually determines the approach or broad outline of research methodology, keeping in mind that clinical professors often work with a number of basic scientists so that dual supervision using a variety of research tools are often a possibility. If the supervisor or cosupervisor is a basic scientist, it is important that they recognize the different background and experience that a clinician will have compared to a nonclinical researcher.

Advice

How to find somebody to supervise your research? Do attend meetings and debates where the supervisor you might consider will be present. It is important to be able to imagine working together. Seek a personal appointment to discuss the option of a project. Speak to previous or present students/clinicians in the department. When the supervisor has approached you, make sure you explore alternatives; this will help to clarify the mind. Be prepared when you are meeting your potential supervisor. Be informed about recent achievements and publications in the department, but also make sure to highlight how you individually could fit in to develop new ideas and projects.

4.5.5 Funding

Research may be funded through successful peer-reviewed grants from funding agencies, which form two large subgroups: (1) state funding (e.g., the various medical research councils, the European Union Research fund, the National Health Service National Institute for Health Research in the United Kingdom, and the National Institutes of Health in the United States) or (2) major charities (e.g., Wellcome Trust, Arthritis Research UK, and Orthopaedic Research UK). Research may be also funded by "soft money" from companies or intradepartmental funds. A period in research requires funding for (1) the salary, (2) the higher degree university fees, and (3) the research consumables for the project. It is essential that research funding is available from the outset; if this is coming from "soft money," it is particularly important to ensure that sufficient funds exist for the duration of the research period. It is common for the prospective researcher to apply for a "research fellowship" to cover the basic salary. For clinicians, it may be possible to be included in the on call rota. Not unusually, the supervisor will have applied for the project to be funded and will advertise this research opportunity. The experimental and laboratory costs will need to be accounted for prior to the commencement of the research project. The application process for a grant will take in the region of 6 months to a year and may need to be completed prior to commencement. Thus, the preparation period for a fully funded time in research will take in the region of 1 to 2 years.

Advice

This is a crucial issue. Nonclinicians are aware of the importance of this topic, but clinicians in training are not exposed to the impact of the availability of funds on an individual's direct progress. The clinician will find that as a researcher, the cost of research will be decisive for one's progress. Enquire about the funds available.

Ideally, make early enquiries and offer to be part of the grant writing team, which will give you an extra insight.

4.6 Conclusion

Spending time in research provides an opportunity to add to the experience of a surgeon/physician by stepping out of the clinical framework. The research project will require a full set of skills that are often new to the clinician. This is true for both clinical research and laboratory research. In both cases, the surgeon will become familiar with technical aspects of the project, which may include the use of clinical outcome instruments, biomechanical measurements, and animal or cell culture experiments. Beyond these technical aspects, there are generic research skills ranging from asking the right question to carrying out a statistical power analysis as well as the ability to interpret and present results. The achievement of submitting a thesis will clearly affirm the successful exposure to such skills.

Last, and by no means least, you might find research is fun. Be prepared to bitten by the bug! Not only the independent way of working and thinking, but also the sense of "finding something new" and being the first to throw new insight onto a problem will make this time worthwhile.

Further Reading

Barker P. Top 1000 scientists: from the beginning of time to 2000 AD. Hove: Book Guild Ltd.; 1999

Bhandari M, Joensson A. Clinical research for surgeons. Stuttgart: Thieme Publishers; 2008

Cryer P. The research student's guide to success. 2nd ed. Buckingham: Open University Press; 2000

King's Biomed on Twitter: https://twitter.com/kingsbiomed; last accessed 23 January 2015

Oxford Science Blog: http://www.ox.ac.uk/news/science-blog; last accessed 23 January 2015

HKU Graduate School - University of Hong Kong. Preparation for a thesis proposal; www.gradsch.hku.hk/gradsch/web/resources/thesis-proposal.pdf; last accessed 23 January 2015

Reis RM. Keeping your research alive. Chron High Educ.

University of Oxford – Support for Researchers: http://www.ox.ac.uk/research/support-researchers; last accessed 23 January 2015

Waugh W. John Charnley: the man and the hip. London: Springer-Verlag London United; 1990

Part 2

Structural Biomechanics

5 Physiological Boundary Conditions for Mechanical Testing

Markus O. Heller

It is widely accepted that the mechanical environment within a bone plays a critical role for the progression and the final outcome of the regeneration and healing processes taking place after sustaining a fracture. However, not only the healing and adaptation processes of the biological tissues, but also the proper function of the implants and hardware used for the stabilization of a fracture depends critically upon the mechanical forces acting within the bone. Detailed knowledge of the loading conditions within the long bones is therefore an essential prerequisite for the successful development of new implants. Moreover, an understanding of how the interaction between the mechanical forces within the bone and the stability provided by an implant define the local mechanical environment at a fracture may allow the development and application of osteosynthesis devices in such a manner that the resulting mechanical environment will at least not hinder, but ideally even promote healing. It is essential that the mechanical loading conditions of a long bone are governed by the forces of the muscles and the contact forces transferred at the joints,[1,2] and this chapter will therefore provide a review of our current understanding of the physiological loading conditions in the human lower extremity.

Key Concepts: Musculoskeletal Loading

The musculoskeletal system provides form, support, stability, and movement to the body. It consists of bones, muscles, cartilage, tendons, ligaments, and other connective tissue. The skeletal muscles are not only the essential active structures that enable us to move our body in a variety of ways and gaits, but they also provide the main contribution to the mechanical loading conditions within our limbs (▶ Fig. 5.1). While muscle forces cannot be directly measured, the development of telemetric implants equipped with technology to measure the forces within the hip, knee, and shoulder joints has resulted in the most detailed and accurate knowledge of the forces acting across the large joints in the human body today.[3]

5.1 In Vivo Loading Conditions at the Large Joints of the Lower Limbs

While previous numerical modeling approaches provided estimates of the forces at the hip as large as 10 times body weight during walking and stair climbing, the in vivo measurements of the joint forces could not confirm these predictions. According to the measurements, the forces at the large joints of the human lower extremities are rather in the range of about 2 to 3.5 times body weight during activities of daily living, with the largest forces at both the hip and knee joints determined during stair descent (▶ Table 5.1).

Although the measurements indicate that there is only little variation in the force magnitudes across activities, and this observation generally holds true also for the three-dimensional orientation of the joint force vectors, there are small yet relevant differences in the quality of loading between walking and, for example, stair negotiation activities. As a result of the increased hip flexion, the muscles of the hip act more in the transverse plane of the femur and hence the anterior-posterior directed component of the hip force vector during stair negotiation can be up to twice as large as during level walking (▶ Fig. 5.2). As a consequence, the torsional moments around the long axis of the femur are also increased during stair climbing (▶ Fig. 5.3). The inclusion of stair climbing loads in the mechanical testing would therefore be particularly important for the development of devices that need to provide adequate stability not only during walking but throughout the spectrum of key activities of daily living.[6]

5.2 Muscle Action Is a Key Modulator of the Internal Loading Conditions

The literature further suggests that specific situations such as stumbling are capable of causing excessively large internal forces.[7] Analysis of musculoskeletal interaction suggests that under these conditions, muscle activity alone is capable of generating extreme joint forces. Similarly, all other bony regions spanned by activated muscles may become excessively loaded during activities such as stumbling. If muscles are activated to their full potential,

Table 5.1 Typical Joint Force Magnitudes (in Multiples of Body Weight) During Activities of Daily Living

Joint	Walking	Stair ascent	Stair descent	Rising from a chair
Hip[4]	2.38	2.51	2.60	1.90
Tibiofemoral[3]	2.61	3.16	3.46	2.46
Patellofemoral[5]	0.76	2.80	–	3.10

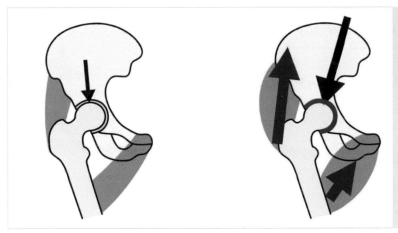

Fig. 5.1 The forces due to weight and inertia represent only a small fraction of the overall forces acting at the joints and within the long bones during activities of daily living (*left*). Here, the forces of the muscles that are required to move our body and/or to stabilize the joints create the largest contribution to the internal forces acting on the bones and articular cartilage (*right*).

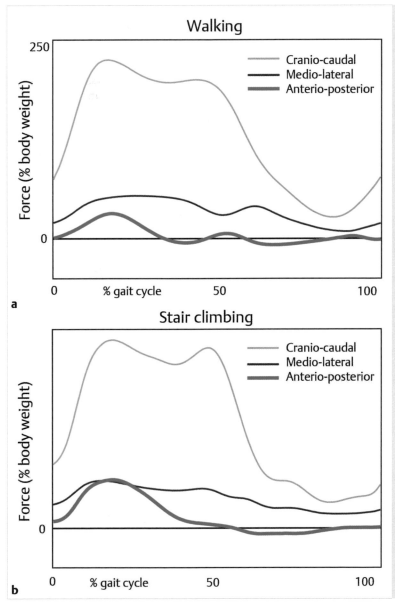

Fig. 5.2 Magnitudes of the three components of the hip contact force vector during a full cycle of normal walking (**a**) and stair climbing (**b**). Although the craniocaudal (axial) force components are very similar, the anteroposterior-directed force component during stair climbing is considerably larger than during walking. The forces determined for a typical subject[4] are given here as percentage of body weight. Please refer to Bergmann et al[4] for further details regarding the coordinate system in which the force components are provided.

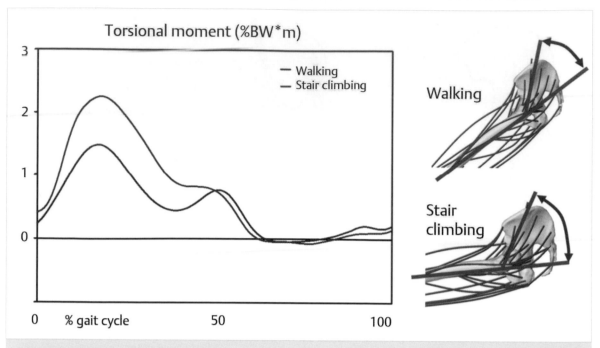

Fig. 5.3 During walking, the muscles at the hip are more aligned with the long axis of the femur than during stair climbing, where the hip is more flexed. This results not only in increased anteroposterior-directed hip contact forces during stair climbing, but also increased torsional moment acting around the femoral shaft.

they may produce not only maximal forces at the joints and extreme compression forces in the bone, but also excessive bending and shear forces. Furthermore, experimental evidence suggests that attempts to unload the fracture site by controlling the external force might not be effective.[8] Taken together, these results suggest that in patients who received osteosynthetic treatment after bone fracture and exhibit unsecure gait patterns, it is likely that unusually large forces or relatively larger shear loading conditions exist, conditions that are particularly detrimental to the secure fixation of bone screws and can limit the longevity of the implants.

5.3 Loading Conditions within Long Bones

While telemetric implants provide excellent insight into the forces acting at the large joints, the mechanical loading conditions throughout the bones are modified by the action of the muscles and therefore differ from those observed directly at the joints. Although ethical considerations discourage the use of invasive methods for determining the coordinated action of all muscle forces in vivo by direct measurement in humans, computer models provide a powerful, alternative means to study the complex distribution of muscle forces in detail.

While early numerical analyses used to overestimate joint forces, recent modeling approaches demonstrate that analytical methods are able to predict the measured in vivo loads within an approximately 15% error in patients with telemetric hip or knee implants (▶ Fig. 5.4). In order to obtain this high degree of accuracy, the key features of the individual musculoskeletal anatomy, accurate skeletal motion data, and information on the external loads are required.[5]

5.4 Organ Level Loading Conditions: Forces and Moments

As such validated models determine the muscle and joint forces throughout the entire lower limb, they are not limited to the study of the internal loading conditions at single locations such as the hip or knee, but rather provide access to the internal loading conditions throughout the entire bones. From such analyses, we understand that the internal loading of the femur is generally characterized by axial compression (F_z), with small shear forces directed mediolaterally (F_x) and anteroposteriorly (F_y) (▶ Fig. 5.5). As a result of the activity of the abductor muscles during gait, compressive and shear forces are largest at the

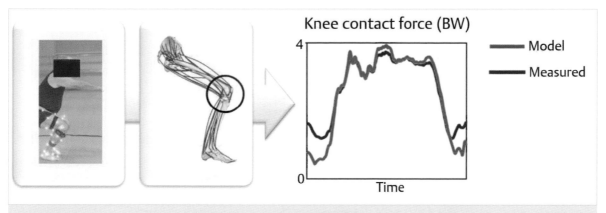

Fig. 5.4 Driven by accurate gait analysis data describing the skeletal motion and external forces during a squat, the analytical model that captures the individual patient anatomy is able to accurately predict the tibiofemoral contact forces, as evidenced by direct comparison of the model predictions to the in vivo measured joint forces.[5]

femoral head and decrease distally toward the diaphysis during walking. Under physiological loading, the bending moments in the femur are dominated by the frontal plane bending moment (M_y), whereas the torsional moment (M_z) is the smallest of all. Even though individual gait characteristics resulted in some variations of the patterns over a cycle, load magnitudes are comparable between patients during walking and stair climbing (▶ Fig. 5.5 and ▶ Fig. 5.6).

Of note, however, are the considerable differences in the magnitude of the compressive forces acting down the femur (F_z). During stair climbing, forces peaked in the diaphysis because of contraction of the quadriceps muscles. The importance of considering the muscle contribution when analyzing long bone mechanical loading is further underlined by the fact that the bending moments determined were considerably smaller than those predicted by previous analyses, which neglected muscle forces.

5.5 Tissue Level Loading Conditions: Bone Strains

Musculoskeletal loading generates stresses and strains within the bone tissue. For implant design and evaluation, it is essential that locally high or low strain values that potentially affect clinical outcome are identified. Finite element analysis provides a convenient way to determine strains within a bone, given that adequate loads are applied. The femur, for example, experiences a rather homogeneous strain distribution, characteristic of frontal plane bending superimposed with axial compression when loaded with all thigh muscles (▶ Fig. 5.7). The use of simplified load cases, however, led to a considerable overestimation of bending moments distally. This occurred because the effect of muscle contraction that

compensates for shear forces and bending moments developed within bone was not included. Very similarly for the tibia, the analysis under physiological-like and simplified loading conditions revealed that only under a fully balanced system of muscle, ligament forces, and joint contact forces the straining of the bone was more or less homogeneous. The prevalence of compressive strains at the posteromedial cortex and the relative tension of the anterolateral cortices suggested a combined loading consisting of axial compression superimposed onto bending in the midsagittal plane. Under simplified loading, the bone strains were overestimated, especially in the distal tibia. In addition to an overestimation in strain magnitude, the strain pattern found under simplified loading also differed substantially from the one under physiological-like loading as it overemphasized bending in the distal portion of the tibia. These studies therefore demonstrate that if major muscles are neglected, tensile and compressive strains are overestimated, while torsional effects tend to be underestimated. These effects may significantly influence the predicted osteosynthesis performance and limits the extrapolation of experimental results to the in vivo situation.

5.6 Application of Physiological Loading Conditions during Mechanical Testing

The previous sections of this chapter explained the particular importance of the muscles in defining the physiological loading conditions at the joints and throughout the long bones. More than 20 muscles at the hip alone work together in a highly orchestrated manner to enable

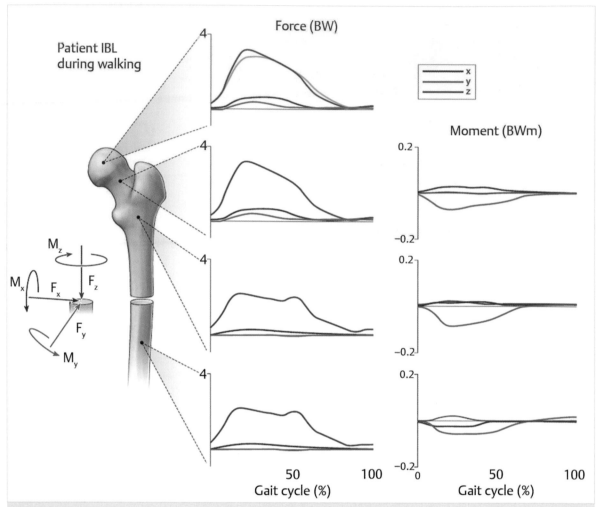

Fig. 5.5 Internal loads at four levels of the femur during the walking cycle (starting with heel strike of one subject). Forces are given in multiples of body weight (*BW*), moments in body weight meters (*BWm*). F_x is the shear force from medial to lateral, F_z is the shear force from anterior to posterior, and F_z is the axial compression force from proximal to distal. M_x is the backward-acting bending moment in the sagittal plane, M_y is the inward-acting bending moment in the frontal plane, and M_z is the torsional moment in the transverse plane. The moments at the head center are zero. The in vivo measured hip contact force component F_z is shown in *gray*. All signs are reversed for the proximal sides. (Fig. 2–2 in Berry DJ, Liebermann J [eds.]. Surgery of the hip. Amsterdam: Elsevier, 2013; Redrawn from Heller MO, Bergmann G, Deuretzbacher G, et al. Influence of femoral anteversion on proximal femoral loading: measurement and simulation in four patients. Clin Biomech [Bristol, Avon] 2001;8:644–649.)

flawless execution of the many motions required during activities of daily living. Although the previous presented modeling approaches capture a considerable degree of the anatomical complexity involved here, translation of these findings into mechanical testing of implants presents major challenges. The following sections of this chapter will deal with two key aspects: firstly, the challenge of reduction in complexity of the load configuration while maintaining key characteristics of physiological long bone loading, and secondly, the challenge to successfully apply physiological load levels in vitro.

5.7 Adequate Reduction of Complexity

The physical space limitations and reduced complexity that can be realized during in vitro testing require a simplification and reduction of the number of muscle fibers down to the essential minimums. Further research, therefore, focused on developing a concept that allowed simplifying the complex representation of the hip musculature with over 30 different lines of muscle action to a reduced number of muscle fibers but maintained the key

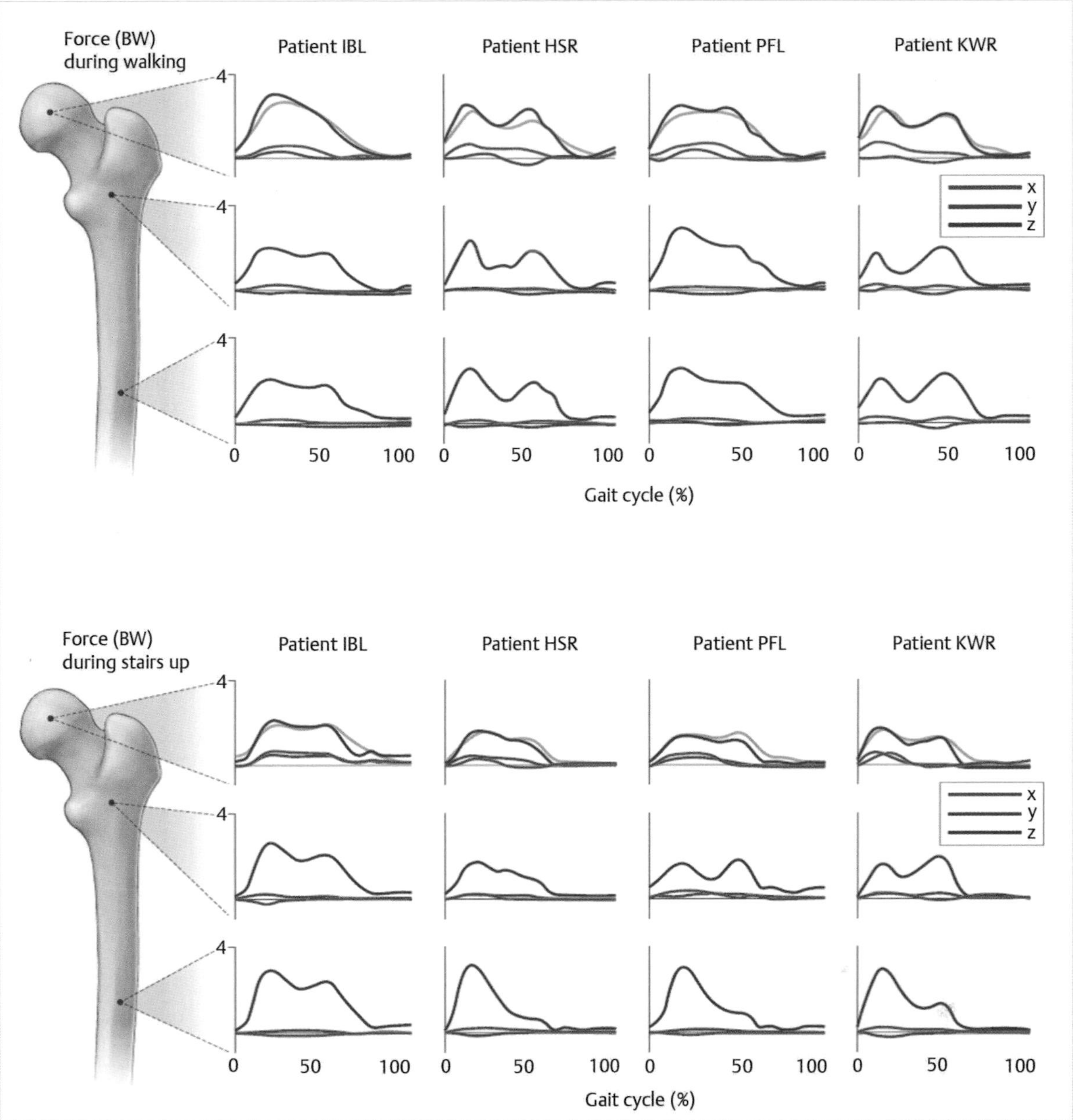

Fig. 5.6 Internal forces (in body weight [*BW*]) during walking (**a**) and stair climbing (**b**) at three levels of the femur. Results are shown for four patients. (Combination of Figs. 2–3 and 2–4 in Berry DJ, Liebermann J (eds.). Surgery of the hip. Amsterdam: Elsevier, 2013; Redrawn from Heller MO, Bergmann G, Deuretzbacher G, et al. Influence of femoral anteversion on proximal femoral loading: measurement and simulation in four patients. Clin Biomech [Bristol, Avon] 2001;8:644–649.)

characteristics of physiological loading.[2] Here, all fibers of the gluteus muscles with a similar function (gluteus maximus, medius, and minimus) were grouped into one simplified "abductor muscle" with a single attachment site. A similar process was applied to the adductor muscles (adductus brevis, magnus, and longus), yielding a resultant "adductor muscle." In an attempt to further reduce the number of muscles included in the model to the lowest feasible total, joint contact forces were calculated for a series of different configurations in which muscles with small forces (i.e., muscles from the group of the lateral rotators) were progressively removed from the model to a point beyond which unphysiological hip joint loading was calculated (► Fig. 5.8).

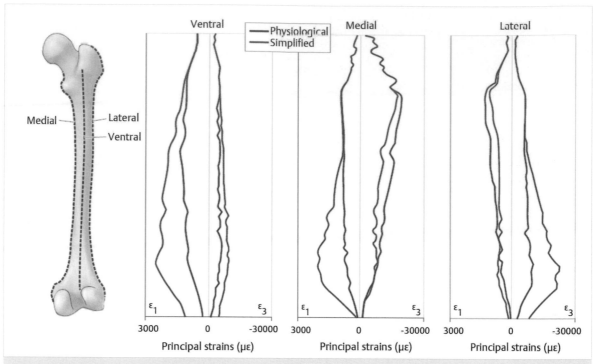

Fig. 5.7 Principal strains ε_1 (maximal) and ε_3 (minimal) along lines on the ventral, medial, and lateral aspects of the human femur at 45% gait cycle with all thigh muscles included (*dark lines*). For comparison, strains are given for simplified load regimes with only the hip contact, abductors, and iliotibial band included (*light lines*). (Fig. 2–8 in Berry DJ, Liebermann J (eds.). Surgery of the hip. Amsterdam: Elsevier, 2013; Redrawn from Duda GN, Heller M, Albinger J, et al. Influence of muscle forces on femoral strain distribution. J Biomech 1998;9:841–846.)

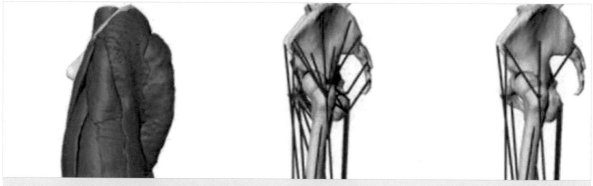

Fig. 5.8 While medical image–based modeling techniques enable detailed modeling of the structures of the musculoskeletal system (*left, center*), a certain degree of simplification (*right*) is necessary before physiological-like loading conditions adequate for mechanical in vitro testing can be derived.

The final load profile for the proximal femur was taken as the most simplified muscle configuration that resulted in physiological-like joint loading throughout the gait cycle at the instances of maximum in vivo measured hip joint contact forces for both walking and stair climbing.

For these two instances, three (walking) and four (stair climbing) muscles of the derived model exerted forces at the proximal femur (▶ Table 5.2). The instance of maximum hip contact force during stair climbing coincided with the peak anteroposterior force and also represented

Table 5.2 Load Profile Developed for the Preclinical Testing of Implants at the Proximal Femur

Walking (body weight = 836N)				
Force	x	y	z	Acts at point
Hip contact	-54.0	-32.8	-229.2	P0
Intersegmental resultant	-8.1	-12.8	-78.2	P0
Abductor (1)	58.0	4.3	86.5	P1
Tensor fascia latae, proximal part (3a)	7.2	11.60-	13.2	P1
Tensor fascia latae, distal part (3b)	-0.5	-0.7	-19.0	P1
Vastus lateralis (4)	-0.9	18.5	-92.9	P2
Stair climbing (body weight = 847N)				
Force	x	y	z	Acts at point
Hip contact	-59.3	-60.6	-236.3	P0
Intersegmental resultant	-13.0	-28.0	-70.1	P0
Abductor (1)	70.1	28.8	84.9	P1
Ilio-tibial tract, proximal part (2a)	10.5	-3.0	12.8	P1
Ilio-tibial tract, distal part (2b)	-0.5	-0.8	-16.8	P1
Tensor fascia latae, proximal part (3a)	3.1	4.9	2.9	P1
Tensor fascia latae, distal part (3b)	-0.2	-0.3	-6.5	P1
Vastus lateralis (4)	-2.2	22.4	-135.1	P2
Vastus medialis (5)	-8.8	39.6	-267.1	P3
Coordinates				
Point	x	y	z	z
P0	0.00	0.00	0.00	
P1	-67.83	-12.04	-35.45	
P2	-49.40	-5.01	-79.52	
P3	-18.79	8.82	-106.23	

the load profile for maximum torsion acting on the shaft of the implant. While these two activities can represent only a fraction of the total activity of a typical patient, the selection seems to be appropriate within the context of standardized preclinical testing of implants, especially considering the load magnitudes, the type of loading, the frequency of the activities, and therefore the number of load cycles to which an implant will be exposed.

In order to obtain the musculoskeletal loads for a preclinical test, two concurring requirements should be met: Firstly, only a limited complexity in terms of the number of muscles included is acceptable in order to realize those conditions within an experimental setup. In addition, however, the loading should result in a mechanical environment that closely resembles the physiological loading conditions. A simplified model of the hip muscles can be obtained from a complex model of the human lower extremities that had been validated against in vivo data. Importantly, the simplified model was also able to capture the muscle activity in the abductor to adequately describe the anteroposterior joint contact force component at the hip during stair climbing. The load profile specified in the study may therefore help to reproduce in vitro loading conditions that are closer to the peak load situations in vivo and could therefore be a key element in the mechanical testing of implants under a more realistic approximation of the musculoskeletal loading conditions.[6]

5.8 Application of Physiological-like Muscle Loading in Vitro

While physiological-like muscle loading can be more readily applied to composite bones, a difficulty associated with the use of cadaver bones is the adequate connection of the muscle–tendon complex to the mechanical apparatus that provides the forces in vitro. When using standard fixation techniques, this connection most often presents the weakest link that fails before physiological force levels can be reached. A further limitation is that physiological muscle force directions are often difficult to apply accurately due to interference from the somewhat bulky attachment devices that could allow for adequate fixation when multiple muscle forces are considered concurrently. To address these issues, an extension hull, comparable to the "finger trap" used to discharge the radiocarpal joint in fracture repositions, is applied over the muscle together with suitable suturing, forming a linear elongation of the tendon. Using the extension hull technique, the muscle forces of a simplified load profile for the patellofemoral joint (which was developed following the general concept as previously described for the hip) then enabled the application of the computationally determined in vivo muscle force magnitudes through the muscle–tendon complex, allowing an adequate simulation of physiological musculoskeletal loading conditions also at the knee.[9]

Jargon Simplified: The Extension Hull

The extension hull (e.g., Lancier Cable GmbH, Münster, Germany) consists of a wire netting made of electroplated steel, open at one end and closing in a sling at the other end. Under tension, the extension hull constricts and the pull is transformed into a compressive force. Before applying the extension hull, the muscle–tendon complex is wrapped taut with gauze bandage, beginning at the bony insertion. The wrapped muscle–tendon complex is then inserted into the hull and pulled tight. Finally, the wire netting is sewn onto the wrapped muscle–tendon complex using Fiberwire (a suture that has a core consisting of polyethylene and is coated with polyester; Arthrex, Inc., Naples, FL). The extension hull is more compact than other clamping techniques, has a flexible diameter, and is available in various lengths. It allows clamping to different muscle–tendon complexes, even in biomechanical setups where the tendon is relatively short (e.g., the rotator cuff). Furthermore, the technique enables the user to accurately define the force direction, offering a wire buckle as an optimal anchorage point.[10]

5.9 Conclusion

The mechanism of load sharing between bone and fracture fixation device influences the longevity and success of the osteosynthetic treatment. High stresses and fatigue due to repetitive loading within the fixation device can lead to its technical failure. A better understanding of the loading of the implant as well as the strain distribution within the bone is essential in determining the appropriateness of a fixation system for safe use in the clinic. While studies that assess osteosynthetic devices in compression, bending, and torsional loading modes in isolation can provide insight into the overall stability of the implant–bone complex and the stiffness and fatigue behavior of the devices, such tests do not permit a reliable assessment of the appropriateness of a fixation device in vivo. In order to assess the chances for a failure of implants that are to be used for different fracture locations, the in vivo performance of an implant can only then be reliably determined if appropriate physiological-like loading conditions are used in mechanical tests. Here, it is important to understand that the internal musculoskeletal loading, but also the specifics of the load sharing between implant and bone, are determined by the action of the muscles. These internal loading conditions might vary considerably with the activity performed but also between, for example, more proximal, metaphyseal, or diaphyseal fracture locations. An understanding of the essential mechanisms that influence and modulate the mechanical loading environment at a fracture site in vivo will allow appropriate consideration of the contribution of muscle and joint forces when devising mechanical tests for the development and optimization of new, targeted therapeutic approaches for the treatment of fractures.

References

[1] Taylor WR, Heller MO, Bergmann G, Duda GN. Tibio-femoral loading during human gait and stair climbing. J Orthop Res 2004; 22: 625–632
[2] Heller MO, Bergmann G, Kassi JP, Claes L, Haas NP, Duda GN. Determination of muscle loading at the hip joint for use in pre-clinical testing. J Biomech 2005; 38: 1155–1163
[3] Kutzner I, Heinlein B, Graichen F et al. Loading of the knee joint during activities of daily living measured in vivo in five subjects. J Biomech 2010; 43: 2164–2173
[4] Bergmann G, Deuretzbacher G, Heller M et al. Hip contact forces and gait patterns from routine activities. J Biomech 2001; 34: 859–871
[5] Trepczynski A, Kutzner I, Kornaropoulos E et al. Patellofemoral joint contact forces during activities with high knee flexion. J Orthop Res 2012; 30: 408–415
[6] Kassi J-P, Heller MO, Stoeckle U, Perka C, Duda GN. Stair climbing is more critical than walking in pre-clinical assessment of primary stability in cementless THA in vitro. J Biomech 2005; 38: 1143–1154
[7] Bergmann G, Graichen F, Rohlmann A. Hip joint contact forces during stumbling. Langenbecks Arch Surg 2004; 389: 53–59

[8] Duda GN, Bartmeyer B, Sporrer S, Taylor WR, Raschke M, Haas NP. Does partial weight bearing unload a healing bone in external ring fixation? Langenbecks Arch Surg 2003; 388: 298–304

[9] Goudakos IG, König C, Schöttle PB et al. Stair climbing results in more challenging patellofemoral contact mechanics and kinematics than walking at early knee flexion under physiological-like quadriceps loading. J Biomech 2009; 42: 2590–2596

[10] Schöttle P, Goudakos I, Rosenstiel N et al. A comparison of techniques for fixation of the quadriceps muscle-tendon complex for in vitro biomechanical testing of the knee joint in sheep. Med Eng Phys 2009; 31: 69–75

Further Reading

Bergmann G, Graichen F, Rohlmann A et al. Realistic loads for testing hip implants. Biomed Mater Eng 2010; 20: 65–75

Heller MO, Bergmann G, Deuretzbacher G et al. Musculo-skeletal loading conditions at the hip during walking and stair climbing. J Biomech 2001; 34: 883–893

Heller MO, Kassi JP, Perka C, Duda GN. Cementless stem fixation and primary stability under physiological-like loads in vitro. Biomed Tech (Berl) 2005; 50: 394–399

6 Static, Dynamic, and Fatigue Mechanical Testing

Christian Kaddick

Mechanical testing is one of the most reliable and established methods in experimental research. The insight gained when seeing specimens move, bend, break, and in some cases, explode during data acquisition is unmatched in comparison to other available methods (i.e., computer simulation). In addition to handling the metals, plastics, and bone under investigation, the experience of seeing structures under load addresses the professional interest of almost any mechanical engineer or biomechanically interested medical doctor.

This chapter aims to provide an overview of material behavior under different loading conditions as well as an overview of the equipment used for static, impact, and dynamic medical device testing. Theory will be combined with examples derived from real tests showing how typical results are derived from test data. The selection of the tests may be biased and represents only a fraction of the infinite possibilities used in mechanical testing. Whenever the following pages pass on the enthusiasm all experimental researchers share, the intention of this chapter is more than achieved.

6.1 Static Testing

During a static test, loads are typically applied only once rates are at or below 1 Hz. As such, these tests are often referred to as "quasistatic" and are independent of time and inertial effects. The focus of a quasistatic test is to investigate the behavior of a structure under external forces and/or moments while maintaining equilibrium. Static tests are the most common biomechanical experiments used to answer questions about how implants interact with biological structures, as well as to detect "weak points" of complex implant designs. Typically, implants do not fail under a single loading event but rather under fatigue loading conditions. As such, the value of quasistatic testing for performance analysis of in

vivo loaded implants is often overestimated; in vivo performance/fatigue analysis is addressed by dynamic testing as described in Chapter 6.3. There are certain considerations that should be kept in mind when designing a quasistatic test such that it yields meaningful results. In particular, test results should be independent of loading history, or all effects related to loading history, such as viscoelastic behavior, should be saturated prior to taking final measurements.

In theory, elastic materials behave like springs, as shown in ▸ Fig. 6.1 (*left*). Given that the yield load is not reached, loading and unloading will follow one straight line. In reality, we see this type of curve only once: in books. There are a number of factors contributing to the initial setting phase and hysteresis of materials, as depicted in ▸ Fig. 6.1 (*right*). The initial deviation from linear behavior is primarily related to fixtures and adaptors required for load application. In other words, small gaps and interface displacements will need a certain load to become closed. Some of the initial setting may also be related to surface effects between the load applicator and the contact area of the specimen. This effect becomes more apparent for porous surfaces (such as cancellous bone) featuring local contact points in comparison to homogeneous contact areas.[1] There are two methods for addressing these issues: One might simply define a preload as a starting point for any further calculation, or one might measure displacements directly at the specimen surface. To do so, there are special tools such as extensometers; these can be attached directly to the specimen or can be noncontacting (i.e., video). These methods provide valuable information about the displacement of a complete section of the test setup. Further, whenever the focus of the experiment requires greater detail, strain gauges offer an additional measurement alternative. The nature of strain gauges leads us to another important topic when designing a test: material behavior. The

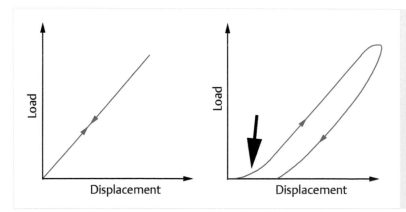

Fig. 6.1 Load versus displacement for an elastic material in theory (*left*) and in reality (*right*).

output of a strain gauge is, as the name suggests, "strain." One might simply calculate stress by multiplying the strain signal by the material's Young modulus (which is a constant). This approach is sufficient for isotropic and homogeneous materials such as most metal and nonreinforced plastic, but will become less reliable for biological structures such as bone or tissue, which often have oriented material properties and are composites. As such, great care must be given when performing data analysis of any test series to ensure accurate and meaningful results.

At this point, it becomes important to clearly distinguish between stress/strain as well as load/displacement. Stresses and strains are given for an infinitesimal small cube of material, whereas loads and displacements are the values that apply to the whole construct. To calculate the lengthening of a segment of bone under tensile load, it is necessary to multiply the measured strain by the segment length. Of note, when performing such calculations it is important not to confuse the Young modulus, which indicates the stiffness of the material itself, with the structural stiffness of the entire implant. For example, a bulky hip replacement manufactured from a low modulus material might result in a much stiffer implant in comparison to a thin or hollow implant manufactured from a high modulus material (such as a cobalt chromium alloy).

As indicated earlier, the straight line of the load versus displacement curve will "yield" at a certain load level (▶ Fig. 6.2). This point primarily indicates when plastic deformation of the material occurs; if yield occurs by plastic deformation, the test status changes from nondestructive to destructive. The yield point (E) is determined using an offset line to the load-displacement curve. The offset value (distance between point C and D—see *black arrow*) is given as a percentage of a reference length, which is often the free length between test fixtures, and is typically 0.2 or 2%. The linear portion of the curve (point A and B) is then defined; this is typically straightforward for some tests but depends largely on the "good judgment" of the test engineer. Linear regression using the least square method is often used to establish a well-

defined line. The yield point is thereby easily calculated by the intercept between the offset line (defined by the same slope as the linear portion of the curve offset by the offset distance) and the load versus displacement curve. It is important to note that the determined "yield" point may also result from slippage within the fixtures of the test setup. Moreover, the effect of reaching the yield point is of particular importance if examining a second load cycle, as it will show an even longer straight line as the material properties may be altered by the so-called work hardening process (a process used to increase the hardness and strength of metals).

The following test example summarizes all effects discussed so far. The test standard ASTM F382 defines the test used to characterize the bending properties of bone plates, as seen in ▶ Fig. 6.3 left with the expected test results shown in ▶ Fig. 6.3 right. At point a shown in ▶ Fig. 6.3 (right), the complete test setup is approaching full contact: Roller bearings are (slightly) self-adjusting,

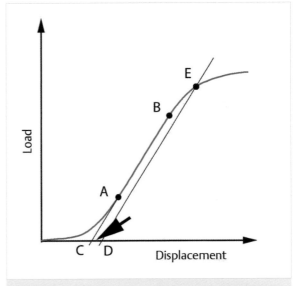

Fig. 6.2 Yield of an elastic material. See text for definition of *points A to E.*

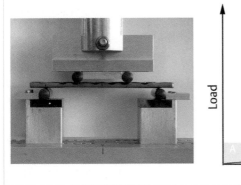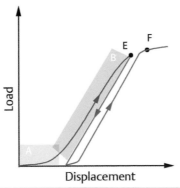

Fig. 6.3 Bending test of a bone plate with interruption after having reached the yield point. The test setup is displayed on the *left*. See text for definition of *points A to F.*

adaptors and load cell connectors are closing small gaps, and small surface irregularities are compressed. Point *A* to point *B* is the reversible nondestructive portion of the test followed by the yield point (*E*), which is the "point of no return." The test operator, for the sake of this example, decided to stop the test at this point and unload the implant for his lunch break. After returning to work, he restarted the test. The second attempt indicates yield at a higher load level (*F*) than seen before (work hardening has occurred). The test was stopped after the operator started to feel uncomfortable about the large displacement and the fact that the load curve did not show any distinct peak (ultimate) load. This behavior is typical for ductile materials as used for bone plates. Of course, it is important not to use the maximum force measured in this test for any calculations, as these values have affected the decision to stop the test (and the subsequent work hardening affects).

The operator would have seen a well-defined fracture load if testing brittle materials such as ceramics.

Moving toward investigating more complex material behavior, we might produce the bone from a plastic material such as polyetheretherketone. The load displacement curve will now show three additional features: creep, hysteresis, and loading rate dependence. Creep of a material is characterized by continuous displacement under constant load. Creeping, or viscoelastic behavior, is typically logarithmic in nature. The benefit of this is that most of the effect is saturated within a short time such that this can be accounted for by defining a "hold period" in our experiment. The bad news is that the material does have its own memory for loading history, so we will have to wait a certain time (in theory forever) before repeating the test. It is important to keep in mind that viscoelastic behavior is temperature dependent, which should be a controlled parameter for any test. The second effect is hysteresis of the material. In material mechanics, hysteresis is present whenever the unloading curve does not follow the path of the loading curve. This effect was discussed previously (unloading after yield) in the example of the metallic bone plate. By definition, the area enclosed by the loading and unloading curve is the dissipated energy (i.e., heat generation of dynamically loaded structures). This effect is also known as "damping" of the material and is often confused with the structural stiffness of implants. For example, a hip stem designed with a reduced structural stiffness will behave like a soft spring generating more displacement at a given load. In this case, the temperature of the implant will not increase ("damp") when being cyclically loaded below the yield point. That is, as the implant is considered to behave as a linear-elastic spring, the loading and unloading curve will be identical with no energy being dissipated. As such, damping, which results in dissipated energy, is not analogous to low structural stiffness. The third and last effect is the impact of the loading rate on the load displacement curve. Typically, the higher the loading rate, the stiffer and stronger the material will behave. Again, this effect is temperature dependent.

For the sake of completeness, it should be noted that the area under the force versus displacement curve (integral) represents the total energy to failure.

Finally, when establishing a quasistatic test, correctly defining the degrees of freedom is of paramount importance. In the personal opinion of the author, this is the source of most errors that render a time- and cost-intensive biomechanical test useless. The inexperienced researcher might start with a slightly more time-consuming but straightforward procedure: any rigid body has six degrees of freedom, three translations, and three rotations. The question is: How many of those degrees can be "released" while keeping the test setup valid? The starting point will be to imagine the specimen being rigidly fixated at the base plate of the test frame as well as at the load application (no degrees of freedom released). Beginning with the translations at the point of load application, one might now remove constraints of the setup until it becomes unstable. One might proceed with the rotational constraints at the point of load application and then move to the specimen fixation at the base plate.

Key Concepts: Constraining Forces

Constraining forces prevent translational and rotational motions and must be compared critically to in vivo loading conditions.

One simple example might explain this principle in detail: A researcher attempts to load a femur in a universal test frame (▶ Fig. 6.4a). He first embeds the bone into a fixture and places it directly beneath the actuator of the test frame (▶ Fig. 6.4a, *left*). This results in a number of obvious (over)constraints: The femoral head is not able to translate in x, y, or z directions, and the distal femoral fixation is not able to rotate around the x, y, or z axes, thereby affecting the applied loads that would be experienced in vivo. There are also some hidden constraints to consider: Our researcher relies on the assumption that the femoral head will rotate around the x, y, and z axes when being loaded. In reality, friction between the load applicator and the femoral head will restrain this motion. The correct test setup therefore requires an update as shown in ▶ Fig. 6.4a (*right*). The friction between the load applicator and the femoral head is minimized by the use of a ball bearing. In addition, the rotational motion (bending moments) at the specimen fixation are released by the use of a steel ball.

To set up a biomechanical test, it is important to envision the expected motions of the construct under load and consider whether this motion will be constrained by the setup. A typical error in doing so is our lack of

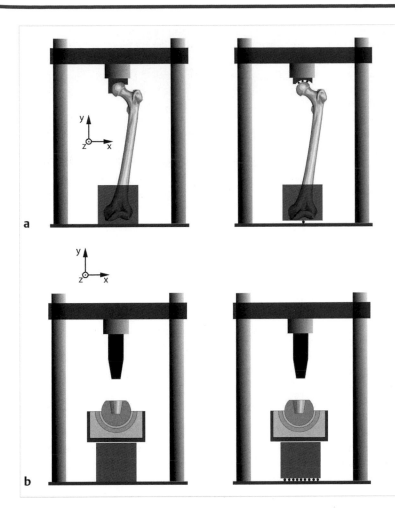

Fig. 6.4 (a) Femur in a universal test frame. The image on the *left* displays overconstrained test conditions; the *right* image displays valid test setup conditions. (b) Hip cup in a universal test frame. The image on the *left* displays overconstrained test conditions, whereas the image on the *right* displays valid test conditions.

imagination when dealing with small motions: Whenever a system is obviously over constrained, we tend to trust in the alignment of fixtures. This would be an adequate approach in a perfect (and unloaded) world, but even extremely small deviations in combination with stiff experimental setups will generate large internal loads, most of which are not recorded by the test frame sensors.

For the test setup displayed at the *left side* of ▶ Fig. 6.4b, the technician trusts in the perfect alignment between the rigidly fixed taper at the load sensor and the rigidly fixed bore of the hip ball at the baseplate of the test frame. In reality, small deviations in the x or z direction will generate large, erroneous forces. To solve this issue, ball bearings as shown in the *right side* of ▶ Fig. 6.4b will allow for self-alignment of the components.

At the very end, a correct test setup will produce accurately measured, meaningful values with lower standard deviations, and furthermore, prevent damage to load cells/sensors by removing unnecessary bending moments.

Electromechanical test frames, often referred to as universal test frames, are used for static testing and cover a wide range of test forces ranging from some mN to upwards of hundreds of kN. Higher test loads will require static hydraulic systems. Typically, more than one load cell will be required per test frame to achieve the precision needed for a given load range. When selecting a load cell, robustness against nonaxial loads should be considered. Modern, but unfortunately expensive, load cells offer a large insensitivity against bending moments. Nevertheless, these readily available technologies make performing static testing widely accessible.

6.2 Impact Testing

The dynamic nature of in vivo loading and some surgical procedures (such as impaction of a bone staple) requires dynamic in vitro testing of implantable devices. Biomechanical questions raised during forensic investigations are also heavily rooted in impact analysis.

Before setting up an impact test, the researcher should carefully consider the need for doing it as well as the anticipated results. For example, some materials behave differently at high loading rates, accelerations generate forces opposite to the acceleration vector (inertia), and crack propagation rates might be sufficiently small such that failure prior to unloading the construct is undetected. That is, some impact tests can be adequately performed under quasistatic load conditions representing a worst case scenario. This approach offers superior control of the applied load. Such control is of great importance when dealing with impact energy (typically defined by a weight dropping from a certain height). The force generated at the test setup is dependent on the overall stiffness, which is not exactly known for most biomechanical applications. An example that may clarify this practically is the determination of the impact force when implanting a total endoprosthesis hip stem. The force generated will depend on the personal feeling about a "good" hammer blow, the weight of the hammer, and most importantly, the stiffness of the femur-patient system. For example, implanting hip stems into a cadaver femur in a biomechanics laboratory using a bench vise does differ dramatically from a lightweight patient lying under anesthesia in the operating theater.

Impact tests are predominantly conducted in drop-test machines. A weight is released from an adjustable height and the subsequent impact results in an energy transfer to specimen (measured in Joules). Whereas smaller weights might be simply lifted and adjusted by hand without the use of a test frame, larger weights and tests demanding greater precision require guidance of the falling weight by low friction/aerodynamic drag mechanisms. Further, the drop weight must be released without external forces (there are multiple engineering solutions for doing so—a cheap and reliable solution is to burn the rope the drop weight is attached to).

Specific impact tests (i.e., beam impact) require standardized test equipment.[2]

Piezoelectric force sensors are typically used for impact testing. These allow for very fast and accurate measurement up to some tens of kHz and provide very stiff force sensors sufficient to capture most (biomechanical) impact phenomena. Strain gauges in combination with high sampling rates provide reliable readings up to some kHz and have also been used successfully in our labs, whereas high-speed cameras are often used synchronized with load data to obtain a deeper understanding of materials and structures deforming under impact conditions[3] (▶ Fig. 6.5).

6.3 Fatigue Testing

The primary focus of fatigue testing is to determine the number of applied load cycles before causing failure (test to failure). Furthermore, the dependency of any structural characters such as material properties, geometry, etc., on the number of applied load cycles can be of interest. Fatigue loads are predominantly applied above 1 Hz up to the kHz range.

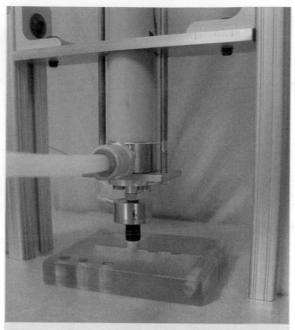

Fig. 6.5 Cartilage under impact load. (Copyright: Kang RW, Friel NA, Williams JM, Cole BJ, Wimmer MA. Effect of impaction sequence on osteochondral graft damage: the role of repeated and varying loads. Am J Sports Med 2010;38:105.)

Fatigue testing, often referred to as "dynamic" testing, is typically performed to prove safety of an implant up to a given number of cycles under predefined load conditions. The so called run-out cycles are defined by the number of cycles a fatigue test is stopped and the implant is considered to have not failed. The corresponding maximum load during such a fatigue test is often referred to as "run-out load." The value for a run-out cycle will depend on the type of medical product. Whereas osteosynthesis implants might become almost unloaded after some weeks of bone healing, cardiovascular implants may need to withstand hundreds of millions of cycles over the lifetime of the patient.

Materials used for medical devices typically possess a logarithmic fatigue behavior (▶ Fig. 6.6). This implies that after a certain number of cycles, the run-out load determined will only change slightly. Determining sufficient test duration is paramount—stopping a test after an appropriate number of cycles will not only reduce costs, but may also allow for more samples to be tested, thereby increasing the significance of each test series.

The mechanical principles of setting up a dynamic test are the same as those discussed in Chapter 6.1. In addition, there are two more factors that must be considered: The type of test fluid used might impact the test results due to degradation effects,[4] and the thermodynamic (heat) effects that result from the dynamic loading regime might alter the material properties.

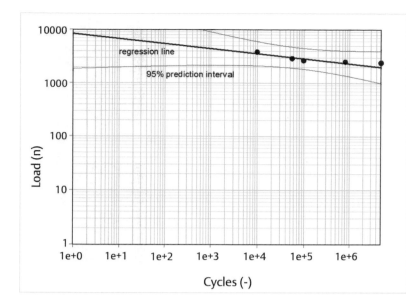

Fig. 6.6 Load versus number of cycles for a hip stem. The test is stopped after 5 million cycles if no failure occurs.

When examining failed specimens, observation of a fracture surface typically shows two distinct areas[5]: a fatigue zone typically with beachmarks and an instantaneous (fast fracture) zone. After onset at the fracture origin point, the fracture propagates and generates progression marks, also referred to as fatigue arrest marks or beachmarks (▶ Fig. 6.7, *zone 1*) until a critical remaining cross-section is reached. Failure of the specimen will then occur within a single load cycle generating the overload zone (*zone 2*).

Whenever the complete fracture of the test sample is defined as failure criteria, this becomes a simple and straightforward test method. As an alternative, the displacement signal of the test frame might be used to detect onset of fatigue fracture. However, depending on specimen geometry and material properties, it might become difficult to differentiate between the displacement under standard load conditions and onset of fracture. Crack propagation gauges may be helpful whenever the fracture site is known and does offer sufficient space for application. As an alternative, acoustic emission is also an appropriate method for determining fracture propagation.[6]

The statistical analysis of fatigue data is often limited by the low number of samples. The test standard ASTM E739[7] shows how to calculate the confidence interval for a given dataset. To be 95% certain that the best fit regression line is contained, the 95% confidence interval is calculated. This is often confused with the term "95% prediction interval," which is the area in which you expect 95% of all data points to fall. A second important consideration when assessing the fatigue performance of an implant is the difference between *attributes* and *values*. A specimen reaching the run-out cycles without failure has the *attribute* "OK" and not the *value*, for example, "5 million." In other words, this specimen is interesting

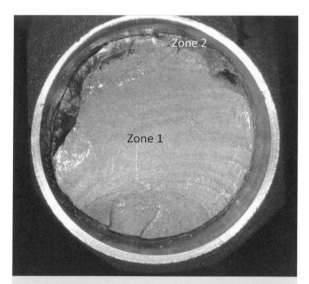

Fig. 6.7 Surface of the taper of a titanium hip stem fatigue fracture. The fracture initiated from the bottom and propagated toward the top. Image provided by courtesy of Prof. Steinhauser, Munich.

but worthless for the statistical analysis of a fatigue test based on values. One way around this would be testing of run-out specimens only (test to success) but much larger numbers of samples are needed for this method when compared to the "value" test (test to failure).

A brief description of the "up-and-down" test method strategy sometimes used for small sample sizes can be found in ASTM STP731.

Technical specifications of the equipment used for dynamic testing depend on the required test loads and test frequency. High test frequencies of up to some kHz can be applied by moving magnet actuators. These types of motors are, for example, used during stent testing. Piezoelectric actuators offer high frequencies at low load levels and small displacements. Whenever high loads in the kN range become necessary, hydraulic or pneumatic actuators become first choice. Of note, friction effects resulting from internal seals prevent testing at lower load levels (mN), such as those required in cartilage research. Heat and noise generation as well as power consumption should also be considered before investing in such systems. Electromechanical systems intended for static testing might be used for some hundreds of load cycles at low test frequencies, but typically are not designed for fatigue testing.

6.4 Conclusion

Today, highly sophisticated test equipment is widely available for almost any type of biomechanical research.

Performing such testing requires a profound knowledge of materials science and technical mechanics. In fact, a test result given to the precision six decimal places does not necessarily indicate a meaningful test setup. First, the researcher should be aware of the simplifications made to reproduce the complex in vivo conditions (i.e., multiple forces acting on a construct under varying directions or aggressive body fluids impacting the performance of a device). After having done so, material-related properties such as heating under dynamic loads and setup-related parameters such as overconstraining should be considered.

Keeping those principles in mind will generate valid test results to enhance our knowledge about fascinating and complex in vivo biomechanics, as well as provide implant safety for the benefit our patients.

References

[1] Kelly N, McGarry JP. Experimental and numerical characterisation of the elasto-plastic properties of bovine trabecular bone and a trabecular bone analogue. J Mech Behav Biomed Mater 2012; 9: 184–197

[2] ISO 179–2. Plastics–Determination of Charpy impact properties–Part 2: Instrumented impact test. 1997

[3] Pascual Garrido C, Hakimiyan AA, Rappoport L, Oegema TR, Wimmer MA, Chubinskaya S. Anti-apoptotic treatments prevent cartilage degradation after acute trauma to human ankle cartilage. Osteoarthritis Cartilage 2009; 17: 1244–1251

[4] Eliaz N. Degradation of implant materials. New York, Springer; 2012

[5] Neville W, Sachs PE. Understanding the surface features of fatigue fractures: how they describe the failure cause and the failure history. J Fail Anal Prev 2005; 5: 11–15

[6] Laonapakul T, Otsuka Y, Nimkerdphol AR, Mutoh Y. Acoustic emission and fatigue damage induced in plasma-sprayed hydroxyapatite coating layers. J Mech Behav Biomed Mater 2012; 8: 123–133

[7] ASTM E739–91: Standard Practice for Statistical Analysis of Linear or Linearized Stress-Life (S-N) and Strain-Life (e-N) Fatigue Data

Further Reading

Mow C. Basic orthopedic biomechanics. Philadelphia: Lippincott Raven; 1997

Box GE. Statistics for experimenters. Hoboken: Wiley & Sons; 2005

Kline J. Handbook of biomedical engineering. San Diego: Academic Press; 1988

7 Use of Human and Animal Specimens in Biomechanical Testing

Robert James Wallace

In order to investigate the effect of aging, disease, treatments, and injury on the mechanical properties of tissues, it is required to perform mechanical testing on biological tissues. While the primary aim of this research will be to obtain knowledge about the effects of these properties on human tissue, it is not always possible to obtain a supply of the required tissue at the desired quality and in sufficient quantity to allow testing to be performed if only human tissue is to be used. Therefore, it is required that alternative materials are used for testing. Although man-made biomaterials have been produced, they do not mimic closely enough the wide range of material properties that are present in true biological tissues. Therefore, in lieu of using human tissue, animal tissue is widely used as a substitute. While it is recognized that there are differences between species, in both the geometry and material properties, these still provide a suitable surrogate for biomechanical testing. In addition to the greater availability of animal sources of tissue for biomechanical testing, there are less legal and ethical restrictions to their use for this purpose. However, the guidelines relating to the ethical treatment of animals for research purposes must be strictly adhered to.

7.1 Use of Animals for Biological Research

It can often be easier to obtain animal material of sufficient quantity and of a reliable quality than to use human bone. Additionally, in the earlier stages of research into a treatment method or drug, it is prohibited to test on humans until the required testing has first been carried out in an animal model. If animals are to be used for research, it is imperative that they are treated humanely. This applies to animals that are used purely as a source of material for testing in vitro or whether a treatment method or drug is to be investigated and the effect studied in vivo. In the United Kingdom, relevant governance is provided by "The Animals (Scientific Procedures) Act 1986."[1] It should be noted that the European governance provided by "Directive 86/609/EEC"[2] must also be complied with (when the research is carried out in the European Union where this law is applicable, along with any individual requirements of the member state).

7.1.1 Biological Variability

Bone is known to be an heterogeneous and anisotropic material (see Chapter 9); therefore, the properties

derived from mechanical testing, even from the same animal, depend on the type (e.g., rib, femur, tibia), the location (e.g., anterior, medial, distal, etc.), and the orientation of testing with respect to the bone (e.g., longitudinal, transverse, radial).

> ### Jargon Simplified: Loading Direction
>
> The terms longitudinal, transverse, and radial should refer to the normal loading axis of the bone. In most cases, the long axis of the bone can be considered the longitudinal axis, the transverse axis runs at 90 degrees to this, and the radial axis runs from the endosteal to periosteal surfaces, as shown in ▶ Fig. 7.1.

As well as variations from anatomical location and between different animals of the same species, there can be considerable interspecies differences in mechanical properties. ▶ Table 7.1 shows the range of mineral volume fraction (MVf), the volume of mineral in parts per thousand, Young modulus (E), ultimate tensile strength (σ_{ult}), ultimate tensile strain (ε_{ult}), and work to failure (W) for a selection of animal species.[3] This shows the wide range of values for these properties that can be encountered.

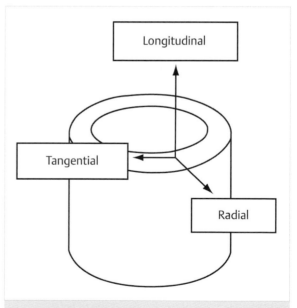

Fig. 7.1 Longitudinal, tangential, and radial axis with respect to the long axis of the bone.

Table 7.1 Mechanical Properties of Various Bony Tissues[3]

Species and tissue	MVf (ppth)	E (GPa)	σ_{ult} (MPa)	ε_{ult} (mm/mm)	W (MJ/m³)
Red deer, immature antler	281	10	250	0.109	15.6
Red deer, mature antler	287	7.2	158	0.114	9.3
Narwhal, tusk cement	331	5.3	84	0.060	3.0
Narwhal, tusk dentine	340	10.3	120	0.037	3.7
Fallow deer, radius	360	25.5	213	0.019	2.1
Human, adult, femur	362	16.7	166	0.029	2.8
Bovine, tibia	364	19.7	146	0.018	1.8
Leopard, femur	375	21.5	215	0.034	3.4
Brown bear, femur	377	16.9	152	0.032	2.3
Donkey, radius	381	15.3	114	0.020	1.6
Flamingo, tibiotarsus	382	28.2	212	0.013	1.4
King penguin, radius	394	22.1	195	0.010	0.8
Horse, femur	395	24.5	152	0.008	0.5
Bovine, femur	410	26.1	148	0.004	0.3
Polar bear (7 years), femur	414	22.2	161	0.020	1.7
King penguin, ulna	421	22.9	193	0.011	1.2
Axis dear, femur	428	31.6	221	0.019	2.4
Fallow deer, tibia	430	26.8	131	0.006	0.4
Wallaby, femur	437	21.8	183	0.009	0.8
Fin whale, bulla	560	34.1	27	0.002	0.02

Abbreviations: MVf, mineral volume fraction; E, Young modulus; σ_{ult}, ultimate tensile strength; ε_{ult}, ultimate tensile strain; W, work to failure.

It is important to bear in mind these differences in material constitution and mechanical properties when examining the results from mechanical testing, especially if comparisons are being made between specimens from different species.

7.1.2 Microstructural Differences

Bone is classified into two broad types, cortical and trabecular bone; the distinctions between these two types and their biomechanical properties are discussed in Chapter 9. However, "cortical" bone can also be classified into different types according to the structure of the mineralized fibrils. These different types of bone all look like cortical bone to the naked eye; however, they are different on a microstructural level. These differences in microstructure result in different material properties and can be attributed to the hierarchical makeup of bone.[4]

Woven bone (primary bone tissue) has an irregular arrangement of collagen fibers. This type of bone contains less mineral and a higher proportion of osteocytes than lamellar bone.

Haversian or lamellar bone (secondary bone tissue) is mature bone where the collagen fibers are arranged in the primary axis of the bone. The fibers are arranged in lamellae, which in trabecular bone are parallel and in cortical bone are arranged concentrically around the haversian (vascular) canals (as shown in ▶ Fig. 7.2). Almost all bone tissue in human adults is haversian.

Parallel fibered bone can be thought of as a stage in between woven and lamellar bone. The bone is arranged into organized mineralized fibers that run parallel to the main axis of the bone or organized into a plywood-like arrangement.

These differences in microstructure give rise to the anisotropy of bone, and small differences in composition throughout the components that make up the material hierarchy[4] (see ▶ Fig. 7.2) can give rise to alterations in the material properties. Therefore, it is recommended that numerous samples are used when testing in order to

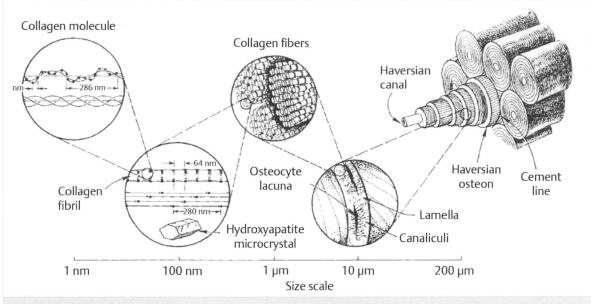

Fig. 7.2 The hierarchical nature of bone from collagen molecule to lamellar bone.[4]

be able to draw firm conclusions from experimental results.

7.2 Use of Human Tissue in Biological Research

The use of human tissues in biological research is governed by strict legal and ethical requirements. Efforts must be made to minimize cosmetic damage to the body during extraction and to perform testing within a specified time period to allow the tissues to be returned to the body for burial.

The use of human tissues and cells is governed by the European Directive 2006/86/EC.[5] If research is carried out in countries in the European Union, the guidelines outlined in this document must be adhered to along with any local requirements of the member state in which the work is carried out. For example, if the research is carried out in the United Kingdom, the relevant requirements are given in the Human Tissue Act 2004.[6]

7.2.1 Health Risk

Risk of infection or disease is greater when working with human tissue than with animal specimens (e.g., hepatitis B and human immunodeficiency virus). It is recommended that two pairs of gloves are worn when working with human tissue in order to provide additional protection. Two pairs of gloves also facilitate the easy change of the outermost pair in order to ensure that optimum hygiene is maintained. Additionally, it is vital to ensure that only sharp scalpels are used when working with human tissue as these will cut cleaner and with less force than when the tool has become blunted, minimizing the risk of accidents. Therefore, frequent change of scalpel blades is recommended to ensure that the work is carried out safely.

Each research institute will have its own health and safety protocol when working with human tissue, and the researcher should become familiar with this before commencing work. It is likely that the researcher will have to ensure that all relevant inoculations are up to date and confirmed with the local occupational health department. In the event of an injury, it is recommended that this should be reported immediately and treatment is carried out in line with the health and safety practices of that institute.

7.2.2 Bone Quality

When human bone is available for use in medical research, it is usually from either a deceased person who has donated the remains to science (cadaver bone) or is from discard material obtained when a patient has undergone surgery, such as a total hip replacement. Proper ethical consent must be gained from the patient before surgery is performed in order for discard material to be used for research purposes. It should be noted that human tissue obtained in this way is likely to come from elderly donors and therefore could be of reduced quality. This can be advantageous if studying the effect of diseases or aging bone quality, but can create difficulties when attempting to compare results to a control group.

When cadaver bone is used, specimens may be available from younger donors than are found from discard material sources. When using specimens from a cadaver, it is important to ensure that the cause of death will not affect the quality of the bone or tissue investigated.

7.2.3 Preservation of Specimens

Because there is both a requirement to test a number of specimens (to account for variability) and the often time-consuming nature of harvesting these specimens, it is often more practical to perform the testing as a two-stage process, where stage one involves the harvest and preparation of the specimens and stage two involves the actual mechanical testing. It is therefore required to preserve specimens prior to testing. The most popular methods of specimen preparation are freezing and embalming.

It has been demonstrated that freezing bone to a temperature of −20°C allows for storage up to a year without any effect on the mechanical properties. If the storage temperature is reduced to −80°C then it follows that the bone can be safely stored for a substantial period of time. If freezing is to be used as a method of preservation, the number of freeze/refreeze cycles should be minimized, ideally with the specimen being frozen once after harvest and defrosted only when required for testing. This method of preservation is known as fresh-frozen and can be considered the gold standard method of specimen preservation.

An embalming fluid, such as formaldehyde, is commonly used to preserve specimens at room temperature. This has the advantage of allowing the specimens to be conveniently handled and therefore is a useful method of preservation where there is a requirement for a practical "hands on" nature, such as in the teaching of anatomy. However, this method of preservation can result in a significant change in the stiffness and strength of bone. Some researchers have shown an increase in these properties, while others have found a decrease. This method of specimen preservation directly affects the collagen present in the tissue by increasing cross-linking. The effect this has on the mechanical properties is to reduce the ultimate strain and toughness.[7] In impact (dynamic) experiments, it was found that the effect was greater.[8] Therefore, caution should be taken when interpreting results of dynamic testing involving embalmed tissues, or where work to failure, toughness, or ultimate strain are examined. Fixation of the tissue can also remove the risk of pathological infection when handling human tissues. The additional safety that this method provides should be considered when deciding on the method of preservation, especially if human tissue is to be handled.[9] The duration of embalming also has an effect on the change in material properties of the specimen, with a greater effect found with increasing duration. Therefore, if embalming is to be used, perhaps for the benefit of reduced infection risk, then the duration should be minimized in order to curtail the influence on the mechanical

properties. If fixation is used as a means of specimen preservation, it is recommended that after fixation the samples of tissue be rinsed and stored in phosphate buffered saline (PBS) in order to remove any excess fixation media left in the tissue.[8]

7.2.4 Preparation of Specimens for Testing

When testing larger bones, care must be taken when removing soft tissue to ensure that the underlying bone is not marked. It would be preferential to have a small amount of muscle or connective tissue remain on the bone than to try to remove this with a scalpel and create small scratches in the bone. Even scratches that are barely visible to the naked eye can create significant stress concentration factors.

> **Jargon Simplified: Stress Concentration**
>
> When there is a sharp change in cross-section, such as is found around a notch or scratch, the area around this feature can experience a much greater stress than surrounding materials. This can result in most of the specimen experiencing a stress below the yield point whereas the area immediately next to the sharp radius exceeds the ultimate allowable stress, causing the scratch to grow into a crack, which can lead to fracture of the bone.

When testing small bones, such as those from a mouse or rat, it is acceptable to leave the soft tissue on the bone while testing due to the dangers outlined previously when removing soft tissues unless tensile testing is to be performed. The risk of creating small scratches is increased due to the difficulty in handling bones of this size, and the influence of any scratch would be greater due to the larger relative depth of scratch to bone. Cutting the soft tissue in a way that it can no longer contribute to the load path would be acceptable preparation for tensile testing.

It should be noted that if performing a bending test on a sample of bone with soft tissue present, the soft tissue must first be deformed locally at the point of contact with the testing apparatus before the bone carries the load. This will result in an increased offset along the displacement axis of the loading graph due to this deformation. Additionally, there will be an offset on the force axis, due to the force required to deform the soft tissue surrounding the bone. Both of these offsets should be accounted for when deriving mechanical properties.

The presence of soft tissue can be especially useful if there is a callus present on the bone. In addition to removing the risk of damage to this delicate part of the structure, where even slight contact with a sharp scalpel would cause significant damage leading to nonrepresentative results, the soft tissue can preserve the structure of a bone/callus specimen that has been destructively tested allowing further examination to be carried out by histological methods. Therefore, it is recommended that when investigating a specimen where there is a bone callus, the soft tissue around this area should not be removed.

7.2.5 Testing Temperature

It has been shown that tissue temperature has an effect on the mechanical properties. At room temperature, bone is stiffer, while at body temperature it has a greater toughness. Therefore, the temperature of testing should also be considered when performing mechanical testing. While it may be considered ideal to test the specimens in the laboratory in as similar a condition to their natural state, the practicalities of maintaining body temperature during testing mean that samples are often tested at room temperature. It is therefore important that the testing conditions are detailed in the write-up of the study to inform the reader.

7.2.6 Tissue Moisture Content

The moisture content of biological tissues also has an effect on the mechanical properties. It has been shown that when a bone is tested in a dry condition, the stiffness and ultimate strength increase and the toughness and strain at failure decrease.[10] In order to obtain representative results, it is important to ensure that the sample is kept moist throughout testing. This can be achieved by ensuring the sample is suitably hydrated in an isotonic solution such as PBS before testing, and if necessary, continuous application of PBS during testing. This could be achieved by use of a saline spray or dispenser. However, most single loading–phase tests do not occur over a length of time where there will be any significant loss of moisture from the sample, and it can be considered adequate to provide no further hydration during testing, as long as the sample was suitably hydrated before commencing.

When performing fatigue testing, preventing dehydration is highly important to ensure that the measured results are not simply due to a change in moisture content of the sample. Because fatigue tests can involve considerable testing time, it is not advised to use manual methods of application in order to prevent dehydration. Therefore, a mechanized method that employs the action of the testing machine or an independent device to continually apply a spray or flow of liquid to the sample would be advantageous. It is important to ensure that any automated way of hydrating the sample adequately covers the entire specimen, as localized drying will change the material properties of that section, thus influencing the overall test. Testing could also be performed with the sample entirely submerged in solution. It should also be noted that the mechanical properties of soft tissues will be altered both quicker and to a greater extent if not kept suitably hydrated.

7.2.7 Size Effects

When performing mechanical testing on biological tissues, it is important to bear in mind the effect that specimen size could have an influence on the results, especially when investigating fracture properties. If bones from a small animal are to be used, it is normally the case that these will be tested whole. Testing performed on specimens from a larger animal often facilitates smaller samples to be machined from these, allowing multiple testing to be carried out on the sample bone. (It should be noted that although this method of sample preparation removes sources of variability from different animals and from different bones in the animal, it cannot remove the influence of different local mechanical properties that result from subtly different microstructure around the bone.)

7.3 Conclusion

When preparing specimens for biological testing, considerations must be given to the type of tissue used and also how this is stored before mechanical testing is carried out. Freezing is considered to be the gold standard method for preserving mechanical properties; however, chemical fixation reduces risk of infection and should therefore not be discounted. Biological tissues have natural variability and care must be taken during sample preparation and with testing conditions to ensure that the results are representative. When working with biological specimens, whether from human or animal sources, all ethical and legal requirements must be met.

References

[1] The animals (scientific procedures) act 1986. London: The Stationery Office; 1986

[2] Directive 2010/63/EU of The European Parliament and of the Council of 22 September 2010 on the protection of animals used for scientific purposes. OJ L L 276/33

[3] Currey JD. Bones: structure and mechanics. Princeton, NJ: Princeton University Press; 2002

[4] Lakes R. Materials with structural hierarchy. Nature 1993; 361: 511–515

[5] Commission Directive 2006/86/EC of 24 October 2006 implementing Directive 2004/23/EC of the European Parliament and of the Council as regards traceability requirements, notification of serious adverse reactions and events and certain technical requirements for the coding, processing, preservation, storage and distribution of human tissues and cells. OJ L 294/32

[6] Human tissue act 2004. London: The Stationery Office; 2004

[7] Boskey AL, Cohen ML, Bullough PG. Hard tissue biochemistry: a comparison of fresh-frozen and formalin-fixed tissue samples. Calcif Tissue Int 1982; 34: 328–331

[8] Currey JD, Brear K, Zioupos P, Reilly GC. Effect of formaldehyde fixation on some mechanical properties of bovine bone. Biomaterials 1995; 16: 1267–1271

[9] Cavanaugh JM, King AI. Control of transmission of HIV and other bloodborne pathogens in biomechanical cadaveric testing. J Orthop Res 1990; 8: 159–166

[10] Currey JD. The effects of drying and re-wetting on some mechanical properties of cortical bone. J Biomech 1988; 21: 439–441

Further Reading

Rho J-Y, Kuhn-Spearing L, Zioupos P. Mechanical properties and the hierarchical structure of bone. Med Eng Phys 1998; 20: 92–102

Turner CH, Burr DB. Basic biomechanical measurements of bone: a tutorial. Bone 1993; 14: 595–608

Weiner S, Wagner HD. The material bone: structure-mechanical function relations. Annu Rev Mater Sci 1998; 28: 271–298

8 Whole Bone Biomechanics

Grace Kim and Marjolein C. H. van der Meulen

A primary function of the skeleton is to bear loads, supporting the body and allowing for motion. As such, the structural behavior of the entire bone is of interest, as are the determinants of this behavior. Three main factors determine whole bone mechanical behavior: tissue quantity, geometry, and material properties, all of which can be experimentally quantified (▶ Fig. 8.1). Bone mass and geometry can be determined directly by measuring weight and size or by using imaging modalities such as computed tomography (CT), dual X-ray absorptiometry or microCT. Material properties can be determined from machined specimens of cancellous or cortical bone. Whole bone mechanical tests examine the culmination of all three contributing factors and the overall behavior of whole bone as a structure.

8.1 Overview of Testing Methods

The theory and methods presented in this chapter will focus on testing methodology and the resulting outcome measures of structural tests of whole bones. Whole bone mechanical testing is performed by applying a monotonically increasing load to a bone using fixtures in conjunction with a materials testing machine while recording the resulting displacement and applied load. The applied load can be axial (tension or compression), bending, or torsional. Relevant structural outcome measures such as stiffness and maximum load are calculated from the load-displacement data.

The load-displacement graphs for all whole bone testing methods have similar features, regardless of the loading mode (▶ Fig. 8.2). Key parameters obtained from the data include the structural stiffness and yield, ultimate, and failure loads. Initially, load and displacement vary linearly, and the linear slope is related to the structural stiffness of the bone sample. The structural stiffness for a given loading mode again depends on the three factors bone mass, bone geometry, and the material properties of the bone tissue. If the sample is loaded beyond the linear portion, the sample yields and retains some permanent deformation. A precise definition of yield is difficult

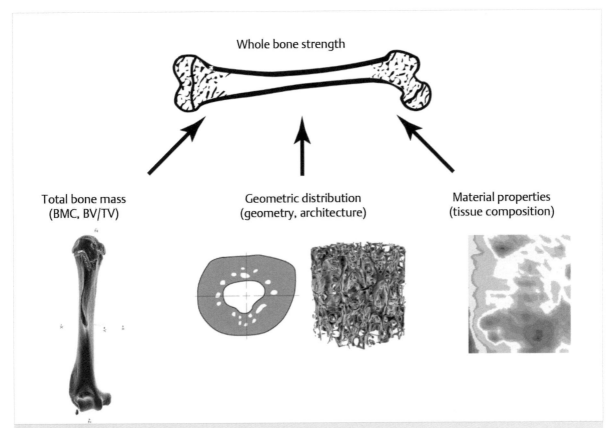

Fig. 8.1 Factors contributing to whole bone strength include total bone mass, bone geometry, and material properties of the bone tissue. BMC, bone mineral content; BV/TV, bone volume/trabecular volume.

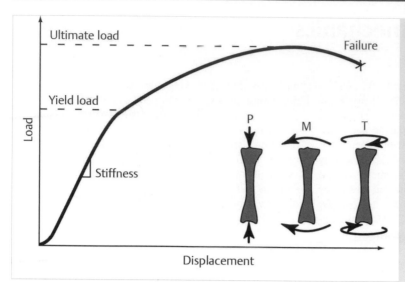

Fig. 8.2 A general load-displacement curve from whole bone mechanical testing with schematics of axial (*P*), bending (*M*), and torsional (*T*) loading configurations. The stiffness is the slope of the initial linear portion. The yield load marks the beginning of plastic deformation. The ultimate load is the maximum load. The failure load is the load prior to catastrophic failure.

and therefore several methods have been suggested to determine the yield point. Because yield is associated with flattening of the load displacement curve, the yield load can be defined by the point where the slope of the linear portion of the curve decreases by 10%.[1] Yield can also be defined as the point where a line with 95% of the stiffness intersects the load-displacement curve.[2] Frequently, an offset yield point is defined by shifting the line of stiffness by a certain amount and determining the intersection between the shifted line and the load-displacement curve. The maximum load value attained during the test is called the ultimate load or somewhat colloquially the strength of the bone sample. The failure load is the load value prior to catastrophic failure of the sample, indicated by an abrupt drop in load with very little change in displacement. Depending on the specifics of the bone sample and testing mode, the yield, maximum, and failure load can overlap. Respective displacements of the yield, maximum, and failure load can also be reported by identifying the corresponding displacement at which the respective loads occur.

Mechanical tests on whole bone samples should ideally be performed immediately after harvesting. If immediate testing is not possible, bones can be wrapped in gauze soaked with phosphate-buffered saline, placed into sealed containers or evacuated plastic bags, and stored at −20°C or below.[3] Frozen samples must thaw in a hydrated state and equilibrate to the prescribed testing temperature prior to testing. To eliminate the effect of temperature and loading rate on mechanical outcomes, all samples should be tested at the same ambient temperature and load rate. The sampling rate of the displacement and load must be high enough such that a sufficient number of data points are available for the test duration.

The following sections review commonly used whole bone testing methods and associated outcome measurements. Key decisions to be made prior to testing whole bone samples include the loading mode, sample preparation, and specific test parameters including the loading rate, fixture geometries, and temperature.

8.2 Axial Loading

Axial loading tests are commonly performed in compression on bone specimens that would also physiologically experience axial loading such as whole vertebrae or lower limb bones.[4] In this testing mode, the applied load is a monotonic compressive load applied along the cranial-caudal axis of the bone. For example, in an axial compression test of a vertebral body, the loading fixture is composed of two circular loading platens with diameters approximately equal to the vertebral endplate (▶ Fig. 8.3). To minimize bending moments during the test, the endplates of the samples can be embedded in bone cement or shaved with a scalpel to make the loaded surfaces parallel to each other. A pin is secured to the lower platen and inserted through the vertebral foramen to consistently align the samples. The vertebral body is then secured at the caudal endplate with a thin layer of cyanoacrylate glue. The compressive load is applied at a constant load or displacement rate until the load drops abruptly, indicating failure. After failure, if loading is continued, the load will eventually increase indefinitely as the crushed vertebra is loaded again and compacted. During testing, the load and crosshead displacement are recorded.

The load-displacement curve represents the compressive load (*P*, in units of Newtons) plotted against the axial displacement (δ, in micrometers or millimeters). The compressive stiffness is the structure's ability to resist deformation due to a compressive load and is often

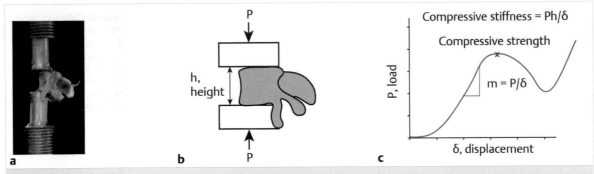

Fig. 8.3 (a) A rat vertebra loaded in axial compression along the anteroposterior axis with cylindrical platens. (b) Schematic of axially loaded vertebra where P is the applied load and h is the vertebral body height. (c) Representative load-displacement data obtained from an axial compression test. Compressive stiffness is calculated from P/δ.

expressed as the ratio of applied load P and displacement δ, resulting in a value of compressive stiffness in N/mm. However, as the resistance of a sample strongly depends on the size of the sample, it is recommended to calculate the compressive stiffness by adjusting the load/displacement ratio by the specimen size:

$$\text{Compressive Stiffness} = \frac{P}{\delta} \cdot h \qquad (8.1)$$

where P/δ represents the slope of the load displacement curve and h is the height of the sample. The maximum load is often referred to as the compressive strength. Another factor that directly determines the compressive properties is the cross-sectional area of the specimen, which can be estimated by the cross-sectional area of the sample. However, as bone specimens are very rarely solid but contain trabecular bone or bone marrow and are furthermore irregularly shaped, the adjustment for cross-sectional area often is inadequate.

8.3 Bending Loading

Bending tests of whole bones are generally performed in three different bending configurations: cantilever bending, three-point bending, or four-point bending. For whole bones, these tests primarily measure the mechanical behavior of the cortical diaphysis and do not capture any contribution from cancellous bone tissue.

8.3.1 Three-Point Bending

Three-point bending tests are typically performed on long bones with large length-to-width ratios such as the femur, humerus, radius, and tibia.[5] Though no bones have constant cross-sectional geometries or homogeneous and isotropic material properties, which

are the underlying assumptions required for beam theory, analysis of bending tests of long bones are based on engineering beam theory. As the name suggests, three points contact the bone: two fixed supports on one side, and a single load point centered between the two supports on the opposing side (▸ Fig. 8.4). As a rule, the span, or distance between the support points, is commonly half the bone length, but this can be increased if the bone ends are potted and stability of the bone on the supports is not compromised. The load point is actuated using a constant load or displacement rate. The bone must be consistently oriented in the loading fixture, such that the loads are always applied in the same anatomic plane, as the cross-sectional shape of the diaphysis rarely is axisymmetric.

The three-point bending configuration induces a moment on the bone that varies linearly along the length of the bone, but it is the moment at the center of the span we are interested in. Given the load (P) at any time during the test, the resulting moment at any point located between the supports (x) can be calculated using beam bending theory:

$$\text{Moment} = M = \frac{Px}{2} \qquad (8.2)$$

The moment ranges from zero at the supports to a maximum value at the center load point where $x = L/2$ and therefore the maximum moment $M_{max} = PL/4$.

The outcome measures are analogous to those of other loading modes. The slope of the load-displacement curve is commonly reported in literature for bending tests (units of N/mm). However, this stiffness cannot be compared with other studies that use different span widths and is not the true resistance of the sample to bending. The bending stiffness should always be reported and accounts for testing geometry, intrinsic material stiffness, and specimen geometry. The slope of the linear portion

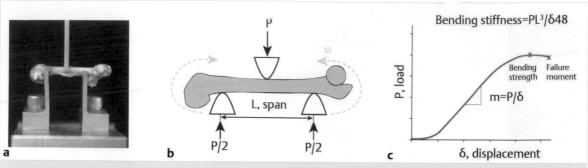

Fig. 8.4 (a) Rat femur tested in three-point bending in the anterior-posterior direction. (b) Schematic of a femur loaded in three-point bending with a span width (*L*), load (*P*), and the resulting moment (*M*) indicated by the *arrows*. (c) Representative load-displacement graph obtained from a three-point bending test. Bending stiffness is calculated as $PL^3/\delta 48$.

of the moment-displacement curve (*P*/δ) is related to the bending stiffness:

$$\text{Bending Stiffness} = \left(\frac{P}{\delta}\right)\frac{L^a}{48} \qquad (8.3)$$

where *L* is the span length. The yield, maximum, and failure moments are calculated using the respective load values and equation (8.2).

The deflection of any point along the beam depends on the applied load (*P*) and the position along the span length (*x*). Like the moment, the maximum deflection occurs at the midpoint of the span. Maximum deflection can be calculated using beam bending theory:

$$\text{Displacement} = \delta_{max} = \frac{PL^a}{48EI} \qquad (8.4)$$

However, this approach requires estimating the Young's modulus (*E*) of the bone sample and the moment of inertia (*I*), or geometric resistance to bending. The maximum displacement of the bone at midspan can be directly measured by the displacement of the actuator or from a linear variable displacement transformer (LVDT) placed at the bottom surface of the bone. When possible, the LVDT approach is recommended. While the addition of an LVDT can make testing more complicated, errors due to local crushing at the load point are eliminated.

In addition to material properties and microstructure of the bone tissue, the geometric parameter that influences bending outcome measures is the moment of inertia. The moment of inertia, also referred to as the second moment of area, takes into account the cross-sectional area and shape of the cross-section. The moment of inertia can be estimated by approximating the cortical cross-section to be a circular tube:

$$\text{Moment of Inertia} = I = \frac{\pi}{64}\left(D_o^4 - D_i^4\right) \qquad (8.5)$$

where D_o is the outer and D_i is the inner diameter of the bone. The moment of inertia can also be estimated by approximating the cortical cross-section as an elliptical tube:

$$\text{Moment of Inertia} = I = \frac{\pi}{64}\left(AB^3 - ab^3\right) \qquad (8.6)$$

where *A* is the major outer diameter, *B* is the minor outer diameter, *a* is the inner major diameter, and *b* is the inner minor diameter. Approximating the cross-section as a hollow circle or ellipse is not ideal, and more accurate values of the moment of inertia can be directly calculated from CT or microCT scans of the bones prior to testing.

8.3.2 Four-Point Bending

Four-point bending is similar to three-point bending except that the load is applied by two load points equally spaced between the supports (▶ Fig. 8.5a).[6,7] This loading configuration creates a length of bone between the inner load points with a constant bending moment, ensuring that the bone fails at the weakest section between the two load points, rather than at the point of maximum applied load. This configuration is advantageous for tests in which one would prefer not to apply a central load to the sample, such as healing fractures. However, the bone sample must be sufficiently long to accommodate the additional loading points.

Similar to three-point bending, the bone must be consistently oriented as the geometry, and thus the moment of inertia, differs about anatomic axes. A constant load or displacement is applied to the bone through the load points until the bone fails while the load and displacement are recorded.

The moment between the two load points is constant and equal to:

$$\text{Moment} = M = \frac{Pa}{2} \qquad (8.7)$$

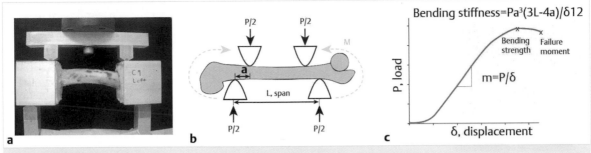

Fig. 8.5 (a) Potted sheep femur in four-point bending. (b) Schematic of a femur loaded in four-point bending with an outer support span width (*L*), distance between outer support and load point (*a*), total applied load (*P*), and resulting moment (*M*) indicated by the arrows. (c) Representative load-displacement data. Bending stiffness is calculated as $Pa^3(3L-4a)/\delta12$.

Using equation (8.7), the load displacement data can be converted into a moment-displacement curve. The slope of the linear portion of the moment-displacement curve (*P/δ*) is related to the bending stiffness by the test geometry:

$$\text{Bending Stiffness} = \left(\frac{P}{\delta}\right)\frac{a^3}{12}(3L - 4a) \qquad (8.8)$$

where *L* is the span width and *a* is the distance between adjacent lower supports and upper load points (▶ Fig. 8.5). The maximum moment calculated from the maximum load and equation (8.7) is known as the bending strength. The yield and failure moments are calculated from the respective load values using equation (8.7). Again, the factors that influence structural outcomes of a four-point bending test are the moment of inertia and material properties of the bone tissue.

In four-point bending, the displacement of the middle of the bone is not the same as the crosshead displacement. The maximum deflection can be calculated using beam bending theory,

$$\text{Displacement} = \delta_{max} = \frac{Pa}{EI4}\left(\frac{a^2}{3} - \frac{L^2}{4}\right) \qquad (8.9)$$

where *a* is the distance between the inner and outer support, *P* is the load applied to the inner load points, and *L* is the distance between outer supports (▶ Fig. 8.5). Similar to three-point bending, Young's modulus and the moment of inertia need to be estimated to calculate the displacement using beam theory. Therefore, use of an LVDT to measure midspan deflection is recommended.

Cantilever bending is very rarely employed as it requires the bone sample to be thoroughly fixed at one end and thus produces an extreme stress concentration at the point of fixation. For completeness, the bending stiffness of a cantilever beam of length *L* that is loaded by the load *P* at the free end can be calculated by

$$\text{Bending Stiffness} = \left(\frac{P}{\partial}\right)\frac{L^3}{3} \qquad (8.10)$$

8.4 Torsional Loading

Another testing mode well suited for long bones is torsion testing, whereby a torsional moment is applied about the long axis of the bone (▶ Fig. 8.6). One end of the bone is completely fixed while the other end is rotated about the long axis of the bone applying a torque using either a constant rotation rate or torque rate. The ends of the long bone must be potted to fix the sample and apply the loads. Alignment jigs are generally used to ensure central positioning of the bone and consistent alignment of the potting fixtures at each end of the bone. Because during rotation of the sample, the sample tends to shorten, the axial forces of the load frame should be controlled and it might be necessary to compensate for axial constraining forces. The angle of rotation (rotational displacement) and the torque (torsional load) are recorded during the test. For a given torque, the angle of rotation depends on the length of the bone, L.

From the torque angle of rotation graph, the torsional stiffness and torsional strength can be calculated. The torsional stiffness is related to the slope (*T/θ*) of the linear region.

$$\text{Torsional Stiffness} = \left(\frac{T}{\theta}\right)L \qquad (8.11)$$

The torsional strength is the maximum torque value withstood by the bone. In torsion, minimal postyield deformation occurs, thus the yield, maximum, and failure torque are often indistinguishable. Factors that contribute to torsional behavior include the bone material properties and polar moment of inertia. The polar

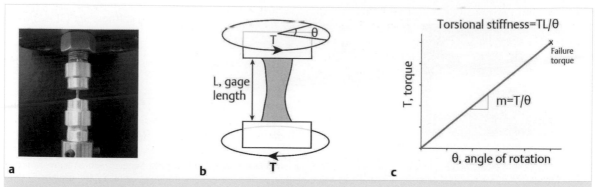

Fig. 8.6 (a) Photograph of a potted mouse femur tested in torsion. (b) Schematic of a femur tested in torsion with gauge length (*L*), applied torque (*T*), and angle of rotation (θ). (c) Representative torque-angle of rotation graph obtained from a torsion test of a long bone. Torsional stiffness is calculated as *TL/θ*.

moment of inertia (*J*) is a measure of the geometric resistance to torsion. If CT or microCT images of the bones are not available, the polar moment of inertia can be estimated by assuming a circular tube geometry and using the following equation:

$$\text{Polar Moment of Inertia} = J = \frac{\pi}{64}\left(D_O^4 - D_i^4\right) \quad (8.12)$$

where D_o is the outer and D_i is the inner diameter of the bone. The polar moment of inertia can also be estimated by approximating the periosteal and endosteal surfaces as similar ellipses using the following equation:

$$\text{Polar Moment of Inertia} = J$$
$$= \frac{\pi}{64}\left[AB\left(A^2 + B^2\right) - ab\left(a^2 + b^2\right)\right]$$
$$(8.13)$$

where *A* is the major outer diameter, *B* is the minor outer diameter, *a* is the inner major diameter, and *b* is the inner minor diameter.

8.5 Calculating Stress and Strain

As previously mentioned, whole bone mechanical behavior depends on bone mass, geometry, and tissue material properties. The outcome parameters calculated from mechanical tests thus far depend on all three factors. However, specific diseases and genetics can cause concurrent changes in material properties and bone geometry, making it difficult to identify the cause of changes in whole bone mechanical behavior. The ability to measure the intrinsic material properties of the bone tissue by accounting for sample geometry in whole bone tests is a valuable tool to understand the mechanisms through which whole bone mechanical behavior changes.

Key Concepts: Stress and Strain

When a force is applied to a whole bone, internal forces are generated within the bone material itself. These internal forces are known as stresses. Specifically, the stress is the average force acting on a specific surface of the bone. This force can be decomposed into two components: axial stress acting normal to the surface and shear stress acting parallel to the surface. The deformation of a volume of material normalized by its original length is known as the strain. Similarly to stress, this deformation can be decomposed into normal and shear components. Both stress and strain are fundamental characteristics of a given material when loaded.

Although material properties can be calculated from whole bone mechanical testing data by accounting for geometry, the irregular geometry of bones and inaccuracy in calculated strains can introduce error into calculated values for Young's modulus and stresses. Thus testing machined samples with regular geometries to evaluate material properties is recommended. However, the following section reviews calculations of stresses, strains, and elastic constants from whole bone tests.

8.5.1 Axial Loading

For axial tests, the load (*P*) is divided by the cross-sectional area (*A*) to determine the resulting tensile (positive) or compressive (negative) stress. The axial stress, σ_{axial}, is assumed to be uniformly distributed across the sample cross-section:

$$\text{Axial Stress} = \sigma_{\text{axial}} = \frac{P}{A} \quad (8.14)$$

The maximum value of stress calculated from the maximum load is the ultimate stress, commonly referred to as the strength. The yield and failure stresses are calculated from the respective load values. The axial strain, ε_{axial}, is calculated by dividing the displacement of the bone by the original gauge length (L):

$$\text{Axial Strain} = \epsilon_{axial} = \frac{\delta}{L} \tag{8.15}$$

The slope of the elastic region of the stress-strain curve (the initial linear region) is the Young's modulus, E:

$$\text{Young's Modulus} = E = \frac{\sigma_{axial}}{\epsilon_{axial}} \tag{8.16}$$

8.5.2 Bending

In bending, the stress, σ_{bend}, varies linearly through the cross-section for stresses lower than the yield stress. The bending stress depends on the applied moment (M), moment of inertia (I), and the position of the point of interest with respect to the neutral axis (c):

$$\text{Bending Stress} = \sigma_{bend} = \frac{Mc}{I} \tag{8.17}$$

The neutral axis is the plane that experiences no stress and is the transition from compressive to tensile stress in the sample. The maximum stresses occur at the periosteal surfaces of the bone, compressive on top and tensile on the bottom for the loading setup, as shown in ▶ Fig. 8.7b. The yield and failure stresses are calculated from the respective moment values using equation (8.17).

The strain at a given location in a bone subjected to three point bending, ε_{3bend}, is

$$\text{Three Point Bending Strain} = \epsilon_{ebend} = \frac{12c\delta}{L^2} \tag{8.18}$$

The strain at a given location in a bone subjected to four point bending, ε_{4bend}, is

$$\text{Four Point Bending Strain} = \epsilon_{4bend} = \frac{6c\delta}{a(3L - 4a)} \tag{8.19}$$

where c is the distance from the neutral axis, δ is the displacement, L is the span width, and a is the distance from adjacent support and loading points. Measuring strains for bending directly using strain gages is preferable to calculation using beam bending theory. The Young's modulus of a bone can be calculated from bending tests by dividing the bending stress by the bending strain.

8.5.3 Torsional Loading

Torsion induces shear stresses and strains, in contrast to the normal stresses and strains induced by compression and bending. Like bending stress, the shear stress (τ) at a given point in a bone cross depends on its position from the axis of rotation (r), applied torque (T), and the polar moment of inertia (J) (▶ Fig. 8.8):

$$\text{Shear Stress} = \tau = \frac{Tr}{J} \tag{8.20}$$

Thus the maximum shear stress occurs at the periosteal surface of the bone. The shear strain (γ) also varies with radial distance from the rotational axis (r), the angle of rotation (θ), and the gauge length of the bone (L).

$$\text{Shear Strain} = \gamma = \frac{\theta r}{L} \tag{8.21}$$

The shear modulus, G, relates the shear stress and strain prior to plastic deformation and is calculated as:

$$\text{Shear Modulus} = G = \frac{TL}{J\theta} \tag{8.22}$$

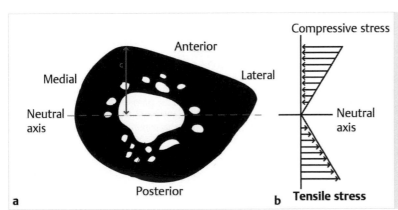

Fig. 8.7 (a) Schematic of a long bone cross-section with distance from the neutral axis (c) indicated. (b) Stress distribution for a beam in bending; the neutral axis does not necessarily coincide with anatomic directions. In the linear region, before the yield stress is reached, the stress varies linearly with distance from the neutral axis through the cross section.

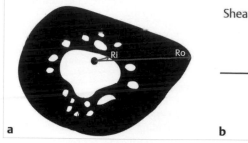
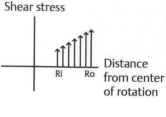

8.5.4 Stiffness in Terms of Material Properties

The structural stiffness for the different loading modes, described in equations (8.1), (8.3), (8.8), and (8.9), can be expressed in terms of sample geometry and elastic moduli:

Axial stiffness = EA

Bending stiffness = EI

Torsional stiffness = GJ

These relationships are based on the same assumptions previously described for each test.

8.6 Test Selection

A variety of considerations contribute to the selection of a specific test, including the research question, replication of physiological loading conditions, bone geometry, and ease of testing. Although no bones are perfectly suited for mechanical testing, bones with minimally varying cross-sections and minimal curvatures reduce errors in calculated strengths and stiffnesses. Geometric factors such as cross-sectional area, moment of inertia, and polar moment of inertia are needed to calculate stresses in samples. However, if the geometry of the bone changes drastically along its length, the values used for these geometric parameters will be inaccurate. In compression, a curved bone will introduce a bending moment in addition to the axial load, leading to errors in the calculated stress. Curved long bones in bending alter the stress and strain variations with respect to the neutral axis. In torsion, curvature increases the distance from the center of rotation, thus increasing the shear stress.

The testing setup of torsion tests allows the bone to fail at the weakest point along the entire gage length, unlike three-point bending. Additionally, torsion tests are not sensitive to cross-sectional orientation, whereas bending tests are sensitive to loading direction, for example anterior-posterior or medial-lateral. When possible, four-point bending tests are recommended as the bone will fail at the weakest point within the loading points, unlike three-point bending for which the maximum moment and maximum shear force occur at the midpoint of the span.

If postyield behavior is of interest, bending tests are recommended rather than torsional tests. Load-displacement curves from torsion tests are usually linear until failure with minimal nonlinear behavior making differences in postyield behavior difficult to elucidate.

8.7 Conclusion

Whole bone mechanical testing measures bone structural behavior, a key measure related to bone function in vivo. By quantifying changes in bone mass, geometry, and material properties, the mechanism through which the structural behavior of bone is changed can be hypothesized. Whole bone testing provides a practical method of evaluating changes in whole bone mechanical behavior due to aging, disease, pharmaceutical treatment, and genetics. Concurrently, identifying changes in bone mass, geometry, and material properties provides further insight into the mechanisms whereby these factors affect whole bone mechanical behavior.

References

[1] Jepsen KJ, Goldstein SA, Kuhn JL, Schaffler MB, Bonadio J. Type-I collagen mutation compromises the post-yield behavior of Mov13 long bone. J Orthop Res 1996; 14: 493–499

[2] Silva MJ, Brodt MD, Ettner SL. Long bones from the senescence accelerated mouse SAMP6 have increased size but reduced whole-bone strength and resistance to fracture. J Bone Miner Res 2002; 17: 1597–1603

[3] Pelker RR, Friedlaender GE, Markham TC, Panjabi MM, Moen CJ. Effects of freezing and freeze-drying on the biomechanical properties of rat bone. J Orthop Res 1984; 1: 405–411

[4] Tommasini SM, Morgan TG, van der Meulen MCh, Jepsen KJ. Genetic variation in structure-function relationships for the inbred mouse lumbar vertebral body. J Bone Miner Res 2005; 20: 817–827

[5] Schriefer JL, Robling AG, Warden SJ, Fournier AJ, Mason JJ, Turner CH. A comparison of mechanical properties derived from multiple skeletal sites in mice. J Biomech 2005; 38: 467–475

[6] Uveges TE, Kozloff KM, Ty JM et al. Alendronate treatment of the brtl osteogenesis imperfecta mouse improves femoral geometry and load response before fracture but decreases predicted material properties and has detrimental effects on osteoblasts and bone formation. J Bone Miner Res 2009; 24: 849–859

[7] Jepsen KJ, Pennington DE, Lee YL, Warman M, Nadeau J. Bone brittleness varies with genetic background in A/J and C57BL/6J inbred mice. J Bone Miner Res 2001; 16: 1854–1862

Further Reading

Burstein AH, Frankel VH. A standard test for laboratory animal bone. J Biomech 1971; 4: 155–158

Turner CH, Burr DB. Basic biomechanical measurements of bone: a tutorial. Bone 1993; 14: 595–608

9 Biomechanics of Trabecular and Cortical Bone

G. Harry van Lenthe and Pinaki Bhattacharya

The skeleton provides support for the body and protection for vital organs. Hence, the bones that form the skeleton must have the right combination of stiffness, strength, and toughness to be able to withstand the forces imposed upon it. The inability to do so may impact substantially on an individual's quality of life. Bone's stiffness and strength are not natural constants. It is one of the fascinating aspects of bone that it can adapt its structure and composition to match the mechanical demands being placed upon it. These mechanical demands may differ from bone to bone and from anatomic location to anatomic location. As a consequence, strong site- and subject-specific variations have been found in the mechanical characteristics of bone. The quantitative evaluation of bone mechanical competence can provide important information in clinical diagnosis, treatment, and follow-up (e.g., in osteoporosis and other metabolic bone diseases). Furthermore, it is important from a scientific point of view for addressing hypotheses concerning biological aspects of bone, like growth, homeostasis, and aging.

Material properties at one length scale are dependent on the architecture of the underlying length scale and on the accompanying material properties of that length scale; for example, the mechanical properties of a human long bone will depend on the material properties of cortical and trabecular bone when measured at a length scale of 5 to 10 mm, and the three-dimensional structure of that bone. In turn, the material properties of trabecular bone depend on the specific trabecular bone architecture and the properties of the material that makes up the trabeculae. In a kind of recursive fashion, one can zoom in further and quantify bone tissue properties as a result of the microstructure within a single trabecula (osteocyte lacuna, cement lines, etc.) and the properties of the materials within that trabecula, such as bone with differing degrees of mineralization and corresponding differences in Young's modulus.

It is the aim of this chapter to provide insight into the considerations underlying the mechanical characterization of bone tissue as opposed to the characterization of whole bone mechanics (see Chapter 8).

9.1 Mechanical Testing

The gold standard to determine bone mechanical properties is through experimental mechanical testing. In itself, direct mechanical testing is a straightforward procedure. Yet, bone, and in particular trabecular bone, is a difficult material to test. Standard test geometries, like defined in mechanical testing standards, can rarely be used for trabecular bone, because it is often too fragile and too inhomogeneous to machine. As a consequence, sample preparation needs dedicated care. Compression testing is the most popular measurement technique, using test specimens that are cylindrical or cubic. Care must be taken in interpreting the outcomes of a mechanical test, as they are influenced by anatomic site and loading direction; furthermore, they can be influenced to a large extent by end artifacts. It also has to be realized that the quantification of bone strength is limited by its destructiveness; a sample can only be fractured once, making it physically impossible to assess the direction-dependent failure characteristics on single specimens.

Similar to mechanical testing of whole bones, the main outcome of a mechanical test on a bone specimen is a force-displacement curve (▶ Fig. 9.1a). The stiffness of the specimen is derived as the slope of the initial linear regime of the force-displacement curve. The area under the curve represents the energy (also strain-energy or work) taken up by the specimen until fracture.

Given that the sample dimensions are known, the force-displacement curve can be transformed into a stress-strain curve (▶ Fig. 9.1b) where stress is defined as

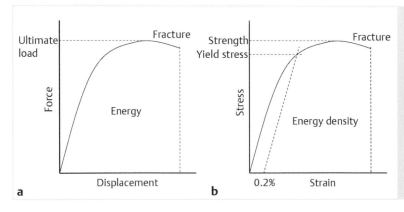

Fig. 9.1 **(a)** A typical force-displacement curve indicating an initially linear-elastic behavior followed by non-linear deformation and subsequent failure. **(b)** The stress-strain curve is derived from the force-displacement curve by normalizing the force by area and the displacement by specimen length.

force divided by the cross-sectional area of the specimen and strain as displacement divided by specimen length. Parameters that can be derived from the stress-strain curve are Young's modulus, yield point, strength, and energy density. The yield point is defined as that particular stress or strain level at which the specimen deviates from the initial linear response; it is typically determined following the 0.2% offset rule (▶ Fig. 9.1b). Strength is defined as the maximum stress level that can be sustained. Toughness can be determined by quantifying the area underneath the stress-strain curve; it represents the mechanical deformation energy per unit volume prior to fracture.

Note that the measures as derived from the stress-strain curve are representative of the bulk material; hence, they are independent of bone geometry. Yet, they include the effects of features with a smaller length scale, such as porosity, the three-dimensional arrangement of trabeculae, osteon composition, and their orientation. In order for the mechanical properties to be representative for the entire specimen, the specimen could be considered to be made up out of one homogeneous material. Trabecular bone can be considered as a continuum material when viewed at a length scale of 5 mm or more.[1] Thus, this finding puts a lower limit to the sample size, which should be at least 5 mm cubes. Ideally, the sample size should be larger because of boundary artifacts (next section); typically, specimen dimension is between 5 mm and 10 mm.

Mechanical testing is most commonly performed as a uniaxial test, performed in the direction of the main trabecular orientation, which is the stiffest direction. For that purpose, specimen preparation is typically performed according to the anatomic orientation. For anatomic sites with a complicated trabecular architecture, X-ray imaging prior to specimen preparation can serve as a guide in defining the proper cutting planes.

9.2 On Boundary Conditions and Preconditioning

Mechanical testing of trabecular bone is potentially subject to large systematic errors.[2] During specimen preparation, some of the trabeculae at the specimen surface might get damaged or even fractured. But even in the case of a perfect extraction of the specimen, substantial boundary artifacts will occur because the trabeculae at the boundaries of the specimens become "free" at one end, and will behave much more flexible than when contained in the trabecular architecture. This causes the boundary layer of the specimens to be softer than the inner portion of the sample; as a consequence the specimen as a whole will behave softer than the same bone specimen in situ. It will be obvious that

this effect is larger for specimens with long, not well-connected trabeculae, hence, typically specimens with low bone volume fraction. The use of endcaps and/or polymethyl methacrylate embedding are good means in reducing this error. The use of a ball joint in the testing setup will reduce the error that could originate from the fact that the surfaces of the specimen are not precisely parallel.

When a sample is taken from bone and tested, it will generally not give the linear-elastic response for low strains, but will show a so-called toe-region (▶ Fig. 9.2). This toe-region is an artifact, the origin of which lies in the creation process of the sample when surface irregularities can form. When the test is started, it is important to have good contact between the platens and the specimen in order to avoid artifacts from fluids on the surfaces and to allow for some alignment and seating of the specimen. The use of a number of preconditioning cycles in which the specimen is loaded within its linear elastic range (e.g., up to 0.1 to 0.2%) will largely remove the toe-region and variability associated with it. In addition, the final experimental test is typically started with a small preload, as to ensure contact between the specimen and the mechanical testing apparatus.

When a toe-region is present, a correction procedure should be applied in order to obtain proper values for the mechanical parameters. Specifically, the linear portion of the stress-strain curve is to be extended such that this line crosses the zero-stress axis. This point on the axis represents the "zero-strain" point from which all strains must be measured.

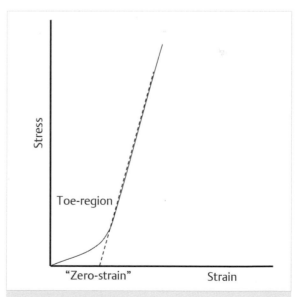

Fig. 9.2 The linear-elastic material behavior, represented by a linear relationship between stress and strain, can be preceded by a non-linear toe-region.

9.3 Experimental Findings

Key Jargon: Anisotropic Material Properties

An **isotropic** material has identical properties in all directions. In contrast, for an **anisotropic** material, the material properties depend on the direction in which they are measured. Special forms of anisotropy are orthotropy and transverse isotropy. An **orthotropic** material has two or three mutually orthogonal axes of rotational symmetry. Its mechanical properties are different along each axis. A **transverse isotropic** material has material properties that are symmetric about an axis that is normal to a plane of isotropy. Cortical and trabecular bone exhibit orthotropic material behavior.[3,4] The extent of its mechanical anisotropy can range from basically 1 (no preferential orientation) to over 10 (10-fold difference in different directions) for both stiffness and strength.

Mechanical testing has shown huge heterogeneity in bone mechanical properties across sites and specimens. The variation is largely related to the amount of bone present in the sample. Yet, the anatomic location also plays a role and has led to defining site-specific density-elasticity relationships; hence, bone samples with the same bone quantity but taken from different anatomic sites will typically have different Young's moduli (▶ Fig. 9.3). The tissue modulus (i.e., the modulus of the material constituting an individual trabecula) appears to be identical for each site; hence, the site specificity appears to be solely due to site-specific variation in trabecular architecture.

9.4 Quantification of Tissue-Level Properties

A direct method to obtain information about local bone tissue properties is through nanoindentation. In short, a hard tip of a material whose mechanical properties are known is pressed into a sample whose properties are unknown. The load placed on the indenter tip is increased as the tip penetrates further into the specimen. After reaching a user-defined value, the load is held constant for a period and then removed. After unloading, the area of the residual indentation in the sample is measured; from the applied load and the indentation area, the hardness can be computed. The elastic modulus of the material can be obtained from the indentation response using the Oliver-Pharr method and by comparing it with a known material; fused silica often serves as a reference.[4] Successive indentations can be made on the same specimen, but they must be separated by about 20 indentation diameters to prevent interference. A disadvantage of nanoindentation is that it requires very smooth surfaces for which substantial specimen preparation is required. Sections, in the order of 100 μm, are progressively ground and finally polished with a diamond suspension to achieve surface roughness below 1 μm. Though it is known that tissue hydration can significantly

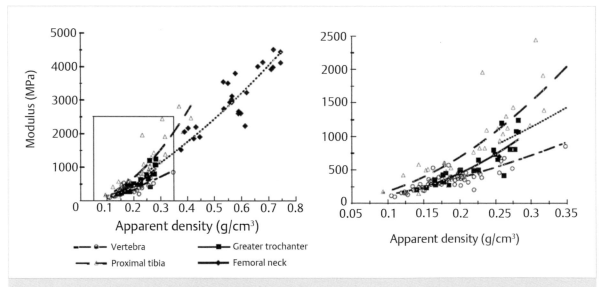

Fig. 9.3 Regressions between apparent modulus and apparent density for each anatomic site. While no differences in power law exponents were found among sites, differences were found among leading coefficients. At a given apparent density, specimens from the proximal tibia and trochanter had higher moduli than those from the vertebra, and those from the femoral neck had lower moduli than those from the proximal tibia. (Taken from Morgan EF, Bayrakta HH, Keaveny. Trabecular bone modulus–density relationships depend on anatomic site. J Biomech 2003;36(7):897–904.)

modify elastic properties, technical challenges exist in conducting nanoindentation on wet bones. Typically, biopsy specimens are fixed in 70% alcohol, dehydrated in absolute alcohol, and then embedded in methyl methacrylate. Fixing in resins remains a concern, because the process can alter mechanical properties. For a more in-depth analysis of nanoindentation and for practical guidelines, see Lewis and Nyman[5] and Oyen and Cook.[6]

An interesting recently developed technique for the quantification of cortical bone properties is the reference point indentation (RPI) method.[7] RPI is essentially a depth-sensing indentation; it works by pushing a thin probe into a material at a known force and measuring the microscopic distance that the probe travels into the material. From the force-displacement data, measures of bone mechanical quality can be derived. In essence, the technique is similar to micro- and nanoindentation; the main difference is that it uses two coaxial probes instead of a single indenter. The inner probe indents the surface, whereas the outer probe, which rests on the adjacent and unindented surface, serves as a reference for displacement of the inner probe. Because the instrument senses depth without the need of an optical measurement of the indented surface, associated systematic errors are avoided. Surface preparation is thereby less demanding; as a result, RPI can even be used in vivo.

The indentation distance increase is the most commonly reported outcome parameter in an RPI procedure. Indentation distance increase is defined as the increase in the indentation distance in the last cycle relative to the indentation distance in the first cycle. It is a measure of the ability the bone to resist additional deformation with repetitive loading (i.e., a local post-yield measure).

9.5 Visualization of Bone Under Load

Whereas biomechanical testing provides detailed information on bone material properties, it fails in revealing local properties such as local deformations and strains. By combining mechanical testing with imaging methods, it has become possible to visualize and quantify bone deformations under load on various levels of structural organization. For trabecular bone samples, several deformations modes were found in human vertebral bone; some trabeculae bend, others buckle, and some are compressed (▶ Fig. 9.4). Fracture initiation and progression can also be visualized and quantified in a nondestructive and three-dimensional fashion (▶ Fig. 9.5). Specifically, the combination of mechanical testing with synchrotron radiation-based computed tomography revealed that microcracks initiated at canal and at bone surfaces, whereas osteocyte lacunae provided guidance to the microcracks. This technique, referred to as image-guided failure assessment, has been validated as compared to classical continuous mechanical testing.[8]

The local strains can be calculated using strain mapping approaches. Strain mapping is a mathematical technique to calculate how a bone or bone sample has deformed between two loading steps. An example of such an approach where deformable registration was applied to cylindrical aluminum foams is shown in ▶ Fig. 9.6. Specifically, digital volume correlation was used to align regions of the images. For a finer and more localized alignment of the images, the "Demons" deformable image registration algorithm was implemented.[9] Based on the Gaussian filtered displacement field, the Green-Lagrange strain tensor was calculated. Where traditional mechanical tests

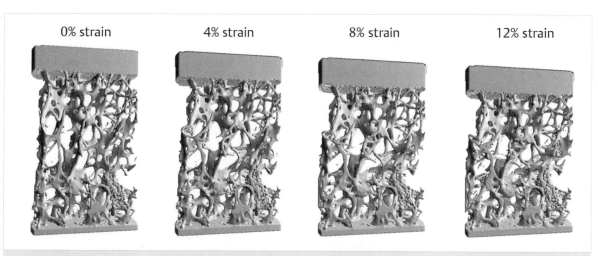

| 0% strain | 4% strain | 8% strain | 12% strain |

Fig. 9.4 Image-guided failure assessment in a human spine sample using time-lapsed tomographic imaging. The images show compression, imaged in steps of 4% strain. Note that only half of the specimen is depicted here, which is possible due to the noninvasive character of the image-guided failure assessment technique. (Copied from van Lenthe GH, Muller R. CT-based visualization and quantification of bone microstructure in vivo. BoneKEy 2008;5(11):410–425.)

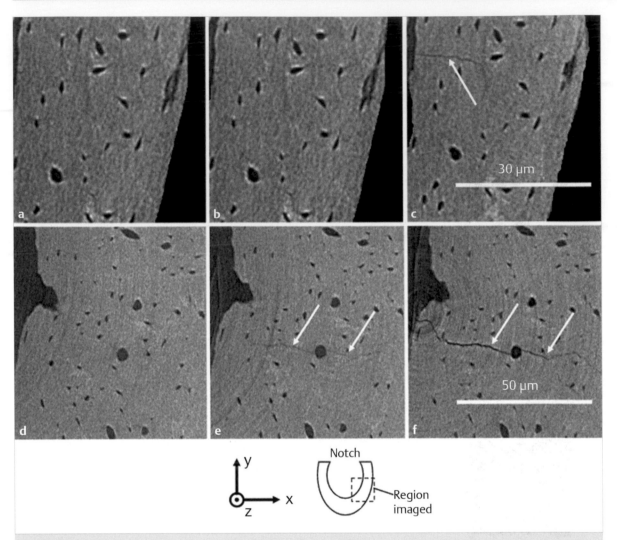

Fig. 9.5 Microcrack initiation and propagation in the femoral middiaphyseal reduced cross-section. (**a**) No visible microcracks at 0% apparent strain for the B6 specimen. (**b**) No visible microcracks at 1% apparent strain for the B6 specimen. (**c**) Microcrack initiation (*arrow*) at 2% apparent strain for the B6 specimen. (**d**) No visible microcracks at 0% apparent strain for the C3 H specimen. (**e**) Microcrack initiation (*arrows*) at 1% apparent strain for the C3 H specimen. (**f**) Microcrack propagation (*arrows*) at 2% apparent strain for the C3 H specimen. Data were assessed using synchrotron radiation computed tomography at 700 nm nominal resolution. (Copied from Voide R, Schnieder P, Stauber M, et al. Time-lapsed assessment of microcrack initiation and propagation in murine cortical bone at submicrometer resolution. Bone 2009;45(2):164–173.)

would only have revealed strength and toughness characteristics, the combination with imaging and computational strain analyses revealed the location of the microcracks and how they propagated through the bone. The strain mapping procedure was used to quantify the strain in the bone volume close to the microcrack (▶ Fig. 9.7).

9.6 Computational Assessment of Bone Competence

Although not an experimental technique per se, computational modeling is widely used in the quantification of

bone mechanical properties. A detailed description of finite element (FE) analysis is beyond the scope of this chapter. Its principles and its application in bone mechanics will be treated in Chapters 20 to 22. Here we will discuss only one application of FE because of its relevance in quantifying tissue material properties.

Microstructural FE (μFE) models allow performance of "virtual experiments" on computer reconstructions of bone. The interesting aspect of μFE in the quantification of bone material properties is that it can accurately quantify the role of the bone structure, leaving the tissue modulus as the only unknown. Tissue modulus can then be quantified as the ratio between the stiffness as measured

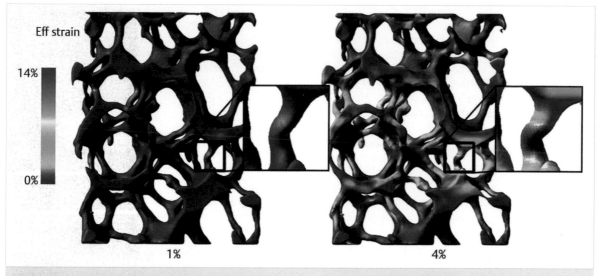

Fig. 9.6 Effective strains in a trabecular bone analog as determined from strain-mapping for applied strains of 1% (*left*) and 4% (*right*). (Image courtesy of D. Christen, ETH Zürich, Switzerland.)

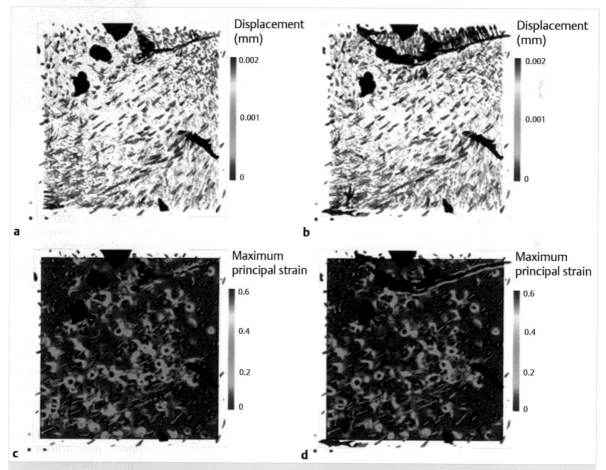

Fig. 9.7 The resulting displacement map (**a, b**) and strain map (**c, d**) for the second load step after the initiation of the first visible microcracks (**a, c**) and the last step prior to failure (**b, d**). There are distinct regions in the transversal plane with the osteocyte lacunae (*yellow*) homogeneously distributed and aligned in which the microcrack (*green*) is propagating along the same direction of orientation. Furthermore, the accumulation of canals (*red*) is causing a stress concentration and consequently, a deflection of the microcrack. (Copied from Christen D, Levchuk A, Schori S, Schneider P, Boyd SK, Muller R. Deformable image registration and 3D strain mapping for the quanitative assessment of cortical bone microdamage. J Mech Behav Biomed Mater 2012;8:184–193.)

in an experimental test and the stiffness as calculated by the virtual experiment, a procedure first described by van Rietbergen et al.[10] It has been demonstrated over and over again that for linear deformation conditions, comparison between biomechanical compression tests on excised trabecular bone samples and μFE show very good agreement ($R^2 = 0.92$) when one single homogeneous, isotropic tissue modulus is applied[11]; this holds true for normal as well as for osteoporotic bone.[12] This "inverse" analysis to quantify tissue properties has become an accepted method to quantify tissue modulus.[13] However, care must be taken in interpreting the outcomes, because the calculated tissue moduli are likely to depend on the specific image resolution with which the specimen was reconstructed. In a way, this mirrors the hierarchical evaluation seen in experimental tests for which it is also well known that material properties depend on the length scale of investigation.

9.7 Conclusion

Experimental mechanical testing is considered the gold standard to determine bone competence at all length scales. Mechanical testing is a straightforward approach; however, testing of bone samples remains challenging because boundary effects can largely determine the outcome of a mechanical test.

In combination with nondestructive, three-dimensional imaging, bone material properties can be derived that go beyond those of traditional measures. More specifically, it has been demonstrated that the combination of imaging and mechanical testing allows the visualization and quantification of local bone deformation and failure characteristics such as crack initiation and propagation. Strain mapping techniques even allow quantification of the local mechanical milieu in terms of strain, directly from the experimental data.

Computational models of whole bone behavior can be developed by combining bone microarchitecture imaging with assessment of bone tissue constitutive properties. Advances in nondestructive three-dimensional imaging point toward a promising future for integrative approaches like functional microimaging. Image-based FE analyses have been demonstrated as great research tools in separating out the combined effects of structure and tissue mechanical properties. Furthermore, due to improvements in computational methods and capabilities of modern computing hardware, it has become possible to perform "virtual experiments." Taken together, the combination of experimental testing with functional imaging and computational analyses hold great potential for a hierarchical approach in unraveling bone mechanical properties from the whole bone down to the cell. The recent introduction of RPI has opened the way for the characterization of bone tissue properties in vivo. It holds promises for a more refined assessment of bone quality in patients.

References

[1] Harrigan TP et al. Limitations of the continuum assumption in cancellous bone. J Biomech 1988; 21: 269–275

[2] Keaveny TM, Pinilla TP, Crawford RP, Kopperdahl DL, Lou A. Systematic and random errors in compression testing of trabecular bone. J Orthop Res 1997; 15: 101–110

[3] Keaveny TM, Morgan EF, Niebur GL, Yeh OC. Biomechanics of trabecular bone. Annu Rev Biomed Eng 2001; 3: 307–333

[4] Oliver WC, Pharr GM. An improved technique for determining hardness and elastic-modulus using load and displacement sensing indentation experiments. J Mater Res 1992; 7: 1564–1583

[5] Lewis G, Nyman JS. The use of nanoindentation for characterizing the properties of mineralized hard tissues: state-of-the art review. J Biomed Mater Res B Appl Biomater 2008; 87: 286–301

[6] Oyen ML, Cook RF. A practical guide for analysis of nanoindentation data. J Mech Behav Biomed Mater 2009; 2: 396–407

[7] Diez-Perez A, Güerri R, Nogues X et al. Microindentation for in vivo measurement of bone tissue mechanical properties in humans. J Bone Miner Res 2010; 25: 1877–1885

[8] Nazarian A, Müller R. Time-lapsed microstructural imaging of bone failure behavior. J Biomech 2004; 37: 55–65

[9] Pauchard Y, Mattmann C, Kuhn A, Gasser JA, Boyd SK. European Society of Biomechanics S.M. Perren Award 2008: using temporal trends of 3D bone micro-architecture to predict bone quality. J Biomech 2008; 41: 2946–2953

[10] van Rietbergen B, Weinans H, Huiskes R, Odgaard A. A new method to determine trabecular bone elastic properties and loading using micromechanical finite-element models. J Biomech 1995; 28: 69–81

[11] Kabel J, van Rietbergen B, Dalstra M, Odgaard A, Huiskes R. The role of an effective isotropic tissue modulus in the elastic properties of cancellous bone. J Biomech 1999; 32: 673–680

[12] Homminga J et al. The dependence of the elastic properties of osteoporotic cancellous bone on volume fraction and fabric. J Biomech 2003; 36: 1461–1467

[13] van Lenthe GH, Voide R, Boyd SK, Müller R. Tissue modulus calculated from beam theory is biased by bone size and geometry: implications for the use of three-point bending tests to determine bone tissue modulus. Bone 2008; 43: 717–723

Further Reading

An YH, Draughn RA. Mechanical testing of bone and the bone-implant interface. Boca Raton, FL: CRC Press; 1999

Cowin SC. Bone mechanics handbook. Boca Raton, FL: CRC Press; 2001

Donnelly E. Methods for assessing bone quality: a review. Clin Orthop Relat Res 2011; 469: 2128–2138

10 Biomechanics of Fracture Fixation

Peter Augat

The basic requirements for successful treatment of bone fractures have long been identified by Lorenz Böhler: reposition, retention, and rehabilitation. The fixation of the fracture has to respect these requirements and has therefore to provide sufficient biomechanical stability. Persistent retention of the fracture requires adequate fixation of the fracture fragments under full or partial load-bearing activities. Therefore, first of all the mechanical characteristics of the fracture fixation technique have to assure the retention of the fracture. Rehabilitation is required to maintain joint mobility but also to introduce some mechanical loading of the fracture. Mechanical loading of the fracture is a prerequisite for a successful healing progress. Certain amounts of motion at the fracture site (interfragmentary movements) induce callus formation and stimulate bridging of the fracture gap. Thus, the second requirement of the fracture fixation is to provide sufficient interfragmentary movement to promote healing. Finally, the fracture fixation technique has to transfer the load between the fracture fragments until the fracture has completely united. To endure the healing time without failure or loosening, the fracture fixation device has to have sufficient fatigue strength.

Measuring the biomechanical properties therefore should include assessment of (1) the quality of retention under load, (2) the stability of the osteosynthesis construct described by the stiffness and the interfragmentary movement, and (3) the strength of the osteosynthesis described by load at failure and fatigue strength.

> ### Jargon Simplified: Fracture Fixation Construct
>
> A fracture fixation device (plate, nail, or screw) can be mechanically tested by itself to assess its inherent mechanical performance, which typically includes fatigue testing. However, much more appealing is the mechanical test of the fixation device when it is applied to a fractured bone specimen or to a bone fracture model. The biomechanical testing of such a fracture fixation construct mimics the mechanical performance for a certain fracture situation and will have much more clinical relevance.

10.1 Design of Experiment

In order to appropriately design a biomechanical experiment on fracture fixation constructs (FFCs), it is essential to formulate a testable study hypothesis. The study hypothesis will define the mechanical characteristic that

will be assessed and will also specify which type of FFC will be studied. The study conclusion will have to describe the clinical implications of the mechanical performance. Although the aim of most studies is to demonstrate some sort of mechanical superiority, it should be taken into consideration that the mechanical superiority does not necessarily correspond to similar clinical advantages. In the contrary, superior mechanical properties may eventually lead to inferior clinical outcome.[1]

10.2 Choice of Load and Load Application

One major challenge in testing of FFCs is the fixation within the frame of the testing machine and the choice of an appropriate loading condition. Ideally, the applied load configuration mimics the physiological load situation as closely as possible. In particular, the direction and contact point of the resulting load vector should simulate the in vivo loading situation. For most of the major joints, the in vivo loading situation are well described,[2] and mechanical testing should consider this expertise. The load frame of the material testing device will have to simulate the resulting load by applying the load to one end of the FFC while the other end is somehow fixed to the machine frame.

Although uniaxial loading is the most frequent form of load application, it may not adequately simulate the in vivo load situation during gait or limb movement. Because it is not a priori known which of the loads occurring in vivo puts the highest challenge on the FFC, several load scenarios or combined load scenarios will have to be realized. The individual load scenario may realize a particular physiological situation or may be just a generic load case (i.e., torsion, shear, bending).

The load application by the testing machine usually simulates a single joint reaction force or the force resultants. Sometimes, it might be necessary to apply additional forces that would be generated from muscles or ligaments in order to simulate physiological loading situations. Such combined loading scenarios can be realized by multiaxial loading devices, lever arm constructs, special pulleys attached to dead weights, or by additional load cylinders (▶ Fig. 10.1).

Fixation of the FFC in the testing frame will always be an approximation of the in vivo loading scenario, but the aim should be to mimic physiological loading as closely as possible. In reality, the fixation in the frame will always be a compromise between providing stable fixation and allowing all necessary degrees of freedom. Ignoring compensatory adjustments can generate very considerable

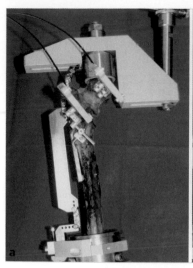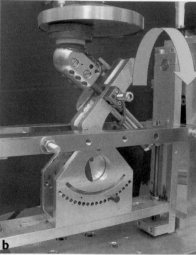

Fig 10.1 Examples of experimental realization of multidirectional load cases. (a) The forces of the tractus iliotibialis and the hip joint reaction are induced by the machine load applicator and a lever arm.[7] (b) Variation of the direction of the hip joint reaction load vector during walking by rotation of the hip axis.[8]

constraining forces and extensive unphysiological load components that may even dominate the overall load. Compensatory adjustments can be realized by using cardanic joints, hinge joints, or linear bearings. This will not only induce defined loading conditions in the FFC but will also spare the load cells of the testing machine from harmful shear forces.

10.3 Testing Conditions

In a biomechanical experiment on an FFC, typically a certain load is applied and the resulting deformation is measured. An important feature is the time characteristic of the loading curve. Loading can be applied "quasi-"statically, dynamically, or cyclically. For the assessment of stability, loading should be applied statically, whereas for the assessment of fatigue strength and retention, cyclic loading should be applied. Dynamic loading can be employed if a sudden catastrophic failure scenario (fall or impact) needs to be simulated.

For "quasi-"static loading, usually several preconditioning cycles (load level less than 10% of failure load) will be performed to avoid settling artifacts and increase reproducibility. The static test itself is performed at relatively slow loading rates reaching the load at failure at around 1 minute. One major direct result from static testing is displacement of the fracture or displacement of the joint surface and deformation of the FFC in specific directions. Stiffness of the FFC is evaluated from the slope of the linear portion of the load-deformation plot with deformation measured in the direction of the applied load (▶ Fig. 10.2). Deformation should be directly measured on the FFC with extensometers, displacement transducers, or optical trackers. If deformation is measured indirectly using the displacement transducer of the testing machine, the stiffness result is biased by the stiffness of the testing frame, testing setup, and intrinsic stiffness of

the load cells. The FFC stiffness will be considerably underestimated if stiffness measurement is not accounting for system stiffness. If static loading is continued until failure, the load at failure and the failure energy can also be determined from the load-deformation plot.

> ### Key Concepts: Considering System Stiffness
>
> The compliance of the machine frame, test setup, and load cell can significantly contribute to measured displacement if measurement is performed with the machine transducers.
>
> The correct stiffness of the FFC S_{FFC} can be obtained by correcting the measured total stiffness S_{total} by adjusting for intrinsic system stiffness S_{System} according to:
>
> $$S_{FFC} = \frac{S_{total} \cdot S_{System}}{S_{System} - S_{total}}$$
>
> The system stiffness S_{System} can be determined by replacing the FFC with an extremely stiff dummy device, for example a solid steel cylinder.

Cyclic loading of an FFC more closely simulates the physiological loading conditions and therefore is the preferred test method to assess failure properties of the FFC. One major challenge in cyclic testing is to identify a load magnitude that is physiologically relevant and also leads to some sort of failure within a reasonable time frame. If the static failure load of the FFC is known, a reasonable load magnitude to start with is about 60 to 80% of the static failure load. The problem with identifying the load magnitude is that a low load will result in run outs (no failure occurs during the intended number of load cycles), whereas a high load magnitude might not obtain reasonable numbers of load cycles. The number of load cycles

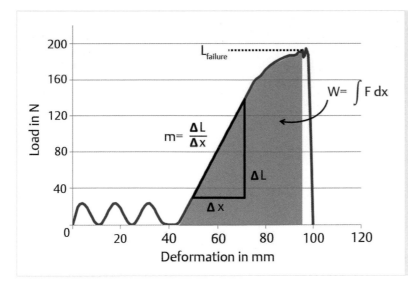

Fig. 10.2 Load-deformation diagram for a static loading experiment. Three preconditioning cycles minimize settling effects. The stiffness m can be determined from the slope of the linear region of the load-deformation diagram, ideally by performing linear regression analysis. Load at failure ($L_{failure}$) is the highest load level prior to the first load minimum, which is not necessarily the overall maximum load level. The energy to failure W can be determined by calculating the area under the load-deformation curve. The point at which the curve levels off and plastic deformation begins to occur is called the yield point, for which several definitions exist.

for FFC constructs should simulate realistic time periods of fracture healing, which is anywhere between 3 and 6 months. This corresponds to approximately 250,000 load cycles and should be sufficient to evaluate osteosynthesis products.[3] However, depending on the complexity of the test setup, loading rates that allow accurate force control will rarely exceed 1 to 2 Hz. Thus, cyclic fatigue testing that simulates reasonable fracture healing times can easily last up to 70 hours. While testing over these time periods is feasible with bone surrogate materials, FFC constructs with fresh frozen bone material will suffer from considerable deterioration and decay. An effective method to reduce testing time is the progressive increase of the load magnitude (▶ Fig. 10.3). Such a staircase protocol should employ a small stepwise increase of the load magnitude (< 5% of failure load) and a limited number of load cycles (< 1,000) at each load step.[4] By adjusting the magnitude of the steps and number of cycles per step, fatigue can be observed within reasonable time frames. Furthermore, run outs are avoided as the load magnitude continues to increase until failure. The results of staircase loading can be analyzed by comparing failure loads, deformation values, or number of load cycles until failure. It is also possible to report the survival by presenting the results in a Kaplan–Meier survival plot.

10.4 Bone Screws

Mechanical tests on bone screws or on bone screw constructs are frequent. It is important to differentiate between tests on the screw itself, on the connection of the screw with a plate or a nail, and on the screw in contact with its bony interface. If the screw itself is the focus of the mechanical assessment, the mechanical test should be performed according to the normative testing procedure defined by the American Society for Testing and

Materials (ASTM). The ASTM F543–07 describes in detail axial pull out and torsional tests on medical bone screws.

Tests on the connection between a bone screw and a metallic implant became important with the development of locked devices in which the screw is mechanically connected with the nail or the plate. Tests on these constructs are mainly focused on the fatigue behavior of the mechanical connections. To simulate physiological loading, the screws are cyclically tested in a cantilever configuration or in torque with or without a superimposed momentum. These tests either result in catastrophic failure of the locking mechanism between screw and implant or in loosening of the screw from the implant. Both scenarios may have considerable clinical relevance.

Finally, the most frequent test scenario on bone screws is evaluating the connection of the screw with the bone. These tests are usually performed on isolated bone screws but can also be performed on complete FFCs evaluating the bone screw interface. As highlighted before, the test setup should aim for a physiological load configuration; although screw pull out is an easy and straightforward testing setup, it sometimes may be of limited clinical relevance as it does not really reflect the in vivo loading situation. Combined loading scenarios introducing tension, compression, shear, and/or bending might be more appropriate to imitate the combined toggling and pulling mechanism of bone screws in a clinically relevant scenario.

10.5 External Fixators

Mechanical testing of external fixator constructs can be excessively complex due to the inherent variability of fixator constructs. The mechanical performance largely depends on the exact configuration of the pins, placement of the bars, and the anatomic mounting plane of

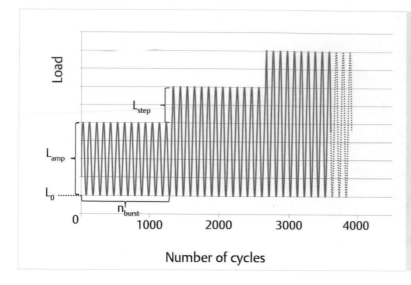

Fig. 10.3 Cycling loading protocol with progressive load levels to prevent run outs. After a certain number of load cycles (n_{burst}), the load level is increased by L_{step}. Depending on the requirements of the test design, either the lower load level L_0 can be held constant with an increase of the load amplitude (as shown) or the load amplitude L_{amp} can be held constant with an increase of the lower load level. With $n_{burst} = 1$, the load level is continuously increased.

the frame. A dominant factor for the mechanical response is the preload on the bone and on the pins or wires. Furthermore, a single value for the mechanical performance is not sufficient to describe the relationship between fragment movement and external loading. Only a comprehensive description of fixation stiffness allows prediction of interfragmentary movement and differentiation between fixation devices and their various configurations. A complete description of the mechanical performance can be obtained by determining the 6×6 stiffness matrix representing the linear relationship between the external loads (three forces and three moments) and the resulting six interfragmentary movements.[5]

10.6 Plate Fixation

The largest number of FFC biomechanical tests is performed on plate constructs. The recent development of plates with various options to lock the screw into the plate have further increased the interest in mechanical performance of bone plate fixation constructs. Testing of the mechanical performance of the plate itself is described in the normative testing procedures defined by the ASTM (F382 and F384). While these test are important for the accreditation of the medical product and to guarantee safe application of the device, they will provide very limited information with respect to their clinical performance.

FFCs with bone plates are assessed biomechanically to compare different plate designs, plate configurations, or plate modifications. Some plate constructs are biomechanically tested to expand their indications or to demonstrate their superiority in specific applications such as osteoporotic bone or periprosthetic fractures. Typically, these investigations are comparative (i.e., two or more different FFC groups are compared to each other). It is of key importance to choose the FFC groups according to the

hypothesis to be tested and to minimize covariates that may affect the test result. For example, if you want to test the hypothesis that a certain locking plate provides larger stiffness compared to a conventional plate, it would be advantageous to match all other parameters (screw numbers, screw diameter, screw configuration, plate thickness, plate length, etc.) as closely as possible within both groups.

Jargon Simplified: Locking Screws

The concept of locking screws was introduced to provide additional stability for plate fixation of fractures. In locked plating, the screws are fixed to the plate by various locking mechanisms and provide angular and axial stability of the screw. Angular stability prevents tilting of the screw, whereas axial stability prevents gliding (pull out). Recently, the concept of locking has also been applied in intramedullary nailing.

If plate constructs are tested to failure, it is important to define what will be considered as failure and also to exactly report failure type. Failure can occur as catastrophic breakdown of one of the components of the FFC. FFC components that typically fail include the bone or the bone surrogate material, the plate, the screws, or the interfaces between plate, screw, or bone. Failure can also be defined as a certain amount of deformation or angulation that will be exceeded during the mechanical test. For example, plates with a large working length may not fail during loading but may lead to complete closure of the fracture gap with associated angulation between the distal and proximal fragment. The amount of deformation or angulation that is defined as failure should refer to clinical values that would not be acceptable or would be a univocal indication for reoperation. Representative photographs of the different failure modes simplify the literal description of the failure. It is also important to discuss these failure modes with respect to their clinical relevance. Ideally, the failure modes that result from biomechanical testing mimic those observed in clinical practice.

10.7 Intramedullary Nailing

Fracture stabilization by intramedullary nailing relies on the jamming or guidance of the intramedullary implant within the bone and on the fixation by the locking bolts to the bone. Clinically relevant mechanical testing protocols will therefore have to address both features of nail fixation. Oversimplification of the model by using surrogate bone cylinders or only the bone ends needs thoughtful justification. To overcome these issues, cadaveric bone specimens or complete surrogate bones will have to be employed.

Typically, intramedullary FFCs are extremely rigid in axial direction and relevant deformations occur only if torsion, bending, or shear is induced. If the axial load is oriented along the long axis of the bone, the intramedullary implant will mainly see compressional forces for which the nail itself has very high resistance. Most of the deformation under axial loading will then occur within the locking bolts. As soon as torque or bending is added, relevant deformations start to occur in the nail. In particular, torsional loads may considerably twist the nail construct between the distal and proximal locking bolts.[6] The design of the load setup therefore has to carefully consider nonaxial load components because they are most likely to challenge the nail component in the intramedullary FFC.

10.8 Fracture Models

For biomechanical testing of an FFC, some sort of discontinuity has to be generated in order for the fracture fixation device to be tested. The discontinuity is typically produced by cutting bone specimens or bone surrogates with saws. In order to guarantee high reproducibility, it is highly recommended to use sawing templates or exact and comprehensible definitions of the sawing planes. Creating a more realistic fracture situation by breaking the bone specimens can result in unacceptable variability of the actual fracture situations and will then require larger sample sizes. The variability can be slightly reduced by perforating the bone along the intended fracture plane by predrilling.

Overall mechanical performance and mechanisms of failure will vary for different fracture models. Depending on the fracture type to be simulated, the fracture situation can be realized with or without a fracture gap. The absence or presence of a fracture gap will dramatically affect the results of mechanical testing of the FFC

construct. In the absence of a gap, deformation of the FFC will be limited and load will be transferred through the bone. This will spare the fracture fixation device from excessive loading and might not be suitable for testing the strength of the fixation device. In the presence of a fracture gap, the gap deformation can be used to monitor the stiffness and describe the response of the FFC under different loading modes. The closure of the fracture gap can be used as an abortion or failure criterion of the FFC construct.

10.9 Bone Model

In order to simulate an FFC, a material has to be chosen that adequately mimics bone. The most important choice is to decide between cadaver material and substitute material. The clear advantage of cadaver material is that it most accurately represents the anatomic and mechanical properties of the in vivo condition. Furthermore, cadaveric bone specimens represent the variations in bone geometry, bone structure, bone mineral density, and bone material properties that have to be expected in the real-life situation of fracture treatment. This enables one to also look for the effects of bone density, size, sex, etc., on the mechanical stability of the FFC. Therefore, if cadaver bone is employed, it is highly recommended to determine the physical properties of the specimens and use these measures for grouping of the specimens or for adjusting the results. This allows for example to match the test groups with respect to bone density (determined by dual X-ray absorptiometry or quantitative computed tomography) or to evaluate the screw pull out force with respect to cortical thickness.

> ### Key Concepts: Bone Mineral Density
>
> Measures of bone mineral density are employed to describe the quality and osteoporotic status of bone material. Dual X-ray absorptiometry measures the areal density in g/cm^2 and quantitative computed tomography the volumetric density in g/cm^3. The measurements can be used to compare bone mineral density values within the solitary experiment. Comparison to other experiments or to clinical measurements of osteoporosis is usually hindered by lack of a clear definition of the region of interest to be measured. In addition, dual X-ray absorptiometry measurements on explanted bone specimens can be falsified by the lack of soft tissue coverage in explanted bone specimens.

The variability in the physical properties of cadaver material presents the challenge that it will inherently potentiate the variability of the mechanical testing results. The sample size required to find statistical differences increases with the increasing variability (= standard deviation) of the data. Tests on cadaver bones therefore require typically more specimens than tests on bone surrogate material. Further limitations of cadaveric bone include its limited availability and its need for preservation. Although formalin embalming effectively preserves bone tissue from degeneration, it also severely affects its mechanical properties, particularly its tensile and fatigue properties. The most effective way of preservation before mechanical testing is freezing below −20°C, which has minimum effects on bone material properties. Prior to testing, the bones have to be completely thawed and have to be kept moist with physiologic saline solution until and during the testing procedure. Finally, the use of biologic material requires certain clean laboratory conditions and precautionary measures for prevention of infection.

Bone surrogate models are easily available, have very reproducible geometric and material properties, and are much easier to handle compared to cadaver material. Various surrogate bone specimens with defined material properties are commercially available. With the increasing need for FFCs in osteoporotic or otherwise softened bone, surrogate specimens with variable material properties are being developed to meet these demands. While these surrogate bone models are ideally suited to investigate the performance of the osteosynthesis device itself, they have very limited informational value on the interface between the device and bone. Thus, findings from screw pull out, cut out, loosening, etc., of the osteosynthesis device from surrogate bone cannot be directly transferred to the clinical setting.

References

[1] Bottlang M, Doornink J, Lujan TJ et al. Effects of construct stiffness on healing of fractures stabilized with locking plates. J Bone Joint Surg Am 2010; 92 Suppl 2: 12–22

[2] Bergmann G, Graichen F, Rohlmann A et al. Realistic loads for testing hip implants. Biomed Mater Eng 2010; 20: 65–75

[3] Morlock M, Schneider E, Bluhm A et al. Duration and frequency of every day activities in total hip patients. J Biomech 2001; 34: 873–881

[4] Bottlang M, Doornink J, Fitzpatrick DC, Madey SM. Far cortical locking can reduce stiffness of locked plating constructs while retaining construct strength. J Bone Joint Surg Am 2009; 91: 1985–1994

[5] Duda GN, Kirchner H, Wilke HJ, Claes L. A method to determine the 3-D stiffness of fracture fixation devices and its application to predict inter-fragmentary movement. J Biomech 1998; 31: 247–252

[6] Augat P, Bühren V. [Modern implant design for the osteosynthesis of osteoporotic bone fractures.] Orthopade 2010; 39: 397–406

[7] Krischak GD, Augat P, Beck A et al. Biomechanical comparison of two side plate fixation techniques in an unstable intertrochanteric osteotomy model: Sliding hip screw and percutaneous compression plate. Clin Biomech (Bristol, Avon) 2007; 22: 1112–1118

[8] Born CT, Karich B, Bauer C, von Oldenburg G, Augat P. Hip screw migration testing: first results for hip screws and helical blades utilizing a new oscillating test method. J Orthop Res 2011; 29: 760–766

Further Reading

Gardner MJ, Silva MJ, Krieg JC. Biomechanical testing of fracture fixation constructs: variability, validity, and clinical applicability. J Am Acad Orthop Surg 2012; 20: 86–93

Tencer AF. Biomechanics of fixation and fractures. In: Buchholz RW, Heckman JD, Court-Brown C., eds. Rockwood and Green's fractures in adults. 5 ed. Philadelphia: Lippincott Williams & Wilkins; 2006:3–41

Thakur AJ. The elements of fracture fixation. 2 ed. New Delhi: Elsevier; 2007

11 Biomechanical Assessment of Fracture Repair

Peter Augat

The healing of a bone fracture is a continuous process in which the fracture ends reunite directly under stable mechanical conditions or form a stabilizing extra- and intramedullary callus under flexible mechanical fixation conditions. Typically during the process of healing, the mechanical stability of the healing bone steadily increases, eventually exceeding the mechanical stability of intact bone. The time for union varies anywhere between 8 weeks and 40 weeks depending on numerous factors including type of bone, kind of fracture, mode of fracture fixation, and most importantly on the definition of fracture union. Currently, there is no such thing as a gold standard for the definition of when a fracture is healed. Moreover, the different methods available for healing assessment do not correlate very well because they all assess different features of fracture healing.

Particularly in research settings, there is the need for objective measures of bone healing to monitor treatment and compare treatment methods. Although there is no consensus on when a fracture is actually healed, clinical studies as well as individual patient assessment require some sort of definition of a measurable end point of fracture healing. In orthopedic clinical studies, fracture healing often is one of the most important outcome variables and can be described by dichotomous (healed/not healed), multilevel ordinal (scoring system), or continuous variables. Healing is typically assessed at predefined time points at which the completion of the healing process is expected. On the other hand, a reliable indicator for the completion of the healing process (or the lack thereof) can also be of importance for the diagnosis of the individual patient. Such an indicator could guide decisions on cast or implant removal or could determine the need for further treatment or operation to achieve healing.

A fundamental problem in quantitatively assessing the healing status of a fracture is the fracture fixation system being used to stabilize the fracture. The purpose of fracture fixation or osteosynthesis is to stabilize the fracture fragments and enable the healing process but also to allow function and usage of the fractured extremity or body part. The mechanical stability of the fixation system always obscures the mechanical stability of the fracture itself. The challenge for biomechanical assessment of fracture healing therefore is to somehow eliminate or correct for the stabilization effect of the osteosynthesis system. The most appealing option is to temporarily remove the fracture fixation system. This, however, is restricted to external fixation systems such as plasters, casts, or perhaps external fixators. A second challenge is patient safety and compliance that limits any repeated measurement to noninvasive, inoffensive, and practical methodologies.

11.1 Direct Measurement Methods

Direct measurement methods directly assess a mechanical quality of the bone that changes during the course of the fracture healing process. It can be distinguished between methods assessing the structural integrity of the whole bone as compared to methods assessing local tissue properties. The structural integrity of healing bone is typically assessed by measuring the integral stiffness of the extremity by static or dynamic load application. Static loading deforms the extremity in relation to the amount of load applied. In dynamic deformation, the vibrational response of the extremity depends on the propagation of the induced oscillations, which are primarily determined by the overall mechanical integrity of the bone. Instead of measuring the overall integrity of the healing bone, direct measurements of mechanical properties can also focus on the site of fracture healing. Thus, measurement of local tissue properties at the fracture site directly reflects the mechanical changes of the healing tissue in the fracture gap and in the periosteal fracture callus.

11.1.1 Direct Measurement Methods: Stiffness

The most frequently assessed mechanical characteristic in fracture healing assessment is the overall stiffness of the fracture. Stiffness measurement requires simultaneous determination of the applied load and the resulting deflection generated by the load. The load can be applied manually by the investigator, by a defined weight that is put on the limb or by the patient itself. The amount of load is measured by a load cell. As a result of the load application, the limb deforms with most of the deformation occurring at the site of the fracture. The deformation needs to be measured as a function of the applied load. There are various methods to measure the deformation of the limb. One way is to directly measure the limb deformation. This can be done with goniometers attached to the skin surface, which measure the relative angulation between the distal and proximal fracture fragments. Alternatively, optical markers can be glued on the skin surface and their movement can be tracked by infrared or optical video capturing. If the fracture is stabilized by external fixation, the fixator pins or fixator bars can be used to track the deformation of the limb. Similarly, goniometers or optical trackers can be attached to the fixator frame and their movement can be measured as a function of the applied load. In patients who are treated by external fixators or by cast, the fixation device can be temporarily removed, providing direct access to the mechanical integrity of the fractured extremity. In the case of internal fixation with plates or intramedullary nails, direct measurement of mechanical integrity of the healing fracture is extremely challenging. The stabilizing effect of the osteosynthesis device completely conceals the instability of the fracture and renders deformation measurements on the skin surface useless. Therefore, the deformation needs to be measured directly at the fracture site with very high local resolution. One possibility is the use of instrumented implants, which employ biocompatible strain gauges directly attached to the osteosynthesis device[1] to measure the deformation of the implant. Alternatively, the deformation can be measured by radiography or fluoroscopic images acquired at the loaded and unloaded situation, respectively.

The loading mode for measuring the integrity of the healed bone can be bending, axial compression, or torsion. For the bending test, the bone to be tested is placed between two supports with the fracture located centrally between the supports. Three-point bending is created by loading the bone at the fracture site, either directly or via the external fixator frame (▶ Fig. 11.1). This three-point bending setup has been frequently used in clinical studies to monitor the healing process in tibial fractures.[2] In most of these studies, a fracture stiffness of 15 Nm/degree was considered as an indicator for successful healing and guided the treatment decisions in further studies in which stiffness was measured. It has to be noted that this stiffness value was obtained in patients with casts or with external fixators, when the cast or fixator was temporarily removed or released.

Jargon Simplified: Composite Stiffness

If the stiffness of a healing bone has to be determined with the implant (fixator, plate) in place, the measured stiffness is composed of the stiffness of the implant and the stiffness of the fracture callus. In such a parallel composite construct, the deformation under an applied load is nearly identical for the implant and for the bone. However, the load is shared between both and is primarily transmitted by the stronger composite. Thus the composite stiffness during the early phase of healing is primarily determined by the stiffness of the implant. During the course of healing, an increasing amount of the load will be carried by the bone, reflecting its increase in stiffness. The stiffness of the healing bone can be calculated from the measured composite stiffness S_{Total} and the stiffness of the implant $S_{Implant}$ using:

$$S_{Total} = S_{Implant} + S_{FractureCallus}$$

Accordingly, the load share (LS) is the percentage amount of load carried by the implant during external loading and is determined by

$$LS = \frac{S_{Implant}}{S_{Total}} = \frac{S_{Implant}}{(S_{Implant} + S_{FractureCallus})}$$

The stiffness of the implant has to be approximated by preceding calibration measurements.

Axial loading by the weight of the patient is a relatively straightforward procedure and can be performed with force plates or even electronic scales. In patients with external fixators, the deformation can be directly measured between individual fixator pins. For calculating the

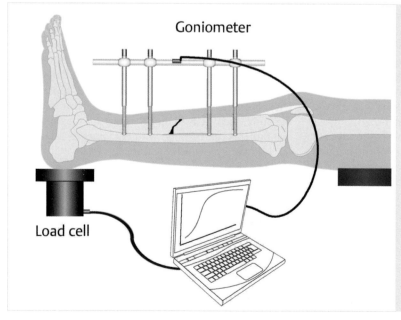

Fig. 11.1 Three-point bending procedure to determine mechanical stiffness of the tibia after fracture. Load is typically applied manually at the level of the fracture. The resulting load to the limb can be determined by a load cell and the deformation is measured with a goniometer either attached to the fracture fixation device or the surface of the skin.

stiffness of the fracture, the *composite stiffness* of the fixator itself and the fracture has to be considered. The deformation measurement can also be expressed as a relative value related to the measurement at the initial time of measurement. The subsequent measurements can then be expressed as a percentage of the initial value. In case of uneventful healing, the measurement signal should demonstrate a continuous decrease over time until the fracture is united.[3] Finally, the load on the fracture can be induced as torsion between the proximal and distal part of the fracture. This method may provide the advantages of maintaining the bone axis and minimizing the risk of bone misalignment during the bone healing process but requires a dedicated measurement device.[4]

An alternative way to directly assess the progress of fracture healing is the determination of the load share between the implant and the healing fracture (▶ Fig. 11.2). The implant and the healing fracture constitute a composite structure sharing the loads between each other. The determination of the load share ratio between the implant and the healing bone requires the load through the implant to be measured while the composite structure is loaded. This can be performed by inserting load cells in the path of load transmission of the implant. Realistically, this can only be performed in the case of external fixation implants in which some of the rods can be temporarily replaced by load cells. Measuring the load share directly enables access to the amount of load that can be supported by the healing fracture and provides direct access to the load-bearing capacity of the fracture. However, the method is extremely complex, time-consuming, and not without risk for the patient as the fixation device has to be temporarily removed.[5]

A general limitation of direct measurement of fracture stiffness is the exact knowledge of the load at the fracture site. If external loads are applied (by weight bearing),

internal loads are generated by the muscles that superimpose the external loads and act at the site of fracture. Because it is almost impossible to control muscle activity of the patient during the measurement, the forces acting at the level of the fracture are not exactly known and consequently are a source of inaccuracy of the measurement. Another important source of measurement inaccuracy is loosening of fixator pins, which are either used to measure the deformation of the bone or to transfer load to the fixator body.[3]

11.1.2 Direct Measurement Methods: Vibration

An alternative technique for direct assessment of the mechanical properties of a healing fracture is vibration analysis. Vibration analysis is frequently employed to detect the loosening of metallic implants in bone, particularly maxillofacial and dental implants. To conduct a vibration analysis for assessing fracture healing, some sort of dynamic mechanical signal has to be introduced into the bone and then transmitted across the fracture site. The analysis of the transmitted signal can be performed as analysis of the wave propagation or by resonant frequency analysis. In resonant frequency analysis, the bone is excited with mechanical signals and the frequency response is determined. Changes in resonant frequency have been shown to depend on the length, the density, and the structural stiffness of the bone. This facilitates the detection of temporal changes of mechanical properties during fracture healing. Vibrational excitement can be induced by a shaker or by an impulse hammer, and the response can be measured by accelerometers or adequately tuned microphones. The natural frequencies at which long bones resonate are at

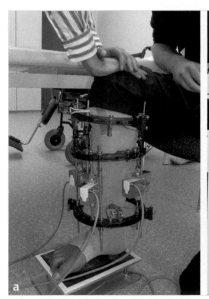
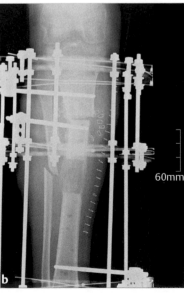

Fig. 11.2 Measurement of load share. The amount of loading is measured by an electronic scale while simultaneously the forces through the external fixator are measured by temporarily inserted load cells.

the lower end of the audible spectrum (100 to 500 Hz). The intensity of a propagating sound wave decreases after a fracture and sounds dull and muffled in fractured bones compared to contralateral intact bone. When the frequency and intensity of the fractured bone coincides with that of the uninjured bone and approaches natural frequency of intact bone, the patient can be considered to have reached full healing. The technique, however, appears to be unable to monitor the healing of hairline fractures as the shift in natural frequency is too small for detection.[6]

Although vibrational techniques are relatively easy to perform, they have not been widely accepted or used for the assessment of fracture healing, and it remains very much a research tool. This is probably related to the problems of coupling the vibrational signal to the bone through the skin and the tremendous effect of metallic implants on mechanical wave propagation. Skin and soft tissues surrounding the bone considerably affect the waveform of applied impulses and thus confound the analysis and interpretation of the data. Most striking is the effect of intramedullary nails and osteosynthesis plates, which are directly connected to the bone. Most of the wave propagation will be deflected from the bone to the metallic implant. The sensitivity of the method to detect changes at the fracture site is then minimized.

11.1.3 Direct Measurement Methods: Ultrasound

Ultrasound (US) waves are frequently employed for the detection of cracks or material irregularities in engineering structures. Propagation of US waves is strongly affected by the mechanical properties of the propagation medium, in particular by sudden changes such as cracks or passages between media with different densities. While the velocity of a US wave is primarily affected by local material properties (elastic modulus, density), the attenuation is largely influenced by structural properties (porosity, connectivity, anisotropy). A fracture in bone is ideally suited to be detected by US waves. Moreover, changes in both material density and structural integrity during fracture healing are reflected in changes in US velocity and attenuation, respectively.

The propagation velocity of a US wave is easily determined by using two US transducers, one being the US emitter and the other the US detector (▶ Fig. 11.3). Characteristically, the US transducer emits signals in the 0.2 to 2 MHz frequency domain. The ratio of the distance between the two transducers and the time of flight of the first arriving signal is the propagation velocity. Similarly, the attenuation of the US signal can be determined by calculating the ratio of the signal intensity of the first arriving signal by the intensity of the emitted signal. The transducers need to be placed as close as possible to the bone surface and need to be coupled to skin by US gel. As thick layers of skin and soft tissue attenuate the US signal, the medial aspect of the tibia is ideally suited to perform measurements with the US technique.

After a fracture in bone, the velocity of the US wave is significantly reduced and is much lower than in the intact bone. Attenuation on the other end increases steeply after the fracture, because the US wave is partly reflected and dissipated at the fracture surfaces. During healing, the attenuation slowly decreases as the tissues in the fracture

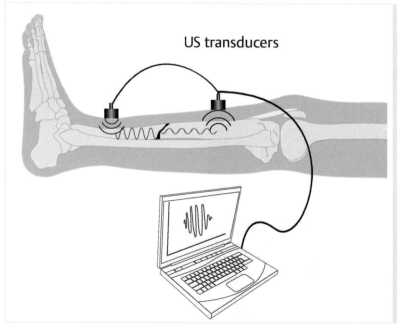

Fig. 11.3 Measurement of ultrasound (US) propagation through a long bone.

gap and in the fracture callus increase material density and approach density values (or more correctly impedance values) of intact cortical bone. By placing the transducers accordingly, US is capable of detecting changes in local material properties and not only the overall fracture integrity. Changes in US properties during fracture healing can be detected much earlier than changes observed by standard radiography.[7]

A big advantage of US measurements for fracture assessment is its ease of use. US devices are readily available and portable, and the measurement values (time of flight and attenuation) can be easily interpreted. However, the attenuating effect of surrounding soft tissues limits its applicability to long bones with thin soft tissue coverage. Furthermore, US signals are typically insensitive to changes in the late phase of healing and are also not capable of differentiating completed healing from asymmetric bone formation or incomplete bone bridging.

11.2 Surrogate Measurements

Surrogate measurements for the assessment of fracture healing employ features of the healing bone that indirectly reflect its mechanical integrity. Most of these surrogate measures make use of X-ray radiation in standard radiographs or in computed tomography (CT), because these methodologies are readily available in all trauma or orthopedic settings. The attenuation of X-rays in bone tissue strongly depends on the amount of mineral that has to be penetrated by the X-ray beam. The increasing calcification of the fracture callus and the fracture gap during the progress of healing can therefore be observed by an increase in X-ray attenuation.

11.2.1 Radiography

If radiographs are produced in a standardized manner, they can be used for quantitative measurements. The amount of bone tissue formed at the site of fracture determines the appearance of the fracture gap and the fracture callus. The most straightforward way of quantifying the healing process is by scoring the appearance of the fracture area. The Radiographic Union Score for Tibial fractures (RUST) assigns a score to a given set of anteroposterior and lateral radiographs based on the assessment of healing at each of the four cortices visible on these projections. Each cortex receives a score of 1 point if it is deemed to have a fracture line with no callus, 2 points if there is callus present but a fracture line is still visible, and 3 points if there is bridging callus with no evidence of a fracture line. The individual cortical scores are added to give a total for the set of films with 4 being the minimum score indicating that the fracture is definitely not healed and 12 being the maximum score indicating that the fracture is definitely healed.[8]

If healing of the fracture is dominated by periosteal callus formation, changes in the amount of the fracture callus indicate the progress of healing. Thus measuring the size of the callus on projectional radiographs is an indicator for healing. The easiest way of estimating the amount of callus formation is the calculation of the callus index. First, the diameter of the periosteal callus is measured at its widest appearance. This value is then normalized by dividing it by the diameter of the long bone adjacent to the fracture site. With digital radiography, a more accurate quantification of the size of the periosteal callus formation is relatively straightforward by quantifying the amount of the projected periosteal callus. Using modern imaging tools, the callus quantification can be performed with very limited user interaction and large reliability.[9] Although an increase in the amount of periosteal callus is often associated with an increase in callus stiffness, it does not always reflect the mechanical integrity of the healing fracture. Particularly in delayed healing, a large fracture callus may be formed that does not necessarily reflect mechanical integrity in the absence of bone formation in the fracture gap.

11.2.2 Absorptiometry

X-ray absorptiometry is a noninvasive method to provide a very reliable quantification of the amount of mineral in bone. These methods are frequently employed to diagnose bone diseases that affect the mineral status of bone such as osteoporosis (see Chapter 26). Application of these methods to fracture healing, however, remains rare. A projectional technique that provides measures of areal mineral density is dual X-ray absorptiometry. Dual X-ray absorptiometry has a very high reproducibility and has the advantage that measures of bone mineral density are not very much affected by adjacent metal hardware such as osteosynthesis plates or nails. True volumetric density of mineralized tissue, however, requires quantitative CT, which provides a three-dimensional dataset of X-ray attenuation coefficients. Calibration of the attenuation coefficients against phantoms containing known concentrations of bone mineral equivalents enable the calculation of volumetric bone mineral densities. The presence of osteosynthesis hardware massively distorts CT images. Modern correction algorithms can correct for the presence of the hardware and reconstruct almost flawless images; however, the quantitative information on bone mineral density remains misrepresented.[10] Both techniques, quantitative CT as well as dual X-ray absorptiometry, expose the patient to a minimal radiation dose if appendicular bones are investigated. The advantages of this noninvasive procedure—high precision, instant availability results, and minor user interactivity—make it a reliable tool for the quantification of the process of fracture healing.

Besides providing quantitative information on mineral densities, these techniques may play an important role in the reduction of total radiation dose to the patient if frequent imaging is essential as, for example, during limb-lengthening procedures.

Quantitative bone mineral measurements can be helpful in estimating the mechanical stability of a healing long bone. Among the various density measurements available, the amount of calcified tissue at the location of the fracture gap is probably the best predictor of fracture stability. Increase of calcified tissue at the level of the fracture gap is highly associated with an overall increase of mechanical stability. The strong association of fracture rigidity with the amount of calcified tissue in the fracture gap as compared to the periosteal region emphasizes the importance of a bridged fracture gap for the mechanical integrity of the healing fracture.[11] In contrast, a weak association between fracture rigidity and the amount of periosteal callus challenges its use as an indicator of the healing status. Although the formation of periosteal callus enables the process of fracture stabilization by increasing the load-bearing area, the size of the periosteal callus is not quantitatively related to the fracture stability. A large callus might rather indicate an exuberant proliferation of periosteal tissue caused by inadequate fracture fixation, premature weight bearing, or an inappropriate micro-movement might be an indication for pseudarthrosis. In metaphyseal regions, fracture healing often occurs without any periosteal callus formation and radiographic changes are very difficult to observe or actually quantify. Moreover, as fractures around the joint are typically treated by internal plate fixation, radiographic evaluation is further obstructed by the presence of metal hardware.[11]

11.3 Function and Performance

The progress of fracture healing and the associated advancement of mechanical integrity of the fracture is paralleled by improvements in function and performance. Thus, parameters that access function should be capable of assessing fracture healing status. For fractures of the lower extremity, one possible option could be the assessment of gait in the course of fracture healing. Parameters with potential sensitivity are the amount of load bearing on the fractured extremity, the self-selected speed of walking, and the harmonization of the gait between the injured and the contralateral limb. The progress of healing is also related to the amount of activity being performed by the patient. This can be measured with body-worn devices for monitoring activities of daily living such as pedometers or accelerometers.

Although these changes in function and performance during fracture healing appear to be obvious, there are only very few studies that were able to demonstrate them in real patient populations. A major problem again is the protection of the fractured area by the fracture fixation device, particularly for internal osteosyntheses. Other factors that obscure the functional improvements include individual pain sensitivity and movement restrictions due to joint and soft tissue injuries. For upper extremity injuries, in particular for monitoring healing after wrist fractures, grip strength measurements can be performed. Again, although this appears to be an objective tool to measure function and performance, it is highly compliance dependent and typically requires measurements of the contralateral site for normalization.

11.4 Conclusion

While direct measures of fracture's mechanical properties provide explicit evaluation of the quantity of interest, their applicability is often difficult and limited to experimental research or research in animals. Surrogate measures, on the other hand, provide often easy access and have also demonstrated strong association with direct mechanical properties of healing bone. Radiographic measures are most widely employed but lack sensitivity in metaphyseal fractures and in the presence of metal hardware. Measures of function and performance are directly related to mechanical integrity but are strongly compliance dependent and pain sensitive.

References

[1] Seide K, Aljudaibi M, Weinrich N et al. Telemetric assessment of bone healing with an instrumented internal fixator: a preliminary study. J Bone Joint Surg Br 2012; 94: 398–404

[2] Richardson JB, Cunningham JL, Goodship AE, O'Connor BT, Kenwright J. Measuring stiffness can define healing of tibial fractures. J Bone Joint Surg Br 1994; 76: 389–394

[3] Claes L, Grass R, Schmickal T et al. Monitoring and healing analysis of 100 tibial shaft fractures. Langenbecks Arch Surg 2002; 387: 146–152

[4] Windhagen H, Bail H, Schmeling A, Kolbeck S, Weiler A, Raschke M. A new device to quantify regenerate torsional stiffness in distraction osteogenesis. J Biomech 1999; 32: 857–860

[5] Aarnes GT, Steen H, Ludvigsen P, Waanders NA, Huiskes R, Goldstein SA. In vivo assessment of regenerate axial stiffness in distraction osteogenesis. J Orthop Res 2005; 23: 494–498

[6] Wong LC, Chiu WK, Russ M, Liew S. Review of techniques for monitoring the healing fracture of bones for implementation in an internally fixated pelvis. Med Eng Phys 2012; 34: 140–152

[7] Eyres KS, Bell MJ, Kanis JA. Methods of assessing new bone formation during limb lengthening. Ultrasonography, dual energy X-ray absorptiometry and radiography compared. J Bone Joint Surg Br 1993; 75: 358–364

[8] Whelan DB, Bhandari M, Stephen D et al. Development of the radiographic union score for tibial fractures for the assessment of tibial fracture healing after intramedullary fixation. J Trauma 2010; 68: 629–632

[9] Lujan TJ, Madey SM, Fitzpatrick DC, Byrd GD, Sanderson JM, Bottlang M. A computational technique to measure fracture callus in radiographs. J Biomech 2010; 43: 792–795

[10] Firoozabadi R, Morshed S, Engelke K et al. Qualitative and quantitative assessment of bone fragility and fracture healing using conventional radiography and advanced imaging technologies—focus on wrist fracture. J Orthop Trauma 2008; 22 Suppl: S83–S90

[11] Augat P, Merk J, Genant HK, Claes L. Quantitative assessment of experimental fracture repair by peripheral computed tomography. Calcif Tissue Int 1997; 60: 194–199

Further Reading

Claes LE, Cunningham JL. Monitoring the mechanical properties of healing bone. Clin Orthop Relat Res 2009; 467: 1964–1971

12 Biomechanics of Cartilage

Lutz Dürselen and Andreas Martin Seitz

Diarthrodial joints are covered with hyaline articular cartilage (AC) enabling the transmission of high loads at low friction. Hence, AC plays a very important mechanical role in our musculoskeletal system. Unfortunately, AC can degenerate idiopathically or due to trauma or joint misalignment leading to osteoarthritis with a potential need for joint replacement. For decades, methods have been investigated to heal or regenerate AC with different strategies. To evaluate such methods, it is important to understand the biomechanical way of functioning of AC. Its complex functionality is accomplished by the biphasic composition of this tissue. It contains chondrocytes, which secrete an extracellular matrix with the main constituents collagen and proteoglycans. Besides this solid matrix, AC possesses a high water content as its fluid component. While collagen is mainly responsible for the mechanical strength of the solid matrix, the proteoglycans are able to store water by osmotic swelling providing the resistance to compression and creating the time-dependent behavior, which results in creep and relaxation phenomena. Any change in composition of the extracellular matrix resulting from trauma or degenerative processes leads to changes in biomechanical properties. Therefore, the biomechanical characterization of AC is an important and useful tool to assess its functional quality and can be used in any kind of research on AC such as basic questions on the functionality of AC, degenerative processes, repair, and tissue engineering aiming to replace destroyed cartilage. A variety of different test methods for the biomechanical characterization of AC are available depending on which properties are of interest regarding a special research question. This chapter gives an overview of practical methods to assess the compressive and time-dependent properties including friction of AC.

12.1 Unconfined Compression and Tensile Testing

The simplest way to determine the material properties of AC is unconfined compression or tensile testing of geometrically standardized specimens. From such experiments, parameters can be derived such as stiffness (K in N/mm), deduced from the force-elongation diagram, and Young's modulus (E in N/mm^2 or MPa), determined from the stress-strain diagram. Although both tensile and unconfined compression testing lead to the same parameters, the results are different, depending on the sample and test conditions. For example, the cartilage tensile modulus has been reported to be one to two orders of magnitude greater than the corresponding compressive modulus.[1] Testing AC under compressive loads commonly involves cylindrical specimens, which can be easily harvested by punches or hollow drills, or cubic specimens, whereas for tensile tests mostly rectangular strips or dumbbell-shaped samples are used, which are more complicated to create. A beneficial attribute associated with the compressive testing method is its comparatively simple test setup (▶ Fig. 12.1a) where a flat-ended rod is used to compress the specimen to a previously defined load, stress, deformation, or strain. Due to the varying Poisson's ratio of different soft tissues, the cross section of the cartilage specimen changes differently during compressive ($v = 0.2$)[2] and tensile ($v > 0.5$)[1] loads. Compared to unconfined compression, tensile testing is more elaborate, because it implies the problem of clamping soft tissue, which is a general pitfall in soft tissue biomechanics. Therefore, the test setup for tensile testing (▶ Fig. 12.1b) commonly consists of two clamps to ensure adequate fixation of the samples during tensile loading.

During testing, it should be considered that both test methods do not intend to represent physiological or in vivo loading conditions. This involves the integrity of the cartilage sample with respect to the loading characteristics, as well as the ambient conditions (e.g., temperature, nutrition, and moistness). Due to its anisotropic and biphasic material behavior, AC shows a typical strain-rate–dependent response during unconfined compression and tensile loading where an increased strain rate is associated with strengthening

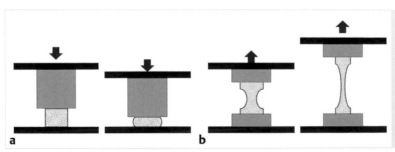

Fig. 12.1 Unconfined compression of a cubic cartilage specimen (**a**) leading to a change in its geometric shape and cross-sectional area, and tensile test of a dumbbell-shaped cartilage specimen (**b**) leading to thinning of its cross-sectional area under tensile loads.

the transient stiffness and Young's modulus[3,4] (► Fig. 12.2a). Another phenomenon can be observed when loading the cartilage specimen to a certain point with instant unloading, leading to a so-called hysteresis loop, which is common for biphasic soft tissues like cartilage[5] (► Fig. 12.2b).

Jargon Simplified:

- Load (F in N): Usually results in a deformation of the tested material.
- Stress (σ in N/mm^2 or MPa): Measure of the internal force acting on a material. Defined as the measure of the force that is applied via a certain area.
- Deformation (Δl in mm): Change in the dimensions of a material to external forces or stress.
- Strain (ε in %): Deformation of a material related to its initial length or height.
- Poisson's Ratio (v): Tapering or bulging ratio of a material in the direction perpendicular to the applied tensile or compressive stress, relative to its initial state.

12.2 Creep/Relaxation and Dynamic Compression

Jargon Simplified

- Aggregate Modulus (H$_A$ in N/mm^2 or MPa): Modulus of a biphasic material in its equilibrium state reflecting the properties of the solid matrix. Can be calculated by dividing the equilibrium stress ($\sigma_{t \to \infty}$) by the corresponding strain (ε):

$$H_A = \frac{\sigma_{t \to \infty}}{\epsilon}$$

- Hydraulic Permeability (k in m^4/Ns): Parameter to describe the fluid flow through a porous material.

When repeating the previously introduced hysteresis loop several times, their characteristics will change in a way that the differences of the loading and unloading curve start to converge (► Fig. 12.3a). Additionally, when using a time-resolving illustration of the stress

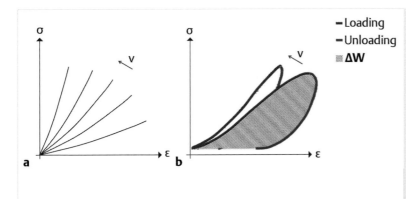

Fig. 12.2 The Young's modulus of articular cartilage samples is dramatically influenced by the loading rate during compression or tensile testing (a): With increasing loading rate (v) the initial resistance, and therefore the Young's modulus, significantly increases. The same phenomenon can be observed when loading and immediately unloading the specimen, resulting in a so-called hysteresis loop (b). Common for biphasic materials like cartilage, the hysteresis loop indicates dissipated energy (ΔW), which is defined as the area embedded between the loading and unloading curve. This area is also loading-rate (v) sensitive.

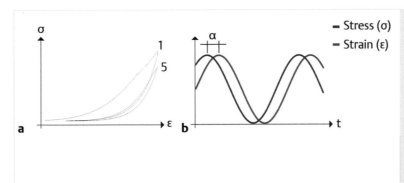

Fig. 12.3 (a) Alternating hysteresis loop: The initial hysteresis loop indicates a bigger difference between the loading and unloading curve leading to a more distinct amount of dissipated energy, compared to the fifth hysteresis loop. (b) Typical phase shift (α) during cyclic loading of cartilage: For a biphasic material, like cartilage, the strain follows the stress. In contrast, a purely elastic material will not have any phase shift, whereas a purely viscoelastic material will have a phase shift of 90 degrees, which means that the highest deformation would be observed at the lowest applied force level and vice versa.

and strain curves of these loading and unloading ramps, a characteristic phase shift of the material response could be observed (▶ Fig. 12.3b). This phase shift also happens during sinusoidal or other alternating loading schemes.

In addition, the characteristic time-dependent properties of AC could be assessed using two more loading tests:

- Creep: Loading of a cartilage sample with a constant load. The samples thickness diminishes by fluid efflux until an asymptotic thickness is reached.
- Stress-relaxation: Compression of a cartilage sample until a desired strain is reached. The applied strain is kept constant over time, whereas the applied load decreases until an asymptotic equilibrium force is noted.

Both load methods are able to reveal the viscoelastic behavior of cartilage over time. However, to gain the aggregate modulus (H_A in MPa or kPa) and hydraulic permeability (k in m4/Ns), each test routine could be conducted in two different ways:

- Indentation test (▶ Fig. 12.4a). Here, a flat indenter is pushed into the cartilaginous surface. The respective decrease of thickness (creep) or load (relaxation) is then measured over time. There is no need for preparing complex, geometrically standardized cartilage samples, because the whole specimen could be mounted into the testing rig, while ensuring adequate positioning. However, the cartilage thickness must be determined in another test (e.g., needle test), because without knowing the sample thickness the application of a certain strain level and relative loading rate is impossible.
- Confined compression testing (▶ Fig. 12.4b). A coplanar, geometrically defined cartilage disk is compressed to a

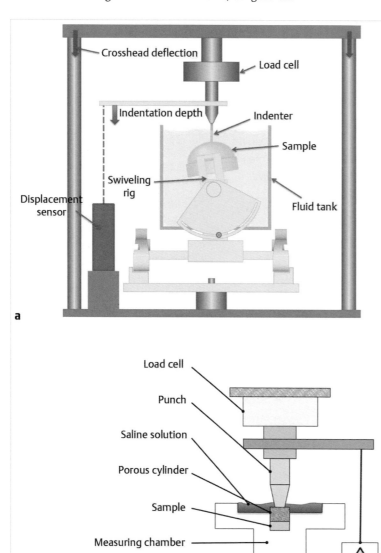

a

b

Fig. 12.4 (a) Setup for indentation testing: An indenter is adapted to a load cell applying a defined load perpendicular to the cartilage surface, which is inserted in an adjustable measuring chamber, filled with saline solution. The indentation depth is measured using an accurate displacement transducer. (b) Schematic drawing of a test setup for a compression test under confined conditions: The geometrically defined sample is radially constrained allowing fluid flow only in the axial direction. The load is applied via a punch and a porous cylinder, which is connected to a load cell. The strain is accurately measured using a high-precision laser displacement transducer.

certain load or strain level and held constant until an equilibrium state is reached. In contrast, the test setup is more complex as it must be ensured to constrain the samples in their radial direction while allowing an adequate fluid flow in the axial direction.

When determining the viscoelastic material parameters, various constitutive mathematical models could be used to solve their according equations.[6,7,8] However, it should be kept in mind that each test method and each mathematical model can lead to different results for the time-dependent, viscoelastic parameters, because mathematical models mostly are simplified models and do not necessarily match reality 100%. Therefore, care must be taken when comparing results with already existing results in literature.

12.2.1 Example for the Experimental Characterization of the Viscoelastic Properties of Articular Cartilage: Stress-Relaxation under Confined Compression

After harvesting a coplanar cartilaginous disk (thickness: 1 mm; Ø: 5 mm), the sample could be tested using a special measuring chamber providing confined conditions (▶ Fig. 12.4b). This means that the cartilage sample cannot extend in the radial direction and no fluid can flow through the sides of the cartilage disk. The measurement chamber is filled with saline solution to prevent dehydration. The load is applied via a porous Al_2O_3 cylinder allowing adequate fluid flow through the surface of the sample.

During testing, it is important to measure the deformation, especially the strain, directly at the surface of the cartilage sample as, for example, measurement errors

related to deflection of the crosshead of a materials testing machine or of the load cell should be avoided. A dedicated external displacement sensor with high accuracy can be used for this critical issue.

The viscoelastic properties strongly depend on the extent of the applied compression. Therefore, it is recommended to perform a test routine with incremental steps, for example increasing the strain stepwise from 5 to 20% of its initial thickness (▶ Fig. 12.5a). The decrease of load is recorded for about 10 minutes or at least until the equilibrium state of each strain step is reached. As previously mentioned, the strain rate during the compression phase of the test also considerably influences the peak load occurring directly after reaching the desired strain step. Therefore, the strain rate must be kept constant over the whole test series of the experiment. Thus it is recommended to use a strain-dependent loading rate (e.g., 10% $*h_0$/min [h_0 = initial height of the specimen]) to load each specimen equally.

For data analysis, the modulus (H) indicating a combined modulus of both the fluid and the solid phase of the viscoelastic material and the hydraulic permeability (k) can be extracted in a first approximation from the measured relaxation curves by fitting the data to a diffusion equation by using a least square fitting algorithm using the following equation[6,7]:

$$\sigma_{(t)} = \sigma_{(t=\infty)} + 2 \cdot H \cdot \frac{\Delta l}{d} \cdot e^{\left(-\left(\frac{\pi^2}{4}\right) \cdot H \cdot k \cdot t\right)} \tag{12.1}$$

where $\sigma_{(t)}$ is the present stress in MPa, $\sigma_{(t=\infty)}$ the equilibrium stress in MPa, H the above-mentioned combined modulus in MPa, $\Delta l/d$ the applied strain level, d the sample thickness in mm, and k the hydraulic permeability in m^4/Ns. The determination of the values for H and k can be performed by any statistical software (▶ Fig. 12.5).

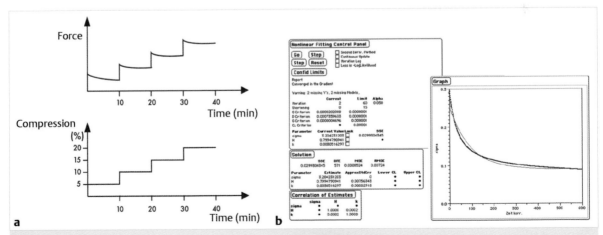

Fig. 12.5 (a) Force-time-graph (*top*) and related compression time graph (*bottom*) of stress-relaxation test with four defined compression states. (b) Screenshot (JMP V.3.2; SAS Institute GmbH, Germany) of the results of the modulus (*H*) and hydraulic permeability (*k*), based on first approximation from fitting the previously measured data to a diffusion equation by using least square fit algorithm.

The exemplary results of the nonlinear curve fitting, calculated with JMP (V.3.2; SAS Institute GmbH, Germany) indicate an H of 0.79 MPa and k = 3.05 * 10 to 15 m⁴/Ns. Furthermore, the graph (▶ Fig. 12.5) shows that the adaptation of the model equation to the measured data is good, but not optimal. This means that the real process does not exactly follow the chosen diffusion model, which does not reflect the dynamic behavior of the cartilage sample directly after application of the load. Therefore, an adequate number of measured data points must be excluded from the fitting process until the correlation coefficient is sufficiently high (e.g., 0.95).

Key Concepts: Mathematical Modeling of Articular Cartilage

Due to the anisotropic behavior of cartilage, there are plenty of mathematical descriptions of the response of cartilage to a various number of external loads and environmental conditions. After measuring the in vitro response of articular cartilage, an adequate mathematical model must be chosen to determine the required material properties. Usually, the model parameters are then varied until the model converges with the experimental data. For this purpose, statistical software can be used providing a variety of fitting algorithms (e.g., least-square, Levenberg-Marquardt, Gauss-Newton). After running the fitting algorithm, the mathematical model results in a best possible representation of the experimental data. This could be checked using the Pearson correlation coefficient and setting its accuracy limit, for example, to r = 0.95.

properties of articular surfaces are of major importance for appropriate joint function. It has been shown in numerous studies that cartilage friction is multifactorial and extremely complex. It is time-dependent (i.e., friction increases with the time of axial load exposure) and also depends on other parameters like compressive stress, strain, lubricant, and sliding velocity (▶ Fig. 12.6).

A variety of lubrication theories such as fluid-film lubrication[9] and interstitial fluid pressurization[10] have been described to characterize the tribological characteristics of AC, none of which is able to explain the entire complexity of cartilage tribology. Hence, it has been speculated that not one specific mechanism alone is responsible for it.[11]

Key Concepts: Transient Friction Properties of Cartilage

One of the most plausible explanations for the time-dependent friction of cartilage was given by Krishnan et al.[10] They measured the fluid pressure under constant unconfined compression and found a load support by the fluid of 88% at the moment of load application while the friction coefficient was at a minimum. Then the fluid load support decreased over time until it reached 9% at equilibrium with the friction coefficient being maximal. Hence, they found a negative proportional relationship between fluid load support and friction coefficient, which means that at the beginning of load application, the fluid is mainly responsible for the low friction and at equilibrium, when the fluid pressure reduces to zero, the solid matrix determines the friction.

12.3 Friction

Joints transfer high forces and at the same time enable low-friction motion. Although these requirements seem contradictory, the special biphasic composition of AC grants this in an ingenious way. Hence, the tribological

The friction coefficient is the most frequently assessed parameter to characterize cartilage tribological behavior. This coefficient μ is simply determined by dividing the friction load F_{Fr} acting in the direction of motion by the normal load F_N that is acting perpendicular to it (▶ Fig. 12.7a). Several experimental setups have been

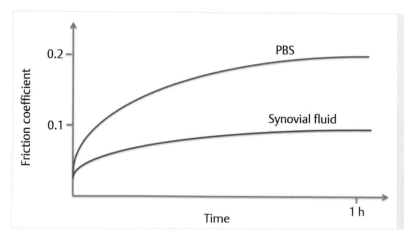

Fig. 12.6 The friction coefficient of articular cartilage typically increases with time and is very sensitive to the type of lubricant. PBS, phosphate buffered saline.

described to measure the friction coefficient. Pendulum testers are used to test, for example, the friction resistance of whole joints.[12] More often, so called pin-on-plate or pin-on-disk setups are used. Here, a cartilage specimen slides under a defined load or strain over a rotating (pin-on-disk) or a translating (pin-on-plate) counter surface (▶ Fig. 12.7b,c). In such experiments, the forces acting in the direction of motion and in the direction of the normal load are recorded and the friction coefficient calculated. The pin-on-disk arrangement provides the possibility of infinite test duration without the need for a change of sliding direction, which is necessary for the pin-on-plate test, where the direction of motion has to be changed after a certain stroke length. The pin-on-disk arrangement is especially helpful when testing cartilage against cartilage samples, because there are not many locations in joints with a long flat surface, which could be used as sliding partner.

12.3.1 Practical Guide for Friction Testing of Cartilage

Due to the complex nature of cartilage tribology, it is not easy to measure the friction coefficient of AC as a number of testing parameters have to be taken into account. Hence, it is difficult to compare results with literature data due to varying test setups and experimental conditions. However, to gain valid results when comparing, for example, two groups of specimens with different treatments, one should be aware of the following parameters that can influence the friction measurement.

1. Sliding partners: Many studies have used glass plates as a counter sliding surface for AC specimens due to the difficulty of harvesting large flat cartilage samples. For example, microscope slides are useful for this purpose and provide a very smooth reproducible surface. In case there is a need for testing cartilage on cartilage, one can use either a pin-on-disk assembly with one cylindrical specimen larger than the other or for a pin-on-plate tester one small cylindrical sample (e.g., 5-mm diameter) and one larger flat specimen. In bovine knee joints, there is a relatively flat surface at the backside of the patella and at the corresponding articular surface at the trochlea. However, any deviation from flatness may result in accelerations in normal direction and thus to a change in friction coefficient.

2. Preparation and geometry of specimens: It is important that the specimen's surface is coplanar with the counter sliding surface. Therefore, when harvesting a cylindrical specimen from a joint, care should be taken to extract it from a location where the drill or punch direction is perpendicular to the joint surface and that this location is as flat as possible.

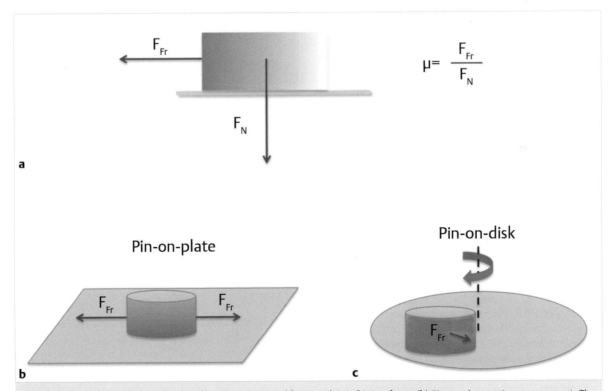

Fig. 12.7 (a) Definition of the friction coefficient. F_N is normal force, and F_{Fr} is friction force. (b) Pin-on-plate testing arrangement: The specimen is sliding linearly over a counter surface. (c) Pin-on-disk testing arrangement: The specimen is sliding over a rotating counter surface.

3. Load or strain controlled: Friction coefficients can vary depending on how the load is applied. A constant load results in a creep experiment with increasing strain over time; a constant strain will lead to stress relaxation with a decaying force. So, one should decide for either load or strain control. Load control is probably the easier way because it can simply be realized by putting on a dead weight. For a strain-controlled procedure, a translation mechanism similar to the crosshead of a material testing machine is needed (which—if available—could indeed be used for this purpose). Whichever method one decides to use, it should be kept in mind that the friction coefficient can also vary at different load or strain levels. Therefore, it is recommended to carry out the tests with stepwise increasing load (stress) or strain.

4. Sliding velocity: It could be shown that the relative motion between sliding partners influences the friction coefficient. Depending on the entire set of boundary conditions, friction can either increase or decrease with raising sliding velocity. Therefore, one should ensure that the sliding velocity is constant throughout the test and especially in a comparative study or at best repeat tests with different velocities. Sliding speeds of 0.1 to 20 mm/sec have been reported in related studies.

5. Stroke length: In a pin-on-plate arrangement, the sliding table must change its direction of motion periodically until equilibrium is reached. In consequence, the friction force changes its direction accordingly. When testing against glass, one can choose a rather large stroke length, which is only limited by the capability of the translation table to move and the length of the glass surface. When testing against cartilage, the stroke length is limited by the length of the counter cartilage surface. However, the longer the stroke length, the more lubricant is needed, which can also be of limited availability in the case of synovial fluid.

6. Duration of test: As mentioned previously, friction increases with time. Initially, the friction coefficient is very low and rises until equilibrium is gained. This can take 1 hour or even more. To achieve comparable results of equilibrium friction coefficient, one should therefore test always until no considerable change in friction occurs.

7. Lubricant: AC friction is extremely sensitive to the lubricant that is present in between both sliding partners. Usually, the lowest friction occurs in the presence of synovial fluid compared to phosphate buffered saline or other physiological solutions. To obtain synovial fluid in considerable amounts is not always feasible. Slaughterhouse or experimental animal facilities are a possible source. In principle, large amounts could be harvested from aspirates from effused knee joints. However, it is unknown whether inflammatory cytokines in such synovial fluid can alter its lubricative

capability (which could be a nice question to investigate). So, for many comparative purposes, phosphate buffered saline can be used as an adequate surrogate with the limitation of a higher friction coefficient.

8. Calculation of friction coefficient: ▶ Fig. 12.6 shows a typical course of a friction coefficient–time curve. The easiest way to characterize it is to determine first the instantaneous friction coefficient μ_0 right after the application of the load and second the friction coefficient μ_{eq} at equilibrium. When testing at different loads or strains and at various sliding velocities, it is possible to create a so-called Stribeck surface, which shows the friction coefficient in a three-dimensional diagram depending on sliding velocity and load/strain.[13]

▶ Fig. 12.8 shows an example of a pin-on-plate tribometer, which allows both the application of a constant load by a dead weight and, alternatively, the compression of the sample at constant strain.

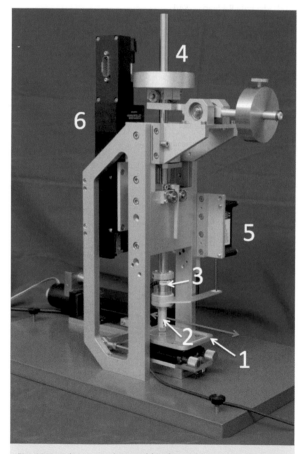

Fig. 12.8 Tribometer designed by the authors. *1*, sliding table; *2*, specimen holder; *3*, multidirectional load cell; *4*, dead weight for the application of a constant load (creep experiment); *5*, laser displacement sensor to accurately measure the deformation of the cartilage sample; *6*, vertical linear motor for the application of a constant strain (stress relaxation experiment); *blue arrow*, sliding direction.

12.4 Conclusion

Cartilage is a soft tissue of complex biphasic structure, which results in its viscoelastic mechanical behavior. The biomechanical characterization strongly depends on many influencing factors as, for example, confining conditions and loading rate. To facilitate the comparison of the results of different studies or to enable others to replicate them, it is therefore of utmost importance to precisely describe the testing conditions. This chapter communicates common test methods to characterize the biomechanical properties of cartilage and clarifies the most important parameters that have to be considered when generating valid biomechanical data.

References

[1] Elliott DM, Narmoneva DA, Setton LA. Direct measurement of the Poisson's ratio of human patella cartilage in tension. J Biomech Eng 2002; 124: 223–228

[2] Kiviranta P, Rieppo J, Korhonen RK, Julkunen P, Töyräs J, Jurvelin JS. Collagen network primarily controls Poisson's ratio of bovine articular cartilage in compression. J Orthop Res 2006; 24: 690–699

[3] Langelier E, Buschmann MD. Increasing strain and strain rate strengthen transient stiffness but weaken the response to subsequent compression for articular cartilage in unconfined compression. J Biomech 2003; 36: 853–859

[4] Oloyede A, Flachsmann R, Broom ND. The dramatic influence of loading velocity on the compressive response of articular cartilage. Connect Tissue Res 1992; 27: 211–224

[5] Park S, Nicoll SB, Mauck RL, Ateshian GA. Cartilage mechanical response under dynamic compression at physiological stress levels following collagenase digestion. Ann Biomed Eng 2008; 36: 425–434

[6] Frank EH, Grodzinsky AJ. Cartilage electromechanics—I. Electrokinetic transduction and the effects of electrolyte pH and ionic strength. J Biomech 1987; 20: 615–627

[7] Frank EH, Grodzinsky AJ. Cartilage electromechanics—II. A continuum model of cartilage electrokinetics and correlation with experiments. J Biomech 1987; 20: 629–639

[8] Mow VC, Kuei SC, Lai WM, Armstrong CG. Biphasic creep and stress relaxation of articular cartilage in compression? Theory and experiments. J Biomech Eng 1980; 102: 73–84

[9] Roberts BJ, Unsworth A, Mian N. Modes of lubrication in human hip joints. Ann Rheum Dis 1982; 41: 217–224

[10] Krishnan R, Kopacz M, Ateshian GA. Experimental verification of the role of interstitial fluid pressurization in cartilage lubrication. J Orthop Res 2004; 22: 565–570

[11] Katta J, Jin Z, Ingham E, Fisher J. Biotribology of articular cartilage—a review of the recent advances. Med Eng Phys 2008; 30: 1349–1363

[12] Teeple E, Elsaid KA, Fleming BC, Jay GD, Aslani K, Crisco JJ, Mechrefe AP. Coefficients of friction, lubricin, and cartilage damage in the anterior cruciate ligament-deficient guinea pig knee. J Orthop Res 2008; 26: 231–237

[13] Gleghorn JP, Bonassar LJ. Lubrication mode analysis of articular cartilage using Stribeck surfaces. J Biomech 2008; 41: 1910–1918

Further Reading

Ateshian GA, Mow VC. Friction, lubrication, and wear of articular cartilage and diarthrodial joints. In: Mow VC, Huiskes R, eds. Basic orthopaedic biomechanics & mechano-biology. Philadelphia: Lippincott Williams & Wilkins; 2005:447–493

Mow VC, Kuei SC, Lai WM, Armstrong CG. Biphasic creep and stress relaxation of articular cartilage in compression? Theory and experiments. J Biomech Eng 1980; 102: 73–84

Woo SL-Y, Buckwalker JA, eds. Injury and repair of the musculoskeletal soft tissues. Park Ridge, IL: American Academy of Orthopaedic Surgeons; 1987

13 Biomechanics of Joints

Richard van Arkel, Bidyut Pal, Hannah Darton, and Andrew A. Amis

This introduction to biomechanics aims to show the reader how bioengineers approach the analysis of human joints. It shows particularly that the forces acting on our joints and other internal structures are usually very much larger than the external forces imposed when we interact with the outside world. A clear example of this is that the forces in the joints of the lower limbs when walking are several times larger than our body weight. It is important for the orthopedic surgeon to have an understanding of the mechanical principles that govern the working of the musculoskeletal system, because only that will allow an informed basis for many aspects of orthopedic practice. Although one may "muddle through" on the basis of common sense, a more scientific basis leads to a deeper understanding. This is needed for evaluating the design or fixation of novel joint prostheses, or the design of fracture fixation devices—What loads must they withstand? How best to maintain reduction of a bone fragment? Is the material strong enough?—for example, so that the surgeon has a solid basis on which to choose the best way to treat the patient.

13.1 Basic Concepts

13.1.1 Joint Classification and General Structure

> **Jargon Simplified: Joint Range of Motion**
>
> Both active and passive ranges of motion (ROM) of joints are used: The active ROM is caused by muscle contractions, whereas the passive range is found by an examiner moving the limb. The passive ROM is usually larger, because the muscles remain flaccid and so they do not impinge between the bones as early as actively contracting muscles when the limit of motion is approached. A person's flexibility is joint specific and so high flexibility in one joint does not guarantee the same amount of flexibility in all other joints.
>
> ROM is measured in degrees, and there are several techniques used to measure the ROM of a joint: Optical, electromagnetic, and inertial sensors can be used, but the most common technology in use is goniometers, which work much like a large protractor with extended arms to improve accuracy.

The joints of the body can be classified as: diarthoses, which are freely movable, amphiarthroses, which are semimovable, and synarthroses, which are nonmovable.

This chapter will focus on the most common of the human joint classifications: the diarthrodial joints. These joints are often referred to as synovial joints and can be further classified depending on their shape and the types of movement they allow (▶ Fig. 13.1). Regardless of their subclassifications, all synovial joints share common structural features (▶ Fig. 13.2).

13.1.2 Static Analysis of Joints

The musculoskeletal system can be thought of as a set of connected links, with the bones acting as beams and the joints as the links between them. Considering this analogy, the movement around the joints can be analyzed much like any other mechanical system. With static analysis, the forces and moments acting around a joint are balanced (that is, they are in both rotational and translational equilibrium) and there is assumed to be no acceleration component to the forces. The concept of static analysis of joints is best explained using an example.

▶ Fig. 13.3 shows an outstretched arm of mass 3 kg (≈30 N weight) supporting a dumbbell of mass 5 kg (≈50 N weight). The center of mass of the arm will be approximately 40% between the point of rotation and the end of the arm (x_1). The corresponding free body diagram is also shown, where R_X and R_Y represent the reaction forces acting onto the head of the humerus in the horizontal and vertical directions, respectively, and *JRF* is the compound joint reaction force. F_M is a muscle force, W_L is the weight of the limb (30 N), and W_D is the weight of the dumbbell (50 N). The distances of each force away from the center of rotation of the shoulder are shown by x_1 and x_2 are 0.24 m and 0.6 m, respectively, and *MA* is the muscle moment arm. Note that the muscle moment arm is perpendicular to the muscle force, F_M, which is at an angle of θ from the horizontal limb. While in this static example, θ is constant at 20 degrees, if the arm was moving this angle would continually be changing as would the muscle moment arm.

> **Jargon Simplified: Moment**
>
> A moment is when a force creates a rotating or pivoting action, and is defined as the product of a force and moment arm (perpendicular distance of the line of action of the force from the pivot point). A moment balance is the sum of all the moments acting about a point; for equilibrium, all anticlockwise and clockwise moments must be equal and opposite.

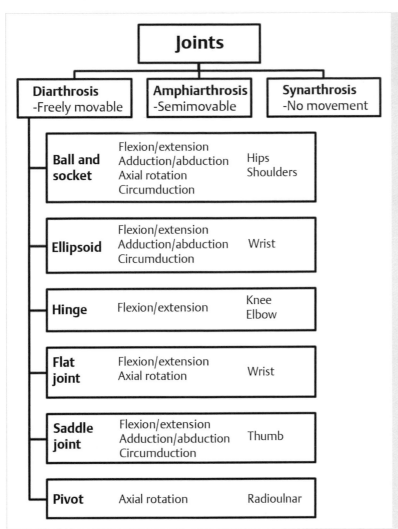

Fig. 13.1 Classification of joints with the most common subcategories for diarthrotic or synovial joints. Subcategories include the most common modes of joint movement and an example.

Joints			
Diarthrosis -Freely movable	**Amphiarthrosis** -Semimovable	**Synarthrosis** -No movement	

Ball and socket	Flexion/extension Adduction/abduction Axial rotation Circumduction	Hips Shoulders
Ellipsoid	Flexion/extension Adduction/abduction Circumduction	Wrist
Hinge	Flexion/extension	Knee Elbow
Flat joint	Flexion/extension Axial rotation	Wrist
Saddle joint	Flexion/extension Adduction/abduction Circumduction	Thumb
Pivot	Axial rotation	Radioulnar

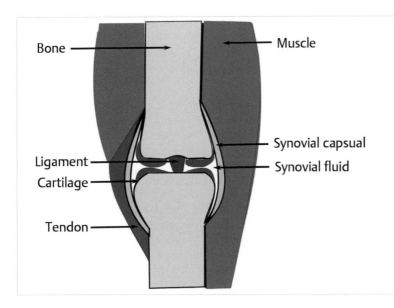

Bone

Muscle

Ligament

Synovial capsual

Cartilage

Synovial fluid

Tendon

Fig. 13.2 Common structures of a synovial joint.

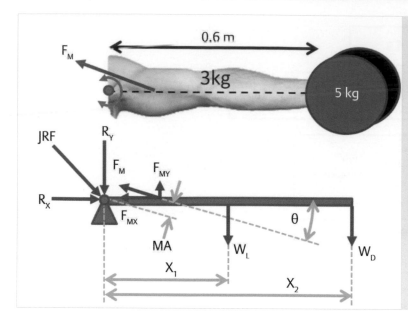

Fig. 13.3 An arm outstretched holding a dumbbell weight and the corresponding free body diagram. Static analysis of the forces and moments required to stabilize the shoulder joint. For details, see text.

In order to calculate the reaction forces and moments at the joint, force and moment equilibrium balances are performed.

$$\text{Moment Balance} = F_M MA = W_L x_1 + W_D x_2$$

$$F_M = \frac{W_L x_1 + W_D x_2}{MA} = \frac{30 \times 0.24 + 50 \times 0.6}{MA} = \frac{37.2}{MA}$$

If

$$MA = 0.2m$$

then

$$F_M = 186N$$

If,

$$MA = 0.02m$$

then

$$F_M = 1860N$$

It can be seen that the muscle force required to support the arm depends greatly on the size of the muscle moment arm. In general, most muscles are attached close to the joint and so they have a small moment arm, which requires a large muscle force in comparison to the external force at the hand. The example will continue assuming a typical human muscle moment arm of 50 mm giving a muscle force F_M = 744 N.

Resolving Forces: The muscular force acts at an angle to the horizontal and thus has both a vertical, F_{MY}, and horizontal F_{MX}, component. These components can be found using simple trigonometry:

Muscle Force Vertical Component : $F_{MY} = F_M \times \sin\theta$
$= 744 \times \sin 20 = 254N$

Muscle Force Horizontal Component : $F_{MX} = F_M \times \cos\theta$
$= 744 \times \cos 20 = 699N$

Force balance: The vertical forces and horizontal forces are independent of each other and so are summed separately.

Vertical Balance : $R_y = F_{MY} - W_L - W_D = 254 - 30 - 50$
$= 174N$

Horizontal Balance : $R_X = F_{MX} = 699N$

The joint reaction force is the resultant reaction force at the joint and can be found using the Pythagorean theorem:

$$JRF = \sqrt{R_X^2 + R_Y^2} = \sqrt{699^2 + 174^2} = 721N$$

The joint reaction force is the equal and opposite reaction to the sum of all the other forces and hence the gleno-humeral joint in this example is under 721 N of compression.

The majority of muscles in the body have small moment arms, and thus joint reaction forces are very high in vivo, often up to 15 times the external load (in the example, the 50 N weight gave a joint reaction force of 721 N!). This effect is magnified when additional muscle actions are needed to maintain joint stability, which is accomplished by using opposing agonist and antagonist muscles. An example might be the addition of a triceps tension during elbow joint flexion, which is an antagonist to the biceps and brachialis, adding to the force onto the humeral trochlea.

13.1.3 Dynamic Analysis of Joints

Joint motion occurs when the clockwise and anticlockwise moments about the joint are not equal. The difference between these moments results in an accelerating torque that acts in the direction of the greater moment. The analysis methods are similar to that for a static analysis, with an additional torque variable in the moment balance that is directly proportional to the joint acceleration. This type of dynamic analysis requires use of data such as the inertial properties of the limb segments, and is necessary if accuracy is needed when analyzing movements such as walking (see Chapter 15, "Musculoskeletal Dynamics").

13.1.4 Joints and Moment Arms

The geometric structure of the bones that surround and make up a joint provide an increased distance between where the muscle force acts and the joint's point of rotation. This creates mechanical advantage and reduces the amount of muscle force required for movement. An example of this is the patella in the knee (▶ Fig. 13.4). The reduced moment arm of the extensor mechanism about the center of rotation after a patellectomy means that a larger muscle tension would be needed to obtain the same knee extension moment. This is one of the reasons why patellectomy is discredited: It makes it very difficult to rise from a chair, for example.

13.2 Kinematics

Clinically, the movements of joints are described in relation to the major body planes and axes (▶ Fig. 13.5).

However, movement of the body can be difficult to describe as it does not always take place in single planes and often the center of rotation of a joint can change depending on its orientation. For ease of interpretation of results where the exact degree of rotation is reported, it is recommended that the International Society of Biomechanics definition of joint coordinate systems[1] is used.

Key Concepts: Degrees of Freedom

The degree of freedom (DOF) of a mechanical system is the number of independent parameters that define its configuration. Different joints of the body have different numbers of DOF up to a maximum of six: three translations and three rotations. An example of this is the knee joint where movements can be related to three principal axes: the tibial shaft axis (superior-inferior), the epicondylar axis (medial-lateral), and the anterior-posterior axis, which are mutually perpendicular to each other. Three translations are possible along these axes, and three rotations are possible around these axes (▶ Fig. 13.6). Most physiological motions do not occur in one isolated DOF; at the knee, flexion-extension is accompanied by small tibial internal-external rotations. These occur automatically, and so are termed "coupled" rotations.

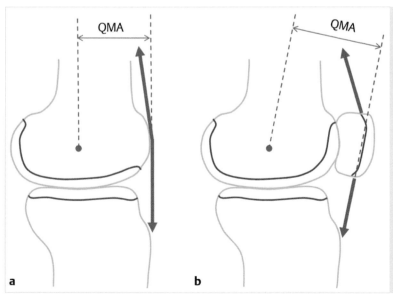

Fig. 13.4 (a) A knee joint without a patella. (b) The human knee (with patella). It can be seen that the extension moment arm of the quadriceps (*QMA*) is significantly increased by the patella. This means that less muscle force is needed to extend the knee joint. With a smaller muscle force, the knee joint contact force is reduced, which helps protect the cartilage from excessive loading (see section in the text titled "Contact Stress: The Effects of Loads on the Joint").

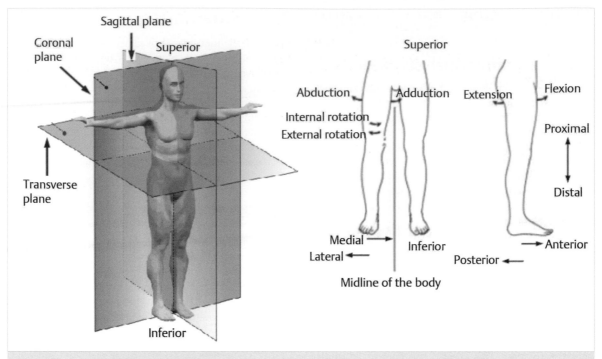

Fig. 13.5 Sketch showing anatomic planes of reference and anatomic directions and movements of the hip joint.

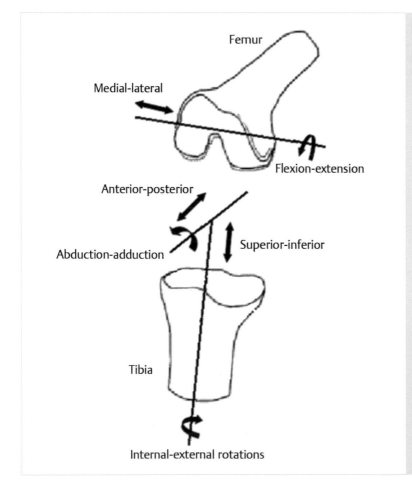

Fig. 13.6 Schematic diagram showing six degrees of freedom for human knee joint movement.

13.3 Joint Loads

Detailed data on the loading of the joint is important for investigations of joint function, injury, and disease. The musculoskeletal loading for any particular joint varies largely between different subject groups (based on age, weight, gender, race, and also activity being undertaken). The joint loads are usually summed together to give a single force (magnitude and direction) known as the joint reaction force (or contact force).

13.3.1 Measuring Joint Loads

The current gold standard for joint contact forces comes from instrumented implants. While these measurements can only be made in selected patients who have undergone arthroplasty and have received special instrumented implants, they provide accurate measurements of in vivo forces. A database of contact forces during daily activities recorded by instrumented implants is available for the hip, knee, spine, and shoulder.[2,3]

While it is possible to accurately measure the joint reaction force with an instrumented prosthesis, ethical considerations discourage invasive methods to quantify in vivo muscle forces. Instead, researchers use mathematical optimization algorithms to estimate the complex distribution of in vivo muscle forces (see Chapter 5, "Physiological Boundary Conditions for Mechanical Testing," and Chapter 19, "Inverse Dynamics"). These methods are validated by summing computed muscle loads to find the joint reaction force and comparing this against in vivo contact forces.

13.3.2 Loading at the Hip

The hip joint reaction force depends on multiple factors, such as position of the "center of gravity" of the body relative to the line joining two hip joint centers, abductor moment arm that is dependent on offset (distance of the center of the femoral head from the shaft axis), and the neck-shaft angle of the femur (varus, neutral, or valgus).

The magnitude of the joint reaction force on each femoral head during upright two-legged standing consists of a body weight contribution (approximately one-third of body weight) and stabilization from the iliofemoral ligament (which limits extension of the hip). The resulting force is low, around 60 to 70% of body weight,[3] and requires little muscle activity to maintain posture. However, slight movements away from this neutral position require muscle activity to maintain balance and thus the joint reaction force increases in proportion to the amount of muscle activity.[4] Typical daily activities can result in forces that are four to five times body weight.

During stair climbing and gait, the hip contact force acts from the surface of the femoral head at approximately 17 degrees with the vertical in the frontal plane (i.e., points superiorly and 17 degrees medially). The abductor muscles make a significant contribution to this force. For example, the abductor muscle forces at the instant of peak hip contact force during walking and stair climbing are 104% and 113% of body weight, respectively.[5]

13.3.3 Loading at the Knee

The line from the center of the mass of the body to the foot contacting the ground passes medial to the knee joint.[6] This medial offset of the path of the ground reaction force produces an adduction moment during activity that causes the medial compartment of the knee to carry a higher load than the lateral compartment (▶ Fig. 13.7).

The adduction moment not only causes the asymmetric loading, it also opens the joint laterally. The iliotibial band and the ligaments of the posterior-lateral corner of the knee and the lateral collateral ligament

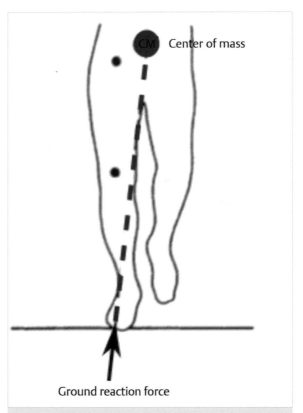

Fig. 13.7 The line of action from the center of mass to the foot passes medial to the knee, producing an adduction moment during walking. This moment produces an asymmetric loading distribution at the knee.

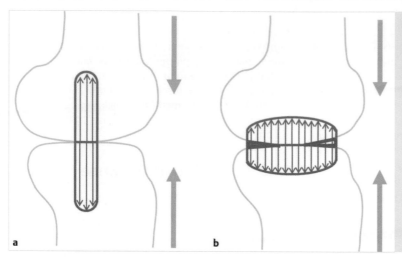

Fig. 13.8 A sagittal section of the lateral compartment of the knee under compressive load. (a) Without the meniscus, the contact area (*red arrows*) between the articular cartilage on the femur and tibia is low, resulting in high contact stresses. (b) The knee meniscus (*blue wedge*) increases the contact area (*red arrows*) between the femur and tibia and thus the same force results in much lower contact stresses.

provide the most resistance to the adduction moment and lateral joint opening. A few other specific muscles such as quadriceps, gastrocnemius, and hamstrings also resist the adduction moment during normal activity.[7] The adduction moment has been correlated with the progression of medial compartment osteoarthrosis and is reduced by medial opening high tibial osteotomy.

13.3.4 Contact Stress: The Effects of Loads on the Joint

The forces from daily activities, such as the walking, running, or stair climbing, create compressive forces across the joint. These compressive forces create stresses in the articular cartilage, the low friction surface that enables sliding between bones. Cartilage provides natural resistance against compressive forces through its biphasic (solid and fluid) behavior, but high contact stresses can be damaging. This is particularly concerning in cartilage because it is avascular and has little regenerative capacity.

The magnitude of contact stress depends on two factors: the magnitude of the applied force and the area over which the force is distributed. To prevent failure from high stresses, the joint can protect itself in two ways: by minimizing the contact force or maximizing the contact area. The contact force can be reduced through increasing muscle moment arms (see section "Static Analysis of Joints" for more details). The contact area can be increased by fibrocartilage structures such as the knee meniscus and the glenoid or acetabular labrum. These structures provide a cross between cartilage and ligaments, and are made of a hydrophilic matrix reinforced with collagen fibers and so provide resistance to tension and compression as well as providing a low friction surface.

13.3.5 The Knee Meniscus

The knee menisci are two crescent-shaped fibrocartilage wedges that follow the outside edge of the medial and lateral compartments of the knee. The menisci increase the contact area between the femur and tibia and hence reduce the contact stresses in the cartilage (▶ Fig. 13.8).

The fiber orientations in the meniscus allow it to deform under compressive joint loads in such a way that it increases the contact area in the joint: The central portion of the meniscus has relatively low collagen fiber content, and these fibers are orientated radially. This means that under compressive load, the meniscus deforms, readily filling the gap between the condyles and increasing the contact area. Conversely, the periphery of the meniscus contains large amounts of circumferentially orientated fibers, which resist the tendency of the joint load to extrude the meniscus radially out of the joint space, and thus take the load (▶ Fig. 13.9).

13.4 Stability

Joint stability is the ability of the joint to return to its original state when displaced. A classic example of stability is given in ▶ Fig. 13.10.

For joints, stability can be achieved passively or actively. Passive stability comes from the joint shape, joint ligaments, and fibrocartilage structures such as the glenoid labrum and knee meniscus. The advantage of passive stability is that it requires no energy expenditure to achieve. Conversely, active stability, which requires muscular forces to control the joint, is energy intensive.

13.4.1 Joint Shape

Congruent joint shapes are naturally more stable. At the hip, the femoral head is almost entirely congruent with the acetabulum creating a closely fitting ball and socket

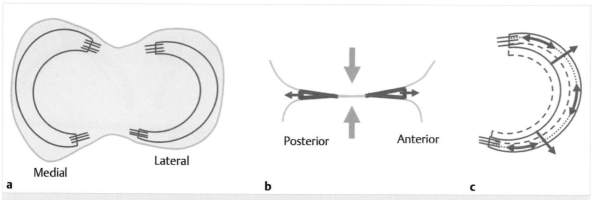

Fig. 13.9 (**a**) A transverse view of the tibial condyles, showing the medial and lateral menisci (*blue*). The lines at each end of the menisci indicate the fibers of the insertional ligaments that link the meniscus horn to the underlying tibia. (**b**) A sagittal view of the lateral femoral and tibial condyles under joint compression; the meniscus is compressed by the joint force (*green arrows*) and extrudes from between the condyles (*red arrows*). (**c**) This extrusion of the meniscus (a radial expansion—the straight red arrows—that results in an increased meniscus circumference) is resisted by tension in the circumferential fibers in the periphery of the meniscus—the curved red arrows.

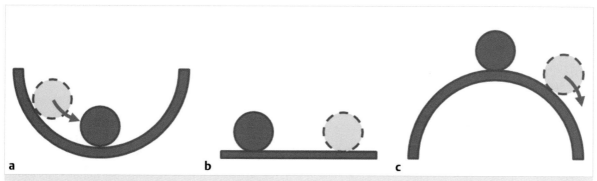

Fig. 13.10 (**a**) Stable: When the ball is moved it returns to its original place. (**b**) Neutral: When the ball moves, it neither returns to its original position nor moves farther. (**c**) Unstable: A small displacement causes the ball to rapidly accelerate away from its original location.

joint that provides a lot of natural stability, similar to that shown in ▶ Fig. 13.10**a**.

At the knee, the femoral condyles are both convex. The medial tibial condyle provides a marginally concave articular surface, giving small amounts of stability. Conversely, at the lateral tibial condyle, the surface is slightly convex, meaning that the joint shape of the lateral part of the tibiofemoral joint is inherently unstable, as is the case in ▶ Fig. 13.10c. The knee joint maintains its stability through its soft tissue architecture and muscle tensions, despite the incongruent shapes. The fine-tuned joint shape at the knee allows complex joint movements about the knee that enhance its function.

13.4.2 Ligaments

Joint ligaments contain large amounts of axial collagen fibers and thus provide resistance against tensile forces. The ligaments provide passive stability to the joint; as a ligament is stretched, it becomes taut and thus creates an elastic returning force that resists the displacement and hence provides stability (▶ Fig. 13.11).

For joints with natural shape stability, such as the hip, these ligaments are slack for most movements and only become taut at the limits of the range of motion. However, in joints such as the knee, they play a key role throughout the entire range of motion.

Ligaments frequently have multiple functions and can provide primary stability in one direction, while assisting another ligament by providing secondary stability against a different translation/rotation.

Example: Anterior Cruciate Ligament

The anterior cruciate ligament (ACL) attaches anteriorly on the tibia and posteriorly on the femur. A simple description of its function is that it prevents the tibia from sliding anteriorly under the femur (or the femur posteriorly over the tibia).

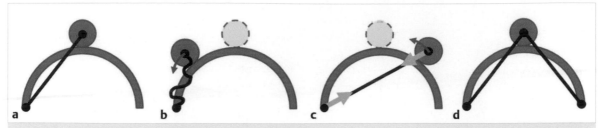

Fig. 13.11 (a) An unstable joint shape with a ligament in its neutral position. (b) The ligament can only act in tension so a displacement to the left causes the ligament to slack and the joint is still unstable. (c) A displacement to the right creates tension in the ligament providing a restoring force and thus the joint is stable with regards to translations to the right. (d) A joint stabilized passively by two ligaments.

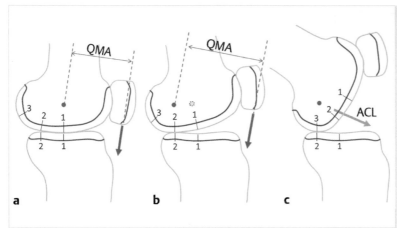

Fig. 13.12 Anterior cruciate ligament (*ACL*) function. (a) During extension, the ACL is tense and the contact point is centrally located between the femur and the tibia. (b) As the knee flexes, the femur rolls posteriorly over the tibia; similarly, the flexion/extension axis of rotation shifts posteriorly increasing the quadriceps moment arm (*QMA*). (c) The joint kinematics change as ACL tension prevents further posterior translation of the femur over the tibia. Now the rolling movement of the femur becomes a sliding movement as the joint continues to flex (i.e., the knee flexes while the contact point on the tibia remains unchanged).

The ACL becomes taut in knee extension, which increases the stiffness and hence stability of the knee. The advantage of this is that less muscle expenditure is needed to maintain stability when standing upright and similarly at heel strike in the gait cycle. It also results in central contact between the femur, meniscus, and tibia, increasing the contact area and hence decreasing the contact pressure during heel strike.

The ACL has a key function during flexion of the knee. As the knee flexes, the ACL becomes less taut due to the action of muscle forces that allow the femur to roll backwards and move posteriorly over the tibial plateau. This is advantageous as the posterior rolling motion of the femur results in a posterior shift of the axis of rotation of the knee and hence increases the moment arm of the quadriceps muscles[8] (▶ Fig. 13.12a,b). This means that less muscle tension is required from the quadriceps to extend the knee (when the moment arm increases, the same torque is produced by a lower muscular force, see Chapter 13.1.4).

However, this posterior rolling motion is controlled by the ACL, which causes the rolling motion to change to a combined rolling plus sliding motion, preventing the femur from dislocating from the tibia while still allowing further knee flexion (▶ Fig. 13.12c). The posterior cruciate ligament acts in a reciprocal manner during knee extension, and deficiencies here cause problems with instability after total knee arthroplasty.

13.5 Trauma

13.5.1 Anterior Cruciate Ligament Trauma

The ACL can tear during traumatic events such as sporting injuries and car crashes. Surgical techniques have been developed to treat ACL tears; however, the clinical performance of these reconstructions is not always successful and some patients experience poor functional outcomes leading to accelerated joint degeneration.

Recent research has emphasized the importance of the separate fiber bundles that make up the ACL.[9] Anatomic double bundle ACL repairs have been developed to mimic this natural ACL morphology, and this advanced treatment has been shown to help restore the rotation kinematics associated with healthy ACL function. This provides an example of how research into the biomechanics of joints may help with trauma care.

13.5.2 Trauma and the Knee Meniscus

The meniscus is commonly torn during trauma to the knee. These tears are painful and can lead to clicking and joint locking. Surgeons traditionally treated meniscal tears by resecting the tissue to alleviate the immediate pain, but the long-term results for many patients were poor as the increased cartilage contact stresses led to rapid joint degeneration and premature osteoarthritis. Now surgeons aim to preserve the knee meniscus where possible, either repairing the tissue or only partially resecting the damaged area.

Biomechanical research has shown that the majority of the collagen fibers are in the peripheral third of the meniscus and thus a partial meniscectomy that completely cuts these fibers could functionally represent a complete meniscectomy and lead to subsequent joint degeneration. It has also been shown that the interactions between the meniscus and the meniscal ligaments govern the tissue's complete function, but further research is needed to fully understand these mechanics and their implications for surgical treatments of meniscal tears.[10]

13.5.3 Long-Term Effects of Joint Injury

Pathology or injury of the soft tissues, which alters the normal gait pattern, is often regarded as the reason behind the genesis and progression of knee osteoarthritis. If there is significant damage to the ligaments/tendons/muscles surrounding the joint, it becomes unstable during activity, leading to an abnormal gait pattern and hence an altered loading distribution within the joint. Over time, this unusual loading may cause severe damage to the cartilage layer that provides a smooth articulation of the joint.[11] Abnormal alignment and musculoskeletal weakness of the joint may also lead to abnormal loading pattern.[9]

13.6 Conclusion

This chapter has provided a brief introduction to the biomechanics of human joints, showing how to perform a simple analysis of the equilibrium between the internal and external forces, so that the loads imposed on internal structures can be estimated. In reality, of course, the body is a three-dimensional structure, and so engineers move rapidly into simultaneous analyses of loads acting in different directions. There also arise complications such as how to decide how groups of cocontracting muscles will share the load, or how their actions when walking might be optimized to save energy.

The section describing the manner in which the menisci act to reduce the tibiofemoral articular contact stresses also shows the initial approach to understanding the behavior of specific tissue structures, and that leads into much work that relates the collagen and mineralized microstructures to the material properties, and how those properties are adapted to best handle the loads imposed in activities of daily life. An understanding at that level is needed if phenomena such as bone loss around implant fixation, caused by "stress-shielding" are to be predicted and avoided by better implant design. The authors hope that a grasp of the biomechanical principles that underlie many of the working practices in orthopedic surgery may lead to an improved understanding of how treatments have been or can be designed and, thus, ultimately to the better treatment of patients.

References

[1] Wu G, Siegler S, Allard P et al. Standardization and Terminology Committee of the International Society of Biomechanics International Society of Biomechanics. ISB recommendation on definitions of joint coordinate system of various joints for the reporting of human joint motion—part I: ankle, hip, and spine. J Biomech 2002; 35: 543–548

[2] Bergmann G, Deuretzbacher G, Heller M et al. Hip contact forces and gait patterns from routine activities. J Biomech 2001; 34: 859–871

[3] Bergmann G. OrthoLoad. Charite – Universitaetsmedizin Berlin. 2008. http://www.orthoload.com/

[4] Nordin M, Frankel VH. Basic biomechanics of the musculoskeletal system. 3 ed. Baltimore: Lippincott Williams & Wilkins; 2001

[5] Heller MO, Bergmann G, Deuretzbacher G et al. Musculo-skeletal loading conditions at the hip during walking and stair climbing. J Biomech 2001; 34: 883–893

[6] Andriacchi TP, Stanwyck TS, Galante JO. Knee biomechanics and total knee replacement. J Arthroplasty 1986; 1: 211–219

[7] Shelburne KB, Torry MR, Pandy MG. Contributions of muscles, ligaments, and the ground-reaction force to tibiofemoral joint loading during normal gait. J Orthop Res 2006; 24: 1983–1990

[8] Williams PL, Warwick R, Dyson M, Bannister LH. Gray's anatomy. 37 ed. London: Churchill Livingstone; 1989

[9] Amis AA. The functions of the fibre bundles of the anterior cruciate ligament in anterior drawer, rotational laxity and the pivot shift. Knee Surg Sports Traumatol Arthrosc 2012; 20: 613–620

[10] Masouros SD, McDermott ID, Amis AA, Bull AMJ. Biomechanics of the meniscus-meniscal ligament construct of the knee. Knee Surg Sports Traumatol Arthrosc 2008; 16: 1121–1132

[11] Hart JM, Ko JW, Konold T, Pietrosimone B. Sagittal plane knee joint moments following anterior cruciate ligament injury and reconstruction: a systematic review. Clin Biomech (Bristol, Avon) 2010; 25: 277–283

14 Spine Biomechanics

Hans-Joachim Wilke, David Volkheimer, and Thomas R. Oxland

Preclinical evaluation is necessary to prove the safety and efficacy of new spinal implants. Besides pure mechanical testing, which is required for approval, in vitro tests are essential to investigate the mechanical functionality of an implant in its natural environment. In vitro experiments allow the measurement of the initial postoperative stability from quasistatic flexibility measurements, or long-term performance of a device (e.g., subsidence or screw loosening), from cyclic tests of an instrumented specimen. Concomitantly to the mechanical testing, finite element calculations may provide an "insight" into different structures. As a final step, animal and clinical studies may address the requirements of the biological environment in situ.

In the first decades of spine surgery, the main goal of a spinal system was to provide enough stability to allow fusion of the treated segment. Despite good or excellent clinical results regarding fusion rates and patient satisfaction, several studies have shown unintentional alterations in the segments adjacent to the fusion site, the so-called adjacent segment degeneration. This finding led to the development of motion preserving devices with the theoretical goal of a reduction or elimination of adjacent segment degeneration. Due to the high degree of innovation of new spinal implants, biomechanical spinal research needs to address this dynamic process. This requires adapting the test requirements to specific implant types in order to provide surgeons with a good basis to choose the appropriate, indication-specific implant.

14.1 Basic Biomechanical Concepts

Biomechanical tests can be performed on intact or on defect specimens. An intact specimen consisting of fresh cadaveric material without severe diseases or structural damage is often used to obtain normative values for the test setup. Injured or defect specimens are spinal segments with an existing or a created disturbance of the ligaments, bony tissues, or disks. Each testing sequence in mechanical testing of spinal segment includes some sort of preconditioning. Preconditioning is used to minimize the viscoelastic behavior of the spinal structures and to allow the implant to settle into the surrounding tissues.

14.2 Rigidity/Stability and Flexibility/Instability

The goal of a fusion implant is to provide stability to the treated segment. A fusion system reduces the motion and decreases flexibility, whereas a flexible system allows greater motions and increases flexibility in comparison to the intact specimen.

The term "stability/instability" should be used solely in the context of the in vivo environment. In this system, an instability (e.g., abnormally large intervertebral motions seen in spondylolisthesis) is thought to be caused by a dysfunction of the stabilizing structures (active, passive, and neural).[1]

Jargon Simplified: Functional Spinal Unit

Two adjacent vertebrae with the intervening intervertebral disk, ligaments, and joint capsules intact represent a functional spinal unit or motion segment. It is the smallest biomechanical unit representing the overall behavior of a specific spinal region.

Jargon Simplified: Construct

A construct is considered a cadaveric or surrogate specimen instrumented with an implant or with a combination of implants.

In the field of spinal biomechanics, a right-handed coordinate system with the following axis orientation is used: The positive x axis is pointing ventrally, the positive y axis to the left lateral side, and the positive z axis cranially. The transverse plane corresponds to the x-y plane, the sagittal plane to the x-z plane, and the frontal plane to the y-z plane (▶ Fig. 14.1).

14.3 Biomechanical Test Methods

In contrast to the strength tests required for approval of a spinal implant or implant system, biomechanical test methods evaluate the characteristics of a device in conjunction with its natural mechanical environment.

These methods can be subdivided into two main categories:
- Test for fatigue to measure the mechanical durability of a construct (failure of the implant, as well as the biological structures).
- Flexibility test to measure the multidirectional primary stability provided by the spinal device at the treatment site.

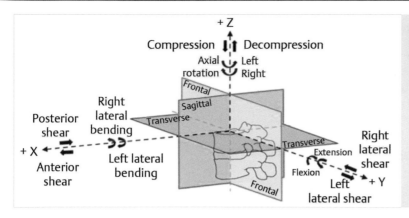

Fig. 14.1 Definition of the three-dimensional coordinate system with illustration of all load and motion directions.

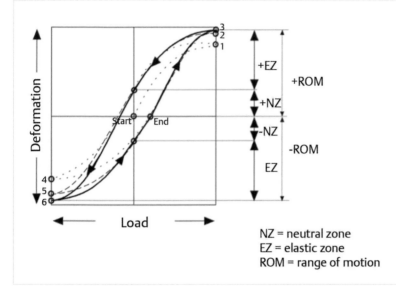

Fig. 14.2 Typical hysteresis curve with definitions of the parameters neutral zone, elastic zone, and range of motion (modified from Wilke, Wenger, and Claes[3]).

NZ = neutral zone
EZ = elastic zone
ROM = range of motion

14.3.1 Quasistatic Testing

Two principal quasistatic test methods can be distinguished: the stiffness and the flexibility protocol. In the stiffness method, the specimen is rigidly fixed at the caudal end while the upper vertebra is moved to a predefined amount; the resultant forces and moments are measured. In the flexibility test, the caudal end is constrained and a load is applied to the cranial vertebra while the motion of the specimen is recorded.[2] This allows for a more unconstrained and therefore more physiological behavior of the specimen. Nowadays, the flexibility test protocol is considered as "gold standard" when the primary stability of a construct is measured.

Because of its nondestructive character, the flexibility test allows the comparison of varying defect situations and implant configurations within one specimen and therefore represents a sensitive indicator for an implant's mechanical behavior in situ. The specimen can be tested in different loading modes, which can be adapted to the individual characteristics of an implant. This test method

is of huge clinical importance because it indicates the potential for rapid healing and fusion.[2]

> **Jargon Simplified: Range of Motion, Neutral Zone, and Elastic Zone (Fig. 14.2)**
>
> The range of motion is the maximal deflection a specimen reaches in a single motion direction. The neutral zone describes the deflection reached with minimal resistance of the specimen. It is a good indicator for the laxity of a specimen. The elastic zone describes the elastic behavior of a specimen between the end of the neutral zone and the point of maximal deflection.

14.3.2 Spinal Loading Simulator

To physiologically simulate the motion of a spinal specimen, a custom-built apparatus, modified materials testing machines, as well as industry robots can be used.

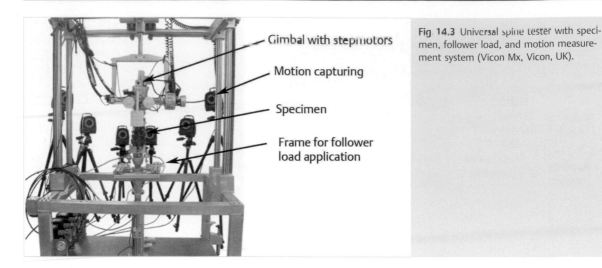

Fig. 14.3 Universal spine tester with specimen, follower load, and motion measurement system (Vicon Mx, Vicon, UK).

- Gimbal with stepmotors
- Motion capturing
- Specimen
- Frame for follower load application

Independent of the simulator, several basic requirements should be fulfilled (▶ Fig. 14.3):

- The apparatus must enable the specimen to move freely in all six degrees of freedom.
- The simulator shall be capable of simulating the six loading components separately.
- Loading shall be applied either continuously or in stepwise fashion.[3]

14.3.3 Motion Measurement System

At the early stages of spine biomechanics, the motion of the whole specimen was often recorded by angular transducers measuring the motion of the cranial vertebra of a specimen. If the mobility at the fusion site was the parameter of interest, the specimen length was limited to a single motion segment. With the emergence of more flexible and more powerful measurement systems using ultrasonic or optical detectors, the motion of each vertebra can be recorded separately, enabling the measurement of multisegmental specimens.

14.3.4 Intradiskal Pressure

Sometimes it can be useful to measure the intradiskal pressure with a pressure transducer implanted centrally into the nucleus pulposus of the disk. This allows a comparison of different implants or defects on the exposure of the intervertebral disk of the treated segment (as long as the disk remains intact) or adjacent segments, which is thought to be a good indicator for the development of accelerated degeneration. To check the validity of the loads applied to the specimen, the data can be compared with in vivo measurements during varying activities.[4,5]

14.4 Specimens

It is widely accepted that fresh unfixed human specimens represent the "gold standard" for biomechanical testing. Formalin fixation strongly stiffens the specimens and leads to a complete loss of viscoelastic behavior. Thiel fixation, on the other hand, rather increases the range of motion (ROM) and may possibly be used for screening tests. Due to the poor availability of human specimens, in very few cases specimens of other species (e.g., calf or sheep spines) can be accepted if the primary parameter of interest is ROM.[3] It is recommended to make anatomical and biomechanical comparisons to human specimens to validate the relevance of the results.

14.5 Loading Scenarios

The majority of in vitro test protocols lack an adequate simulation of muscle forces, because the loads acting on the spine are complex and the load magnitudes exerted by muscles remain widely unknown. Several protocols have been introduced to find a compromise between clinical quality of biomechanical in vitro data and the complexity of the test setup. Independent of the protocol used, the loads (forces and/or moments) should be chosen in a way that the specimen reaches the physiological in vivo ROM without the risk of damage. This allows multiple testing of different implant configurations within one specimen, which can be benchmarked against the intact condition or the specific clinical "gold standard."

It is widely accepted that the use of pure moments is the most appropriate loading scenario, because it guarantees the application of known loads in the treated segment, enabling a comparison between research groups and implants. A compressive follower load can be applied additionally to pure moment testing.

14.6 Pure Moment

To guarantee comparability of biomechanical data, it is important that the load magnitude is constant along the specimen (i.e., the moment applied to the segment of interest is known). This requirement can be fulfilled when a pure moment is applied at the upper vertebra of the specimen while the caudal end is rigidly fixed (► Fig. 14.4). The physiological magnitude depends on the region and the condition (e.g., bone mineral density) of the spinal specimen. The magnitude applied varies between research groups within a moderate range, but as a guideline pure moments of ± 7.5 Nm should be used for the lumbar, ± 5 Nm for the thoracic, and ±2.5 Nm for the cervical spine (with exception of C1-C2 [± 1 Nm]).[3]

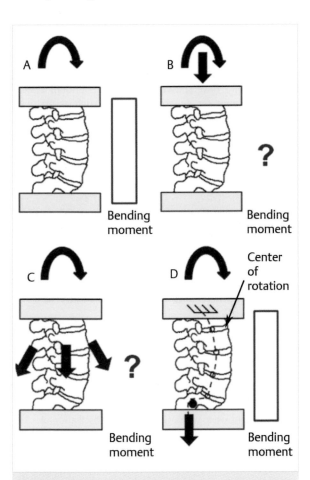

Fig. 14.4 Bending moment diagrams for four types of load application. (a) Pure moment produces uniform bending moment. (b) Pure moment + axial preload results in a variable bending moment when the specimen deflects. (c) Pure moment + muscle forces produces variable bending moment when the specimen deflects. (d) Pure moment + follower produces uniform bending moment.

14.6.1 Pure Moment Plus Axial Preload

To simulate the compressive effect of musculature, a combination of pure moments and axial preload can be used. If the axial preload is applied in a way that the line of action passes through the center of rotation, the bending moment along the length of the specimen is uniform as long as the specimen stays straight. If the specimen is not straight or buckling, an undefined bending moment results. This makes it impossible to compare the results across different tests and/or specimens.

14.7 Muscle Simulation

To achieve a more realistic motion of the specimen, muscle forces can be simulated using tensioned cables. Load cells can be used to measure the forces exerted by the simulated muscle groups. Due to the high complexity of the muscle system, simplifications have to be made regarding the number of muscles, force magnitude, and insertion points. Several in vitro studies with varying muscle groups have shown the stabilizing effect of muscle forces, which led to a decrease in ROM and neutral zone (NZ).[6] However, this finding is highly dependent on the muscle simulation layout. Until now, no consensus has found how muscles can be simulated in a physiologically reasonable way.

14.8 Follower Load

To overcome the disadvantages of a missing simulation of muscle forces when using solely pure moments and the high complexity of simulating the major musculature, Patwardhan et al[7] published an intelligible approach to achieve a more physiological testing condition. To simulate the stabilizing effect of musculature on the spine, a compressive follower load is used. In contrast to a vertical load, which was shown to generate buckling of the spine at low magnitudes (100 N for the lumbar spine and 40 N for the cervical spine), the path of the follower load is guided through the center of rotation of each vertebra. This can be achieved by guiding loading cables along a line that connects the center of rotation of each motion segment. This follower load creates pure compression of the motion segments, and therefore increases the load-carrying capacity of the specimen. It was shown that the lumbar and cervical spine support high loads (1,200 N and 250 N, respectively) without buckling.[7] Due to the strong, unphysiological influence of the follower load on lateral bending and axial rotation, this test mode is solely applicable in flexion and extension.

14.9 Influence of Specimen Length

In general, the length of a specimen should match the length of the implant together with at least one adjacent segment on either end of the construct. In a flexibility test with sheep spines, Kettler et al[8] have shown that the length of the specimen has an important quantitative influence on ROM, NZ, as well as coupled motions. The ROM of the same motion segment was smaller when tested in polysegmental than in monosegmental specimens. NZ and coupled motions showed an inverse behavior with the largest values in polysegmental and the smallest values in monosegmental specimens.

Therefore, the length of specimens should be kept constant within an experiment and results of specimens with varying lengths should be compared only qualitatively.

14.10 Hybrid Testing

Several clinical studies have documented the adverse effect of degeneration at the adjacent segments after fusion. Despite incomplete evidence, it is believed that the motion-preserving devices are capable of reducing or eliminating this effect. The hybrid test method was developed to measure the adjacent segment disease using in vitro tests.[9]

The hybrid test method is based on the flexibility testing with pure moments. At first, the ROM of the intact specimen is measured under application of appropriate pure moments. Subsequently, the specimen is instrumented and the construct is driven moment-controlled until the ROM of the intact specimen is reached. As a final step, the ROM of the adjacent segments is quantified and compared with the intact state. The adjacent segments are thought to develop degeneration if the motion postoperatively exceeds the one of the intact specimen.

Despite high popularity due to a lack of alternatives, this method entails some major drawbacks. The basis of this protocol is the assumption that a patient tries to move the spine after fusion to the same limits as before spinal fixation. Clinical data supporting this thesis are rare and in many studies, no distinct tendency for postoperative hypermobility at the adjacent segments could be found.

It is questionable whether the flexibility test protocol, especially if pure moments are used, basically is capable to detect effects of a fusion on adjacent segments for two reasons. When pure moments are used, the bending moment along the specimen is uniform, independent of the stiffness of the neighboring vertebrae. Assuming that a segment is rigidly instrumented and the specimen is forced to reach the same ROM as the intact specimen, a higher moment is required and therefore the motion of the adjacent segments increases proportionally to the moment. Therefore, a stiffer implantation unavoidably leads to an increase in ROM at the adjacent segments. Additionally, the flexibility protocol does solely represent the primary stability of the spine. Therefore, the effects of healing and remodeling, which may play an important role in the pathogenesis of adjacent segment disease, cannot be simulated and it remains questionable if this protocol can really address adjacent level effects.

14.11 Cyclic Testing

Cyclic tests, whether dynamic or quasistatic, are valid to address the failure modes occurring over time due to repetitive loading. The effect of accumulating fatigue microfractures may lead to a decreasing stability of the construct, resulting in loosening, pull out, migration, or loss of correction of rigid pedicle screw systems if the connection between screw and bone is the weak point, or even screw breakage when the strength of the screw itself is compromised. Most biomechanical fatigue studies are concerned with rigid fusion systems, but clinical follow-up studies have shown that time-dependent effects are also present for dynamic systems, such as artificial disks, where subsidence leads to a loss of disk space, resulting in malalignment of the motion segment or breakage of the implants.

> **Jargon Simplified: Amplitude, Frequency, Period, and Offset (▶ Fig. 14.5 and ▶ Fig. 14.6)**
>
> Amplitude is the maximal oscillation of a signal related to the offset line. It is usually denoted by A.
>
> The frequency of a signal is the number oscillations per unit time. Frequencies are usually denoted by f and the unit is the hertz (Hz); 1 Hz means one event repeats once per second.
>
> The period is the length of time taken by one oscillation. It is denoted by T and is the reciprocal of the frequency f.
>
> Offset describes the mean value of a signal. If the mean value of a signal is zero, there is no offset. An offset of a mechanical signal can, for example, be the static body weight while walking, whereas the oscillation of the force signal (dynamic forces) is represented by the amplitude.

Several clinical studies have reported that these fatigue failures are quite common, especially for osteoporotic patients with compromised bone quantity. To measure the effect of cyclic loading on the stability of a construct, these test protocols can be combined with several test methods, such as flexibility testing after a defined number of loading cycles or screw pull out when fusion systems are evaluated. The effect of subsidence can be

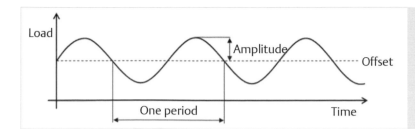

Fig. 14.5 Sinusoidal signal with explanation of amplitude, period, and offset.

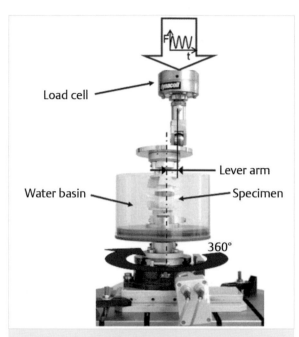

Fig. 14.6 Cyclic loading simulator that allows the application of an eccentric force while the specimen is turning.

detected with height measurements or X-ray imaging. Comparative testing of different devices or implant configurations can help to identify the potential failure modes due to design weaknesses and to support the development of more promising systems.

Depending on the test frequency, one can distinguish between quasistatic and dynamic tests. Quasistatic cyclic tests, characterized by relatively slow frequencies (< 1 Hz), can be conducted using multidirectional flexibility test machines or industry robots, whereas for dynamic testing, usually dynamic materials testing machines are modified according to the specific test modalities.

In most cases, human specimens for biomechanical testing are derived from elderly persons with a high probability of reduced bone mineral density. Several studies have shown that bone mineral density plays an important role in loosening of spinal implants. Therefore, it can be assumed that these specimens are not likely to withstand repetitive loading for long times. To get rid of this drawback, human specimens should be scanned for bone mineral density and only specimens with high bone mineral density should be used. As an alternative, animal specimens or even artificial materials have gained popularity in failure testing. If animal models are used, many authors prefer calf spines due to their particularly geometric similarity and their high bone mineral density.

14.12 Loading Scenarios

To determine the potential of a device to resist failure, a scenario to mimic the loads a spine will face postoperatively has to be elaborated. There are three different parameters to be considered: the number of loading cycles, the magnitude and manner of the load, and the frequency of load application.

Ashman et al[10] have calculated that a spine can undergo more than 1 million loading cycles during a 4-month period of time. It is known that it takes 4 to 8 months for a treated segment to achieve solid bony fusion. Therefore, a loading protocol theoretically should at least contain 1 million loading cycles. Nevertheless, in most fatigue studies, less than 20,000 repetitive loadings were conducted. This discrepancy can be explained by the expenditure of time the simulation of 1 million cycles would require. Wilke et al[3] recommended that an experiment, including preparation, should not exceed 20 hours. To realize 1 million loading cycles within 20 hours (without preparation time), a frequency of almost 14 Hz would be necessary, which is far beyond the common frequencies that can be achieved with rather complex biomechanical testing setups. Furthermore, in vitro fatigue testing does not account for bony healing, which permanently decreases the loads acting on the implant. Additionally, patients are usually protected from excessive loading by limiting their physical activity and it therefore can be concluded that the spine undergoes less repetitive loading than the spine of a healthy person.

To avoid untimely failure of the construct, the chosen load magnitudes are much smaller than the ultimate strength, which depends on the species, spinal region, and bone mineral density of the specimen. For the human lumbar spine, a maximal compressive load of 400 N is commonly used, whereas it can be higher if calf spines are used. Usually, this load is applied eccentrically, causing an additional bending moment. This loading scenario with a combination of compressive force and moment is frequently applied when the specimen is tested dynamically in a materials testing machine with frequencies between 1 Hz and 5 Hz. For the quasistatic fatigue protocols (frequencies smaller than 1 Hz) with universal spine testers, the application of pure moments, eventually combined with an axial compressive preload, can be considered as state of the art.

However, preliminary tests to evaluate the feasibility of the newly elaborated protocols are recommended to prove that the failure modes fit to those seen in clinical practice.

14.13 Conclusion

Preclinical evaluation is required to prove the safety and efficacy of new spinal implants. Besides strength testing that is required for approval, in vitro tests are essential to investigate the functionality and durability of an implant in its natural environment. In vitro experiments allow the measurement of the initial postoperative stability from quasistatic flexibility measurements, or long-term performance from cyclic tests of an instrumented specimen. Concomitantly to the mechanical testing, finite element calculations may provide an "insight" into different structures. As a final step, animal and clinical studies may address the requirements of the biological environment in situ.

References

[1] Panjabi MM. The stabilizing system of the spine. Part I. Function, dysfunction, adaptation, and enhancement. J Spinal Disord 1992; 5: 383–389, discussion 397
[2] Panjabi MM. Biomechanical evaluation of spinal fixation devices: I. A conceptual framework. Spine 1988; 13: 1129–1134
[3] Wilke H-J, Wenger K, Claes L. Testing criteria for spinal implants: recommendations for the standardization of in vitro stability testing of spinal implants. Eur Spine J 1998; 7: 148–154
[4] Nachemson A, Morris JM. In vivo measurements of intradiscal pressure. Discometry, a method for the determination of pressure in the lower lumbar discs. J Bone Joint Surg Am 1964; 46: 1077–1092
[5] Wilke H-J, Neef P, Caimi M, Hoogland T, Claes LE. New in vivo measurements of pressures in the intervertebral disc in daily life. Spine 1999; 24: 755–762
[6] Wilke H-J, Wolf S, Claes LE, Arand M, Wiesend A. Stability increase of the lumbar spine with different muscle groups. A biomechanical in vitro study. Spine 1995; 20: 192–198
[7] Patwardhan AG, Havey RM, Meade KP, Lee B, Dunlap B. A follower load increases the load-carrying capacity of the lumbar spine in compression. Spine 1999; 24: 1003–1009
[8] Kettler A, Wilke H-J, Haid C, Claes L. Effects of specimen length on the monosegmental motion behavior of the lumbar spine. Spine 2000; 25: 543–550
[9] Panjabi MM. Hybrid multidirectional test method to evaluate spinal adjacent-level effects. Clin Biomech (Bristol, Avon) 2007; 22: 257–265
[10] Ashman RB, Birch JG, Bone LB et al. Mechanical testing of spinal instrumentation. Clin Orthop Relat Res 1988; 227: 113–125

Further Reading

White AA, Panjabi MM. Clinical biomechanics of the spine. Philadelphia: JB Lippincott; 1990

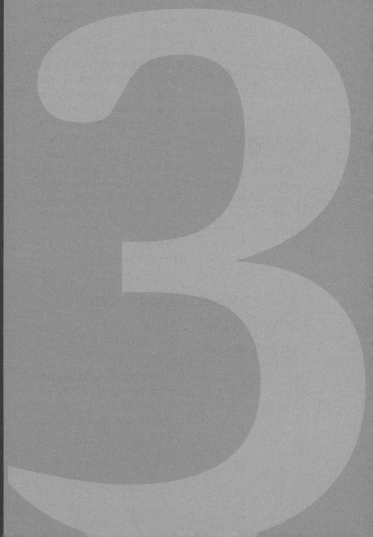

Part 3

Functional Biomechanics

15 Musculoskeletal Dynamics

Jim Richards and James Selfe

In this chapter, we will explore the concepts of open and closed kinetic chains and the methods of assessing upper limb and lower limb musculoskeletal dynamics during a selection of functional tasks. This chapter presents techniques to investigate joint performance and control and provides a framework for functional joint assessment.

This battery of methods can provide useful information in the assessment of joint movement and control; however, as we will highlight, much care needs to be taken to determine which of these methods are appropriate as many parameters and variables could be measured. So the questions that we should ask before any tests are conducted are "What do we need to know?," "What does this method of analysis actually tell us?," and "How does this inform clinical practice?" With these questions in mind, musculoskeletal dynamics may be used to investigate important clinical questions and provide a significant contribution to clinical research.

assessment of therapeutic and surgical intervention. Parameters usually investigated in a laboratory gait analysis include: joint and segment kinematics, kinetics (ground reaction forces), inverse dynamics (joint moments and powers), and electromyography.

Jargon Simplified: Kinematics, Kinetics, and Inverse Dynamics

Kinematics is the study of the motion of the body without regard to the forces acting to produce the motion. The most commonly reported kinematic parameters in gait reports are joint angles, which can give us important information on the functional range of motion of a joint. Less common is the inclusion of joint angular velocities, which can often give us more information about joint control.

Kinetics is the study of forces that act on the body but without any reference to the position of the joints. These are usually assessed using force platforms, which allow the study of ground reaction forces. These are often used to determine abnormal loading and push off patterns, but can also give useful information about the movement of the body over the stance limb and mediolateral stability by considering the center of pressure.

Inverse dynamics combines the study of kinetics and kinematics. This may be used to calculate moments about joints and the power absorption/generation about those joints. This in turn may be used to indicate which muscles are active (e.g., by considering if the moments are trying to flex or extend a joint).

Key Concepts: Kinetic Chains

Before we consider specific functional tasks, it is worth considering the concept of open and closed kinetic chains. A closed kinetic chain occurs when a distal segment meets considerable resistance (e.g., the foot on the ground in stance phase during walking). An open kinetic chain occurs when the distal segment is free to move in space with little or no resistance (e.g., the foot in swing phase during walking or the hand during reaching tasks).[1] There are a number of functional differences between open and closed kinetic chains that include differences in movement patterns and muscle activity. For example, during an open kinetic chain seated leg extension exercise, the proximal tibia rotates around a stationary distal femur and shear forces across the tibiofemoral joint are relatively high. During a closed kinetic chain standing squat, both femur and tibia move simultaneously under compression and shearing forces are reduced. This is an oversimplification as most joints have a significant triplanar motion.

15.1 Closed Kinetic Chain Lower Limb Tasks

15.1.1 Gait

Gait may be described as both closed chain during stance phase and open chain during swing phase. Many of the techniques of studying human gait have been applied to clinical practice leading to more detailed clinical

In addition to external measures, it is also possible to determine which muscles are active during different tasks and the level of electrical activity within the muscles using electromyography, often referred to as motor unit action potential. This, in combination with the kinematic and inverse dynamics data, allows us to determine which muscles/muscle groups are controlling the joint movement and whether they are working concentrically or eccentrically. It is also possible, with careful modeling, to obtain useful estimates of muscle forces.

In addition to the parameters mentioned previously, many other parameters have been identified as being clinically relevant for different patient groups. This has led to the development of modeling joints from considering joints to be simple hinges to more complex methods of considering the movement in six degrees of freedom and from the consideration of the foot as a single segment to multisegment analysis. In all cases, it is vital that clinicians agree on what factors are important for a given patient group and that bioengineers take this into consideration when conducting gait analysis.

Clinical relevance

Human walking allows a smooth and efficient progression of the body's center of mass. To achieve this, there are a number of different movements of the joints in the lower limb. The correct functioning of the movement patterns of these joints allows a smooth and energy-efficient progression of the body. The relationship between the movements of the joints of the lower limb is critical. If there is any deviation in the coordination of these patterns, the energy cost of walking may increase and also the shock absorption at impact and propulsion may not be as effective, possibly leading to dysfunction and pain.

15.1.2 Stairs and Step Down

Stairs were developed over 6,000 years ago to add semi-permanency to steep paths. Stair ambulation is often unavoidable and changes the joint kinematics in comparison to level walking. Stair ascent and descent each present unique challenges from the context of joint kinematics and muscle effort. When ascending, humans are required to raise their center of gravity during the pull up and then actively carry it forward to the next step. This is achieved through concentric muscular contraction, which displaces the center of gravity vertically. When descending, humans must actively carry their center of gravity forwards and then resist gravity during the controlled lowering phase. This is achieved through eccentric muscular contraction, which controls the rate of lowering of the center of gravity by absorbing kinetic energy. Eccentric muscle action predominates during descent, and the quadriceps must provide the majority of muscle force for controlled lowering of body mass while stepping down. If strong eccentric contractions were not employed, the center of gravity would accelerate under the influence of

the gravitational pull of the earth. ▶ Fig. 15.1 shows a comparison of the knee movement between walking, stair ascent, and descent.[2]

Clinical Relevance

The rehabilitation implications for stair ambulation are to restore adequate joint range of motion, motor control, muscle strength, and appropriate balance. The point of greatest instability during stair activities occurs when the support limb moves into single support with all three joints in a flexed position, this is particularly important when descending. Eccentric activity of the quadriceps controls the lowering of the body mass during descent, and any reduction in motor control from arthrogenic inhibition may lead to the person falling. Activities that promote controlled loading of the quadriceps during stair descent should progress gradually in rehabilitation. For example, minisquats and small step ups/downs should be employed prior to introducing the patient to stairs of normal height. Step up/down height can be adjusted until the person has enough strength and muscle control to attempt stair ambulation.

15.1.3 Squats and Dips

Squat exercises are a popular multiple joint workout and form an integral part of most rehabilitation programs. The use of eccentric squat activities for rehabilitation associated with tendinopathy has been well documented.[3] The exact etiology of tendinopathy is unknown; however, evidence suggests that a biochemical and biomechanical combination contribute. The biomechanical factors include an apparent disorganization of the collagen fibers that leads to a general thickening of the tendon. In addition, neovascularization has been identified around the area affected by the tendinopathy. Eccentric exercises have been shown to have a significant effect

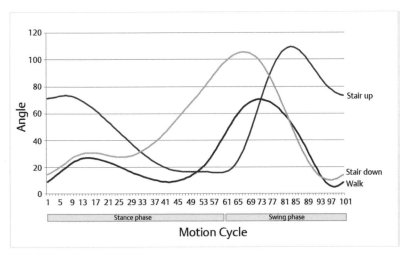

Fig. 15.1 Angulations of the knee joint during walk (*blue*), stair up (*red*), and stair down (*green*) in humans.[2]

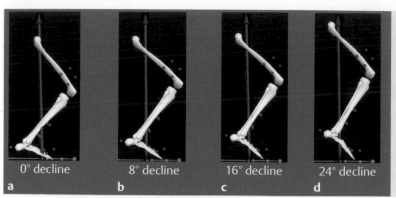

Fig. 15.2 Single limb squat at different decline angles (Richards et al).[7]

0° decline	8° decline	16° decline	24° decline
a	b	c	d

on the rate of recovery from tendinopathy,[4] but the physiological and biomechanical effect of the exercises is somewhat unknown. It has been suggested that the eccentric exercise induced a remodeling within the injured tendon that reduced the neovascularization and realigned the collagen fibers.

Many eccentric exercises and techniques used have little scientific background. Purdam et al[5] identified this as an area for further investigation and proposed a conservative management technique for patella tendinopathy. The technique was based on performing a single limb squat with the eccentrically controlling limb placed on a 25-degree decline. The basis for using a 25-degree decline was that by forcing the ankle into plantarflexion, passive and active calf tensions are reduced, which in turn reduces the work done around the ankle and produces a more focused exercise that targets the knee extensors. However, the reasoning for a 25-degree decline angle was not clearly identified. Zwerver et al[6] confirmed increased knee flexion moments at the deepest point of the squat with increasing angles of declination (up to 30 degree). Richards et al[7] showed the differences between flat squats and squats performed on an 8-, 16-, and 24-degree decline (▶ Fig. 15.2). Richards et al[7] and Zwerver et al[6] determined that the joint moments and muscle work done at the ankle may be controlled by altering the orientation of the foot on the squat platform by changing the angle of declination. By increasing the decline angle, a reduction in the loads and muscle activity were seen at the ankle while increasing the knee moments and muscle activity.

Clinical Relevance

Using a graduated decline squat angle offers a knee rehabilitation that allows a graduated increase in the load applied to the knee and graduated reduction in ankle moments and forces as the decline angle increases. Using a range of decline squat angles allows clinicians to be able to offer a controlled graduated rehabilitation environment for squatting tasks.

15.2 Open Kinetic Chain Upper Limb Tests

Some of the most important open kinetic chain movements are performed by the shoulder and elbow joints. These allow us to perform a huge variety of tasks essential for activities of daily living. However, the full range of tasks is out of the scope of this chapter. We will instead consider the importance and challenges of assessing the shoulder joint during commonly used clinical tasks.

The primary function of the shoulder joint is to place the hand optimally. To allow this degree of mobility, the shoulder joint is unique in having a large humeral head centered over the small socket of the glenoid. This anatomical arrangement predisposes the shoulder to instability, the price it has to pay for being the most mobile joint of the body.

Jargon Simplified: Codman's Paradox

Codman's paradox is the apparent rotation of the humerus during motion following a sequence of angular movements, even though no rotation is primarily performed. To demonstrate Codman's paradox, the arm is first placed in the anatomical position with the open palm facing forwards and the medial epicondyle of the humerus pointing to the midline of the body. The arm is then flexed forwards to 90 degrees. The arm is then abducted by 90 degrees, which brings the epicondyle facing forwards. As the arm is brought back to the side to its original apparent position, the medial epicondyle is pointing forwards rather than medially even though the humerus was never rotated axially. For many years, Codman's paradox was much debated, as the sequence-dependent nature of rotation about the orthogonal axes was not fully appreciated. This paradox has been a source of much frustration and contention; although algebraically complex, it may help in the understanding of many axial rotations during the daily movements of the shoulder.

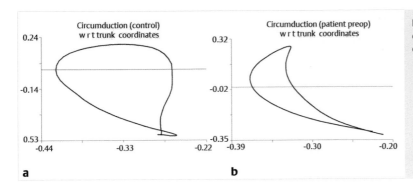

Fig. 15.3 Shape of the right shoulder circumduction trace referenced to the trunk coordinates (Monga et al).[14]

One method of measuring the movement is by using three-dimensional motion analysis; however, it is important to note that the biomechanical model used should be able to measure the complexities of the angular and linear movement in all three planes. By using the calibrated anatomical system technique, it is possible to analyze dynamic motion data of body segments in six degrees of freedom. However, one of the challenges of any method of analysis of the glenohumeral joint complex is Codman's paradox.

In the description of movements of the shoulder joint, it is important that the "sequence" of rotations about various axes is specified. The International Society for Biomechanics has produced recommendations on definitions of joint coordinate systems and of the Cardan sequences to facilitate and encourage communication among researchers and clinicians. However, these recommendations are still challenged by the complexity of some movement patterns such as circumduction (circular limb movement).

One method recently described for analyzing the circumduction movement does not consider the angular movement but instead considers the path traced by the elbow in the different planes as the shoulder performed a circumduction maneuver. The area covered within this imaginary "trace" represents a composite measure of the range of movement of the shoulder complex. To make the area comparable between various subjects of differing arm lengths, the trace can be described as a normalized proportion to the subject's arm length, with the movements of the elbow referenced to the subject's trunk (▶ Fig. 15.3).

15.2.1 Clinical Relevance

It is important with any biomechanical measures to be able to relate these to a perceived patient benefit. Therefore, in any assessment, it is vital to include an assessment of pain and perceived functional benefits. In the case of examining the changes in shoulder joint control, common clinical scores used include the Oxford instability score and the Constant score. Interestingly, in patients with shoulder instability, significant improvements were seen in the shoulder circumduction movement patterns and Oxford instability scores after surgical intervention; however, the Constant score did not change.

15.3 Muscle Testing

The type of muscle contraction affects the resistance that can be controlled, held, or overcome. The three types of muscle contraction are isometric, concentric, and eccentric. Isometric contractions are stabilizing contractions where the muscle length remains virtually constant. Concentric contractions are where the muscle shortens during the activity. These are generally the weakest muscle contractions, requiring more motor unit recruitment than isometric and eccentric for a particular load. Eccentric contractions are where the muscle lengthens during the activity. These are generally the strongest muscle contractions, requiring less recruitment than isometric and concentric for a particular load.

The speed of movement during muscle activation is also an important consideration. There are three ways of classifying speed during exercises: isotonic, isokinetic, and isometric. Isotonic is when a constant load is applied but the angular velocity of the movement may change; this allows an infinite variation in the rate of contraction of a muscle. Although this is closest to real life muscle and joint function, the changing of speed continually affects the amount of force that a muscle can produce and makes the exact muscle function hard to assess. Isokinetic is when the velocity or angular velocity of the movement is kept constant, but the load may be varied. The setting of the speed of working helps improve our assessment of muscle performance, but the speed or velocity of the joints are being restricted to only one set speed at any one time. Isometric relates to the force varying but the joint is held in a static position; therefore, muscle length remains the same as no movement occurs. This tells us what static moment may be supported; however, this does not necessarily relate to the moments that can be produced or supported dynamically.

If we consider the manner in which antagonistic pairings of muscles work, we quickly see that using concentric/concentric muscle torque and power is questionable

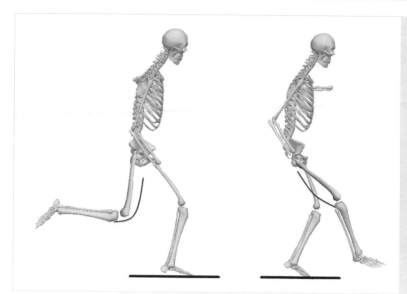

Fig. 15.4 Quadriceps and hamstrings action during kicking.

in its use as a functional comparison. If we take, for instance, the activity of kicking a ball, the quadriceps will be acting concentrically to accelerate the tibia forwards toward extension and therefore generating the power to kick the ball, whereas the hamstrings will be required to act eccentrically to decelerate the tibia to stop the knee going into hyperextension, which could cause ligament and joint damage (▶ Fig. 15.4).

A more functional assessment, therefore, would be to examine the antagonistic pair of muscles by testing the extensors concentrically and the flexors eccentrically, or vice versa, depending on the assessment or the activity being replicated. A far better method of assessing muscle functional capacity of antagonistic pairs of muscles in this situation would be to study concentric quadriceps power and compare this with eccentric hamstrings power. This allows the balance between power generation by the quadriceps and power adsorption by the hamstrings.

15.3.1 Clinical Relevance

Professional soccer is a lucrative international business with large sums of money involved in the movement of players between nations and clubs. Presigning medical assessments are important, both medically and financially, as players exhibit high rates of injury, with thigh strain representing 17% of all injuries; typically, a 25-player squad can expect 10 thigh strains per season.[8] Muscle strength is one of the most important components, in relation to function and injury. In presigning medical assessments, isokinetic testing at speeds of 60, 180, and 300 degrees/second are usually only performed in concentric mode as this is often the first time the player has been tested, and there can be safety issues around understanding and compliance with eccentric testing.

15.4 Assessment of Proprioception

Proprioception is thought to play a significant role in preventing acute injury and in the evolution of chronic injury and degenerative joint diseases. Proprioception has been defined as a specialized sensory modality that gives information about joint position sense, kinesthesia, and vibratory perception. Joint position sense information is provided through a variety of sensory receptors in the periphery, including joint mechanoreceptors, muscle receptors, and cutaneous tactile receptors. In particular, cutaneous tactile receptors are responsible for detecting vibratory information. There is a body of evidence that suggests cutaneous receptors also provide proprioceptive feedback.[9] Three methods for assessing joint proprioception are discussed below.

The passive angle reproduction test was first described by Perlau et al.[10] In this test, the limb is moved passively without resistance to predetermined target angles. For the knee, these are often at 20 degrees and 60 degrees flexion. Slow passive movement is employed often at an angular velocity of 2 degrees/second to limit reflexive muscle contractions. Subjects are instructed not to voluntarily contract their muscles.

The active angle reproduction test is very similar to passive angle reproduction testing; however, following positioning at the predetermined target angle, the subject moves the limb or joint by active muscular contraction at an angular velocity approximating 2 degrees/second and stops when they perceive the target angle has been reached (▶ Fig. 15.5).

Interpretation of passive angle reproduction and active angle reproduction testing can be performed by dichotomizing the results into "good" and "poor" based on the

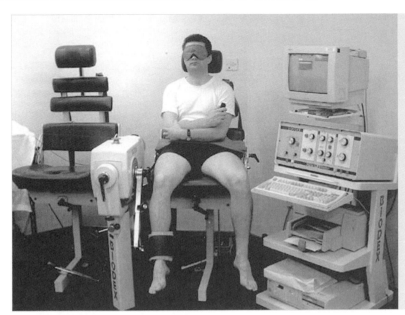

Fig. 15.5 Active angle reproduction test on an isokinetic dynamometer.

accuracy of the scores relative to the target angle. For knee testing, subjects with "good" proprioception are defined as those < 5 degrees away from the target angle, and those with poor proprioception are defined as those ≥ 5 degrees away from the target angle.

Threshold to detection of passive movement was first described by Corrigan, Cashman, and Brady.[11] In this test, subjects are instructed to press a handheld stop button, which "locks" the dynamometer in place, when they feel a sensation of movement or a change in the starting position of the limb or joint. The angle at which the subject locks the dynamometer is recorded from the on-screen goniometer. The usual range of angular velocities is 0.2 degrees/second to 5 degrees/second. However, it should be noted that not all isokinetic dynamometers are capable of slow enough speeds to perform these types of test.

15.4.1 Clinical Relevance

Proprioceptive deficits have been found in anterior cruciate ligament–deficient knees,[11] osteoarthritic knees, knees with chronic effusions, and in patients with patellofemoral pain and patellofemoral dislocation. It has also been suggested that patellofemoral patients with subtle forms of chronic malalignment may exhibit dysfunction of the peripatellar plexus, detectable with proprioceptive testing.[12] These researchers found histological evidence of neuromata and nerve damage to the peripatellar soft tissues, particularly the lateral retinaculum, that suggested altered proprioception. They recommended that proprioception training with tape should form part of a rehabilitation program in patients with these symptoms. The effects of taping and bracing interventions may be mediated through enhancing control mechanisms via

proprioceptive effects. This may partially be explained by Edin, who reported that type III slowly adapting afferents found in the skin around the knee and in the thigh display omnidirectional strain sensitivity, which would make them particularly sensitive to the effects of taping techniques.[9] Functional magnetic resonance imaging has confirmed that the degree to which the brain is activated can be influenced by varying the somatosensory inflow from the skin around the knee.[13]

15.5 Conclusion

The majority of research in clinical biomechanics focuses on gait. In this chapter, we have highlighted some alternative functional tasks, in addition to gait, that are important for a patient's quality of life, and we have suggested appropriate measurement strategies for investigating these tasks. Researchers and clinicians need to be selective in their choice of which tasks and which measures to use to ensure that they are clinically relevant for individual patients. Through an understanding of functional tasks, movement function and dysfunction can be analyzed in great detail in relation to joint function and control, and a holistic view of a patient's movement strategies can be gained.

References

[1] Palmitier RA, An KN, Scott SG, Chao EY. Kinetic chain exercise in knee rehabilitation. Sports Med 1991; 11: 402–413

[2] Richards J, Holler P, Bockstahler B et al. A comparison of human and canine kinematics during level walking, stair ascent, and stair descent. Wiener Tierarztliche Monatsschrift Ascent 2010; 97: 92–100

[3] Stanish WD, Rubinovich RM, Curwin S. Eccentric exercise in chronic tendinitis. Clin Orthop Relat Res 1986: 65–68

[4] Alfredson H, Pietilä T, Jonsson P, Lorentzon R. Heavy-load eccentric calf muscle training for the treatment of chronic Achilles tendinosis. Am J Sports Med 1998; 26: 360–366

[5] Purdam CR, Jonsson P, Alfredson H, Lorentzon R, Cook JL, Khan KM. A pilot study of the eccentric decline squat in the management of painful chronic patellar tendinopathy. Br J Sports Med 2004; 38: 395–397

[6] Zwerver J, Bredeweg SW, Hof AL. Biomechanical analysis of the single-leg decline squat. Br J Sports Med 2007; 41: 264–268, discussion 268

[7] Richards J, Thewlis D, Selfe J, Cunningham A, Hayes C. A biomechanical investigation of a single-limb squat: implications for lower extremity rehabilitation exercise. J Athl Train 2008; 43: 477–482

[8] Ekstrand J, Hägglund M, Waldén M. Epidemiology of muscle injuries in professional football (soccer). Am J Sports Med 2011; 39: 1226–1232

[9] Edin B. Cutaneous afferents provide information about knee joint movements in humans. J Physiol 2001; 531: 289–297

[10] Perlau R, Frank C, Fick G. The effect of elastic bandages on human knee proprioception on the uninjured population. Am J Sports Med 1995; 23: 251–255

[11] Corrigan JP, Cashman WF, Brady MP. Proprioception in the cruciate deficient knee. J Bone Joint Surg Br 1992; 74: 247–250

[12] Sanchis-Alfonso V, Rosello-Sastre E, Martinez-Sanjuan V. Pathogenesis of anterior knee pain syndrome and functional patellofemoral instability in the active young. Am J Knee Surg 1999; 12: 29–40

[13] Callaghan MJ, McKie S, Richardson P, Oldham JA. Effects of patellar taping on brain activity during knee joint proprioception tests using functional magnetic resonance imaging. Physical Therapy 2012; 92 (6):821-30. DOI: 10.2522/ptj.20110209

[14] Monga P. Three-dimensional analysis of shoulder movement patterns in shoulders with anterior instability: A comparison of kinematics with normal shoulders and the influence of stabilization surgery. MD Thesis, 2012. http://clok.uclan.ac.uk/9586/1/9586_Monga_ethesis2013.pdf

Further Reading

Hamill J, Knutzen KM. Biomechanical basis of human movement. 3 ed. Philadelphia: Wolters Kluwer/Lippincott Williams & Wilkins; 2008

Levine D, Richards J, Whittle MW. Whittle's Gait Analysis. 5th ed. London, UK: Churchill Livingstone; 2012

Richards J. Biomechanics in clinic and research. 1st ed. Edinburgh, UK: Elsevier; 2008

Zatsiorsky V, Prilutsky B. Biomechanics of skeletal muscles. 1st ed. Champaign, IL: Human Kinetics; 2012

16 Measurement Techniques

Dieter Rosenbaum

Clinical gait analysis has developed to a well-established method in centers specialized for the treatment of complex movement disorders in children and adults. With a set of different tools, the aim is to gain a better understanding for the human movement disorders of a patient, including the individual reasons and underlying causes for functional limitations that may have been caused by developmental disorders, diseases, or traumata.

While gait analysis requires considerable instrumental and personnel efforts, its value and efficacy is still subject to discussion. More recent reports underline the applicability for quality control issues as well as the importance for influencing clinical decision-making and planning of surgical interventions.[1,2]

The following clinically relevant aims may be addressed or achieved with clinical gait or motion analysis:

- Support of diagnostic possibilities
- Choice of the appropriate conservative or operative therapy
- Quality control of therapeutic interventions
- Follow-up of the course of the disease or healing process
- Prediction of the outcome of the chosen treatment option
- Objective outcome assessment in clinical trials

16.1 Methods and Technologies

16.1.1 Instrumented Three-Dimensional Gait Analysis

The standard tool for clinical movement analysis is the instrumented three-dimensional gait analysis. With the help of kinematic and kinetic parameters, it describes the gait characteristics of individual patients in detail and identifies potential gait asymmetries or movement impairments (i.e., it describes the quality of gait).

In instrumented gait analysis, the movement of a subject is typically being captured by an array of cameras that record the position of body-attached markers. The markers are applied at specific positions of predefined marker models (e.g., the two traditionally used Helen-Hayes (▶ Fig. 16.1) or Cleveland Clinic marker sets that have been described and extensively validated).[3,4] Recently, new models were proposed in order to prevent the known limitations or uncertainties of the traditional models by anatomically or functionally improved calibrations.[5]

> ### Key Concepts: Markers to Detect Body Movement
>
> Passive markers usually use reflective spheres that are attached to defined anatomical landmarks with adhesives and do not require any energy supply. Advantage is the cable-free attachment, disadvantage is that markers cannot be unequivocally identified (i.e., markers can be confused inadvertently).
>
> Active markers are usually light-emitting diodes that need an energy supply and are therefore cable-bound and more obstructive. However, due to a predefined order or frequency of the light signals, markers can always be identified unequivocally.

More recently, new approaches have been introduced that try to prevent the limitations that are involved in the use of markers by development of markerless tracking solutions. With standard video cameras, the outline of the moving object is automatically recognized against the invariable background of the image, and various directions of view eventually allow for a combination into a three-dimensional shape recognition of the moving subject.[6] The expectation was to use fairly low-cost instrumentation and apply it in normal environments (i.e., not necessarily laboratory-based) but to date, these systems are just beginning to appear on the commercial market.

The kinematic information obtained from image- or marker-based analysis can be combined with the assessment of ground reaction forces that describe the interaction between the human body and the environment during ground contact. The combination of kinematic or movement data with external loads enables the determination of the kinetic information. The external loads imposed on the body can be combined with the known position of the joint centers and the body's inertial properties (mass and moment of inertia) to calculate or estimate the joint moments and powers in the hip, knee, and ankle joint by using the inverse dynamics approach. For each phase of the gait cycle, the size and direction of the force vector as well as the location of the joint center are known and can be used to determine the external moments. Using optimization algorithms (see Chapter 19), the internal (muscular) moments can also be computed. This approach works typically very well in the sagittal (flexion/extension moments) and frontal (abduction/adduction moments) plane but usually not in the transverse plane.

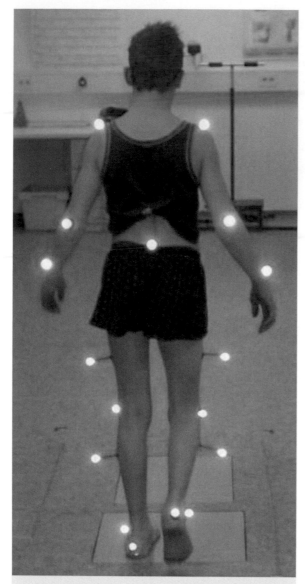

Fig. 16.1 Juvenile subject equipped with passive markers for instrumented gait analysis. Shown here is the ground contact with the left foot on the first of two ground reaction force plates for recording a complete gait cycle.

16.2 Advanced Technologies

Highly interesting data were obtained by in vivo measurements of patients equipped with instrumented prostheses of the hip and knee joint, and more recently also of the shoulder or spine implants. By telemetric transmission of strange gauge data imbedded in the prosthetic component, the information of implant loading during daily life activities, physiotherapy exercises, and sports was recorded from within the body and gave detailed insight based on direct measurements rather than model-based assumptions[7,8] so that comparisons between

calculated and measured hip joint contact forces were possible.[9]

Further methods allow for a more detailed description of the movement of the joint components but usually require some kind of imaging that may mean potentially harmful exposure to ionizing radiation. The imaging is being used to create a three-dimensional model of the joint partners. In fluoroscopic images, the outline of the bone or joint prosthesis is being detected and matched to the three-dimensional model for each captured image. This technology was initially developed for the assessment of knee joint replacements and relied on the engineering data of the prosthetic components, but it can now be used with computed tomography or magnetic resonance imaging of the anatomical joints (e.g., Chen et al[10]). Here, two fluoroscopic images with different views are necessary to recreate the exact joint position in space. These systems are mostly used for measuring kinematics of the knee joint or knee replacement, with recent approaches being developed for foot and ankle assessments. A limitation is the temporal resolution of the fluoroscope as well as the limited space that either restricts measurements to detecting only one step/movement cycle or requires a treadmill for stationary recording of a sequence of steps.

The modeling world is trying to advance from general models (often based on data on the Visible Human Project) toward developing personalized neuromuscular-skeletal models, also based on imaging, which can be used for predictions (e.g., Viceconti et al[11]). However, this very elaborate approach is probably quite some distance away from being easily incorporated into something like a clinical routine application.

16.3 Pedobarography

A specific kinetic assessment tool is the measurement of plantar pressure distribution during standing or walking, the so-called pedobarography. This can either be used for barefoot loading assessment with pressure distribution platforms or for shod walking with in-shoe measurements using insoles between foot and shoe or orthotic. Barefoot measurements (▶ Fig. 16.2) are used to evaluate the basic foot function during static and dynamic loading, whereas in-shoe measurements can be used to evaluate the effects of shoes or orthopedic devices.

In contrast to ground reaction force measurements, measurement of pressure enables only the vertical component of the force to be assessed. However, the spatial resolution provided by pedobarographic devices has the advantage of providing local information on the distribution of the force. Thus, the loading of different foot regions or anatomical structures can be differentiated. In essence, it is a local force measurement; with the knowledge about the size of the sensing element, the locally acting pressure can be calculated. Therefore, it is

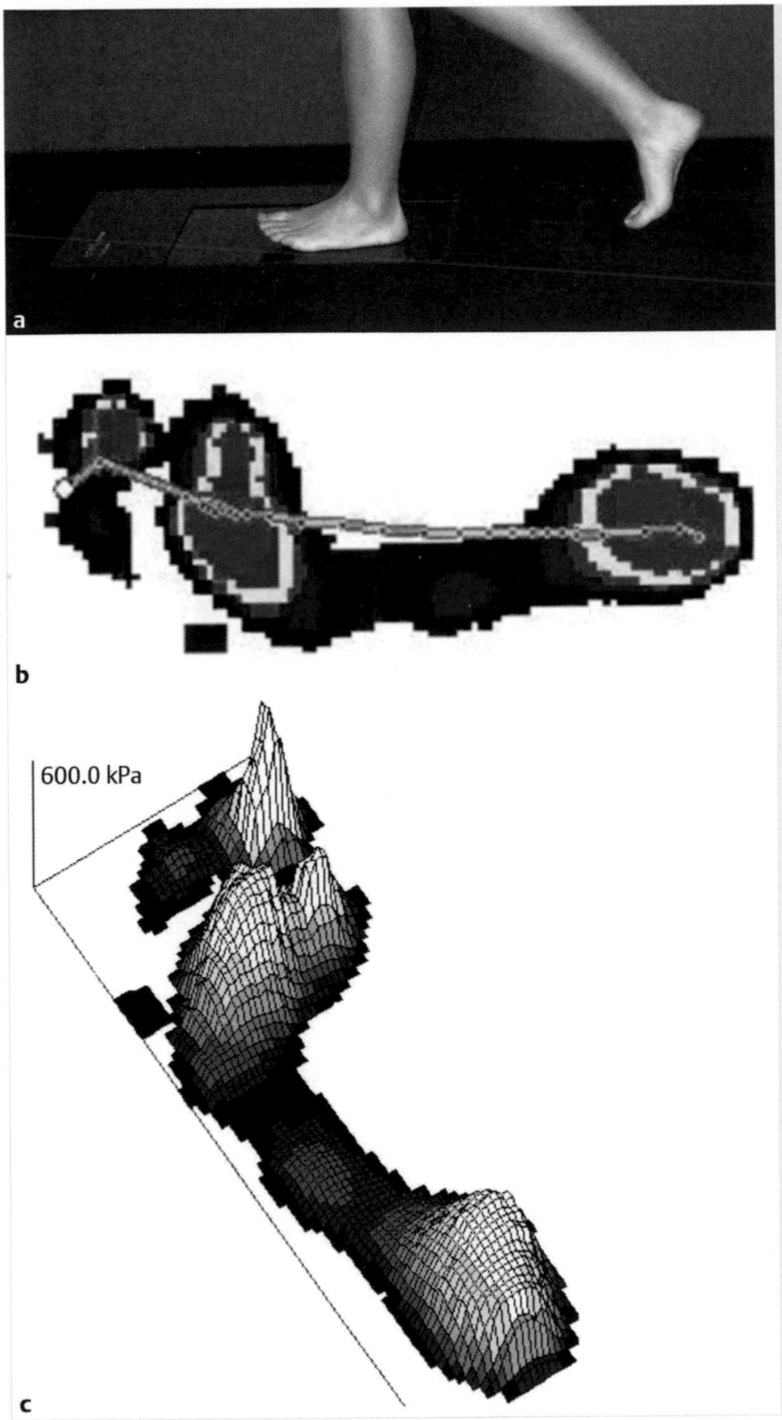

Fig. 16.2 (a) Subject during barefoot pedo-barography on the Emed ST-4 platform (novel GmbH, Munich, Germany), contacting the sensor area with the left foot. The result of the measurement is the pressure distribution underneath the foot. Shown here is a color-coded image, the so-called maximum pressure picture (b), and the three-dimensional, gray-scaled "pressure mountain" representation (c).

comprehensible that the higher the spatial resolution, the more detailed pressure differences can be detected; with larger sensor sizes, the actual pressure is distributed over a larger area and usually tends to be lower than with smaller sensors.

The information obtained with pressure distribution measurements can be used to analyze foot-related problems caused by nonphysiologically increased pressure peaks or excessive loading of foot regions that could be treated (e.g., by redistributing forces by individually shaped orthotics).

16.4 Electromyography

If information about the underlying causes of human movement is required, we need to investigate the muscles as the "effector organs" by means of electromyography.

Key Concepts: Electromyography

Electromyography (EMG) detects the bioelectric activity produced during muscle contractions and converts the fairly low-amplitude signals by amplification and a certain amount of signal processing to electric signals that can be digitally recorded and stored. Surface EMG, which is applicable for larger muscle groups that are just covered by a layer of skin and subcutaneous tissues that are not electrically active, uses electrodes attached to the skin overlying the respective muscle groups. Fine-wire or needle EMG with in-dwelling electrodes that are placed inside the muscle of interest can be applied for smaller and deeper muscles.

Usually, the raw EMG signals are stored and subsequently postprocessed (e.g., with various filtering, rectifying, and averaging techniques). For cyclic movements as in gait analysis applications, repeated cycles of EMG activity can be averaged to obtain a linear envelope that indicates the average muscle activity pattern during the respective activity. For quantitative comparisons, some kind of amplitude normalization is required as the amplitude can vary greatly due to the signal attenuating effect of the subcutaneous tissues. The processed signals can be evaluated with respect to their timing (when is the muscle "on" or "off"), amplitude (how high is the muscle activity in a certain phase of the movement), or frequency content (information about the degree of fatigue within a muscle). A comparison of agonists and antagonists can give insight into the coordination between muscle groups as well as the degree of co-contraction that may indicate a more or less skilled level of motor control. New techniques like principal component analyses or wavelet analyses have been developed and applied to visualize and analyze an even deeper level of information content of the complex stochastic signals when the conventional analyses do not provide enough insights.

16.5 Activities of Daily Living Measurements

Finally, the tools for movement analysis outside a gait laboratory should be mentioned. It has been acknowledged that laboratory-based gait analysis gives insights into the patient's performance under well-controlled conditions. However, it might also be interesting to find out how well patients are able to use their potential in daily life and how (un-)limited mobility and independence might be. This can be assessed by sensors that can be worn by the patients (e.g., at the waist, leg, and/or arm) without causing any restrictions in the activities of daily life. Depending on the chosen monitor, these devices can provide simple, straightforward parameters like the daily number (and intensity) of steps, the activity profile with time periods (or percentages) spent with dynamic activities and in different body postures, or an estimation of the energy expenditure during more or less long-term observation periods of up to several weeks. This kind of information allows objective assessment of the general behavior and physical activity level of patients in their natural environment. It may be used to monitor the healing or rehabilitation process after conservative or surgical treatment; to control the achievement of guidelines with respect to leading a healthy, active lifestyle (comparative data and generally accepted recommendations are available); or as a means of self-controlling by the patients themselves who might want to reach certain activity levels.

In comparison to the laboratory-based assessment of gait quality, these tools may provide information about the gait quantity in daily life.

16.6 Conclusion

The high demand with respect to instrumentation and personnel may have prevented a more widespread application of clinical gait analysis in daily practice. Therefore, the new developments like markerless tracking may come with the prospect for easier and less expensive instrumentation, which would be interesting and applicable also for less advanced and specialized centers. The combination of laboratory-based functional measurements and assessment of physical activities in daily life may offer a valuable level of information about the individual patient's gait quality and quantity, which sheds light on his or her limitations or rehabilitation of gait and mobility after a disease or injury and the respective conservative, medical, or surgical treatment.

References

[1] Wren TA, Gorton GE III, Ounpuu S, Tucker CA. Efficacy of clinical gait analysis: a systematic review. Gait Posture 2011; 34: 149–153
[2] Wren TA, Otsuka NY, Bowen RE et al. Influence of gait analysis on decision-making for lower extremity orthopaedic surgery: baseline data from a randomized controlled trial. Gait Posture 2011; 34: 364–369
[3] Kadaba MP, Ramakrishnan HK, Wootten ME. Measurement of lower extremity kinematics during level walking. J Orthop Res 1990; 8: 383–392
[4] Kadaba MP, Ramakrishnan HK, Wootten ME, Gainey J, Gorton G, Cochran GVB. Repeatability of kinematic, kinetic, and electromyographic data in normal adult gait. J Orthop Res 1989; 7: 849–860
[5] Leardini A, Sawacha Z, Paolini G, Ingrosso S, Nativo R, Benedetti MG. A new anatomically based protocol for gait analysis in children. Gait Posture 2007; 26: 560–571

[6] Corazza S, Mündermann L, Chaudhari AM, Demattio T, Cobelli C, Andriacchi TP. A markerless motion capture system to study musculoskeletal biomechanics: visual hull and simulated annealing approach. Ann Biomed Eng 2006; 34: 1019–1029

[7] Bergmann G, Graichen F, Rohlmann A, Linke H. Hip joint forces during load carrying. Clin Orthop Relat Res 1997: 190–201

[8] Bergmann G, Rohlmann A, Graichen F. In vivo Messung der Hüftgelenkbelastung. 1. Teil: Krankengymnastik. Z Orthop Ihre Grenzgeb 1989; 127: 672–679

[9] Stansfield BW, Nicol AC, Paul JP, Kelly IG, Graichen F, Bergmann G. Direct comparison of calculated hip joint contact forces with those measured using instrumented implants. An evaluation of a three-dimensional mathematical model of the lower limb. J Biomech 2003; 36: 929–936

[10] Chen CH, Li JS, Hosseini A, Gadikota HR, Gill TJ, Li G. Anteroposterior stability of the knee during the stance phase of gait after anterior cruciate ligament deficiency. Gait Posture 2012; 35: 467–471

[11] Viceconti M, Taddei F, Cristofolini L, Martelli S, Falcinelli C, Schileo E. Are spontaneous fractures possible? An example of clinical application for personalised, multiscale neuro-musculo-skeletal modelling. J Biomech 2012; 45: 421–426

Further Reading

Baker R. The history of gait analysis before the advent of modern computers. Gait Posture 2007;26(3):331–342 (Comment: A valuable historical perspective)

Basmajian JV, De Luca CJ. Muscles alive, their functions revealed by electromyography, 5 e. Baltimore, MD: Williams & Wilkins; 1985 (Comment: The classic monograph on electromyography)

Perry J. Gait analysis. Normal and pathological function. Thorofare, NJ: Slack Inc.; 1992 (Comment: A good basic reference for clinical gait analysis)

17 Clinical Assessment of Function

David Hamilton

Orthopedic interventions are assessed on their outcome. Various outcome scores are commonly used to compare prostheses, surgical techniques, postoperative care, and also in auditing departments or individual surgeons. Functional outcome, though imperative to the patient, is only superficially considered in most studies. Survival curves, for example, are the standard long-term evaluation of arthroplasty implant longevity. This analysis is rightly criticized, however, as not adequately defining the failure of the implant or commenting on the function of the patient prior to the diagnosis of failure.[1]

Any structured evaluation of an individual's performance can be a functional assessment. These can be simple questionnaires or complex biomechanical models of gait analysis. The latter situation is not discussed in this chapter, because it is covered elsewhere in this book (see Chapters 15 and 16).

17.1 What Is Function?

Physical function has long been considered an important aspect of the individual's quality of life; indeed, the quote "motion is life" is attributed to Hippocrates. Function, though, is not simple to define as it refers not just to motion, but the ability to perform unaided controlled voluntary and purposeful activity within a social context. This is reflected in the World Health Organization's definition of health as a state of complete physical mental and social well-being—not merely the absence of symptoms. Functional activity encompasses the tasks and activities that a person performs, ranging from fundamental activities such as eating and locomotion through to work, recreational activities, and sport.

17.2 Assessing Function

The difficulty in assessing the function of an individual is in the breadth of the definition of function. There is really no limit to what can be tested: range of joint motion, muscle strength, time taken to perform tasks, posture, balance, proprioception, and motor skills/coordination. This can comprise assessment of walking, running, hopping, kneeling, lunging, pushing, pulling, gripping, and so on. It is vital to consider the context in which function applies to the subject or patient being tested; elderly fracture patients with multiple comorbidities and chronic diseases require a very different type of functional assessment than the young knee arthroscopy patient. It should also be recognized that in a clinical context what we really wish to measure is not function, but dysfunction—or how far removed from the patient's "normal function" the individual is as a result of his or her condition, or indeed our treatment of it.

17.3 Measuring Function

Though there are potentially infinite physical tests, broadly speaking there are two ways in which to assess the function of a patient: Ask them or measure them.

> ### Jargon Simplified: Patient-Reported Outcome Measures
>
> Scoring systems that are assessor-based (i.e., completed by the medical team) clearly carry some subjective bias, and use of these has been criticized.[2] Patients are thought to offer a complimentary perspective to that of the clinician into the effectiveness of health care. Clinicians can make observations as to the patient's impairment and disability, but only the patient can report on his or her quality of life.[3] Advocates of these patient-reported outcome measures say that they provide a remarkably sophisticated measure of whether a treatment has worked in the (important) sense of whether the patient feels better, and how much better.[4]

Self-report assessments are ones in which individuals are asked to report their perceived level of functioning during daily activities described in standardized questions.[5] Broadly, these questionnaires fall into three categories: generic health assessments, disease-specific instruments, and joint-specific tools. Generic scores allow comparison across different disorders and surgeries but may not be sensitive to detect specific functional changes. Disease-specific scores may be more sensitive to change following intervention but lack generalizability across different groups. Another criticism of disease-specific scores is that they cannot isolate the function of individual joints. As such, if one wishes to assess patient function, following joint arthroplasty for example, an arthritis-specific score could be used, but this would assess the overall pain and function of the individual, and be influenced by pain and dysfunction in other joints. Joint-specific scores, then, are the most commonly employed tools following interventions to individual joints. Clearly, however, these apply only to the joint in question. A combination of these scores may then form the best outcome analysis.[2,6] Much has been written about these self-report scores, and a good review can be found in Clinical Research for Surgeons (part of this series) (see Further Reading).

Patient-reported outcome measures are commonly used as they are comparatively cheap, effective at collecting large volumes of data, and do not require fol-low-up clinic visits to achieve this. A disadvantage of these patient report–based scales for assessing postope-rative function is that what they actually measure is the patient's perception of their function and are thus subjec-tive.[6,7] As a consequence, they are thought to be highly influenced by pain, which affects their content valid-ity.[5,6,7] High levels of content validity are required to eval-uate biomechanical aspects of function, and generally, performance-based measures demonstrate this.

17.4 Performance Measures

Terwee et al[5] define a performance measure as one in which the individual is asked to perform an activity that is evaluated in a standardized manner using predefined criteria, such as time taken. Essentially any activity can be a test of function, as long as it is conducted in a reprodu-cible fashion with a defined start and end to the test and some way to quantify the result. Various tests have been proposed and many validated for calculating the limita-tions conferred by specific conditions or for assessing improvement following a particular surgery. Typical examples include simple walking or step tests (measured either in distance or time), or more demanding activity such as treadmill or cycle ergometer protocols. Composite measures that employ assessment of multiple activities are thought to be more valid than those that assess only one aspect of function such as walking tests; an example being patients with mild osteoarthritis who are unaf-fected during walking but may have difficulty in climbing stairs or rising from chairs.[5] There are various multiactiv-ity tests that have been validated for use in specific situa-tions. In general, these are broadly very similar to each other and no one combination has proven more effective than another.

17.5 Activities of Daily Living

Again, a variety of measures are available to the research-er with which to assess the impact of the disease/proce-dure on the patient's daily activity. A simple analysis can be conducted with tools such as the Barthel Index, which assesses the ability of the patient to complete 10 activ-ities of daily living independently, with a score awarded out of 100 (representing complete independence). Activ-ities of daily living include feeding, toileting, bathing, dressing, walking on a level surface, and transferring. Clearly, this is aimed at the more disabled patient, per-haps one on a protracted hospital ward stay following a hip fracture.

Walking ability and exercise tolerance can be readily measured in a laboratory or outpatient setting, but this is often not representative or realistic of the daily activity undertaken at home. Activity diaries have been widely used in a rehabilitation context to try to monitor this,

though they have proven somewhat unreliable. More recently, portable accelerometers have been developed with which to record the patient's movements. Various models are available that can assess the amount of time the patient spends walking, standing, or sitting; daily energy expenditure can be calculated from this. While relatively unobtrusive, because they are generally attached to clothing or worn against the skin with adhe-sive tape, these are of course more expensive and require charging and cleaning between patient uses.

17.6 Muscle Strength

Muscle strength is often assessed as a marker of function-al ability, primarily as wastage or weakness that often accompanies musculoskeletal disorders and is associated with reduced levels of function. Additionally, this is often the focus of rehabilitative efforts following surgery; change in strength can be used as a measure of treatment effect. There are advantages to assessing strength as opposed to function as this is more readily generalizable across groups and can be measured on a continuous scale for ease of analysis. Strength is thought to reflect func-tional ability, particularly in the lower limb where a rea-sonable correlation between strength and walking ability has been consistently demonstrated.[6,8]

17.6.1 Ways to Measure Strength

Muscle strength is actually a complex term. There are dif-ferent aspects of strength and corresponding ways to assess these. Most straightforwardly, strength can be con-sidered in terms of being static or dynamic. Isometric contractions refer to applying or generating force without movement (such as in a clinical exam), whereas isotonic contractions (both concentric, shortening the muscle, and eccentric, lengthening the muscle) involve generation of force throughout movement. Functional activity generally involves both of these types of muscle contraction.

The length of the muscle is directly related to how much force can be generated. Broadly, the maximal force can be applied at the midpoint of a muscle contraction where the largest numbers of actin and myosin filaments are overlapped. Detailed description of the structure and function of muscle is outside the scope of this chapter, though it is well covered in physiology textbooks (see Further Reading).

Even within seemingly specific muscle strength tests, there are a plethora of potential measures: maximal vol-untary contraction, endurance profile, number of repeti-tions at specific weights or percentages of maximal muscle force, coordination, stabilizing function, and many more. Peak values are generally reported, which is useful if the purpose of testing is to assess the maximal force ge-neration; however, the mean value and standard devia-tion are more representative values of "functional ability."

Table 17.1 Scores for the Manual Testing of Muscle Strength Oxford/Medical Research Council Scale

Grade	Description
0	No contraction
1	Flicker or trace contraction
2	Active movement throughout range with gravity counterbalanced
3	Active movement through range against gravity
4	Active movement through range against gravity and some resistance
5	Normal power
Daniels and Worthington	
Normal	Motion through range against gravity and maximal force
Good	Motion through full range against gravity and less than maximal force
Fair	Motion through range against gravity
Fair (−)	Motion through at least half range but not complete against gravity
Poor (+)	Impaired against gravity, but does not reach half the available range
Poor	Motion through full range with gravity diminished
Poor (−)	Motion through partial range with gravity diminished
Trace	Palpable contraction but no movement
Zero	No palpable contraction

17.6.2 Strength Testing

The simplest way to assess strength is by manual muscle testing, as is typically done in a musculoskeletal examination. There are many different scales to categorize findings of manual testing, common scores include the Oxford/Medical Research Council scale[9] and Daniels and Worthington[10] (▶ Table 17.1). These scales test strength through the range that the muscle moves the joint.

These tools rank on an ordinal scale from no contraction through to maximal resistance, which is generally accepted to equal the contralateral limb or another person of the same sex and build age category as the patient. This results in a largely subjective assessment, applying categorical values. The Oxford/Medical Research Council scale records on a linear scale from 0 to 5, though the magnitude of change between grades is not necessarily consistent. There is a lack of sensitivity with very broad categories that has resulted in many applying a plus or minus to subdivide the categories, further questioning the usefulness of this evaluation, because intratester reliability is of particular concern.

Handheld Dynamometry

Patients simply apply a force to the dynamometer, which gives a reading. These are easy to use and provide a more objective assessment of the force generated. Handheld dynamometers are designed to measure isometric force. The subject is asked to apply maximal force by pushing, pulling, or squeezing the device, and the results are recorded via a gauge or digital display that provides a numerical value. Several studies have been conducted to examine the reliability of these instruments, and the general report is of excellent results. Standardization of the test procedure is the main difficulty, especially when testing the large muscle groups that cross multiple joints.

Isokinetic Dynamometry

This is a slightly different form of muscle strength testing. The basic principle of isokinetic dynamometry is that a machine moves a lever arm around a fixed axis at a constant angular velocity but does not apply resistance. The subject tries to push or pull the lever arm as it moves through the range, and torque is measured where the limb attempts to move the arm beyond the preset speed. This allows a muscle group to be maximally loaded throughout the range of motion. Though work, power, or fatigue can be calculated, peak torque is must commonly reported and is defined as the highest point on the generated torque curve (usually expressed in Newton meters). Various studies have shown that age, sex, height, and weight all affect peak torque and should thus be taken into account in any analysis, especially between subjects.

Advantages of this type of analysis are that it is objective and readily quantifiable. Additionally, maximal muscle strength is not restricted by weakest part of range (as it is with concentric through range testing). However, while modern systems are user friendly, they are large, complex, time-restrictive, and expensive. Realistically, only those with access to an existing research facility will be able to utilize such detailed measurement tools. A particular disadvantage of these systems when considering functional assessment is that the movement produced by the machine is artificial, as natural movement does not occur at fixed angular velocities.

17.7 Power Output

Power output (particularly in the lower limb) is thought to be more reflective of function than absolute strength due to the role of velocity of movement in everyday tasks.[8] This is simply the ability to quickly generate force throughout a movement, and it is clearly important in rising from a chair or climbing the stairs.

Devices such as the Nottingham Leg Extensor Power Rig[11] have been widely used in population studies and particularly in orthopedic cohorts. This device is pictured and consists of a chair and pedal connected to a flywheel

(▶ Fig. 17.1). The patient depresses the pedal to full extension of the knee, which turns the wheel. From the velocity, a power output can be determined.

17.7.1 Relationship between Self-Report of Function and Measured Function

Self-report questionnaires and performance measures assess different aspects of physical function. It has been

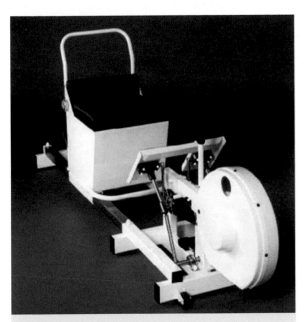

Fig. 17.1 Stock picture of Leg Extension Power Rig from Nottingham University (Nottingham, UK).

suggested that in terms of expressing the difficulty patients have in moving around or looking after themselves, self-report measures provide information concerning the experience associated with doing the task, whereas performance measures confer information about the ability to do the task.[7]

One assessment type should perhaps not be considered preferential to the other, as they provide distinct but complementary information. This is akin to the suggestion that generic and specific patient-reported outcome measures should be employed. The choice of assessment tools depends on a variety of factors relating to the aim of the study, level of detail of observation required, funding, and the context of the study. A theoretical framework for assessing functional outcome in the orthopedic context is displayed, highlighting the way levels of information can be sought.[6] Radiographs assess the mechanical function of the fracture or implant, physical tests assess the function of the limb, and patient report tools confer the wider ability of the individual to function in society (▶ Fig. 17.2).

The specific research question will determine which level of information is required, though for comprehensive analysis, it may be that all should be represented.

17.8 Choosing the Test

In the absence of specific recommendations, the researcher is free to determine which test is performed. In addition to considering the available facilities and the general abilities of the patient group in question, it is often useful to assess the associated literature and consider making the same measurements as other groups, as this facilitates later meta-analysis.

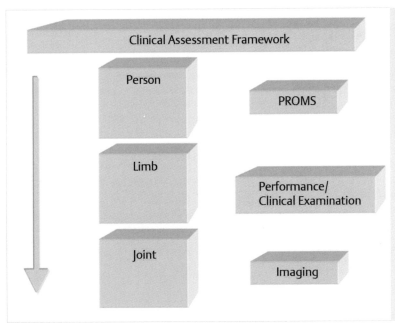

Fig. 17.2 Framework loosely based on the World Health Organization classification of impairment, disability, and handicaps encompassing three levels: the joint, its function within the limb, and its function within the person. Different assessments are required to ascertain information about these different levels. Assessing the implant requires imaging, performance data assesses the function of the limb, and patient-reported data reflects the individual's perception of his or her overall function. PROMS, patient-reported outcome measures.

The key question is whether the proposed test is appropriate to use in the suggested context; is it valid, sensitive, and reliable?

> **Key Concepts: Quality Measures of a Test**
>
> Validity is whether the test actually measures what it pertains to, sensitivity refers to the ability of the test to discriminate the changes that it is trying to detect, and reliability broadly refers to the accuracy and reproducibility of the test—these concepts are well covered elsewhere (see Further Reading). Further questions should be asked regarding the validity of physical tests and performance measures. The validity of the information arising from the test depends on three factors: the patient, the tester, and the instrument.

All patient performance tests rely on voluntary effort. The patient must then understand what is being requested and be willing and able to complete the test. Standardized assessment protocols are required to achieve this, specifying, for example, alignment of the testing device, patient and tester positions, verbal instructions, method of any encouragement given, etc. It is also important to consider any influence of the specific condition being assessed. Common issues in orthopedic research are the influence of pain and of fixed flexion deformities. These can affect the ability of the patient to perform the test and may limit comparison with other patients or the wider literature. Patient groups are likely to have medical comorbidities that must also be controlled for in the analysis.

17.9 Interpretation of Findings

A note of warning: It is easy to overinterpret the findings of functional assessments and assume that the data obtained through a specific test represents the much wider ability of the patient to function in society. The test simply measures the ability of the patient to perform a task in the manner tested at that time—the patient may not be able to repeat it due to pain, comorbidity, or indeed volition. The other concept of particular importance is that of the normal control. For example, comparing the strength of the (operated) left arm against the (uninjured) right depends entirely on the "normality" of that contralateral limb. Previous injury, comorbidity (such as stroke), or even a pronounced dominance may substantially limit the validity of such observations.

17.10 Conclusion

There is no agreement as to which functional tests should be performed for orthopedic clinical analysis or for research purposes. This allows great flexibility for the researcher, but requires an understanding of the possible options to make an informed choice. The only limit to the functional assessments that can be preformed is the researcher's imagination, though standardization of test parameters is vital to ensure validity. If possible, a test already validated for the clinical population in question is preferable. Function is complex to assess, and particular attention must be paid to the appropriateness to the measure chosen to contextualize the functioning of the patient.

References

[1] Price AJ, Longino D, Rees J et al. Are pain and function better measures of outcome than revision rates after TKR in the younger patient? Knee 2010; 17: 196–199

[2] Beard DJ, Knezevic K, Al-Ali S, Dawson J, Price AJ. The use of outcome measures relating to the knee. Orthopaedics & Trauma 2010; 24: 309–316

[3] Black N, Jenkinson C. How can patients' views of their care enhance quality improvement? BMJ 2009; 339: 202–205

[4] Timmins N. NHS goes to the PROMS. BMJ 2008; 336: 1464–1465

[5] Terwee CB, van der Slikke RM, van Lummel RC, Benink RJ, Meijers WG, de Vet HC. Self-reported physical functioning was more influenced by pain than performance-based physical functioning in knee-osteoarthritis patients. J Clin Epidemiol 2006; 59: 724–731

[6] Hamilton DF, Gaston P, Simpson AHRW. Is patient reporting of physical function accurate following total knee replacement? J Bone Joint Surg Br 2012; 94: 1506–1510

[7] Stratford PW, Kennedy DM. Performance measures were necessary to obtain a complete picture of osteoarthritic patients. J Clin Epidemiol 2006; 59: 160–167

[8] Marsh AP, Miller ME, Saikin AM et al. Lower extremity strength and power are associated with 400-meter walk time in older adults: the InCHIANTI study. J Gerontol A Biol Sci Med Sci 2006; 61: 1186–1193

[9] MRC. Aids to the examination of the peripheral nervous system. Memorandum No. 45 HMSO. London: Medical Research Council; 1976

[10] Daniels L, Worthington C. Muscle testing: technique of manual examination. 4 e. Philadelphia: W.B. Saunders; 1980

[11] Bassey EJ, Short AH. A new method for measuring power output in a single leg extension: feasibility, reliability and validity. Eur J Appl Physiol Occup Physiol 1990; 60: 385–390

Further Reading

Bhandari M, Joensson A. Understanding outcome measurement. In: Bhandari M, Joensson A. Clinical research for surgeons. Stuttgart: Thieme; 2009:101–116

Spurway NC. Muscle. In: Maughan RJ. Basic and applied sciences for sports medicine. Oxford: Butterworth-Heinemann; 1999:1–47

Terwee CB, Mokkink LB, Steultjens MPM, Dekker J. Performance-based methods for measuring the physical function of patients with osteoarthritis of the hip or knee: a systematic review of measurement properties. Rheumatology (Oxford) 2006; 45: 890–902

18 Functional Biomechanics with Cadaver Specimens

Camilla Halewood, Punyawang Lumpaopong, J.M. Stephen, and Andrew A. Amis

Cadaver specimens are a powerful tool for biomechanical testing when it is difficult to control or measure the movements or forces of interest in joints or soft tissues in vivo. Donated specimens allow researchers to better understand a vast array of biomechanical themes, including functional anatomy, pathology, joint motion, material properties of human tissue, and consequences of arthroplasty. Cadaver specimens perform a vital role in preclinical testing of new surgical techniques and implant designs, and can be used to validate computer simulations. Pairs of specimens can often be used in conjunction, with one acting as a control. In some cases, it is possible to have intraspecimen controls, where various interventions are performed on the same specimen, making direct and multiple comparisons possible and eliminating some specimen variability.

Key Concepts: Ethical Issues

The use of cadaveric specimens in medical research has been an integral part of increasing understanding of human body mechanics for many years. Ethical approval should be obtained prior to conducting experimental studies on specimens to ensure donated bodies are used in a responsible manner and for a meaningful purpose. Cadaveric specimens for research purposes can be obtained from hospitals directly where informed consent must be sought from family members of the deceased, or through donor banks where individuals donate their body and a fee can be paid to cover processing costs by registered institutions. Legislation regarding the storage and management of cadaveric tissue varies from country to country and is tightly regulated; therefore, individuals should check with local authorities prior to commencing experiments.

18.1 Specimen Management

Human tissue decomposes if left in an open air environment, and therefore cadavers are commonly preserved using two methods: in a fresh frozen state or in an embalmed state. In the frozen state, tissue should be stored below −20°C and be completely defrosted at room temperature prior to use. Defrosting can take 24 hours or more depending on the size of the specimen. Freezing has been shown not to have a significant effect on collagenous tissue properties[1] or on compression and torsional strength of bone. An alternative to freezing is tissue embalming, where formaldehyde is used either alone or in combination with other fixative agents. The fixation process acts by increasing crosslinks within and between collagen fibers, altering the action of defleshing agents

and subsequent tissue decomposition. Although embalming has the potential to prolong tissue usage, there are a number of disadvantages of its use. During biomechanical testing, embalmed specimens have been found to result in loss of range of motion due to tissue stiffening, and there is strong evidence that formalin significantly alters the mechanical behavior of the ligaments and bone, meaning formalin-fixed specimens are not representative of in vivo conditions. Care must therefore be used by the researcher in deciding which preservation method is most appropriate to meet the research objectives of the planned experiment.

Responsible laboratory management of cadavers is vital to prevent tissue decomposition and enable as close as possible comparison to be made with in vivo tissue. Stress relaxation tests have identified that changes in water content influence the viscoelastic behavior of soft tissues, with dehydration found to cause increased stiffness, and overhydration resulting in increased tissue compliance. The effect on creep (the increase in strain with the tissue under sustained or repeated stress) has also been investigated, and although effects were found to be reversible, exposure of ligamentous tissue to sucrose (to cause tissue dehydration) and phosphate buffered saline solutions (to cause tissue overhydration) caused decreased and increased tissue creep, respectively. Water-rich structures such as the menisci and articular cartilage have been found to lose height and thickness following only 1 hour of exposure to air, and the mechanical properties of intervertebral disks have been found to have a significant dependence on hydration. These findings should act as a caution to the researcher to take care when managing tissue in the laboratory setting. A protocol to ensure appropriate monitoring of cadaver tissue hydration is necessary to ensure validity and reliability of experimental results; this may include regular spraying of specimens with a wet solution. If the specimens are thin, testing them in a 100% humid environment may be an option.[1]

18.2 Experimental Design

The correct choice of hardware and measuring instruments for use with cadaveric specimens is crucial and must be done with the objectives of the study in mind. In general, cadaveric biomechanical studies on osteosynthesis are done to determine mechanical properties (e.g., stiffness, fixation strength, the number of load cycles to failure, and the stability of fixation methods). Three experimental stages are usually carried out to compare biomechanical responses: (1) the intact specimen; (2) after osteotomy, fracture creation, or soft tissue resection; and (3) after surgical intervention or repair.

18.2.1 Experimental Hardware

The anatomical part that is to be studied and the objectives of the experiment both play an important role in the design of the test rig. In general, most studies require the design and construction of a new test rig that can best simulate the biomechanics of the anatomical part for a particular experiment. Major design considerations include desirable range of motion and loading conditions: types of loads (static, dynamic, cyclic, etc.); loading direction (axial, torsional, bending, etc.); magnitudes of loads (e.g., physiological or most unfavorable); and loading methods (e.g., direct to the bone or via muscle pulling). Test rigs can be configured to include a newly designed loading apparatus (▶ Fig. 18.1a). The design can vary from a very simple hanging-weight mechanism to more sophisticated mechanisms consisting of several servohydraulic or pneumatic actuators. For studies aiming to determine mechanical properties or those in which load or displacement is to be controlled, test rigs are commonly used on universal materials testing machines (UTMs) (▶ Fig. 18.1b), equipped with load cells for force measurement. With UTMs, loads can be applied to bones at a variety of different rates and magnitudes as desired, either until specimen failure or between preset limits of load or displacement. It must be noted that the selection and use of UTMs and load cells must be done with awareness of their specifications and limitations of use. In particular, they should be able to reproduce physiological strain rates when simulating injuries, because of the rate-dependence of tissue properties. Many university engineering departments will have these machines.

Mounting a specimen in a test rig usually requires custom-designed jigs and fixtures. This is because most standard gripping accessories are not suitable for gripping bone or soft tissues. Bone specimens such as the proximal humerus or distal tibia are usually held in cylindrical or rectangular-shaped metallic pots by means of acrylic bone cement or screws, or a combination of the two. It may also be necessary to make an alignment fixture to ensure that the specimen is mounted with a desired orientation, so that consistent loading conditions are attained as desired. An example of this might be, for example, that a femur is mounted so that the path of an axial compressive load passes from the center of the head of the femur to the center of the knee. Depending on the objectives of the test, mounting blocks can be designed to provide complete immobilization of the socket or to allow socket movements in certain directions (degrees of freedom), depending on allowable motions of each end of the test specimens. This may be important to avoid the mounting "locking-in" unwanted bending effects when the specimen tries to deform under load. In some cases, mounting blocks are also designed so that their positions are adjustable. When designing a test that loads the joint directly, without additional muscle forces (as in

▶ Fig. 18.1b), then data on joint forces that have been obtained from instrumented prostheses in vivo are available to download from www.orthoload.com.

The manner in which muscle forces are implemented in a cadaveric experiment is often important, because most of joint force arises from the muscles, rather than from body weight. The rig shown in ▶ Fig. 18.1a, for example, includes the action of the quadriceps simulated by means of cables attached to the individual muscle heads close to the patella. The cables are tensed by taking them over pulleys to hanging weights, which are simple and accurate for constant loading. The directions and magnitudes of muscle tension must be derived from the anatomy/physiology/biomechanics literature, for example by sharing the forces among a group of co-contracting muscles by using published data on physiological cross-sectional areas, then scaling the tensions by reference to data on the intensity of electromyographic signals during the relevant physical activity in vivo. Variable tensions may be simulated most easily by using pneumatic cylinders with calibrated air pressure regulators. Advice should be sought from a mechanical design engineer, because there are several other ways to load the specimen, including servohydraulic cylinders, springs, or electromagnetic actuators for example, in order to obtain reliable data in the easiest manner.

18.2.2 Measuring Instruments

Intrinsic material properties of tissues and structural responses of specimens are two major groups of parameters usually determined in cadaveric studies (▶ Table 18.1). When using a UTM, mechanical properties such as stiffness, strength, and toughness can be obtained by processing load and deformation data obtained from the integrated load cell. The UTM will most likely output force-displacement information, but that may include artifacts caused by the mounting method. For accurate localized strain information in the tissue, a clip-on or video extensometer, digital image correlation system or strain gauges should be used in conjunction with the UTM. Strain gauges can be used when more accurate strain measurements in a few critical regions are required. Optical strain measurements avoid artefacts caused by attaching instruments to soft tissues.

Measuring mechanical responses usually requires extra instrumentation. For example, custom-designed rigs may require force and/or torque transducers to measure the loads actually exerted on the specimen by loading actuators. Moreover, osteosynthesis studies usually focus on assessment of biomechanical stability of fracture fixation, which relates to the measurement of relative rotational and translational movements between two fracture fragments (interfragmentary motion) or between fragments and implants such as metal plates, screws, and intramedullary nails. For measuring translational and rotational

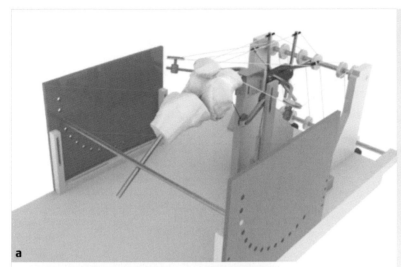

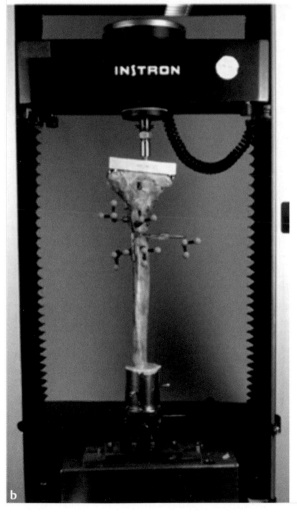

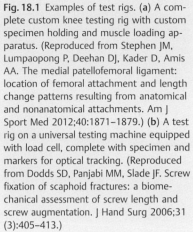

Fig. 18.1 Examples of test rigs. (**a**) A complete custom knee testing rig with custom specimen holding and muscle loading apparatus. (Reproduced from Stephen JM, Lumpaopong P, Deehan DJ, Kader D, Amis AA. The medial patellofemoral ligament: location of femoral attachment and length change patterns resulting from anatomical and nonanatomical attachments. Am J Sport Med 2012;40:1871–1879.) (**b**) A test rig on a universal testing machine equipped with load cell, complete with specimen and markers for optical tracking. (Reproduced from Dodds SD, Panjabi MM, Slade JF. Screw fixation of scaphoid fractures: a biomechanical assessment of screw length and screw augmentation. J Hand Surg 2006;31 (3):405–413.)

Table 18.1 Types of Biomechanical Parameters

Measuring parameters		Measuring instruments
Intrinsic material properties	Young's modulus or stiffness, tensile, or compressive strength	Universal materials testing machine load cell, extensometer, strain gauge(s)
	Toughness	Charpy or Izod impact machine
	Fixation strength, load cycles to failure	Universal materials testing machine load cell
	Load to failure	Force/torque transducer
	Bone strain	Strain gauges, digital image correlation
Structural responses of specimens	Relative motion/stability	Three-dimensional motion capture, linear or rotary displacement transducers, Roentgen stereophotogrammetric analysis
	Contact pressure	Pressure sensors

displacement in one dimension, linear variable differential transformers (LVDTs) and rotary variable differential transformers are normally used. More sophisticated motion measuring systems such as Roentgen stereophotogrammetric analysis (RSA), optical tracking systems, video-optical systems, and computer-based surgical navigation systems are used to obtain spatial motion data. The basic principle of these systems is that they record spatial locations and orientations of markers attached on bones and implants throughout the test cycle. Further data processing is required in order to obtain required relative motions. Apart from the aforementioned measuring instruments, pressure sensors are also used when contact is of interest, for example, in research that studies contact characteristics of prosthetic joints and contact pressure between implants and overlying soft tissues, after bone fracture and osteosynthesis.[2]

It is very important that measuring instruments are correctly calibrated to maintain validity of measurements. Accuracy and precision should be considered when selecting an instrument for a particular experiment. Calibration methods for certain instruments for measuring particular parameters are usually recommended by their manufacturer.

18.3 Functional Testing

There are three main types of functional tests that can be carried out using cadaver specimens and the hardware described in the previous section: mechanical properties testing; assessment of implant, graft, or fracture fixation; and the examination of entire joints. Within each of these is a number of possible tests, some of which will be described here. Proper planning of these types of test is critical, made even more so by the use of donated cadaver specimens. Preliminary testing, using animal cadaver substitutes such as ovine or porcine specimens, is recommended to ensure that every donated human specimen is utilized to its full potential. It may sometimes be possible to use animal tissues instead of human, but care must be taken to ensure their validity. In particular, most animals are put down at a young age, so their tissue material properties may differ significantly from human tissue.

18.3.1 Mechanical Properties

Testing tissues, such as ligament, tendon, bone, or meniscus, in isolation allows the researcher to measure the material properties of the structure in order to better understand its function in vivo and, in the case of those structures being used as grafts, in order to compare their properties to those of the structure being replaced. It is sometimes easy to make a test specimen that consists solely of the material being tested, such as a strip of bone to be bent, or a long tendon to be tensile tested. However, other structures, particularly short ligaments, may be tested most easily by leaving them in situ, then clamping the UTM to the bone at each end of the specimen.[3]

18.3.2 Tensile and Compressive Testing

Tensile testing is used to give load-extension and failure strength information about a material. For this type of materials testing, soft tissue specimens can be clamped in mechanical grips and mounted into a UTM for tensile loading. Care should be taken that there is no relative slip between the specimen and the clamp, and that any extension measured is solely that of the specimen stretching. Cryoclamps, which allow the clamped part of the soft tissue to be frozen, thus preventing any slippage, can also be used.[4] A realistic crosshead speed (i.e., the speed at which the tissue is elongated) should be chosen based on expected mechanism in vivo. A constant displacement rate can be used, independent of the tissue length, or the speed can be chosen based on a percentage of the initial length, giving a constant initial strain rate. Attention must also be given to the line of action of the applied load.

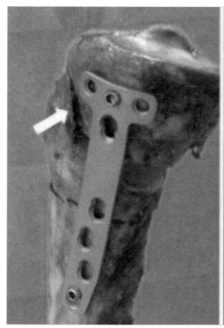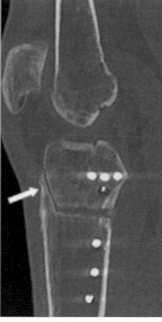

Fig. 18.2 Left: Cadaver tibia with biplanar osteotomy and plate in situ. Right: X-ray showing tantalum beads for Roentgen stereophotogrammetric analysis. (Reproduced from Pape D, Lorbach O, Schmitz C, et al. Effect of a biplanar osteotomy on primary stability following high tibial osteotomy: a biomechanical cadaver study. Knee Surg Sports Traumatol Arthrosc 2010;18(2):204–211.)

Tissues that are commonly subjected to tensile testing include ligaments (with and without bone blocks) or tendons. The opposite of tensile testing, compression testing, examines material behavior when the direction of the load is reversed. In biomechanics, tissues such as bone, articular cartilage, and meniscus are commonly examined under compressive loading.[5] A load is applied at a constant rate, and a force-compressive displacement curve is the output. The researcher must decide whether the specimen will be constrained in the plane perpendicular to the applied load or whether the material will be allowed to extend in all directions as it is squashed. This has a large effect on hydrated tissues, such as articular cartilage, in view of water expulsion when compressed.

18.3.3 Fatigue Testing

The setup for tensile fatigue testing will be very similar to that of straightforward tensile testing in terms of equipment used and specimen type. In this instance, however, the researcher is interested in how the tissue behaves over a period of cyclic loading, rather than just a "one-shot" test to failure. The number of cycles, the maximum and minimum loads, and the rate of testing must be decided prior to testing. The amount of elongation and its location in the soft tissue are of interest. After cyclic loading, if the tissue is still intact, it is common to perform a final tensile test to failure. If a dual-axis UTM is available, torsional fatigue can also be examined.

18.4 Fixation Assessment

Single cadaver bones can be used to assess the fixation of various types of orthopedic devices and procedures. As

with mechanical properties testing, custom-made fixtures and jigs and UTMs are often used for this type of research.

18.4.1 Implant Fixation

Initial fixation of implants such as knee or hip prostheses or osteotomy plates can be assessed using cyclic loading and LVDTs or RSA to measure micromotion.[6] With RSA, sets of small metal beads are placed into the bone on either side of the osteotomy to be monitored, or on the implant and in the surrounding bone, prior to the test (▶ Fig. 18.2). Stereo X-rays are then used to calculate the three-dimensional positions very accurately. Primary fixation is particularly relevant for cementless implants, where good osseointegration is vital to implant success. It is important that the *relative* motion between implant or plate and the bone is measured. When using LVDTs, this is achieved by fixing the LVDT to the bone with the probe resting against the implant.

18.4.2 Graft Fixation

Ligament reconstruction using soft tissue allo- or autografts is a successful procedure, but the fixation of the graft is critical and can cause problems, particularly when the patient becomes active soon after surgery, before the graft has undergone osseointegration. Cadaver specimens can be used to compare different graft fixation methods in two different ways. Either the two bone tunnels, such as femoral and tibial, are analyzed separately, or the entire bone-graft-bone complex is assessed.[7] In both cases, cyclic loading by way of a UTM should be employed to examine slippage of the graft in the bone tunnels. As with the tensile testing described previously, it is crucial that if there is a free end of graft, it is clamped securely so that any extension measured by the UTM is caused by the graft slipping in the bone tunnel, not in the clamp. If there is any doubt about this, then an LVDT or RSA should be used to measure graft-bone motion directly.

18.4.3 Fracture Fixation

Different methods of fixing fractures can be assessed by creating "fractures" in intact specimens. Care should be taken to replicate the fracture as far as possible from specimen to specimen, using cutting guides, and to make the fracture physiologically relevant. The efficacy of the fixation method can be assessed using one of three methods: strength testing, where the fixation is loaded until failure occurs and the failure load is noted; fatigue testing, where the fixation method is cyclically loaded until failure occurs; or nondestructive stability testing, where the fracture is loaded at physiological loads and the micromotion across the gap is measured. As with other fixation assessment, there is a range of measuring devices that could be used, including RSA, three-dimensional optical tracking, or arrays of LVDTs.

18.5 Whole Joint

18.5.1 Kinematic Testing

Understanding three-dimensional motions of human joints is an important part of biomechanical studies. Orthopedic interventions seek to treat injury and pain but must also aim to replicate normal motion and function. As with most of the testing described here, in vitro kinematic testing usually utilizes a test rig and a method of measurement. The Oxford Knee Rig is a well-known and much replicated example of a kinematic testing rig, seeking to replicate full six-degree-of-freedom knee movement during squatting, but there are myriad custom-designed kinematic test rigs being used by biomechanics researchers to assess surgical interventions with cadaver specimens. Measurements should be taken from the intact specimen first, using a three-dimensional motion capture system (most commonly a stereo camera setup that tracks groups of optical markers pinned to each bone) and then repeated after each intervention. Advantages of taking these kind of in vitro measurements include elimination of soft tissue artifact, as trackers can be pinned directly into bone, and comparison of varying types of intervention (e.g., different designs of total knee replacement in one knee, which is not possible in vivo).

18.5.2 Stability Testing

As well as full six-degree-of-freedom movement, it can be useful to measure the mechanical stability of a joint in just one plane. Joint stability usually depends on a number of interacting factors, so it can be hard to measure the contributions of individual structures to the stability of a joint. These contributions can be evaluated by measuring the force required to translate or rotate a joint in a particular direction away from a neutral equilibrium position, then repeating the motion after cutting the structure of interest: the reduction of load corresponds to the contribution of that structure when intact.[8] The effect on joint stability of joint replacement or ligament rupture and reconstruction can also be analyzed. Note that this "mechanical" stability is an objective measurement, usually expressed in terms of N displacing force per millimeter of displacement (e.g., it must not be confused with the subjective feeling of "instability" that patients complain about, although they may well be related).

18.5.3 Contact Mechanics

The contact pressures and patterns inside joints are particularly difficult to measure in vivo due to highly interventional methods. Cadaveric specimens allow pressure measuring films such as Tekscan (Tekscan, Inc., Boston, MA) and Fujifilm Prescale Pressure Indicating Film (Fujifilm, Tokyo, Japan) to be inserted inside joints, permitting the contact to be characterized for the joint of interest before and after various surgical interventions.[9] Care should be taken when using these pressure measurement devices: Calibration for use with cadaveric tissue can be problematic, and the insertion of the pressure films into joints without disrupting the surrounding soft tissue is vital. The thickness of the sensor film may also affect the contact mechanics, if the joint has congruent surfaces, or if the shape of the joint causes the sensor film to wrinkle.

18.5.4 Soft Tissue Strains

The effect of surgical procedures on soft tissue strains can also be examined using cadaver specimens. Length changes between eyelets positioned at the origin and insertion of a ligament can be measured using a monofilament suture, attached to an LVDT, over a range of motion for joints before and after different kinds of surgical procedures.[10] ▶ Fig. 18.3 shows a diagram of a cadaveric knee mounted in an extension rig with sutures attached from the LVDT to the lateral retinaculum and medial collateral ligament.[10] The suture should be fixed at one eyelet (moving relative to the LVDT) and allowed to slide freely through the other eyelet (stationary relative to the LVDT). If both eyelets are able to move relative to the LVDT, then two transducers are required to measure ligament length changes. Local variations of tissue strain can be measured using digital image correlation, in which single or stereo pairs of video cameras track a pattern of speckles sprayed onto a specimen. A simple version of this allows uniaxial tissue strain to be measured using

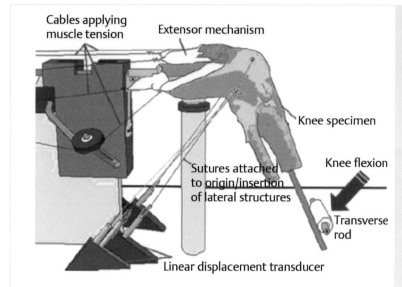

Fig. 18.3 Knee kinematics test rig showing linear variable differential transformer arrangement (Reproduced from Ghosh KM, Merican AM, Iranpour-Boroujeni F, Deehan DJ, Amis AA. Length change patterns of the extensor retinaculum and the effect of total knee replacement. J Orthop Res 2009;27 [7]:865–870.)

video cameras mounted on the UTM, measuring the distance between a pair of marker points on the specimen.

18.6 Conclusion

Used in carefully planned in vitro experiments, cadaveric specimens can be used to deliver a wealth of information about orthopedic surgical techniques, implant performance, and treatment options that in vivo or in silico work cannot solely provide. They are also needed to validate computer models used in predictions of stresses and are an important step prior to clinical use of novel procedures. However, care must be taken to make the experiments as realistic as possible and to avoid artifacts caused by factors such as postmortal tissue changes.

References

[1] Viidik A, Lewin T. Changes in tensile strength characteristics and histology of rabbit ligaments induced by different modes of postmortal storage. Acta Orthop Scand 1966; 37: 141–155

[2] Rosenbaum D, Bauer G, Augat P, Claes L. Calcaneal fractures cause a lateral load shift in Chopart joint contact stress and plantar pressure pattern in vitro. J Biomech 1996; 29: 1435–1443

[3] Race A, Amis AA. The mechanical properties of the two bundles of the human posterior cruciate ligament. J Biomech 1994; 27: 13–24

[4] Pring DJ, Amis AA, Coombs RRH. The mechanical properties of human flexor tendons in relation to artificial tendons. J Hand Surg [Br] 1985; 10: 331–336

[5] Proctor CS, Schmidt MB, Whipple RR, Kelly MA, Mow VC. Material properties of the normal medial bovine meniscus. J Orthop Res 1989; 7: 771–782

[6] Pape D, Lorbach O, Schmitz C et al. Effect of a biplanar osteotomy on primary stability following high tibial osteotomy: a biomechanical cadaver study. Knee Surg Sports Traumatol Arthrosc 2010; 18: 204–211

[7] Scheffler SU, Südkamp NP, Göckenjan A, Hoffmann RF, Weiler A. Biomechanical comparison of hamstring and patellar tendon graft anterior cruciate ligament reconstruction techniques: the impact of fixation level and fixation method under cyclic loading. Arthroscopy 2002; 18: 304–315

[8] Merican AM, Iranpour F, Amis AA. Iliotibial band tension reduces patellar lateral stability. J Orthop Res 2009; 27: 335–339

[9] Lee SJ, Aadalen KJ, Malaviya P et al. Tibiofemoral contact mechanics after serial medial meniscectomies in the human cadaveric knee. Am J Sports Med 2006; 34: 1334–1344

[10] Ghosh KM, Merican AM, Iranpour-Boroujeni F, Deehan DJ, Amis AA. Length change patterns of the extensor retinaculum and the effect of total knee replacement. J Orthop Res 2009; 27: 865–870

Further Reading

Currey JD, Brear K, Zioupos P, Reilly GC. Effect of formaldehyde fixation on some mechanical properties of bovine bone. Biomaterials 1995; 16: 1267–1271

Szivek JA, Gharpuray VM. Strain gauge measurements from bone surfaces. In Mechanical testing of bone and the bone-implant interface. Boca Raton, FL: CRC Press; 1999:305–320

Turner CH, Burr DB. Basic biomechanical measurements of bone: a tutorial. Bone 1993; 14: 595–608

Woo SL, Orlando CA, Camp JF, Akeson WH. Effects of postmortem storage by freezing on ligament tensile behavior. J Biomech 1986; 19: 399–404

Zavatsky AB. A kinematic-freedom analysis of a flexed-knee-stance testing rig. J Biomech 1997; 30: 277–280

Part 4

Numerical Biomechanics

19 Inverse Dynamics

John Rasmussen

Simulation of biomechanical systems by computer is essentially the solution of equations in which one set of information is used to derive another. In other words, something must be known from the outset for simulation to be possible, and the character of this knowledge determines which type of simulation approach is appropriate. In the branch of biomechanics dealing with analysis of forces in muscles, joints, and bones resulting from various movements and activities of daily living, the methods are usually based on the field of rigid body dynamics that again is based on Newton's laws. An understanding of this field is conveniently initiated with a review of Newton's second law:

$$\mathbf{F} = m\mathbf{a} \qquad (19.1)$$

where $\mathbf{F}$ is the sum of forces acting on a body, m is the mass of the body, and $\mathbf{a}$ is its acceleration. $\mathbf{F}$ and $\mathbf{a}$ can have multiple dimensions (i.e., three if the motion takes place in space). Newton's second law is therefore a simple system of equations in which we can find some of the properties if we know some of the other properties. Let us presume that m is known. This leaves us with the following two options:

1. If we know the sum of forces, $\mathbf{F}$, then we can determine the acceleration and thereby the motion.
2. If we know the motion and thereby the acceleration, $\mathbf{a}$, then we can find the sum of forces that must have affected the body in order to generate the motion.

Newton's second law applies to particles and can be extended to rigid bodies if m is interpreted as mass moment of inertia and mass, $\mathbf{F}$ as moments and forces, and $\mathbf{a}$ as angular and linear accelerations.

This leads to a similarly structured but more complex set of equations, the Newton-Euler equations, which can be combined to describe the behavior of mechanisms (i.e., linkages comprising several mutually connected rigid bodies). So even for very complex mechanisms, such as the human body with its hundreds of bones, if we know the forces, we can determine the motion, and if we know the motion, then we can find the forces that caused it.

There is more than an academic difference to the two approaches. Notice that $\mathbf{F}$ is the sum of all forces acting on the body, which in a musculoskeletal system includes the muscle forces, which are experimentally very difficult to determine. On the other hand, well-established methods are available for observing and capturing motions of living organisms, primarily camera-based motion capture systems. It is therefore relatively easy in practice to know the motions and compute the forces, whereas the opposite is tricky. Furthermore, in many practically relevant biomechanical situations, the body is either static or follows a known pattern of movement, for instance in seated postures, pedaling, or lifting.

Analyzing the unknown forces from known motions is called inverse dynamics, and it is the topic of this chapter.

19.1 A Simple Example

Inverse dynamics is very much an engineering approach to biomechanical simulation. Let us consider the simplified example of a foot on an ankle joint shown in the free body diagram of ▶ Fig. 19.1. Despite the anatomical reality, we shall consider the foot as a single rigid segment and the ankle as a hinge joint. In this two-dimensional

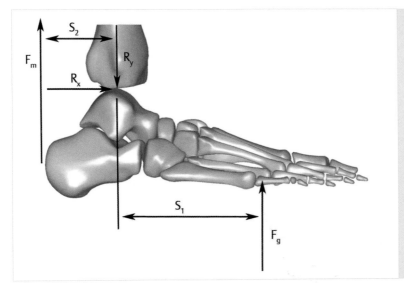

Fig. 19.1 Free body diagram for a foot.

case, two reaction force components, R_x and R_y, are working in the ankle joint. The ball of the foot is loaded by a vertical ground reaction force, F_g. We consider initially only the muscle force, F_m, from the soleus muscle working through the Achilles tendon. The mass of the foot is disregarded.

We start by the moment equilibrium about the ankle:

$$F_g s_1 - F_m s_2 = 0$$
$$\Downarrow \qquad\qquad (19.2)$$
$$F_m = \frac{F_g s_1}{s_2}$$

Horizontal equilibrium quickly reveals that

$$R_x = 0 \qquad\qquad (19.3)$$

All that remains now is to determine R_y from vertical equilibrium:

$$F_m - R_y + F_g = 0$$
$$\Downarrow \qquad\qquad (19.4)$$
$$R_y = F_m + F_g$$

Let us insert some plausible numbers:
$s_1 = 0.1$ m, $s_2 = 0.04$ m, $F_g = 1{,}600$ N
This leads to the following forces in the system:
$F_m = 4{,}000$ N
$R_y = 5{,}600$ N

Please notice that the modest external force gives rise to large internal forces. This is typical for musculoskeletal systems. We are generally unaware of the magnitude of the forces working inside our bodies and the strength of our tissues. When a basketball player ruptures a knee ligament or a sprinter ruptures an Achilles tendon, we can rest assured that really substantial forces are at play. It is not difficult to get an impression of the forces by palpation of the tendons, for instance inside the elbow during elbow flexion.

Key Concepts: Equilibrium

This example has three unknown quantities, namely the internal forces R_x, R_y, and F_m. To determine them, three equations are available (i.e., horizontal force equilibrium, vertical force equilibrium, and moment equilibrium). In other words, identification of the internal forces requires solution of three equations with three unknowns. To simplify matters, we decided to begin with the moment equilibrium about the ankle, which automatically eliminated the unknowns R_x and R_y, providing a single equation from which the muscle force can be isolated.

Despite this example being static, it is in reality inverse *dynamics* in its simplest form: We know the posture and the velocity (in this case the velocity is zero) of the elements in the system, and we also know the external forces acting on the system. With this input, we can compute the internal forces (i.e., the muscle force and the joint reaction force).

In practical use of inverse dynamics, the systems tend to be much more complicated than the simple foot example, so we prefer to have computers solve the equations for us. Computers are generally excellent equation solvers, but they are not very intelligent and not good at making smart decisions about how to form the equations to simplify the solution procedure by decoupling the equations, as we did in the example. Therefore, they generally have to solve many simultaneous equations, and their formation requires a stringent approach. Let us review the structure of the problem in the case where we formulate it as three equations with three unknowns:

$$R_x = 0$$
$$-R_y + F_m = -F_g \qquad\qquad (19.5)$$
$$-s_2 F_m = -s_1 F_g$$

We can cast these equations into a matrix form:

$$\begin{bmatrix} 1 & 0 & 0 \\ 0 & -1 & 1 \\ 0 & 0 & -s_2 \end{bmatrix} \begin{Bmatrix} R_x \\ R_y \\ F_m \end{Bmatrix} = \begin{Bmatrix} 0 \\ -F_g \\ -s_1 F_g \end{Bmatrix} \qquad (19.6)$$

This type of formulation is particularly well suited for computer processing, and there are very efficient numerical methods available for handling of matrices and linear equations. Despite the fact that anatomically realistic models are usually much more complicated than this simple example, it turns out that it is always possible to cast the equilibrium equations into the form of equation (19.6), even in the case of the full human body with 200 bones and three-dimensional conditions. Because of this general feature, it is convenient to introduce a formalism that can be used later:

$$\mathbf{Cf} = \mathbf{r} \qquad\qquad (19.7)$$

where

$$\mathbf{C} = \begin{bmatrix} 1 & 0 & 0 \\ 0 & -1 & 1 \\ 0 & 0 & -s_2 \end{bmatrix}, \ \mathbf{f} = \begin{Bmatrix} R_x \\ R_y \\ F_m \end{Bmatrix}, \ \mathbf{r}$$
$$= \begin{Bmatrix} 0 \\ -F_g \\ -s_1 F_g \end{Bmatrix} \qquad\qquad (19.8)$$

In this system, matrix $\mathbf{C}$ contains only constants that can be found prior to the solution of the problem, $\mathbf{f}$ is a vector representing the unknown internal forces, and $\mathbf{r}$ contains the external forces. The system of equations therefore fundamentally expresses that the external forces on the system must be balanced by internal forces. This is the fundamental mathematical structure of an inverse dynamics problem.

19.2 Redundancy and Muscle Recruitment

Although the basic structure of the equilibrium equations is always as displayed previously, some important complications arise for realistic musculoskeletal systems. One of the problems is redundancy in the system, which arises because the body has many more muscles than degrees of freedom. To illustrate this point, we shall extend the previous example a little, as shown in ▶ Fig. 19.2.

The only difference from the previous example is that we now have two muscle forces, F_{m1} and F_{m2}, performing plantarflexion of the ankle.

With the additional muscle force, the equilibrium equations are:

$$R_x = 0$$
$$-R_y + F_{m1} + F_{m2} = -F_g \qquad (19.9)$$
$$-s_2 F_m - s_3 F_{m2} = -s_1 F_g$$

which in matrix form becomes:

$$\begin{bmatrix} 1 & 0 & 0 & 0 \\ 0 & -1 & 1 & 1 \\ 0 & 0 & -s_2 & -s_3 \end{bmatrix} \begin{Bmatrix} R_x \\ R_y \\ F_{m1} \\ F_{m2} \end{Bmatrix} = \begin{Bmatrix} 0 \\ -F_g \\ -s_1 F_g \end{Bmatrix} \qquad (19.10)$$

The coefficient matrix **C** is now rectangular, indicating that there are more unknowns than equations in the problem. The mathematical consequence of this is that the system of equations does not have a unique solution, but rather infinitely many different solutions. Physically, we can understand this property by noticing that the ground reaction force, F_g, can be balanced by F_{m1} alone, by F_{m2} alone, or by many different combinations of the two

muscle forces, as long as the two muscle forces in concert produce a moment about the ankle joint of the same size and opposite the moment produced by F_g.

For instance, when we walk, we are simultaneously activating several muscles about the ankle joint in a carefully tuned pattern to produce gait of the desired speed and direction, and we have no perception of the fact that we are instantly choosing between an infinite number of possible activations of the muscles. It even turns out that, if we measure the activity in the muscles in cyclic movements by electromyography, the same muscle activation patterns seem to be repeated over and over again, although a perfectly repetitive movement could theoretically be produced by different muscle activation patterns in each cycle. This indicates that the body does not choose muscle activations randomly but employs a rational criterion.

From experimental investigations, some criteria can be identified:

- Muscles spanning the same joint tend to help each other. This phenomenon is called synergism, and muscles helping each other are called synergistic muscles. Referring back to the example, we can therefore rule out the option that only one of the two muscles may be doing all of the work.
- When the externally applied moment over a joint is increased, then so is the activity in all the synergistic muscles.[1]
- Certain muscles can be observed to work "against the movement" (that last phrase is in quotes because it turns out that it is not completely trivial to define precisely what it means). Such muscles are called antagonistic muscles or simply antagonists, and their presence has been recognized for many years and is known as Lombard's paradox.[2]

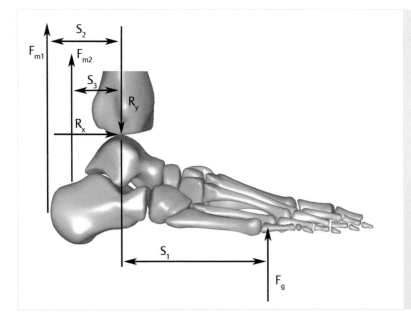

Fig. 19.2 Example with two muscles.

The observation that muscles tend to work in systematic patterns seems logical in an evolutionary thinking, where optimal muscle coordination may have resulted from natural selection (i.e., species and individuals with good muscle coordination have an advantage and may propagate their genes). Mathematically, such an idea can be formulated as an optimization problem, as follows.

$$G\left(f^{(M)}\right) \qquad (19.11)$$

subject to

$$\mathbf{Cf} = \mathbf{r}$$
and $\qquad (19.12)$
$$f_i^{(M)} \geq 0, \; i = 1 \cdots n^{(M)}$$

This is a so-called mathematical program, and its solution is a set of muscle forces, $\mathbf{f}^{(M)}$, that minimize the objective function G, while honoring the constraints. Notice that one of the constraints is the set of equilibrium equations (i.e., feasible solutions must be in equilibrium with the external forces).

Notice that the vector of internal forces, $\mathbf{f}$, has been divided into two parts:

$$\mathbf{f} = \left[\mathbf{f}^{(M)} \mathbf{f}^{(R)}\right]^T \qquad (19.13)$$

The first part, $\mathbf{f}^{(M)}$, contains muscle forces, while the latter, $\mathbf{f}^{(R)}$, contains the joint reactions. This division reflects that muscle forces require metabolism and therefore energetic resources, whereas the joint reactions come for free. It is therefore plausible that the cost function, G, depends on the muscle forces but not necessarily on the joint reactions. Finally, please notice the additional nonnegativity condition for each element of $\mathbf{f}^{(M)}$. This is the mathematical way of requiring that muscles cannot push.

These points all had physiological motivations, but what about the cost function G? Which function is the right one, and what might nature in fact be trying to minimize in its selection of muscle recruitment patterns? The set of possible cost functions is of course endless, so it is useful to limit the scope a little, and this may be done with mathematical arguments. One of the obvious systematizations is to limit the possible objective functions to polynomial sums of muscle forces:

$$G = \sum_{i=1}^{n^{(M)}} \left(\frac{f_i^{(M)}}{N_i}\right)^p \qquad (19.14)$$

If we believe that the right objective function can be found among this class of functions, then the problem is reduced to identifying the normalizers, N_i, and the degree of the polynomial, p. We are fairly certain that large muscles should pull more load than small muscles, and

this indicates that N_i should somehow express the strength of the i'th muscle (i.e., the cross-sectional area of the muscle). There is good experimental evidence for the notion that we will not get realistic predictions of muscle forces if we do not consider the mutual strengths of the muscles in the formulation of the problem.[3]

The degree, p, of the polynomial is more disputable except for the general agreement that $p = 1$ can be ruled out because it does not produce the synergism between the muscles that can be observed experimentally. Any value of $p > 1$ will result in synergy between the muscles and also some extent of antagonistic muscle forces in complex systems. It is possible to show that this antagonism arises as a result of either biarticular muscles or of three-dimensional joints. It is also possible to show mathematically that the amount of synergism between the muscles increases with p. A special case occurs when p goes to infinity ($p \to \infty$). In this case, the muscle recruitment problem becomes equivalent to the following.

$$max_i\left(\frac{f_i^{(M)}}{N_i}\right) \qquad (19.15)$$

subject to

$$\mathbf{Cf} = \mathbf{r}$$
and $\qquad (19.16)$
$$f_i^{(M)} \geq 0, \; i = 1 \cdots n^{(M)}$$

The physiological explanation for this formulation is minimization of fatigue. The objective function focuses on the single muscle in the system that has the largest relative load; all muscles are recruited to minimize this load. This means that all of the muscles end up helping each other as much as possible. Numerical experiments with the different options indicate that smaller values of p, for instance $p = 2$ or $p = 3$ yield good results for submaximal loads, whereas the minimum fatigue criterion is useful for larger loads. However, compared with the biological variation between individuals, all values of $p > 1$ show similar trends in the muscle recruitment, and it is impossible to determine conclusively whether one or the other is the correct criterion,[4] although recent investigations favor the minimum fatigue criterion.[5]

19.3 Muscle Models

As previously mentioned, the factors N_i can be interpreted as a measure of the strength of the i'th muscle. Muscles are complex and remarkable machines, and their strength depends on the working conditions. A mathematical model of this dependency is called a muscle model, and such models play important roles for muscle recruitment. Most practically used models are based on the works of A. V. Hill (1886–1977, Nobel Prize 1922).

These models are phenomenological and not based on a deeper understanding of the mechanisms leading to muscle contraction, but they are efficient and work well unless very detailed modeling of single muscles is desired. Hill models typically take pennation angles (i.e., the angle between the fiber direction and the muscle force direction), fiber composition, passive-elastic tissue, dependency between contraction velocity and strength, and dependency between current fiber length and strength into account. These properties go under the term "contraction dynamics."

A muscle model for inverse dynamics takes as input, in addition to the aforementioned anatomical data, current fiber length, which is a function of the origin-insertion length of the muscle in a given posture, and current contraction velocity, which is a function of the motion of the segments to which it connects. Its output is then the strength of the muscle (i.e., N_i). Choice of an appropriate muscle model for a given problem involves consideration of the nature of the movement. If the movement is fast or has a large range of motion, then it is probably necessary to take contraction dynamics into account. However, Hill models considering contraction dynamics require detailed anatomical parameters that may not be readily available. If data are lacking or the quality is questionable, their inclusion may degrade the accuracy of the simulation rather than improve it.

19.4 Applications

Inverse dynamics has the advantage of numerical efficiency, which enables modeling of very complex and realistic musculoskeletal systems with hundreds of muscles on inexpensive computers. Applications fall into the categories illustrated by the examples in ▸ Table 19.1.

Frequently, the applications of inverse dynamics are characterized by the presence of an object or a device that works in conjunction with the human body (e.g., a medical implant, an orthosis, a piece of furniture, or a tennis racket). Another important characteristic is the presence of multiple closed kinematic loops in the models. The human body in its own right contains multiple closed kinematic chains (e.g., in the shoulder or the forearm), and any connection with an environment that touches the body on multiple points also forms closed kinematic chains. The ability to handle closed kinematic chains and facilities enabling the user to model the environment and its influence on the human body is essential for any practical application of musculoskeletal modelling.

19.4.1 Example: Plexus Brachialis Lesions

Let us illustrate the points of the preceding section with a slightly more detailed example. Lesions in the plexus brachialis nerve occur frequently as the result of traffic accidents, sports injuries, and other incidents of high shoulder impacts. The plexus brachialis can be injured anywhere from its cervical origin to the insertions into the muscles. The practical consequence of the injury and the chances of rehabilitation depend much on the location of the lesion with the more proximal locations being the more serious and with much poorer prognosis. Plexus brachialis injury due to trauma often affects young people used to active lifestyles. Its consequence can therefore be many years of disability (▸ Fig. 19.3).

The typical symptom of a plexus brachialis injury is a drop arm (i.e., inability to maintain the posture of the shoulder girdle, which falls frontally and inferiorly, and inability to move the arm, especially to elevated postures). ▸ Fig. 19.4 illustrates the reason for this disability. It shows the muscle activations in the arm of an able-bodied person putting the hand to the mouth. It is obvious that a complex pattern of muscle activation is required to balance the multiple degrees-of-freedom of the arm, and inability to activate a subset of these muscles can significantly encumber the motion.

In this group of patients, the joints are functioning normally but the muscles are paralyzed and consequently unable to provide the forces necessary to produce articulation. This means that a passive orthosis may be helpful if it can prevent the shoulder girdle from dropping and compensate the upper extremity for the forces of gravity. In this context, a musculoskeletal model of the shoulder complex can be used to investigate a number of important issues:

- Using an anatomical map of the plexus brachialis branches, it can be determined which muscles are paralyzed depending on the location of the lesion. These muscles can now be paralyzed in the model, and it can be investigated which postures are likely unattainable for given lesions because the remaining muscles cannot support them.
- For a patient with a given lesion and inability to reach certain arm postures, the model may determine how much additional passive elasticity is required from an orthosis to enable the remaining muscles to support the posture and the movement leading to it. Subsequently, the model can be used to design an orthosis in terms of elastic properties in different directions to enable maximum mobility for the patient in a range of motions.

As is obvious in ▸ Fig. 19.5, several lesion locations such as C5, C6, and C7 indicated in blue in Fig. 19.3 make it completely impossible to perform the motion because the patient is almost devoid of strength. Others, such as Root, C7, C8, or T1, may be possible with the assistance of a passive orthosis that carries a portion of gravity. To summarize, the musculoskeletal model helps understand the mechanisms of this disability and can subsequently be useful in the design of the intervention. >

Table 19.1 Some Application Fields for Inverse Dynamics

Area	Typical Applications
Orthopedics and rehabilitation. Applications in this field are typically surgical planning, development of orthopedic implants, and design of rehabilitation exercises. The image shows an analysis model for a spinal implant device (muscles on the right side removed for visibility). The influence of the device on the mechanics of the spine and vice versa is analyzed with the model.	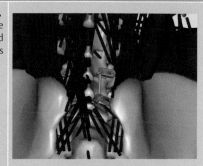
Ergonomics. Many industrial products and workplaces derive their value from their ability to interact with the human body. Working situations involving lifting, pushing, pulling, and/or repetitive movements often lead to injury. Musculoskeletal simulation can identify locations of high load and how they depend on the working conditions. Ergonomic design of workplaces can be significantly improved with this technique.	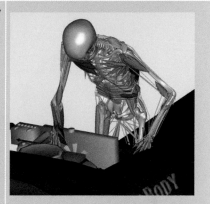
Sports. Many sports performances depend on optimal techniques, for instance kicks, pitches, swimming strokes, jumps, etc. Musculoskeletal analysis makes it possible to analyze the importance of these techniques and perfect them, and to design exercises targeted at particular sports performances. In addition, musculoskeletal simulation can be used to design sports equipment that works optimally for given performances.	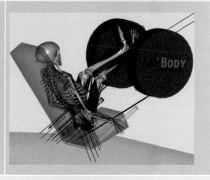

The examples are all developed with the AnyBody Modeling System (AnyBody Technology, Aalborg, Denmark).

19.5 Limitations, Assumptions, and Validation

When computer models are used to make critical decisions, for instance about treatment of patients, the validity and correctness of the model become crucial, and this leads to the desire to validate models (i.e., provide a justification that the model provides sufficiently accurate results to merit the conclusions).

Model validation is a difficult field and possibly inconsistent with the theory of science, which states that models can be falsified but never validated. For instance, Newton's laws were falsified for certain speed and size domains by the theory of relativity by Einstein and later by quantum mechanics. Yet, Newton's mechanics is still accurate enough under most practical circumstances to form the basis of very critical decisions. Although models cannot be validated, failure to falsify them builds confidence that the model works. Recently, Lund et al[6] published a comprehensive review of validation methods for musculoskeletal models concluding that validation is, in the best case, very difficult.

Rather than attempting a top-level validation of a given model that simultaneously proves the validity of all

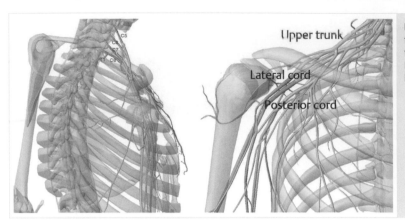

Fig. 19.3 N. plexus brachialis originating from the cervical spine and branching into the upper extremity (image from the Visible Body). The legends indicate typical lesion locations.

Upper trunk

Lateral cord

Posterior cord

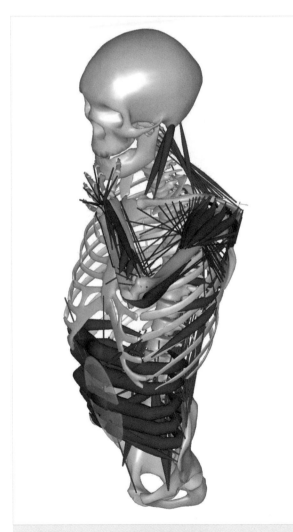

Fig. 19.4 Muscle forces, illustrated by means of bulging, in an able-bodied model lifting the hand to the mouth.

its components and correctness of its algorithms, one may take a bottom-up approach and review the basic limitations and assumptions of the models. Some of the important points are the following:

• Inverse dynamics is based on Newton's laws or more precisely, in the case of the AnyBody Modeling System (AnyBody Technology, Aalborg, Denmark), on the Newton-Euler equations, which describe the dynamics of mechanisms. These equations include all inertia forces such as gravity, acceleration forces, centrifugal forces, gyroscopic forces, and Coriolis forces. Their only major assumption is that the segments are rigid and joints are ideal.

• Some system developers are tempted to make the assumption of open chain models because it simplifies the equations significantly and seems to be compatible with the basic structure of the human body with its trunk and attached extremities. Unfortunately, this is a serious misunderstanding. The human skeleton contains many closed chains, for instance in the shoulder girdle, the forearm, and the thorax, and these cannot be modeled adequately under the assumption of open chains. Furthermore, in typical working situations of double stance or grasping a handle, the human body forms closed kinematic chains with the environment. ▶ Table 19.1 shows several such examples, and they can only be handled if the model does not presume open kinematic chains.

• As discussed earlier in this chapter, muscle systems are redundant and require the assumption of a recruitment objective function. We do not know which function is the "right" one, and this is a fundamental problem facing inverse dynamics. However, the equilibrium equations [see equation (19.12)] stem directly from the Newton-Euler equations and must be fulfilled regardless of the choice of recruitment function. In other words, muscle recruitment does not randomly depend on the choice of recruitment function, and in practice different reasonable choices of recruitment functions typically do not cause radical differences in the result.

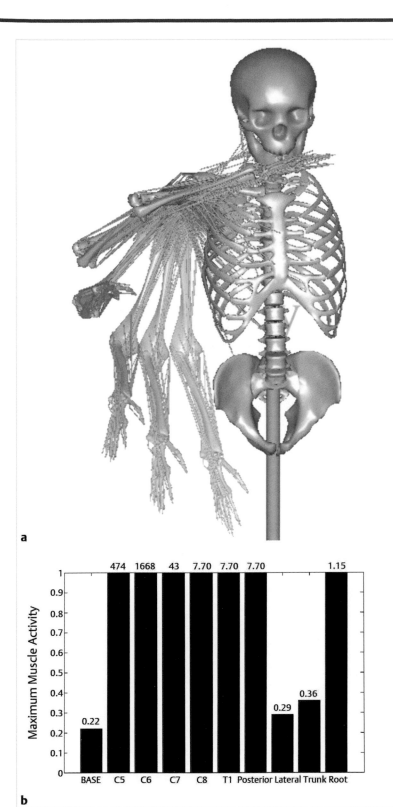

Fig. 19.5 (a) The musculoskeletal model performing an upper extremity motion typical for daily life, namely taking the hand to the mouth. (b) Upper extremity motion typical of daily life and the computed maximum muscle activation levels associated with it. BASE is for the case of no lesion, and the other columns show necessary muscle activity in the presence of the lesions of ▶ Fig. 19.3. Activation above 1 means that the movement is beyond the strength capability of the patient. In the interest of legibility, the columns are cut at activation 1 with the actual values listed on top.

- Musculoskeletal models depend on anatomical data, motion data, and possibly on measured external forces from force platforms and such. All of these are subject to significant uncertainty that may drastically influence the result, and this is likely the single most important challenge facing system and model developers. Consider, for instance, the moment generated about the hip by the ground reaction force in gait. To avoid excessive moments, humans tend to control their gait patterns such that this vector passes not too far from the hip joint center. Unfortunately, this means that a small deviation in measured kinematics or ground reaction force direction may cause the vector to shift to the wrong side of the hip joint center in the model, thus causing recruitment of posterior muscles rather than anterior muscles or vice versa. Such model sensitivity is difficult to manage and may lead to significantly erroneous analysis results.

In conclusion, musculoskeletal modeling by inverse dynamics is a technology with many applications but also requiring users with dual skills in mechanics and physiology to obtain reliable and valid results. In this sense, the technology is similar to more established simulation technologies, such as finite element analysis and computational fluid dynamics. The confidence in this technology will grow, as it has done in other simulation technologies, as models, methods, and software continue to evolve and reach larger audiences.

References

[1] Crowninshield RD. Use of optimization techniques to predict muscle forces. J Biomech Eng 1978;100(2):88–92

[2] Lombard WP. The action of two-joint muscles. Am Phys Ed Rev 1903; 8: 141–145

[3] Prilutsky BI, Gregory RJ. Analysis of muscle coordination strategies in cycling. IEEE Trans Rehabil Eng 2000; 8: 362–370

[4] van Bolhuis BM, Gielen CCAM. A comparison of models explaining muscle activation patterns for isometric contractions. Biol Cybern 1999; 81: 249–261

[5] Ackermann M, van den Bogert AJ. Optimality principles for model-based prediction of human gait. J Biomech 2010; 43: 1055–1060

[6] Lund ME, de Zee M, Andersen MS, Rasmussen J. On validation of multibody musculoskeletal models. Proc Inst Mech Eng H 2012; 226: 82–94

20 Principles of Finite Elements Analysis

Zohar Yosibash

The biomechanical community is challenged by the need to predict the mechanical response of biological tissues as bones, muscle, blood vessels, etc., especially when an intervention is mandatory. For example, the mechanical response is of major interest in the case of insertion of metallic implants in a fractured bone or in the case of stents insertion in an atherosclerotic artery. In such instances, numerical simulations by finite element (FE) methods can provide invaluable information for the clinical community, *if the FE analyses are verified and validated.* This chapter, therefore, provides the principles of FE methods with an emphasis on the concept of verification and validation and its optimal and successful use in biomechanical practice.

Consider as an illustrative example a physical system that is composed of a human femur that is clamped at its distal part and loaded by a given force on its head. If an experiment can be performed on the femur (as shown in ▶ Fig. 20.1), the displacements at any point on the femur's surface as well as the strains may be measured. These are the "physical quantities" of interest, denoted by $\boldsymbol{u}_{Phy}$. To enable the prediction of these quantities of interest without the need to perform an experiment (or when such experiments are impossible to be performed), a mathematical model can be formulated that will provide the solutions $\boldsymbol{u}_{Comp}$. Such complex mathematical models are usually extremely nonlinear and very difficult to formulate. Therefore, *idealization assumptions* are being introduced (generating *idealization errors*) to enable a more simplified mathematical model to be formulated, with a solution denoted by $\boldsymbol{u}_{Simp}$. This simplified mathematical model should be understood to be an idealized representation of the reality and should never be confused with the physical reality that it is supposed to represent. Due to the complex geometry of the domain of interest and the nonlinearity of the problem, even the simplified mathematical formulation cannot be solved analytically. Therefore, a discretization process is applied by which the simplified mathematical problem is reformulated so it can be solved on digital computers. The most frequently applied method of discretization is the FE method. The FE method finds an approximate solution denoted by $\boldsymbol{u}_{FE}$ and the *discretization error* is the difference between the approximated FE solution and the solution of the simplified mathematical problem $\boldsymbol{u}_{Simp}$. Referring again to ▶ Fig. 20.1, one notices that:

$$\boldsymbol{u}_{Phy} - \boldsymbol{u}_{FE} = \boldsymbol{e}_D + \boldsymbol{e}_I + \boldsymbol{e}_C \qquad (20.1)$$

Equation (20.1) implies that if one wishes to determine how well the FE solution represents the physical quantities of interest, then the discretization, the idealization, and the conceptualization errors have to be quantified.

This chapter concentrates on the principles of the FE solution, $\boldsymbol{u}_{FE}$, and on the estimation of the associated discretization error, $\boldsymbol{e}_D$. Estimating $\boldsymbol{e}_D$ is essentially what is meant by *verification*.

The first part of this chapter provides a deeper understanding on the basics and principles of FE methods, and the second part is more practical, discussing the appropriate use of FE analyses and the interpretation of FE

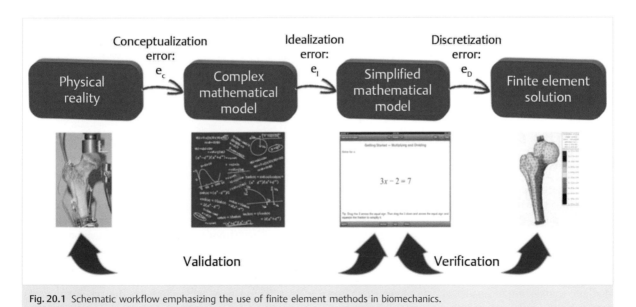

Fig. 20.1 Schematic workflow emphasizing the use of finite element methods in biomechanics.

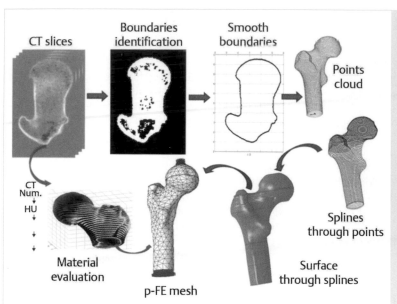

Fig. 20.2 Creating a finite element mesh for a femur (with material properties) from a computed tomography scan.

results. Specific considerations and pitfalls are high-lighted, and a proper process for the verification of the results is detailed.

20.1 The Finite Element Methodology

Let us consider for demonstration purposes the mechanical response of a femur under moderate loads, which after idealization can be considered to behave linearly elastic having isotropic but inhomogeneous material properties. One would be interested in the displacements, strains, and stresses at any point in the femur to determine, for example, if there is a risk of fracture. For this purpose, an FE analysis may be performed that requires three ingredients: (1) the geometric description, (2) a "constitutive model" and material properties that describe the physical phenomenon and the behavior of the material, and (3) boundary conditions (forces and constrains) that are applied.

20.2 The Geometry and Finite Element Mesh

For a patient-specific analysis, the geometry description of the femur may be obtained from a computed tomography (CT) scan, so that the outer and inner contours of the femur can be segmented (▶ Fig. 20.2). After segmentation, the data is manipulated using a computer-aided design software and a solid model of the bone is generated, call it Ω. This solid model of a complex topology can be divided into a collection of smaller, simple geometric shapes such as hexahedral, pentahedral, or tetraherdral elements

— each called a *finite element*. The collection of these elements is called the FE "mesh". Each element is denoted by Ω_ℓ, so that $\cup \, \Omega_\ell = \Omega$.

20.3 The Mathematical Basis of the Finite Element Method

To compute the elastic response of the femur, a set of partial differential equations (the Navier-Lame system,[1] known also as the elasticity system, without body forces) has to be solved in the domain of the femur denoted by Ω:

$$\frac{E}{2(1+v)}\nabla^2 u_x - \frac{E}{2(1+v)(1-2v)}\frac{\partial}{\partial x}\left(\frac{\partial u_x}{\partial x}+\frac{\partial u_y}{\partial y}+\frac{\partial u_z}{\partial z}\right) = 0$$

$$\frac{E}{2(1+v)}\nabla^2 u_y - \frac{E}{2(1+v)(1-2v)}\frac{\partial}{\partial y}\left(\frac{\partial u_x}{\partial x}+\frac{\partial u_y}{\partial y}+\frac{\partial u_z}{\partial z}\right) = 0$$

$$\frac{E}{2(1+v)}\nabla^2 u_z - \frac{E}{2(1+v)(1-2v)}\frac{\partial}{\partial z}\left(\frac{\partial u_x}{\partial x}+\frac{\partial u_y}{\partial y}+\frac{\partial u_z}{\partial z}\right) = 0$$

$$(20.2)$$

Here $\boldsymbol{u}_{Simp} = [u_x(x,y,z),\, u_y(x,y,z),\, u_z(x,y,z)]^T$ is the sought displacement vector, $E(x,y,z)$ (Young's modulus), and $v(x,y,z)$ (Poisson ratio) are the material properties at each point. The elasticity system (20.2) is complemented by traction $\boldsymbol{T}$ or displacement boundary conditions. The analytical solution that solves this problem would be the "classical" or "strong" solution $\boldsymbol{u}_{Simp}$. However, due to the complex domain of the femur, it is impossible to obtain analytically $\boldsymbol{u}_{Simp}$. To obtain an *approximated* solution by FE methods, we first transform the strong form into a "weak formulation" by multiplying the set of equations by a "test function" $\boldsymbol{v} = (v_x(x,y,z),v_y(x,y,z),v_z(x,y,z))^T$, then

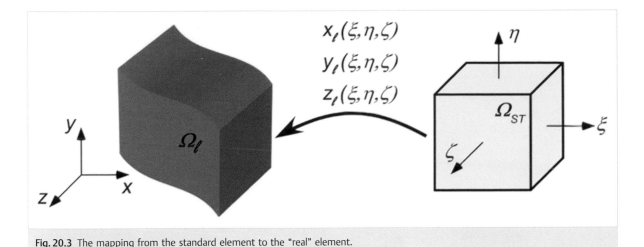

Fig. 20.3 The mapping from the standard element to the "real" element.

integrate over the entire femur and apply the Green's lemma (integration by parts) so we finally obtain the formulation:

Seek $\boldsymbol{u}_{Simp}$ so that $\mathbf{B}(\mathbf{u}, \mathbf{v}) = \mathbf{F}(\mathbf{v}), \quad \forall \boldsymbol{v}$,
where

$$B(\mathbf{u}, \mathbf{v}) = \iiint_\Omega ([D]\mathbf{v})^T [E][D]\boldsymbol{u} \ d\Omega,$$

$$\mathbf{F}(\mathbf{v}) = \iint_{\partial\Omega} \boldsymbol{T}^T \mathbf{v} \ d\Gamma,$$

$$[D] = \begin{bmatrix} \frac{\partial}{\partial x} & 0 & 0 \\ 0 & \frac{\partial}{\partial y} & 0 \\ 0 & 0 & \frac{\partial}{\partial z} \\ 0 & \frac{\partial}{\partial z} & \frac{\partial}{\partial y} \\ \frac{\partial}{\partial z} & 0 & \frac{\partial}{\partial x} \\ \frac{\partial}{\partial y} & \frac{\partial}{\partial x} & 0 \end{bmatrix},$$

$$[E] = \frac{E}{(1+\nu)(1-2\nu)} \begin{bmatrix} 1-\nu & \nu & \nu & 0 & 0 & 0 \\ & 1-\nu & \nu & 0 & 0 & 0 \\ & & 1-\nu & 0 & 0 & 0 \\ & & & \frac{1-2\nu}{2} & 0 & 0 \\ & \text{Symmetric} & & & \frac{1-2\nu}{2} & 0 \\ & & & & & \frac{1-2\nu}{2} \end{bmatrix}$$

$$\text{(20.3)}$$

The weak formulation of equation (20.3) can also be cast into an equivalent formulation, the "minimum potential energy":

Seek $\boldsymbol{u}_{Simp}$ that minimizes the "potential energy":

$$\Pi(\boldsymbol{u}) = \frac{1}{2} B(\boldsymbol{u}, \boldsymbol{u}) - F(\boldsymbol{u}) \tag{20.4}$$

Once $\boldsymbol{u}_{Simp}$ is found, one can easily compute the stress vector by $\boldsymbol{\sigma} = [E][D]\boldsymbol{u}_{Simp}$.

To solve equation (20.4), a major difficulty still exists, namely, one is required to find one displacement field *among an infinite number of displacements* that when inserted into $\Pi(\boldsymbol{u})$ will result in a minimum value. Let us

denote by $\mathscr{E}(\Omega)$ the space of all possible displacements, so we seek for $\boldsymbol{u}_{Simp} \in \mathscr{E}(\Omega)$. From the practical point of view, this is of course impossible, and instead of an infinite number of possible functions, we seek a displacement field within a *finite number of functions* (we denote this finite set of functions $S(\Omega) \subset \mathscr{E}(\Omega)$ that satisfies equation (20.4). This function is the FE solution, $\boldsymbol{u}_{FE}$. Of course, that $\boldsymbol{u}_{FE}$ may not provide the minimum value to $\Pi(\mathbf{u})$, among all possible functions in $\mathscr{E}(\Omega)$, but it is the "closest" to $\boldsymbol{u}_{Simp}$ among all functions in $S(\Omega)$. *The discretization error is introduced because we seek for a solution in $S(\Omega)$ instead of in $\mathscr{E}(\Omega)$.* If one uses hierarchical spaces, that is a family of increasingly larger spaces, each containing the smaller spaces, $S_1(\Omega) \subset S_2(\Omega) \subset S_3(\Omega) \subset \cdots \subset \mathscr{E}(\Omega)$, then the FE solutions $\boldsymbol{u}_{FE1}, \boldsymbol{u}_{FE2}, \boldsymbol{u}_{FE3}\cdots$ obtained are progressively closer to $\boldsymbol{u}_{Simp}$. Of course, as the space $S(\Omega)$ is enriched by more and more functions, then the approximated solutions become closer to the exact solution. The systematic enrichments of the subspaces are called *extensions*, and these are mandatory for estimating the discretization error to quantify how close are $\boldsymbol{u}_{FE1}, \boldsymbol{u}_{FE2}, \boldsymbol{u}_{FE3}\cdots$ to $\boldsymbol{u}_{Simp}$. We will get back to the estimation of the discretization error later on.

Having a mesh, the integral over the entire domain in equation (20.4) is the sum of integrals over the elements, so that equation (20.4) can now be stated as:

Seek $\boldsymbol{u}_{FE} \in S(\Omega)$ that minimizes

$$\sum_l \frac{1}{2} \iiint_{\Omega_l} ([D]\boldsymbol{u})^T [E][D]\boldsymbol{u} \ d\Omega_l - \iiint_{\partial\Omega} \boldsymbol{T}^T \boldsymbol{u} \ d\Gamma_l \tag{20.5}$$

One may observe that we partitioned the overall problem into "elemental problems," and have now to compute the integrals in equation (20.5) over each element. Integrating over different-shaped hexahedra elements, for example, is a complicated procedure. To overcome this difficulty, a standard element is introduced $\Omega_{ST} = \{(\zeta, \eta, \varsigma) -1 \leq \zeta \leq 1, -1 \leq \eta \leq 1, -1 \leq \varsigma \leq 1,\}$ and an

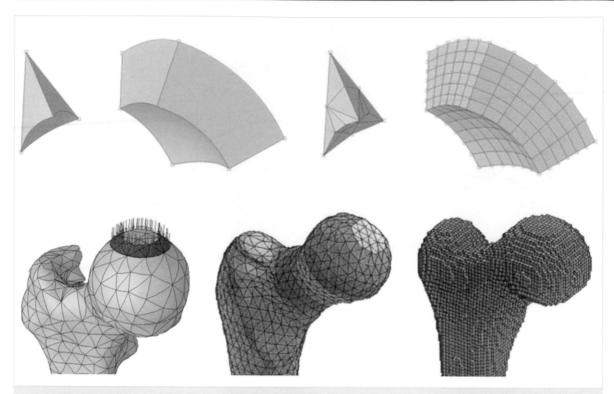

Fig. 20.4 *Top left*: p-extension. *Top right*: h-extension. *Bottom*: FE models of the proximal femur. *Left*: p-finite element method (large fewer elements with curved surfaces). *Middle*: Structural h-finite element method. *Right*: voxel-based h-finite element method.

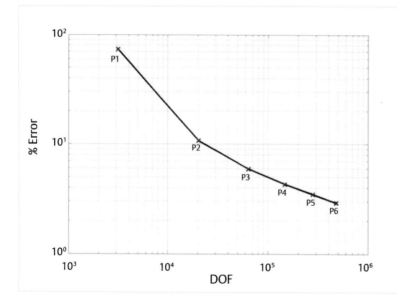

Fig. 20.5 A typical example of the convergence of the relative error in energy norm (algebraic convergence due to clamping without mesh refinement).

associated "mapping" is possible so to "map" the standard hexahedral element into any "real" hexahedral element with curved faces (see ▶ Fig. 20.3) by using the blending function method.[2] In this manner, each integral in equation (20.5) is evaluated over the standard element introducing the Jacobian of the mapping. For example:

$$\iiint_{\Omega_l} ([D]\boldsymbol{u})^T [E]\ [D]\boldsymbol{u}\ d\Omega_l =$$

$$\int_{-1}^{1} \int_{-1}^{1} \int_{-1}^{1} ([D]\boldsymbol{u}(\zeta,\eta,\varsigma))^T [E][D]\boldsymbol{u}(\zeta,\eta,\varsigma)\, J\ d\zeta\ d\eta\ d\varsigma$$

$$(20.6)$$

Because the minimum potential energy formulation has been split into a sum over all elements, and furthermore, all integrations are performed over the standard element, it is only natural to define a basis function on the standard element. In each element, the displacements are represented by a set of basis functions—these are also called shape functions. Let u_{FE} in each element be expressed in terms of elemental M basis functions, which are constructed by monomials, $N_i(\zeta, \eta, \varsigma)$ (spanning a finite-dimensional subspace):

$$u_{xFE}^{(l)} = \sum_{i=1}^{M} a_i^{(l)} N_i(\zeta, \eta, \varsigma)$$

$$u_{yFE}^{(l)} = \sum_{i=M+1}^{2M} a_i^{(l)} N_i(\zeta, \eta, \varsigma)$$

$$u_{zFE}^{(l)} = \sum_{i=2M+1}^{3M} a_i^{(l)} N_i(\zeta, \eta, \varsigma) \tag{20.7}$$

$$\Downarrow$$

$$u_{FE}^{(l)} = \begin{bmatrix} N_1 \cdots N_M & 0 \cdots 0 & 0 \cdots 0 \\ 0 \cdots 0 & N_1 \cdots N_M & 0 \cdots 0 \\ 0 \cdots 0 & 0 \cdots 0 & N_1 \cdots N_M \end{bmatrix} \begin{pmatrix} a_1^{(l)} \\ \vdots \\ a_{3M}^{(l)} \end{pmatrix}$$

where $a_i^{(l)}$ are the amplitudes of the basis functions in element l, and for example $N_1 = \frac{1}{8}(1 - \zeta)(1 - \eta)(1 - \varsigma)$. Seeking for u_{FE} reduces to the determination of the unknowns $a_i^{(l)}$. These are collected from all elements in the FE model and stored in a vector denoted a. The number of entries in the vector a represents the dimension of the space in which u_{FE} is sought and is called the *number of degrees of freedom* (DOFs).

Substituting equation (20.7) in equation (20.6) and thereafter in equation (20.5), then collecting the contribution of all elements (a process named the assembly process), one obtains the set of algebraic equations, which may be stated as:

Find the vector a that minimizes

$$\frac{1}{2} a^T [K] a - a^T r \rightarrow [K] a = r, \tag{20.8}$$

where $[K]$ is denoted stiffness matrix and r is the load vector. The FE solution is obtained by inverting the stiffness matrix and multiplying it by the load vector. In most FE methods, the stiffness matrix is symmetric and sparse, therefore efficient numerical methods exist that invert it (e.g., a problem with a million DOFs can be solved nowadays on a personal computer within less than half an hour).

20.4 Estimation of the Discretization Error—The h- and p-Versions of the Finite Element Method

Obtaining the vector a and using equation (20.7) for determining u_{FE} *for a single FE solution* cannot quantify

the discretization error $e_D = u_{Simp} - u_{FE}$. To estimate e_D, one has to increase the dimension of the FE space (i.e., performing an extension procedure [increasing the number of DOFs]). There are three different possibilities:

- *h*-extension: Refining the FE mesh (i.e., adding more elements), while describing u_{FE} in each element by a small number of shape functions (M in equation (20.7) is small).
- *p*-extension: Keeping the FE mesh fixed and increasing the number of basis functions in each element (M in equation (20.7) is progressively increased).
- *hp*-extension: Changing the mesh and the number of basis functions over individual or all elements.

In ▶ Fig. 20.4, typical h- and p-FE models are presented. In the top row, we show hexahedral and tetrahedral elements that undergo p-extension (*left*: The number of elements in the model does not change, only the number of basis functions is increased by adding polynomials of higher degree) and h-extension (*right*: The basis function over each element remains at low order, while the elements are divided into smaller elements).

The most important and basic quantification of the discretization error is the *error in energy norm* that is associated with the root-mean-square average of the stresses over the entire domain.[2] It can be shown that the error in energy norm can be computed using the potential energy as follows:

$$\| e_D \|_\varepsilon \overset{\triangle}{=} \sqrt{\frac{1}{2} B(e, e)} = \sqrt{\Pi(u_{FE}) - \Pi(u_{Simp})} \tag{20.9}$$

This error measure is a global measure because it is the integration over the entire domain, and unless this measure is under a given tolerance, the FE solution cannot be claimed to be a good approximation of u_{Simp}.

The error estimates are presented as error bounds,[3] and they are expressed in terms of the number of DOFs. For problems with smooth boundaries and continuous boundary conditions commonly encountered in biomechanics, *the use of p-version of the FE method exhibits exponential convergence, which is much faster compared to the algebraic convergence observed by the classical h-version.*

Although the solution u_{Simp} is unknown, by using mathematical relations on consecutive FE solutions having progressively increased DOFs, one may estimate and plot the error in energy norm versus the DOFs. As an example, in ▶ Fig. 20.5 the convergence in energy norm is presented for a p-FE analysis of a femur, increasing the polynomial degree from 1 to 6. At p = 6, there are about 50,000 DOFs in the FE model, and the relative error in energy norm is reduced to about 3%, which is of high enough accuracy for three-dimensional problems.

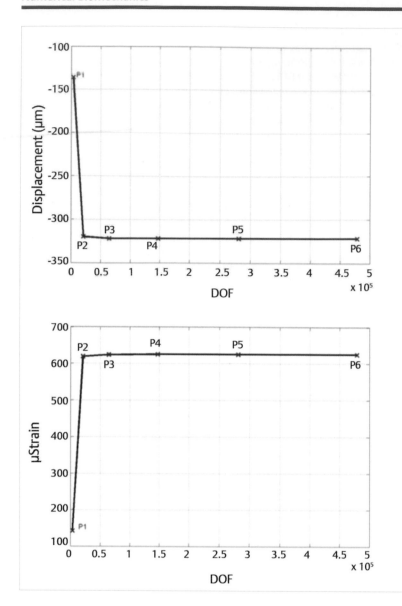

Fig. 20.6 A typical example of the convergence of pointwise displacement (a) and strain (b).

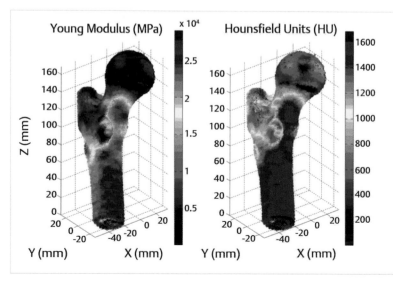

Fig. 20.7 Hounsfield units in a proximal femur (*right*) and corresponding E according to (11) (*left*).

The convergence of the error in the energy norm is a *necessary* condition for extraction of other data from the FE solution, but is not a sufficient condition. Usually the pointwise values of displacements or stresses are of interest, and after error in energy norm is converged one has to consider the convergence of other pointwise entities by inspecting that the extracted values do not change as the number of DOFs is increased. See, for example, such convergence plots for strains and displacements at a specific point in ► Fig. 20.6.

Because most of the analyses on bones have usually smooth solutions, there is an advantage in using p-FE methods for the following reasons:

1. Convergence rates are much faster compared to conventional h-FE methods.

2. Elements may be distorted and have large aspect ratios up to 100, unlike h-FE methods where the aspect ratio of elements is restricted to 4.

3. Tetrahedral meshes do no poses any "stiffening effects" when the polynomial order is increased in p-FE methods, unlike the "overstiff" h-tetrahedral elements.

4. Control of discretization error is inherent in p-FE methods (where many solutions are automatically obtained on same mesh) unlike the tedious work required in h-FE methods to refine the mesh and perform a convergence check over multiple meshes.

20.5 Assigning Material Properties to the Finite Element Model

One major issue associated with FE analyses of bone tissues at the macro scale (order of magnitude of 1 to 2 mm) is the assignment of material properties. Bone is considered to be elastic and inhomogeneous (material properties change from point to point within the bone). Furthermore, the realistic bone tissue is also orthotropic or at least transversely isotropic (the bone behaves differently to loading in different directions). Many studies have demonstrated that there is a strong correlation between material properties and the bone density,[4] and that in many cases long bones such as the femur may be considered to be isotropic. Therefore, the spatial variation of the material properties may be obtained from CT scans by determining the ash density at each point within the bone (with an intermediate density measure named ρ_{EQM}) according to the Hounsfield units (HU):

$$\rho_{EQM} = 10^{-3}(a \times HU - b)\left[g/cm^3\right]$$
$$\rho_{ash} = 1.22 \times \rho_{EQM} + 0.0523\left[g/cm^3\right]$$
$$E_{Cort} = 10200 \times \rho_{ash}^{2.01}\,[MPa]\ \rho_{ash} > 0.6$$
$$E_{Trab} = 5307 \times \rho_{ash} + 469\,[MPa]\ 0.27 < \rho_{ash} \le 0.6$$
$$E_{Trab} = 33900 \times \rho_{ash}^{2.20}\,[MPa]\ \rho_{ash} \le 0.27$$

(20.10)

or,

$$E = 12000\rho_{ash}^{1.45}\,[MPa]$$

(20.11)

► Fig. 20.7 shows a plot of the Hounsfield units on the surface of a femur and the corresponding Young's modulus.

The material properties are required in an FE analysis for the computation of the stiffness matrix (it depends on $E(x,y,z)$ in equations (20.5) and (20.6)). More specifically, the integral in equation (20.6) is computed by numerical integration, thus the integrand has to be evaluated at specific points within the element (Gauss points).

$E(x,y,z)$ at the Gauss points is determined by the CT scan. Instead of computing the material properties at each Gauss point, in many h-FE models an average property is computed from all CT voxels in that element, and this average is assigned to all Gauss points in that element. Although easier to implement, this method, apart from being less realistic, imposes difficulties in the convergence study because the material properties within a given bone change from a coarse mesh to a more refined one, and convergence is difficult to achieve. In p-FE methods, however, the material properties are independent of the underlying FE mesh,[5,6] and each Gauss point has a different material property.

A more realistic representation of the bone tissue is by assigning to it inhomogeneous orthotropic material properties. The major difficulty with this approach is the lack of in vivo knowledge of the material trajectories and the distinct nine material properties (or at least five of them in case of a transversely isotropic material assumption). In these cases, micromechanical approaches may be used to obtain approximated transversely material properties that can be assigned to FE models of femurs.[7]

20.6 Assigning Loading and Constrain Boundary Conditions to the Finite Element Model

The last step required for an FE analysis is the assignment of loading and constrain boundary conditions to the FE model. Choosing the physiological magnitude and direction of the various forces on the femur to mimic a specific motion (like stair climbing, stance position, or walking) is a complicated task[8,9] and is associated with idealization—thus, it will be discussed in subsequent chapters. Here, we address the application of the appropriate set of loadings and constrains on the FE model.

A common conceptual error is assigning a point force (like a nodal force) or a line force (N/m) on the boundary of a three-dimensional domain. Only a traction (force

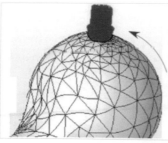
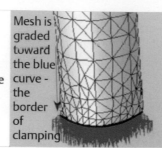

Mesh is graded toward the blue curve - the border of tractions

Mesh is graded toward the blue curve - the border of clamping

Fig. 20.8 Example of mesh refinements toward abrupt changes in boundary conditions (p-finite element mesh).

over an area, N/mm²) is allowed, so even if the force acts on a very small area, it should be prescribed accordingly. Any point or line force will result in an infinite strain energy; therefore, as the number of DOFs is increased, the solution will not converge, but the strain energy will tend to infinity. Similarly, in a two-dimensional analysis, a pointwise force is prohibited, but only a line force is allowed on domain's boundary.

The same conceptual error is associated with the assignment of point and line displacements (or clamping) on the surface of a three-dimensional domain.

20.7 Practical Considerations when Using Finite Element Methods or Interpreting the Finite Element Results

Nowadays, providing FE results (usually with colorful pictures) is not enough and the assessment of the numerical error is of equal importance as the FE results themselves. Thus, each FE analysis has to be accompanied by the estimation of the error in energy norm and the evidence that the data of interest (be they strains, displacements, stiffness, stresses, etc.) are accompanied by a convergence plot (as shown in ▶ Fig. 20.5 and ▶ Fig. 20.6), demonstrating that the results are independent of the discretization parameters as elements' size, type of elements, etc.

To achieve accurate results, it is a good practice to refine the FE mesh where rapid changes in the shape of the geometry occur or at areas where the material properties or boundary conditions change rapidly. Using h-FE methods, one needs to create elements that have aspect ratios less than four, angles as close to 90 degrees as possible, and an element that is not too distorted. These restrictions do not apply usually to p-FE methods. At locations in the FE model where an *abrupt* change in geometry (sharp corners, for example), an abrupt change in material properties at the surface of the domain (at the interface of a metallic device bonded to the bone, for example), or an abrupt change in boundary conditions (where the clamping of the bone ends, for example) occurs, the FE results are usually incorrect, and FE results from elements that are in the first and second layer

around the abrupt change should be avoided. In case these areas are of interest, a local very refined mesh should be used (see examples in ▶ Fig. 20.8).

Another measure easily checked that hints on the *inaccuracy* of the FE results are large discontinuities in strains/stresses at the borders of the elements (the contrary is not true, that is, if the discontinuities are small, it does not hint on the accuracy of the FE results). The FE method only assures that the displacements u_{FE} are continuous across elements' boundaries, but the strains and stresses may, and often do, have discontinuities (jumps) across elements' boundaries (▶ Fig. 20.9). These jumps become progressively smaller as the number of DOFs is increased (i.e., when the discretization error decreases). Most FE commercial programs have a "smoothing algorithm" when plotting the strains/stresses on the domain of interest that "smooth the jumps" by interpolating the strains/stresses through the Gauss points of the elements —these colorful pictures at times mislead the analyst and create a misleading illusion as if the results are converged. Therefore, it is always a good practice to dismiss this smoothing algorithm when plotting stresses or strain results.

Most automeshers (algorithms in preprocessors that assign an FE mesh to a solid model) create by default tetrahedral elements in a three-dimensional domain. Using linear tetrahedral elements is not recommended because of large numerical errors associated with this kind of elements (they produce an "overstiff" response). Therefore, it is always suggested to use hexahedral elements. Furthermore, the less distorted the elements are and the closer the aspect ratio is to one, the higher is the accuracy when h-FE methods are considered. p-FE methods are insensitive to the aspect ratio of the elements and much less sensitive to distortion. The tetrahedral p-FE methods do not suffer from the "overstiff" response if the p-level is increased beyond four.

The FE analyst never has in his or her possession the entire data to the required precision, and in many cases it is not trivial to predict how sensitive the results are to small changes in the FE input data. It is therefore strongly suggested to perform sensitivity checks to determine how much the data of interest change as a result of small changes in the uncertain data available. These sensitivity analyses are especially important if the location of

Principle stress p=2   Principle stress p=4   Uz displacements p=2

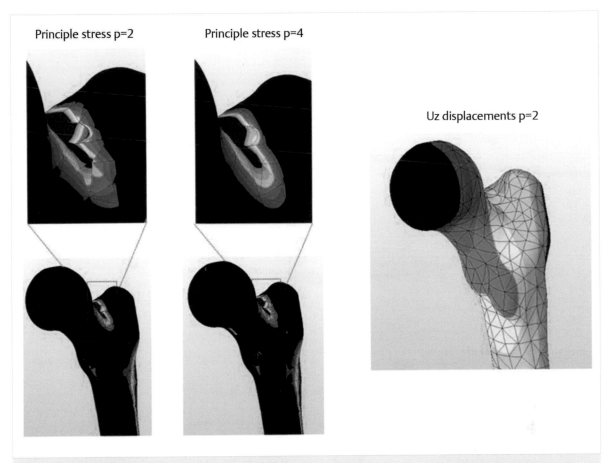

Fig. 20.9 Example of stress "jumps" across elements' boundaries that hint on a finite element solution not yet converged (p = 2), whereas as the p-level increases to p = 4, the jumps are much less pronounced. On the right, the displacements have no jumps.

interest on the bone is close to the displacement boundaries or locations of load application. For example, in many biomechanical experiments, the bone is being "clamped" or positioned into a rigid cast. If the location of interest on the bone is in a close proximity to the application of the boundary condition, then the FE results at this location have to be checked to determine if they change much following small changes in the location and type of the boundary conditions. A large change in the result of interest following a small change in the input data may indicate an ill-posed problem, and thus the FE results may be misleading. An FE model that is oversensitive to parameters that are uncertain may and in fact often does produce erroneous results.

20.8 Finite Element Methods and μFinite Element Methods

When the entire bone is of interest, one uses regular FE models with homogenized material properties, as described previously. For studies on bone samples usually in the trabecular regions, the need of detailed FE methods emerges. This task progressed with the development of μCT scanners, allowing nowadays the creation of FE models with elements having the dimensions of an order of a μmeter—these are termed "μFE models". The μCT scans possess an exquisite level of anatomical detail; however, due to the very high radiation level they cannot be used in vivo. Therefore, only in vitro studies are allowed. μFE models are created by converting each μCT voxel (usually of a typical edge dimension of 10 to 50 μmeter) into a hexahedral element, such that one obtains the trabecular architecture implicitly. For example, a 1 mm^3 of trabecular bone may contain up to 100,000 elements, and the computational resources and computational time may be enormous. This necessitates custom FE codes, parallel algorithms, and high-performance computing that became available in the past decade. A highly automated mesh generator is used to create voxel-based meshes—however, due to the box-shaped elements, the boundary has irregular surfaces that cause significant errors in the strains and stress results, and thus the boundary stresses and strains have to be averaged.

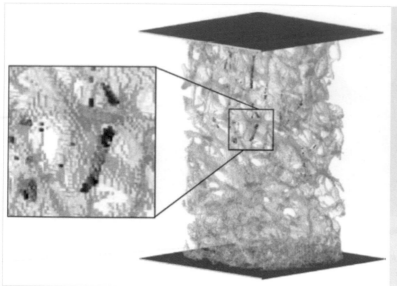

Fig. 20.10 A μ-FEM of a human trabecular bone cylinder (8 mm diameter, 12 mm length) generated from a μ-CT with a 30 μmeter resolution. (Reprinted from Chevalier Y, Pahr D, Allmer H, Charlebois M, Zysset P. Validation of a voxel-based FE method for prediction of the uniaxial apparent modulus of human trabecular bone using macroscopic mechanical tests and nanoindentation. J Biomech 2007;40 [15]:3333–3340, Fig. 3.)

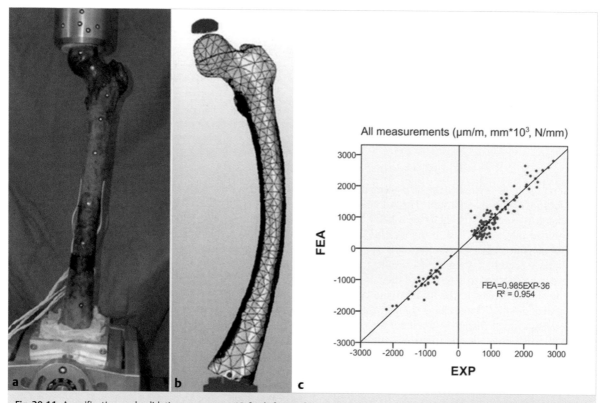

Fig. 20.11 A verification and validation process on 12 fresh-frozen femurs (in vitro experiments and p-finite element analyses that mimic the experiments) and the corresponding match between finite element and experimental results (displacements, strains, and stiffness). (From Trabelsi N, Yosibash Z, Wutte C, Augat P, Eberle S. Patient-specific finite element analysis of the human femur—a double-blinded biomechanical validation. J Biomech 2011;44([9]:1666–1672.)

Although very expensive computationally, the μFE models are valuable in providing an understanding of how changes in trabecular architecture (e.g., trabecular thinning and loss of individual trabeculae) and damage accumulation affect the mechanical behavior. An example of such a μFE model is provided in ▸ Fig. 20.10. One of the main uses of μFE models is to establish relations between the homogenized mechanical properties and the trabecular architecture and lamella's mechanical properties.[10,11] The effect of specific changes in the architecture, due to osteoporosis, for example, on the homogenized material properties may be addressed. Another application of μFE models is the estimation of the stresses and strains (and possible failure at the local level) in response to the load applied at the organ level. Studies have shown that due to the special architecture, the stresses and strains at the lamella level may lead to local damage with implications on spatial heterogeneity in stresses and strains, damage accumulation, and bone adaptation.

20.9 The Concept of Verification and Validation

Patient-specific FE bone models based on quantitative CT scans can be easily generated nowadays, and thousands of papers have been published in the past decade with colorful pictures (the majority without a clear documentation of the verification process that is mandatory for any numerical method). However, for the application of such FE methods in clinical practice, verification is necessary but not sufficient. After the verification, a validation process has to be completed—this means that the FE results (shown to be free of numerical errors) must match closely the experimental findings that the FE model mimics (i.e., a process by which one ensures that the idealization error, e_I, is small). These FE models are usually validated by biomechanical in vitro experiments, and if possible in a double-blinded manner by two different groups to avoid any bias. All measurable data should be addressed, such as strains (measured by strain gauges), displacements, and stiffness of the bone. An example of a verification and validation procedure has been presented in several recent publications[6,7,12,13] and shown in ▸ Fig. 20.11. Details on the validation process and the

advocated synergy between models and experiments are the topic of the next chapter.

References

[1] Sokolnikoff IS. The mathematical theory of elasticity. 2 e. Sykesville, MD: McGraw-Hill; 1956

[2] Szabo B, Babuska I. Finite element analysis. Hoboken, NJ: John Wiley and Sons; 1991

[3] Babuska I, Suri M. The p and h-p versions of the finite element method, basic principles and properties SIAM Rev 1994; 36: 578–632

[4] Keyak JH, Falkinstein Y. Comparison of in situ and in vitro CT scan-based finite element model predictions of proximal femoral fracture load. Med Eng Phys 2003; 25: 781–787

[5] Yosibash Z, Padan R, Joskowicz L, Milgrom C. A CT-based high-order finite element analysis of the human proximal femur compared to in-vitro experiments. J Biomech Eng 2007; 129: 297–309

[6] Yosibash Z, Trabelsi N, Milgrom C. Reliable simulations of the human proximal femur by high-order finite element analysis validated by experimental observations. J Biomech 2007; 40: 3688–3699

[7] Trabelsi N, Yosibash Z. Patient-specific finite-element analyses of the proximal femur with orthotropic material properties validated by experiments. J Biomech Eng 2011; 133: 061001

[8] Bergmann G, Deuretzbacher G, Heller M et al. Hip contact forces and gait patterns from routine activities. J Biomech 2001; 34: 859–871

[9] Heller MO, Bergmann G, Kassi J-P, Claes L, Haas NP, Duda GN. Determination of muscle loading at the hip joint for use in pre-clinical testing. J Biomech 2005; 38: 1155–1163

[10] van Rietbergen B, Weinans H, Huiskes R, Odgaard A. A new method to determine trabecular bone elastic properties and loading using micromechanical finite-element models. J Biomech 1995; 28: 69–81

[11] Verhulp E, van Rietbergen B, Huiskes R. Comparison of micro-level and continuum-level voxel models of the proximal femur. J Biomech 2006; 39: 2951–2957

[12] Trabelsi N, Yosibash Z, Wutte C, Augat P, Eberle S. Patient-specific finite element analysis of the human femur—a double-blinded biomechanical validation. J Biomech 2011; 44: 1666–1672

[13] Cristofolini L, Schileo E, Juszczyk M, Taddei F, Martelli S, Viceconti M. Mechanical testing of bones: the positive synergy of finite-element models and in vitro experiments. Philos Trans A Math Phys Eng Sci 2010; 368: 2725–2763

Further Reading

Szabo B, Babuska I. Introduction to finite element analysis. Formulation, verification and validation. Hoboken, NJ: John Wiley and Sons; 2011

Wriggers P. Nonlinear finite element methods. New York: Springer; 2008

Yosibash Z, Trabelsi N. Reliable patient-specific simulations of the femur. In Gefen A, ed. Patient-specific modeling in tomorrow's medicine. New York: Springer; 2012:3–26

21 Validation of Finite Element Models

Luca Cristofolini

While in natural sciences, empiricism is predominant, mathematical modeling is traditionally limited to inductive models that extrapolate from repeated experimental observations. The extreme specialization of research has slowly separated mathematical modeling skills from experimental skills in most research groups, and it is not rare to see groups where only one of these skills is truly developed. This is a pity: The complexity involved with understanding the biomechanical behavior of the musculoskeletal system is overwhelming; to advance comprehension, one should be ready to use every technique available.

The loading scenarios applied in vitro generally follow two different philosophies that reflect the complexity of the human musculoskeletal system:

1. Individual load components are applied to the bone, with no direct connection to any specific in vivo loading scenario for several reasons. First of all, many bone segments undergo in vivo a number of quite different loading during a variety of motor tasks.[1] Rather than replicating a large number of loading conditions, in some cases it is preferable to separately apply the main load components to the bone. Furthermore, often no details are available about the magnitude and direction of the loads applied in vivo to the bones. When information is scarce or inaccurate, it is preferable to bypass the problem by focusing on a simplified (and better controlled) loading scenario.
2. When adequate knowledge is available and it is necessary to include the complexity of in vivo loading in the in vitro simulation, experimental studies aim at replicating the load components applied during selected motor tasks.[2] In order to represent the physiological range of loading configurations, different motor tasks need to be simulated.[3,4] In general, such in vitro simulations involve a more complex loading system, often including the action of relevant muscle groups.[5,6]

In the past decades, the mechanical behavior of bone structures has been intensively investigated with mathematical models. The most commonly used numerical models in biomechanics are finite element (FE) models. An FE model is a numerical model that enables calculation of selected physical quantities (e.g., stress, strain, risk of fracture) based on discretization of the structure into elements of simple geometry (see Chapter 20). FE models also have been extensively used for the determination of the mechanical stresses that physiological activities, pathological conditions, or surgical treatment induce in bones. FE models can also be used to investigate the mechanobiological phenomena underlying bone adaptation.[7] FE models, if compared to most experimental techniques, offer the advantage of estimating the stress/strain distribution over the whole structure rather than in a few selected points/regions, and enable a time-effective exploration of the effect of relevant study parameters. Subject-specific modeling procedures enable the creation of an FE model of a bone segment from computed tomography (CT) images. This makes it possible to estimate mechanical magnitudes in bones that cannot be measured in vivo without invasive or unethical procedures.

Both numerical models and in vitro experiments are *models* of the physical event under investigation. Therefore, both their relevance and their reliability cannot be taken for granted. A synergistic use of numerical models and in vitro experiments can provide at the same time corroboration to both types of models and a deeper insight into the physical event being investigated. There are a few studies where numerical modeling and controlled in vitro experiments are combined in a single study, mostly using the experiments to corroborate/falsify the numerical models (this process is usually called validation). Validation is a crucial aspect as it is the only procedure that enables quantifying the reliability of a model for a clinical application. Unfortunately, the combination of numerical and experimental approaches is most often restricted to the validation purposes, with no contribution in the opposite direction (from FE models to in vitro experiments). However, the great potential of experimental-numerical integration is the cross-fertilization between the two approaches.

21.1 Weak Points and Needs of Finite Element Models

21.1.1 Limitations of Numerical Models

One should never forget that a model cannot account for something that is totally unknown and unexpected. Mathematical models are fabrications of the human mind and can only know what is already to some extent known. Therefore, numerical models can only be used to investigate known (or at least suspected) scenarios. Besides this primary limitation, there are others related to the specific nature of numerical models. The biggest limitation comes from the process at the root of each model: idealization. We observe the physical reality, and from this observation we develop an idealized representation of the phenomenon of interest, which we describe in mathematical terms. Such an idealization can either be achieved by neglecting certain aspects (Aristotelian idealization) or by assuming true something we know to be false (Galilean idealization; e.g., a massless object). In both cases, this process is associated with some limitations of the validity of the model, which cannot be overcome. For instance, a model where contact is assumed to be frictionless will never be able to elucidate anything useful about frictional abrasion.

A second limitation of numerical models derives from the numerical tools used. Any numerical solution is approximated: Such an approximation defines a "resolution" for our model. Details and events that are finer than this resolution cannot be investigated with that model. Some numerical approximations, such as those caused by finite-precision computing, are usually negligible. However, in the FE method, there are other problems such as the discretization of the integration domain that might induce critical errors (see Chapter 20). For instance, an FE estimate of the contact stresses at the tip of a sharp object (e.g., like the thread of a bone screw) may not be reliable up to two- or three-elements distance.

The third problem with the FE method is the so-called identification of the model. This consists in the determination of the values to be assigned to the model parameters (i.e., Young's modulus, friction coefficient). In general, these values derive from experimental measurements or estimates and are available with limited precision. Such uncertainty in the model parameters propagates to the model predictions. A typical problem is the identification of the boundary condition in validation experiments.

21.1.2 Requirements of Finite Element Models: Definition of the Modeling Scope

As said previously, a model of a given bone segment or anatomical region is not universal and is not capable of addressing any possible biomechanical questions. Therefore, the scope of the model should be defined as clearly and unambiguously as possible. Models can be used simply to represent a phenomenon (e.g., for teaching purposes, for memorization). The modeling scope must be defined with great detail and should include which portion of reality we want to capture, which biomechanical quantities we need to estimate, and under which conditions.

21.1.3 Requirements of Finite Element Models: Idealization and Deployment

A model consists in an idealization of a portion of reality by observing how mechanical/biological quantities are organized in space and time, and how they interact with each other. In scientific modeling, this cognitive

artifact should be expressed in logical terms: Models can be divided into *inductive* models (i.e., regression models, data models), *deductive* models (i.e., models based on the laws of physics), or *abductive* models (i.e., Bayesian models).

The model is now converted into a tool that can be practically used to address the modeling scope. Typically, idealization is captured into mathematical form, which is then solved either analytically or numerically. Due to the complexity of the models involved in biomedicine, most models are solved numerically (i.e., in an approximated form).

21.1.4 Requirements of Finite Element Models: Verification

When a mathematical model is solved numerically, it is important to quantify the accuracy of such an approximate solution. For linear models, it is generally possible to estimate the errors associated with the numerical solution. Post hoc indicators such as the stress error indicator or convergence tests (▶ Fig. 21.1) on parameters, such as potential energy of the entire bone, displacements, and strains at the points of interest, can estimate the error due to the spatial discretization of the domain, which is one of the most delicate aspects of FE modeling (see Chapter 20).

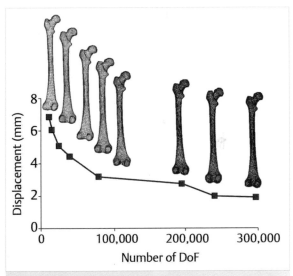

Fig. 21.1 Convergence plot used to check the adequacy of the mesh used to model a human femur. In this instance, the displacement under load at a given point of the bone (the center of the femoral head) shows an asymptote. Similar plots can help assessing a number of indicators such as strain values at most relevant points or the strain energy density. Mesh refinement (which is computer-costly) is stopped when a further increase in the number of elements affects the output by less than an assigned threshold. (Copyright of the VPH-OP consortium; reproduced with permission.)

21.1.5 Requirements of Finite Element Models: Sensitivity Analysis

FE models estimate the state of a system (e.g., the stress/strain distribution) based on a set of initial values. It is important to verify how an uncertainty on such input parameters affects the estimates provided by the model. First of all, because the initial values used for the identification of the model are always associated with an error, we need to ensure that this uncertainty does not excessively affect the conclusions we aim to draw from the model. Secondly, if we notice that the model is hugely sensitive to small variation of some initial values, this can suggest that idealization or its mathematical or numerical deployments are critical. Assuming one has a reliable estimate of the uncertainty associated with each parameter to be used in the model, it is recommended to run a sensitivity analysis to estimate how these uncertainties propagate through the model and affect the model outcome. This can be done with a simpler exploratory analysis such as the *design of experiment* and related simplified Taguchi strategies, or using a more complex Monte Carlo–based statistical FE modeling approach. Sensitivity analysis is the best way to discover truly unforeseeable errors in the model.

21.1.6 Why Do Finite Element Models Need Validation?

The predictive accuracy of a model can be measured by comparing its outcome against matching quantities measured in a controlled physical experiment. Every model is reasonably accurate within certain limits (the modeling scope must be compatible with such limits [i.e., no material behaves linear-elastic indefinitely]). It must be noted that validation (in the sense of determining if a computational model represents the actual physical event with sufficient accuracy) is not even possible.

There is not a single possible approach for validation that applies to all problems. When it is not obvious which mathematical model is best suited for the scope, a *strong inference* approach is advisable. Strong inference consists of having two or more candidate mathematics compete with respect to the results of one or more controlled experiments. One should always remember the Ockham's razor: If two models show similar predictive accuracy, the one with fewer assumptions should be chosen.

21.2 Limitations of in Vitro Experiments

While in vitro experiments can help in addressing some problems of FE models, one should also be aware of the limitations of experimental measurements. First of all, in vitro experiments are time-consuming and require costly strain/displacement/force transducers, including dedicated data loggers. Moreover, experimental measurements are affected by both random and systematic error (▶ Fig. 21.2).

21.2.1 Error Affecting Experimental Measurement: Bias

Systematic error can be induced by a number of factors including:
- Defective preparation/use of the transducers: this can result in largely biased readouts.
- Perturbation induced by the measurement systems (i.e., when a strain sensor is bonded to a bone it reinforces its surface, contributing to load bearing). Therefore, the actual strain distribution is underestimated systematically.
- Ambiguous or ill-defined anatomical reference frames: As such, reference frames often rely upon subjective identification of bone landmarks, and different operators will achieve different alignment of the specimens.
- Poor information about in vivo loads.
- Ill-designed loading setup: In some cases, the loading system results in overconstrained conditions, where additional load components (other than the intended one[s]) are generated within the loading system.

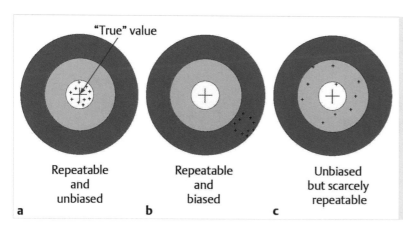

Repeatable and unbiased

a

Repeatable and biased

b

Unbiased but scarcely repeatable

c

Fig. 21.2 Error affecting experimental measurements belong to two categories: systematic and random. An ideal accurate measurement (a) has good repeatability and the average measured value is close to the "true" value. (b) Systematic errors lead to biased measurements. (c) Random experimental noise makes measurements.

21.2.2 Error Affecting Experimental Measurement: Noise

The second type of error is different in nature. Random error (noise) can be induced by:

- Measurement noise: All measurement systems, including mechanical ones, are affected by "noise," including mechanical vibration, electromagnetic interference, etc.
- Uncertainty in the pose of the test specimens: Holding and applying loads to bone segments can be difficult because of the irregular geometry. This results in variability between test repetitions or between specimens.
- Uncertainty in the positioning and alignment of the transducers: If a transducer is randomly misplaced or misaligned, the readout will suffer from an unpredictable error.
- Scarce repeatability of the applied loads: In most cases, material testing machines or dedicated simulators are used. In all such cases, actuators, loading fixtures, and control systems are used that unavoidably introduce some random error.

21.2.3 In Vitro Experiments Are Costly

The addition of any new measured parameter or replication of measurements is associated with the need of using more transducers and more specimens. The availability of human tissue specimens is limited, both for practical and for ethical reasons. For these reasons, in many cases the sample size of in vitro experiments is statistically underpowered. Furthermore, if an in vitro experiment needs to be performed repeatedly under similar conditions (e.g., to test different implantable devices, different loading configurations, different interface conditions, etc.), most of the experimental cost and effort need to be replicated. Therefore, in vitro experiments are not the best tool for performing comparative studies on a large number of conditions, or for performing sensitivity analysis to explore a large number of scenarios.

21.2.4 Guidelines for Designing and Improving an in Vitro Setup

Although this is sometimes not sufficiently appreciated, in vitro experiments are just models of the physical event under investigation. Therefore, the closeness of an in vitro experiment to the physical event under investigation cannot be taken for granted. This should be assessed by comparing the in vitro experiment against some more direct evidence of the physical event: In the case of bone testing, this could be some clinical data of bone fractures or in vivo recording of loads.

When designing an experiment, one must bear in mind that the experiment, like any other model, is capable of capturing only some details of a reality that is much more complex. Therefore, in vitro experiments must be designed with a specific research question in mind. Details that are not relevant to such a research question should be omitted, as they would only reduce the overall control we have on the experiment.

As a prerequisite, reliability of in vitro experiments must be assessed, so that uncertainty is estimated for each measured magnitude. Repeated measurements on the same specimen are crucial to estimate the intrinsic measurement repeatability. At the same time, repetitions on more specimens are necessary to estimate the variability between specimens.

21.3 The Role of in Vitro Experiments in Improving Finite Element Models

Experiments cannot be used to address the limitations of FE models relating to the numerics and computational postprocessing. However, experiments are extremely valuable for feeding FE models with reliable input parameters (identification) and for comparing FE models against reliable reference measurements (validation; ▶ Fig. 21.3). Although mechanical testing can be performed at all dimensional scales, the following examples refer to organ-level models. The underlying principles remain valid also when other scales are involved such as in whole-body modeling or in micro-FE simulation.

21.3.1 Preliminary Identification of Most Relevant Scenarios and Indicators

As stated previously, models can only address known scenarios: If the details of an FE model are chosen to provide most accurate information for a chosen indicator (e.g., bone stress), they might be unsuitable for predicting other magnitudes (e.g., fracture). As in vitro experiments rely upon physical specimens, in a way they are closer to reality and therefore are better capable of capturing aspects of reality that might be completely missed by FE models. Once in vitro tests have identified the relevant mode of failure, or loading scenario, FE models can be specifically designed or tuned to address such a mode or scenario.

21.3.2 Boundary Conditions

The position of the applied loads relative to the bone is a very critical factor determining the output of an FE model. For instance, when the articular force is applied to the femoral head in vitro, it is not possible a priori to determine accurately the position of the resultant force because long bones undergo significant deflection when

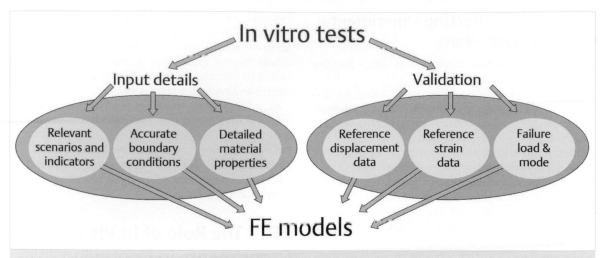

Fig. 21.3 Block diagram showing how in vitro experiments can support finite element (*FE*) models. Two pathways exist: identification of the model parameters, and validation of model predictions. (Copyright of the VPH-OP consortium; reproduced with permission.)

loaded, and the contact area between the bone and the loading device may change during load application. Consequently, it is not possible to predict, a priori, the changing position and direction of the applied force under the applied load. Therefore, even assuming that the position of the applied force is defined in principle (based on biomechanical and anatomical considerations), the problem remains how to accurately measure the actual position of force application in the actual in vitro experiment. Inaccurate identification of the position of the applied force would undermine the comparison between in vitro experiment and FE model, and consequently the accuracy of the FE simulation.

21.3.3 Constitutive Equations and Failure Criteria (Tissue Level and Subtissue Level)

FE models designed to predict structural behavior, organ-level strength, or bone-implant response usually adopt a continuum-level assumption for bone tissue. Continuum-level models require the definition of continuum-level bone tissue mechanical properties. Alternative approaches have been presented where an organ-level model containing information at the tissue-level (and therefore explicitly modeling the trabecular architecture) has been generated. However, because of the need of impressive computational power, and high-resolution imaging (micro-CT), such models cannot currently be associated with clinical applications.

Bone tissue is inhomogeneous, anisotropic, and to some extent viscoelastic in nature. Bone viscoelasticity can be neglected for most biomechanical studies simulating bone stresses as a consequence of physiological loads. However, when strain rate is an important factor (e.g.,

impact), bone viscoelasticity can be accounted for by considering the strain rate effect when assigning the elastic modulus. The modulus of elasticity (Young's modulus) of bone tissue has been reported to vary by over 50% for cortical bone and by over 500% for cancellous bone, depending on anatomical site, direction of loading, and donor's details. Most of this variability can be explained in terms of inhomogeneity. However, in early FE models, bone tissue was modeled as a fully isotropic and homogeneous material. Assigning average elastic constants to the entire bone structure is associated with large errors (of the same magnitude as the uncertainty associated with the Young's modulus). Errors of the order of 10 to 50% are to be expected on average, with local peaks largely exceeding 100%.

More recently, bone inhomogeneity was introduced in FE models of bones deriving bone tissue density from CT scan data and deriving bone Young's modulus from tissue density. The density-elasticity relationships are, however, still associated with a very wide confidence band. Possible improvement, though limited to in vitro validation studies, could consist of testing bone tissue from the same bone specimen that is modeled with FE. Such tests should be performed after organ-level testing has been completed, following an established paradigm for multiscale testing of bone structures.[8] Such tests may include:

• Tissue histomorphometry from micro-CT scanning can improve the assessing of bone structure and its associated anisotropy, which would enrich FE models.
• Material mechanical testing: Tissue specimens of some millimeters can be extracted at selected regions and tested. In this case, directly measured material properties are available for the selected locations and would be available to identify the parameters of each region of the FE model.

- Subtissue microstructure from polarized light microscopy provides clear insight into the microstructural arrangement of bone, including collagen orientation within the lamellae.

All such experimental measurements at the tissue and subtissue level would provide better assessment of the model parameters, thus improving the correct *identification* of the model.

Finally, it must be remembered that the cited density-elasticity relationships can identify the elastic modulus in only one direction (typically, the direction of the largest principal strain). Subject-specific information about bone anisotropy would improve FE models significantly but are scarcely available.

21.3.4 Validation at Last!

Because validation in absolute terms is not possible, it may be acceptable to validate a numerical model with respect to a number of experimental measurements. In most cases, this is the only viable solution. Such experiments obviously represent only a series of individual cases and cannot cover the possibly infinite range of cases applied to the numerical model. Validation experiments are not necessarily designed to represent a specific physiological condition or motor task. In most cases, validation experiments are designed so as to achieve the best control on the experimental conditions and to provide accessible and measurable outputs. It must be clear that the experimental-numerical comparison should be made on quantitative data, and should be one-to-one for each specimen and for each measurement within each specimen.

Some critical issues to replicate the experimental measurements in the numerical models can be identified:

- One-to-one correspondence: To avoid sources of error related to intersubject variability, the FE model being validated must correspond to the same physical specimen tested in vitro.
- Spatial registration: In order to replicate boundary conditions and the position of sensors, the relative pose of the reference system of the FE model has to be established with respect to the in vitro one. A documented procedure to achieve this aim is (1) to digitize the bone segment, plus any relevant points, and the experimental reference frame with a digital coordinate measurement system (▶ Fig. 21.4); and (2) to subsequently use an Iterative Closest Point algorithm, as proposed for solving rigid registration problems, to perform the registration of the acquired points cloud on the bone surface extracted from CT data, and also to find the transformation between the experimental laboratory reference system and the FE model.
- Measurement area: In vitro strains and displacements are measured over a finite sensing area. Given the highly inhomogeneous nature of bone tissue and the possible presence of high strain gradients, the calculated strains/displacements must as well be averaged over the sensing area of each transducer.
- Measurement direction: In case uniaxial strain gauges are used, the gauge direction of the grid should be digitized, spatially registered in the model, and the component of calculated strain in that direction ex-

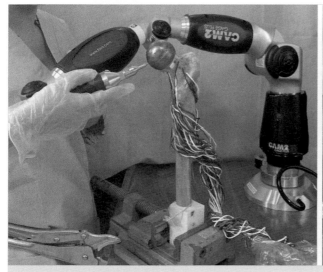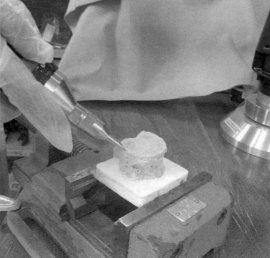

Fig. 21.4 High-precision digitizers can be used to acquire the position of relevant points on the physical specimens so as to identify them in the geometry of the corresponding finite element model. In the *left image*, a digitizer is used to acquire the spatial coordinates of relevant points of a resurfaced proximal femur instrumented with strain gauges. In the *right image*, the endplate of a lumbar vertebra is digitized to identify the boundary conditions of in vitro testing. (Copyright of the VPH-OP consortium; reproduced with permission.)

tracted and compared against the experimental read-out. When triaxial strain gauges are used, two principal strains and their direction are available for comparison with the FE predictions. Similarly, the direction of in vitro measured displacements (after compensation of rigid-body motion artifacts) should be correctly taken into account to enable experimental-numerical comparisons.

Local and global accuracy metrics must be defined to thoroughly and quantitatively validate an FE model. A global accuracy metric can be obtained by plotting the principal strains predicted by the FE model against the corresponding magnitudes recorded experimentally, for a number of loading configurations (▶ Fig. 21.5). The goodness of the prediction can be expressed by the determination coefficient (usually indicated as R^2), and by the slope and intercept of the regression curve. Ideally, one should find a perfectly linear relationship between measurements and predictions ($R^2 = 1$) with unitary slope and zero intercept. However, statistical artifacts may occur when data are clustered in two large clouds, which typically happens when the two principal strain components

are examined (see plot in ▶ Fig. 21.5). In this case, the analysis must be complemented by a local metric, in terms of average error (computed as the quadratic norm error, also known as root-mean-square error), and of peak error.

21.4 How Finite Element Models Can Improve in Vitro Experiments

While the flow of information from experiments to FE models is somewhat obvious, in vitro tests can also benefit from FE models. In fact, the limitations of in vitro experiments in most cases are related to the need for optimization of the experimental setup. In this perspective, FE models can play a very important role in assisting with the optimization of the experimental testing method. This includes (▶ Fig. 21.6) (1) effectively addressing the research question, (2) optimizing the use of experimental resources, and (3) minimizing the sources of error.

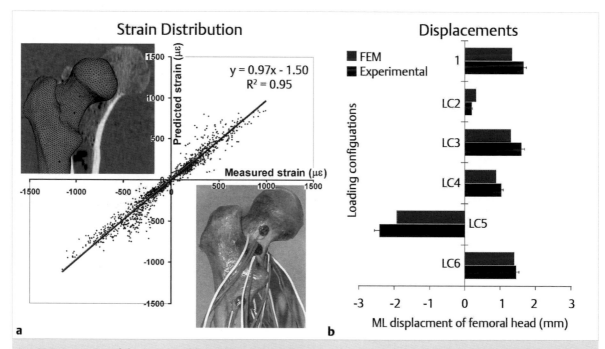

Fig. 21.5 Assessment of the accuracy of finite element (*FE*) predictions when quantitatively compared against experimental measurements. The closeness of the slope to 1.000 and the goodness of fit (R^2 close to 1.000) indicate the ability of the FE model to replicate the displacements and strain patterns measured in the physical specimens. In this instance, eight proximal femurs were investigated using an FE model based on the computed tomography scan of the physical specimens. (**a**) Principal strains were measured (and compared) at 15 locations, for six different loading configurations on all eight femurs. Experimentally measured strain was associated with an error of 0.4% (coefficient of variation between test repetitions on the same specimen). (**b**) Anteroposterior and mediolateral displacements on the femoral head and femoral diaphysis were measured by four displacement transducers for six different loading configurations (LC1 to LC6): In this case, the mediolateral displacements predicted by the FE model are compared against the corresponding in vitro measurements. FEM, finite element method; ML, mediolateral. (Copyright of the VPH-OP consortium; reproduced with permission.)

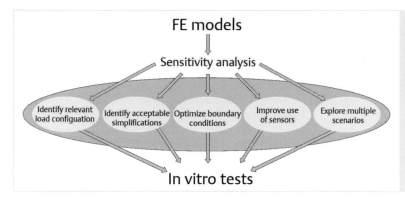

Fig. 21.6 Block diagram showing how finite element (FE) models can be used to improve in vitro experiments. The main tool is that of sensitivity analysis on the parameters affecting the experiments. (Copyright of the VPH-OP consortium; reproduced with permission.)

21.4.1 Identification of Most Relevant Testing Scenarios

One of the most difficult issues when designing a biomechanical simulation (whether in vitro or numerical) is the adequate choice of the loading configuration (direction and magnitude of applied forces). The loading configuration issue is particularly critical in orthopedic biomechanics as a wide variety of loading configurations are exerted during daily activities, depending on the individual lifestyle, on the motor task being performed, and on a number of factors that vary within the same motor task (i.e., motion, speed, environment). In addition, within a given motor task, the magnitude and direction of the applied forces change over time. For these reasons, if the most relevant motor task is not selected, or if the most relevant instant within the right task is not simulated, the in vitro simulation can be misleading. In principle, one could perform a number of in vitro preliminary experiments to determine which of the possible motor tasks is most relevant, and, for the selected motor task, which instant is most crucial. However, performance of such an exploration in vitro can be extremely costly and time-consuming. FE models (even simplified ones) in this phase can be extremely helpful and resource-effective for a preliminary exploration. For instance, the most relevant scenario for spontaneous fractures of the proximal femur[9] was identified using FE models. With a similar approach, the most relevant loading configurations to investigate implant stability of hip stems was identified using an FE model.[10]

21.4.2 Identification of an Acceptable Degree of Simplification

Mechanical loading of skeletal bones derives from articular forces, but also (and often predominantly) from the action of muscles. In most cases, a large number of muscles act simultaneously on the same bone. In vitro simulation of each muscle force requires the use of dedicated actuators and controllers. A compromise must be found between a very complex experimental setup that takes into account a large number of factors, but in most cases suffers from poor control of the testing conditions.

21.4.3 Optimization of Boundary Conditions

Experimental error in in vitro biomechanical testing derives to a large extent from poor control of the boundary conditions and forces applied to the specimen. The point of application and the direction of the forces in vitro are affected by experimental errors. It is often the case that some components of such errors have little effect on the output under investigation (e.g., bone strain or failure load), whereas others propagate to the output in a dramatic way. Sometimes one force component is directly controlled, while others are applied as a consequence, and therefore only indirectly controlled. The use of FE models enables simulating how errors affecting each load component propagate to the measured quantities (e.g., strain or failure load). The experimental setup can be designed to give the highest priority to accurately controlling those uncertainties (e.g., the position of one of the applied forces; ▶ Fig. 21.7) that most severely affects the accuracy of the results using sensitivity analyses supported by FE models.

21.4.4 Optimized Use of in Vitro Transducers

Positioning and alignment of transducers is affected by errors (▶ Fig. 21.7). Such an uncertainty can be estimated with repeated in vitro applications. However, this error cannot be avoided. If a transducer is placed in a region where the measured quantity has a steep gradient, malpositioning or misalignment will affect the output measurement to a larger extent. FE models can be used to assess the distribution of the measured variable so as to avoid placing transducers in areas where such gradients are excessively steep.

Some transducers, such as strain gauges, provide an output that is some average over the area covered by the

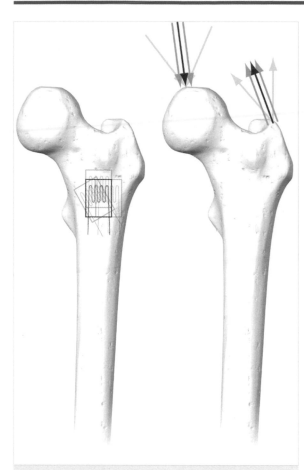

Fig. 21.7 In vitro measurements are affected by positioning and alignment errors of the testing components. *Left*: The alignment and position of the strain gauges used in vitro segment are affected by errors with respect to the intended position. Finite element models can be used to estimate how each of such components of error propagate to the measured output. *Right*: The position, direction, and magnitude of the forces applied in vitro to a bone segment are affected by errors (*gray arrows*) with respect to the intended position (*black arrows*).

21.4.5 Sensitivity Analysis

In many clinical applications, the sensitivity of an output on variation of input parameters needs to be evaluated:

- Different loading conditions are known to affect bones or bone-implant constructs in different ways.
- The effect of bone quality on bone strength is crucial for investigating bone pathologies such as osteoporosis.
- While developing a prosthetic device, the designer needs to know if different prosthetic materials provide better or worse performance when coupled to the host bone.
- Interface conditions between an implantable device and the host bone can be a discriminating factor between failure and success.

In vitro exploration of such variables experimentally would require a large number of experiments and specimens. FE models are definitely more resource-effective in performing this type of sensitivity analyses and greatly complement in vitro experiments.

The prediction accuracy of FE models has improved in the past years through a combined numerical-experimental approach (▶ Fig. 21.8).

Similarly, FE models were used to optimize the experimental setup (▶ Fig. 21.9). In fact, with repeated testing and the support of FE models that replicated the experimental testing conditions, sources of error were assessed. Each source of variability was examined and kept under control as much as possible, focusing first on the strain measurement method, and later on the loading setup. Both the interspecimen repeatability and, most of all, the intraspecimen repeatability that can be achieved with such a support from FE simulations are better than any other value found in the literature (▶ Fig. 21.9).

Such an integrated approach enabled an extremely detailed investigation of the strain pattern in the proximal femur, was and can also extended to the design, optimization, and preclinical validation of hip implants.

21.5 Conclusion

In this chapter, we explored how experimental and numerical methods should be combined synergistically in order to obtain more than the sum of what we would get with each approach in isolation.

In fact, the combination of FE modeling and controlled experiments within the same research team can be exploited to create a virtuous circle where models are used to improve experiments (▶ Fig. 21.6) and experiments are used to improve models (▶ Fig. 21.3), and their combination synergistically increases the knowledge on the proximal femur. This can be achieved under the following conditions:

- A fundamental requisite is the integration of a computational group and an experimental group within the

transducer itself (typically a few square millimeters). This can be beneficial: The transducer operates as an averaging filter, reducing the effect of the position errors described above. However, there is also a negative side effect: Peak values are underestimated because of this smoothening effect. FE models can help define the optimal size of the strain gauge based on the presence of local peaks and on the steepness of gradients.

In addition, mechanical transducers in most cases provide pointwise measurements and do not provide any information about the distribution of the measured variable. FE models can provide a preliminary distribution of the measured magnitude so as to suggest where the transducers should be applied.

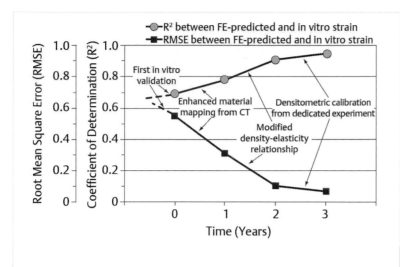

Fig. 21.8 Improvement over time of the finite element (*FE*) models of the human femur developed by our group. The accuracy of the FE-predicted strain was quantified against in vitro strain gauge measurement. Two indicators are plotted: the coefficient of determination (R^2) and the root-mean-square error (*RMSE*; computed over all strain measurement locations, and normalized by the maximum experimental value). R^2 increased over time (an ideal value of 1.000 corresponds to perfect match between experimental and FE-predicted strain). Root-mean-square error decreased over the years (an ideal value of 0.000 corresponds to no discrepancy between experimental and FE-predicted strain). (Copyright of the VPH-OP consortium; reproduced with permission.)

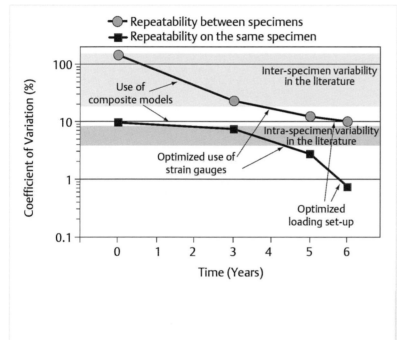

Fig. 21.9 The plot shows how the in vitro experiments on the human femur performed by our group improved over the past years. The repeatability achieved with a support from finite element simulations was better than any previously published study. The coefficient of variation (ratio between standard deviation and average) is plotted over time both for the intraspecimen repeatability (the testing setup was disassembled and reassembled between repetitions) and between specimens. Also indicated is the range reported in the literature for the repeatability between specimens and on the same specimen. The first significant improvement in reproducibility was achieved with the introduction of the composite femur models. Later on, finite element models replicating the experimental testing conditions enabled examining each source of variability. Focusing on the strain measurement method and on the loading setup, experimental error was further reduced. (Copyright of the VPH-OP consortium; reproduced with permission.)

same research team (in association with a multidisciplinary team that is typical of bioengineering laboratories, including physicians, biologists, physicists, engineers, etc.).

- Integration and collaboration between the computational group and the experimental group must be encouraged, with computational researchers spending more and more time in the experimental facilities, and vice versa.
- In vitro experiments must be designed in collaboration with people in charge of numerical simulations, to ensure that the loading conditions and measured variables were suitable for integration also into FE models.

To get a practical sense and have a clearer view of the experimental details, FE researchers must take part in the key phases of the in vitro experiments.

- Researchers carrying out experiments must seek the help of FE researchers to gather as much information as possible through FE-supported sensitivity analysis, so as to optimize the experimental setup.

21.5.1 Acknowledgments

The authors wish to thank a number of coworkers and colleagues: Marco Viceconti, Massimiliano Baleani, Fulvia Taddei, Enrico Schileo, Saulo Martelli, Mateusz M.

Juszczyk, Paolo Erani, and Lorenzo Zani. The artwork is due to Luigi Lena. The European Community (grants: IST-2004–026932 "Living Human Digital Library—LHDL" and #223865 "The Osteoporotic Virtual Physiological Human —VPH-OP") and Regione Emilia-Romagna (Region-University Research Program 2007–2009) co-funded this study.

References

[1] Charite—Universitaetsmedizin Berlin. OrthoLoad. http://www.OrthoLoad.com. 2011

[2] O'Connor JJ. Load simulation problems in model testing. In: Miles AW, Tanner KE, eds. Strain measurement in biomechanics. London: Chapman & Hall; 1992;14–38

[3] Cristofolini L, Saponara TA, Savigni P, Erani P, Viceconti M. Preclinical assessment of the long-term endurance of cemented hip stems. Part 1: effect of daily activities—a comparison of two load histories. Proc Inst Mech Eng H 2007; 221: 569–584

[4] Heller MO, Bergmann G, Deuretzbacher G et al. Musculo-skeletal loading conditions at the hip during walking and stair climbing. J Biomech 2001; 34: 883–893

[5] Stolk J, Verdonschot N, Huiskes R. Hip-joint and abductor-muscle forces adequately represent in vivo loading of a cemented total hip reconstruction. J Biomech 2001; 34: 917–926

[6] Duda GN, Heller M, Albinger J, Schulz O, Schneider E, Claes L. Influence of muscle forces on femoral strain distribution. J Biomech 1998; 31: 841–846

[7] Ruimerman R, Hilbers P, van Rietbergen B, Huiskes R. A theoretical framework for strain-related trabecular bone maintenance and adaptation. J Biomech 2005; 38: 931–941

[8] Cristofolini L, Taddei M, Baleani M, Baruffaldi F, Stea S, Viceconti M. Multiscale investigation of the functional properties of the human femur. Philos Transact A Math Phys Eng Sci 2008; 366: 3319–3341

[9] Cristofolini L, Juszczyk M, Martelli S, Taddei F, Viceconti M. In vitro replication of spontaneous fractures of the proximal human femur. J Biomech 2007; 40: 2837–2845

[10] Stolk J, Verdonschot N, Huiskes R. Stair climbing is more detrimental to the cement in hip replacement than walking. Clin Orthop Relat Res 2002: 294–305

Further Reading

Babuska I, Oden JT. Verification and validation in computational engineering and science: basic concepts. Comput Methods Appl Mech Eng 2004; 193: 4057–4066

Cristofolini L, Schileo E, Juszczyk M, Taddei F, Martelli S, Viceconti M. Mechanical testing of bones: the positive synergy of Finite-Elements models and in vitro experiments. Philos Transact A Math Phys Eng Sci 2010; 368: 2725–2763

Henninger HB, Reese SP, Anderson AE, Weiss JA. Validation of computational models in biomechanics. Proc Inst Mech Eng H 2010; 224: 801–812

Jones AC, Wilcox RK. Finite element analysis of the spine: towards a framework of verification, validation and sensitivity analysis. Med Eng Phys 2008; 30: 1287–1304

Viceconti M, Olsen S, Nolte LP, Burton K. Extracting clinically relevant data from finite element simulations. Clin Biomech (Bristol, Avon) 2005; 20: 451–454

22 Computational Biomechanics of Bone

Pankaj Pankaj

"Computational" mechanics comprises simulating the mechanical response of an object, such as bone, using models created on a computer. The mechanics is incorporated in the computer code and it invariably involves numerical methods or approximations. One of the popular numerical approaches is finite element (FE) analysis. The discussion on computational biomechanics in this chapter is with reference to FE analysis; however, most of the input parameters required for modeling using this approach would be required for other methods as well. The focus here is on the information that we require to conduct a computational analysis of bone and on the type of results that we can expect to obtain from such an analysis.

22.1 Input Parameters

Consider, for example, a femur subjected to loads on the femoral head, as shown in ▶ Fig. 22.1. We may be interested in the deformation or stresses/strains in the bone in the proximal region. We briefly discuss the key input parameters essential for modeling a problem such as this in the following paragraphs and these are considered in greater detail in the following sections.

1. *The geometry:* We need to know the shape and the internal structure (e.g., volumetric regions with cancellous and cortical bone). For FE analysis, the geometry is subdivided into simpler shapes (e.g., tetrahedrons or hexahedrons) called elements.

2. *Material properties:* We need to know, for instance, the elastic properties of bone in different regions of the femur. Further, if the femur is expected to be loaded beyond its elastic capacity, the simulation program will require postelastic properties as well. Furthermore, it is known that bone does not deform immediately on application of loads; its response is time dependent. For some problems, it may be essential to prescribe properties that can describe such time-dependent behavior. It is apparent that the computer code being employed for analysis needs to be capable of accepting and interpreting this complex range of properties.

3. *Boundary conditions:* We need to specify how the object being analyzed is supported or restrained from undergoing rigid body motions (i.e., move without deforming). It is important to note that in the absence of any restraints, the body will simply shoot off in space when subjected to forces. Restraints should be such that the object cannot undergo rigid body translations or rotations. For the femur subjected to forces on the femoral head shown in ▶ Fig. 22.1, a typical approach involves restraining it

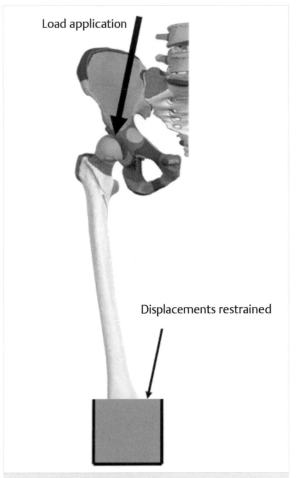

Fig. 22.1 A femur subjected to a load on the femoral head (*arrow*) and restrained from movement distally (adapted from Primal Pictures 2009).

completely in all directions at a distal transverse plane as shown. Clearly, this is not the in vivo support condition, which is far more complex. However, this approach is capable of providing good answers to many clinical questions. Similar support conditions are often employed when conducting physical laboratory experiments.

4. *Loads:* The direction, magnitude, and location of loads need to be specified for a computational analysis. For the example of the femur being considered, the value and direction of the loads as well as the surface region of the femoral head on which these loads act will change with the physiological activity being undertaken. Computational biomechanics offers the opportunity to conduct an evaluation for a wide range of load cases, which is not possible in a laboratory setting.

22.2 Output Results

Once the input has been specified, the FE analysis can be initiated. What can one expect to get out of it? The commonly sought output parameters are deformations, stresses, and strains. Computational biomechanics can provide this information at practically any location. Moreover, it permits evaluation of all components of displacements stresses and strains. These details are impossible to obtain from biomechanical experiments.

It is important to give the output a sanity check before examining the more complex output parameters. Superimposed undeformed and deformed shapes of the geometry (before and after loading) provide the simplest check as normally it is quite easy to visualize how deformation is likely to happen. A second simple check is to examine the reactions at the restrained points in all directions. The algebraic sum of the reactions needs to be equal to the load applied.

Stresses and strains constitute the key features of the output. It is important to remember that each of these has six components. With respect to stress, we have normal stresses σ_x, σ_y and σ_z, and shear stresses τ_{xy}, τ_{yz}, and τ_{zx}. Similarly for strain, we have normal strains ε_x, ε_y, and ε_z, and shear strains γ_{xy}, γ_{yz}, and γ_{zx}. In these, x, y, and z refer to the coordinate directions chosen when providing geometric data. While these values are useful (e.g., we may be interested in finding out how load in a particular direction affects normal stresses in another direction), it is important to remember that these values vary with the choice of the axes; another modeler doing exactly the same problem with a different set of axes will get different absolute values for these coordinate-dependent quantities. It is more useful to examine invariant quantities (i.e., those that do not depend on the choice of the coordinate system). It is always possible to transform the coordinate system at each point such that the stress (or strain) only has normal components and no shear components. These three normal components are called principal stresses (or strains) and are provided by all commercial codes. The principal values provide the largest, an intermediate, and the smallest normal stresses/strains, and are very useful to examine. As per the commonly used sign convention, tension is positive and compression is negative, so maximum principal stress contours can be used to indicate regions experiencing tensile stresses and minimum principal stress contours for compressive stresses. It is, however, important to remember that in general the directions of principal values vary from point to point.

Another stress invariant often used in literature is the von Mises stress (σ_v). This is simply a scalar quantity constructed using stress components as

$$\sigma_v = \sqrt{\frac{\left(\sigma_x - \sigma_y\right)^2 + \left(\sigma_y - \sigma_z\right)^2 + \left(\sigma_z - \sigma_x\right)^2 + 6\left(\tau_{xy}^2 + \tau_{yz}^2 + \tau_{zx}^2\right)}{2}}$$

(22.1)

While von Mises stress is a good indicator of "how much" stress the object is experiencing, it is not able to tell whether these are tensile or compressive. The von Mises stress is a very good predictor of yielding of many metals and is used as their yield criterion. It is not a good indicator for bone yielding or failure, though it has been used in this way (further discussed later in this chapter). As a result, many researchers criticize production of von Mises stress contours for bone. However, von Mises stresses provide a good measure of stress state in bone but should be used in conjunction with principal stress values.

While stress and strain are related, it is important to note that for triaxial problems, the two can provide quite distinct results. Consider, for example, a cube subjected to uniformly distributed compressive load in one direction. As a result, it will experience compressive strains in the direction of loading and tensile strains in orthogonal directions. However, while it will have compressive stresses in the direction of loading, stresses in the orthogonal directions will be zero. Therefore, it is a good idea to examine not only stresses but also strains.

The output can provide a large variety of information, depending on the type of analysis being conducted. It is useful to appraise the variety of output parameters; some may provide much better answers than others on the behavior being examined.

22.3 Defining the Geometry

Biomechanical systems have a complex geometry. However, advances in imaging technologies followed by automated software procedures to convert these images to FE meshes have made defining the geometry of biomechanical systems much easier. For biomechanical analysis, the three-dimensional (3D) geometry is typically developed from computed tomography (CT) or magnetic resonance imaging scans of either cadaveric bone samples or that of real patients. These are then segmented to define regions and provide boundaries for different segments (e.g., soft tissue and bone) of the object. Although research into more reliable automated segmentation techniques is ongoing, it is now possible to create a fairly accurate representation of 3D bone geometry (depending on the resolution of the scan), which can be converted to a FE mesh using specialized packages such as ScanIP (Simpleware Ltd., Exeter, UK) or Mimics (Materialise, Leuven, Belgium). Many FE packages will also generate the mesh from 3D geometry provided to them as a computer-aided design (CAD) file. Such files are often available for implants from their manufacturers.

Similarly, by using high-resolution, µCT, or µ-magnetic resonance imaging scans, even the geometry of the bone microstructure can be constructed. The typical process is illustrated in ▶ Fig. 22.2. It is, however, important to note that a computational analysis of the whole bone with microlevel resolution (as shown in ▶ Fig. 22.2) is rarely conducted, though this is not impossible with the high speed and parallel computing resources available today. For the whole bone analysis, the bone material is mostly assumed to be a solid continuum. The effect of porosity and microstructure is incorporated by varying the material properties of this solid. This aspect is further discussed in the next section.

In recent years, "patient-specific modeling" has been receiving increasing attention.[1] In clinical practice, CT or magnetic resonance imaging scans are not regularly obtained for operations involving joint replacement or trauma. In the absence of volumetric images, patient-specific geometry cannot be readily constructed, though there has been some research on the development of 3D models from planar radiographs.[2]

Imaging technologies have made it possible to generate high-quality 3D geometries. As a consequence, expectations from computational modeling have increased. Unfortunately, it is not always realized that geometry alone does not constitute a model; it requires other input parameters (discussed in the following sections) whose specification can be challenging.

22.4 Defining the Material Properties

For bone, the simplest and most common (though not necessarily accurate) assumption is that it has linear isotropic elastic and time-independent properties. This assumption implies that the mechanical behavior can be described by two material parameters: Young's modulus and Poisson's ratio. In most computational studies with generic bone geometries, it is a common practice to further assume that the material is homogeneous, though distinctly different regions (e.g., cortical and trabecular) may be assigned different properties. In subject-specific studies for which CT data are available, inhomogeneous material properties can be assigned. Typically, CT attenuations (or radiodensity measured using Hounsfield units) at different points are first converted into bone density and then the latter used to estimate the Young's modulus. Conversion of CT data to density has a basis in physics; however, density to Young's modulus conversion is largely empirical. The other constant, Poisson's ratio, required for describing an isotropic material is assumed

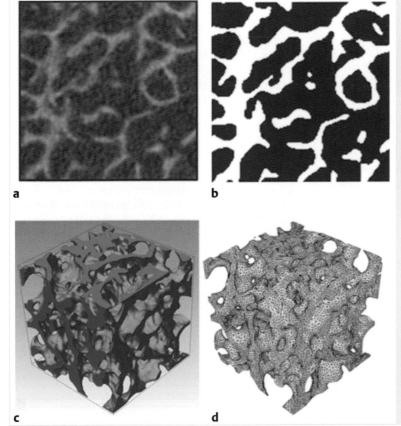

Fig. 22.2 The process of constructing three-dimensional finite element models from µ-computed tomography scans. (**a**) A slice of trabecular bone µ-computed tomography. (**b**) Binarizing the slice into solid and pore. (**c**) Three-dimensional model from binarized slices. (**d**) Finite element mesh. The sample shown is 4×4×4 mm.

to be constant (typically a value of 0.3 is assumed for bone).

Jargon Simplified: Young's Modulus

Commonly denoted by E, Young's modulus is the ratio of stress to strain along the same axis when loaded uniaxially. Consider a cube with edges of length L subjected to a horizontal force P_1 in the x direction as shown in ▶ Fig. 22.3a. If the force is uniformly distributed over a cross-sectional area, A, and causes the cube to stretch by ΔL in the x direction, the normal stress is given by

$$\sigma_x = \frac{P_1}{A}$$

and normal strain is given by

$$\epsilon_x = \frac{\Delta L}{L}$$

The Young's modulus thus is calculated by

$$E = \frac{\sigma_x}{\epsilon_x} = \frac{P_1 \cdot L}{A \cdot \Delta L}$$

Jargon Simplified: Poisson's Ratio

Poisson's ratio, ν, is the negative ratio of transverse strain to axial strain. In ▶ Fig. 22.3a, stretching in the x direction causes a contraction $\Delta L'$ in the y direction resulting in a compressive normal strain

$$\epsilon_y = \frac{\Delta L'}{L}$$

The Poisson's ratio is given by

$$\nu = -\frac{\epsilon_y}{\epsilon_x}$$

An incompressible material has a Poisson's ratio of $\nu = 0.5$, and metals have ν of about 0.3. Poisson's ratios are between 0.2 and 0.5 (average: 0.3) for cortical bone and between 0.01 and 0.35 (average: 0.12) for cancellous bone.

Jargon Simplified: Shear Modulus

Shear modulus, G, is the ratio of shear stress to shear strain. Consider ▶ Fig. 22.3b, in which a force P_2 acts on the top surface with cross-sectional area A. If the bottom surface is restrained, the cube will deform as shown in the figure. The shear strain γ_{xy} is given by

$$\gamma_{xy} = \theta = \Delta L''/L$$

If the force is uniformly distributed over the top surface, the shear stress is given by

$$\tau_{yx} = \frac{P_2}{A}$$

The shear modulus can now be expressed as

$$G = \frac{\tau_{yx}}{\gamma_{yx}}$$

For isotropic materials shear modulus, Young's modulus and Poisson's ratio are related by:

$$G = \frac{E}{2(1 + \nu)}$$

While the assumption of isotropy serves well for many biomechanical studies, it is well recognized that both cortical and cancellous bone are better represented by orthotropic or transverse isotropic elasticity requiring many more properties for relating stresses to strains. These are not easy to obtain but have been evaluated in the laboratory with bone samples using mechanical tests, nanoindentation techniques, and ultrasonic methods. Each of these has limitations and may not be able to provide the full set of elastic constants. Computational techniques, based on converting μCT or μ-magnetic resonance imaging scans to FE models (sometimes referred as μFE models), as shown in ▶ Fig. 22.2d, provide a simple way of evaluating the complete set of elastic constants. In these, the solid or tissue phase is generally assigned isotropic elastic values and the assumption is that anisotropy (or orthotropy or transverse isotropy) at a larger macro scale (also called apparent level) arises due to the microarchitecture. Once μFE meshes have been developed and material properties assigned, six strain states are

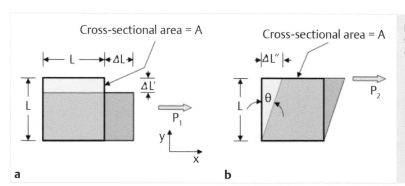

Fig. 22.3 Deformation of a small cube due to the application of (a) a uniaxial tensile force P_1 or (b) a shear force P_2.

computationally applied to each sample: tensile/compressive strain in the x, y, and z directions, and pure shear strain in the xy, xz, and yz planes to simulate mechanical tests. The stress response enables the evaluation of all elastic constants. As with experimental approaches, such an analysis can only provide values for the region being analyzed. It has been suggested that orthotropic elastic constants in cortical bone are related to porosity,[3] providing a simple approach for assigning elastic constants for computational analysis. While this correlation might apply for midshaft cortical regions of long bones, the relationships at other anatomical sites and within trabecular bone are likely to be more complex. Depending on what is being sought from an analysis, inclusion of orthotropy (rather than isotropy) can significantly alter some of the output variables as Young's modulus in one direction can be three times the value in another direction.[3,4]

Jargon Simplified: Linearity and Elasticity

The term elastic implies that any deformation experienced by the material on application of forces is fully recovered when the forces are removed. Addition of the term linear means that the mechanical response (e.g., deformation) is proportional to the load applied (i.e., doubling of the load will double the deformation).

Jargon Simplified: Δ Isotropic, Anisotropic, Orthotropic, and Transverse Isotropic Elasticity

An isotropic material is one that has the same mechanical properties in all directions and requires two elastic constants to relate stresses to strains. A fully anisotropic material has different properties in different directions and requires 21 elastic constants to relate stresses to strains. Orthotropic and transverse isotropic elasticity lie in between and require nine and five constants, respectively. Orthotropic materials have three orthogonal planes of elastic symmetry. Transverse isotropic materials have a plane with identical properties in all directions in that plane but different properties in the direction perpendicular to the plane. These terms should not be confused with homogeneity or inhomogeneity, which refer to properties at different points within the material (and not directions).

Very often, computational analysis is required to provide results for cases that take the bone beyond its elastic limit. In these cases, unloading leaves irreversible deformations or strains. Theories of elastoplasticity (most common) and damage mechanics have been used to model post-elastic behavior. Detailed discussion of these is beyond the scope of this chapter, but we will discuss the key features of the theory of elastoplasticity (or simply plasticity) and follow this up with issues associated with modeling bone using this theory.

Jargon Simplified: Viscoelasticity

Use of elastic properties implies that deformations takes place instantaneously upon load application. This is not true for bone as it is known to demonstrate slow progressive deformation under constant stress. This property is useful in reducing mechanical shocks due to sudden loading. Mathematically, this can be incorporated in computational models using viscoelasticity, a property that permits materials to exhibit both viscous and elastic characteristics and allows inclusion of time-dependent variation of strain on application of stress.

Elastoplasticity of a material is prescribed by specifying its yield criterion and post-yield behavior. The yield criterion specifies the critical stress/strain at which "yielding" is initiated. Post-yield behavior describes the continued loading process that causes both elastic and plastic components of deformation. Post-yield stress-strain relationships need to be based on real material behavior and most commonly relate small increments of strain to increments of stress.

Let us briefly consider the yield criteria for bone. Experiments on bone indicate that it has three key features when yielding if defined in terms of stress. Firstly, it yields at a higher magnitude of uniaxial stress in compression than it does in tension. This is often termed as tension-compression strength asymmetry. Secondly, anisotropic elasticity of bone is accompanied by anisotropy of strength (i.e., it yields at different stresses in different directions). Thirdly, like inhomogeneity of bone's elasticity (elastic constants varying from point to point), its strength is also inhomogeneous.

Many different yield criteria have been used to simulate post-yield behavior of bone. The most widely employed criterion has been von Mises; this is readily available in all computer codes. As per this criterion, yielding is initiated when the stress state σ_v (equation (22.1)) reaches a predefined stress value σ_{yld}, which is the only parameter required to define the material's yield. The criterion is isotropic, and it is really meant for ductile metals; it does not incorporate tension-compression strength asymmetry. In other words, it is actually unsuitable for bone. Some of the simple criteria that require few parameters to define the material and have been employed for bone are the *Drucker-Prager Criterion*, which is isotropic but incorporates strength asymmetry; the *Maximum Principal Stress Criterion*, in which yielding only occurs due to tensile stresses; and the *Tresca Criterion* (or maximum shear stress criterion), which is isotropic and does not include strength asymmetry. Among the more complex criteria, requiring several material parameters, are the *Hoffman Criterion* and the *Tsai-Wu Criterion*. It is important to note that parameters required to define yielding of a material being modeled using a particular criterion need to be determined through experiments, so the more complex the criterion, the greater the experimental effort.

The previous discussion is related to criteria based on stress (i.e., yielding is initiated when a combination of stress components reaches a prescribed value). In recent years, there has been some discussion as to whether the bone yields due to stress or due to strain.[5] Although prior to yielding, stress and strain are related through elastic constants, there are subtle differences between yielding defined using stress and that defined using strain. As mentioned earlier, a cube of material being compressed along one axis will expand in the orthogonal directions (due to Poisson's effect) if there are no restraints or loads applied in these directions; as a result, it will have strains in the unloaded directions but no stresses. There has been some discussion as to whether stress-based or strain-based criteria are better for bone, and recently a consensus appears to be emerging on the superiority of strain-based criteria.

If yielding is defined in terms of strain, then some of the complexities associated with the stress-based definitions disappear. Unlike stress, bone yielding in terms of strain is isotropic (i.e., it yields at the same strain in all directions).[6,7] Also, in terms of strain, yield values of bone are almost homogeneous (different for cortical and cancellous bone, though). This last feature can be explained by simply considering two bone samples, one with high density and the other with low density. The high-density sample will have higher Young's modulus and will undergo lower strains at a given load, whereas the low-density sample will experience higher strains at the same load. In other words, for both samples to experience the same strain (say the yield strain), the high-density sample will need to be subjected to higher loads (or stresses) in comparison to the low-density sample. This is shown in ▶ Fig. 22.4.

Algorithms for a simple yield criterion for bone based on maximum and minimum strains were recently developed.[6,7] These criteria require parameters for defining yield that are based on principal strains or yield strains in different loading directions. Unfortunately, yield criteria based on strain are currently not readily available in commercial codes, but considering that they are finding favor with the bone biomechanics community they are likely to be soon included.

It is now recognized that the mechanical response of bone is not time-independent (i.e., on application of load the deformation does not take place instantaneously but with time).[8] This time-dependent response gives bone a shock-absorbing capability and is often modeled using viscoelasticity. To incorporate viscoelastic behavior in

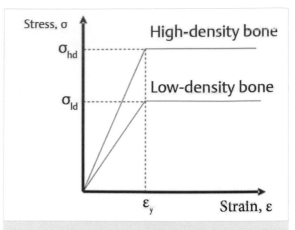

Fig. 22.4 Idealized stress-strain curves for low- and high-density bone. In the elastic regime, the high-density bone has a steeper curve and yields at a higher stress (σ_{hd}) in comparison to low density bone (yield stress, σ_{ld}). Both samples, however, yield at approximately the same strain, ε_y. The post-yield response has been shown here to be flat—this is not really true for bone, which has a complex post-yield behavior.

computer simulations, experimental data to describe time-dependent properties of bone needs to be provided to the FE code (the code needs to have capabilities to simulate such behavior). Two related terms are employed in this respect: *creep* and *stress relaxation*. The first term describes the change in strains with time after load application, whereas the latter refers to change in stresses after initial application of strains or deformation. It has been suggested that inclusion of time-dependent effects is particularly important in assessing differences in fracture risk associated with impact loading events.

22.5 Defining the Boundary Conditions and Loads

Biomechanical simulations aim to reproduce the in vivo scenario as closely as possible. Application of the realistic boundary conditions and loads provide the biggest challenge in this respect. The term boundary conditions relates to describing how an object is restrained from movement as loads (or forces) are applied to it. Bones are supported by muscles and ligaments (and other soft tissue) at the joints, and experience forces through each of these. Muscular, ligamentous, and joint reaction forces acting on the bone vary with the physiological activity being undertaken. It is quite onerous to include all these in a computational model and practically impossible in an in vitro laboratory experiment. In most computer simulations, the effect of muscles and ligaments is widely ignored and the bone is greatly restrained at an appropriate location. For example, in order to evaluate the stresses within the human pelvis due to, say, a single-legged

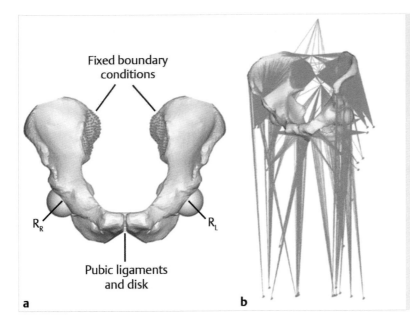

Fixed boundary conditions

R_R R_L

Pubic ligaments and disk

a   b

Fig. 22.5 (a) A model of a pelvis restrained at sacroiliac joints. (b) Pelvis modeled with muscles and ligaments. (From Phillips ATM, Pankaj P, Howie CR, Usmani AS, Simpson AHRW. Finite element modelling of the pelvis: inclusion of muscular and ligamentous boundary conditions. Med Eng Phys 2007;29[7]:739–748.)

stance, we may apply full displacement restraints at the sacroiliac joints, as shown in ▶ Fig. 22.5a,[9] and apply forces to the acetabulum through the femoral head. A more realistic approach comprises inclusion of muscles and ligaments (typically modeled using spring elements); these are attached at appropriate attachment locations on the cortex and restrained at insertion points, as shown in ▶ Fig. 22.5b. The loads may once again be applied at the acetabulum through the femoral head, resulting in fairly uniform stress distribution in the human pelvis.[9] Artificial restraints typically result in stress concentrations and large stress magnitudes at locations close to the restraint. Any restraints employed in modeling should attempt to simulate reality as closely as possible. Studies indicate that despite artificial restraints employed in modeling, the stresses and strains evaluated close to the regions of load application (and away from the restraints) provide good estimates of the mechanical response.

Incorporation of muscles in computational models in the form shown in ▶ Fig. 22.4b is not straightforward because it requires stiffness properties of the muscles to be provided as input parameters. Because muscle stiffness varies with and during physiological activity, this input data cannot be readily provided for simulation. Another approach, for including the effect of muscles and ligaments, is by applying forces emanating from these at the attachment sites.[10] In this case, forces (both magnitudes and directions) and the locations at which they act are required as input parameters. Muscle forces are typically obtained through optimization studies (i.e., it is assumed that muscles share forces in an optimum manner; see Chapter 20). These forces, along with joint reaction forces, should maintain the system in equilibrium. However, in computational simulation, some restraints are still necessary to maintain numerical stability.

Application of loads presents two questions: loads corresponding to which physiological activities should be considered, and what are the values of forces for a particular activity. The answer to the second question is being provided by directly measuring values in patients using smart implants (http://www.orthoload.com). In terms of the choice of physiological activities, most previous studies on the femur and tibia have considered loads during a standing position or peak loads in a walking load cycle. More complex activities, such as getting up from a chair (or from a squat position) or climbing stairs, have received relatively little attention. The reasons for this appear to be lack of data on loads for complex activities and the difficulty in validating the numerical results.

22.6 Conclusion

Computational biomechanics presents challenges and requires a good understanding of the methods. It is far less onerous than an in vitro experimental program and provides greater opportunity to mimic the in vivo situation. It generates a surfeit of information and therefore requires the ability to extract and interpret results. After initial modeling effort has been put in, several additional cases can be run at low cost. As a result, computational biomechanics is particularly useful for conducting parametric studies.

References

[1] Pankaj P. Patient-specific modelling of bone and bone-implant systems: the challenges. Int J Numer Method Biomed Eng 2013; 29: 233–249

[2] Galibarov PE, Prendergast PJ, Lennon AB. A method to reconstruct patient-specific proximal femur surface models from planar pre-operative radiographs. Med Eng Phys 2010; 32: 1180–1188

[3] Donaldson FE, Pankaj P, Cooper DML, Thomas CDL, Clement JG, Simpson AHRW. Relating age and micro-architecture with apparent-level elastic constants: A µFE study of female cortical bone from the anterior femoral midshaft. Proc Inst Mech Eng H 2011; 225; 585–596

[4] Ulrich D, van Rietbergen B, Laib A, Rüegsegger P. The ability of three-dimensional structural indices to reflect mechanical aspects of trabecular bone. Bone 1999; 25: 55–60

[5] Nalla RK, Kinney JH, Ritchie RO. Mechanistic fracture criteria for the failure of human cortical bone. Nat Mater 2003; 2: 164–168

[6] Pankaj P, Donaldson FE. Algorithms for a strain-based plasticity criterion for bone. Int J Numer Method Biomed Eng 2013; 29: 40–61

[7] Bayraktar HH, Gupta A, Kwon RY, Papadopoulos P, Keaveny TM. The modified super-ellipsoid yield criterion for human trabecular bone. J Biomech Eng 2004; 126: 677–684

[8] Johnson TPM, Socrate S, Boyce MC. A viscoelastic, viscoplastic model of cortical bone valid at low and high strain rates. Acta Biomater 2010; 6: 4073–4080

[9] Phillips AIM, Pankaj P, Howie CR, Usmani AS, Simpson AHRW. Finite element modelling of the pelvis: inclusion of muscular and ligamentous boundary conditions. Med Eng Phys 2007; 29: 739–748

[10] Ramos A, Fonseca F, Simões JA. Simulation of physiological loading in total hip replacements. J Biomech Eng 2006; 128: 579–587

Further Reading

Reilly DT, Burstein AH. The elastic and ultimate properties of compact bone tissue. J Biomech 1975; 8: 393–405

23 Numerical Simulation of Implants and Prosthetic Devices

Sebastian Eberle

Implants for fracture fixation and prosthetic devices for joint replacement have very different objectives. Implants for fracture fixation are meant to reduce and to stabilize the fracture fragments of a broken bone, so healing can take place. The final goal of a so-called osteosynthesis is to completely restore the bone's preinjury tissue quality and functionality. Implants for fracture fixation have fulfilled their function after the healing process and are in fact often removed. By contrast, internal prosthetic devices are meant to grow into the bone as the bone grows around the prosthesis and completely replace a joint. The final goal of a total joint replacement is to artificially restore the functionality of an injured or arthritic joint.

However, both types of devices have to endure large loads within the human musculoskeletal system while sustaining their biomechanical functionality. The different aspects of this biomechanical functionality are often subject to biomechanical research studies to identify superior implants and treatment strategies. Most of the time, mechanical in vitro testing is employed to test the functionality of implants for fracture fixation and prosthetic devices (see Chapter 7 and Chapter 11 for details on mechanical testing in structural biomechanics). Yet, not all research questions and hypotheses can be addressed by biomechanical experiments. It is, for example, not possible to determine the strain or stress distribution within an intramedullary nail that is implanted in a bone. Furthermore, some in vivo processes cannot be captured by in vitro experiments (e.g., the biomechanical behavior of an ingrown joint replacement or in vivo loading scenarios with a large number of muscle forces). Finally, biomechanical research on implants by clinical studies is considerably restricted due to ethical reasons.

Numerical simulation methods like the finite element (FE) method have the potential to close these gaps in biomechanical research on implants. The FE method is a numerical method to compute approximate solutions of partial differential equations and integral equations (see Chapter 20 for details on the FE method). If the FE method is applied to solid continuum mechanics, displacements, strains, and stresses of solid structures subjected to load can be computed, which makes it very suitable for structural biomechanics. The application of the FE method is generally termed finite element analysis (FEA). Due to the capabilities of the FE method, the numerical simulation of implants and prosthetic devices by FEA has several advantages over experimental methods:

- Virtual experiments are perfectly repeatable and reproducible. The effect of single parameters on the computed results can be analyzed. Each parameter variation can be computed with exactly the same initial conditions. This is usually not possible in biomechanical experiments.
- Simulation models are completely observable. There is no need for measurement devices at specific locations that could influence the system.
- Simulation models can be more realistic than biomechanical experiments, because they allow the application of physiological boundary conditions in terms of muscle forces and realistic joint kinematics.
- Simulation models allow an "endless" number of parameter variations. Large sensitivity studies can be accomplished much faster and cheaper than with traditional experiments.

But, an FEA computes only an approximate solution and incorporates numerical errors and modeling errors due to simplifications and assumptions regarding the system behavior. These errors need to be verified and minimized to obtain reliable results. This can be accomplished by verification and validation within the process of modeling and simulation (▶ Fig. 23.1). The goal of the modeling and simulation process is to transfer a conceptual model, which is a simplified representation of reality, into a computable simulation model.[1] By the process of verification and validation, it is assessed if the computational model is built right, and if it accurately represents the underlying physics of the problem.[1]

> ### Key Concepts: Verification
>
> Verification is the process of determining that a model implementation accurately represents the developer's conceptual description of the model and the solution to the model."[2] Therefore, verification means to check the single procedures that are necessary to perform a simulation study for errors. Errors could be, for example, transposed digits, erroneous applied boundary conditions, or typos in a custom written code. A very important aspect of model verification in FEA is to check the numerical error of a FE model by mesh convergence analysis. Maxim: "Building the model right."

Due to the process of verification and validation, it is obvious that a single simulation model cannot reliably address an arbitrary number of problems. Simulation studies are meant to solve a particular problem or to address a specific research question or hypothesis. Simulation should not be employed to an end in itself. In the

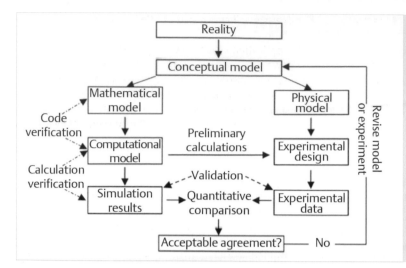

Fig. 23.1 Schematic overview of the verification and validation process. (Figure taken from Anderson AE, Ellis BJ, Weiss JA. Verification, validation and sensitivity studies in computational biomechanics. Comput Methods Biomech Biomed Engin 2007;10 [3]:171–184, with permission.)

end, the application of numerical methods in biomechanical research is similar to the employment of any other scientific method. Therefore, numerical simulation studies have to be planned as any other biomechanical research study.

Key Concepts: Validation

Validation is "The process of determining the degree to which a model is an accurate representation of the real world from the perspective of the intended uses of the model."[2] Therefore, validation means to check if the chosen modeling approach and the made assumptions are appropriate to represent the aspect of reality that is of interest. In biomechanics, validation is usually accomplished by performing experiments and comparing the experimentally determined measurements to the computed values. Maxim: "Building the right model."

23.1 Planning a Simulation Study

When planning a simulation study, two key issues have to be addressed:

1. What am I looking for? Which parameter do I want to compute? What is my research question, or what is the hypothesis I want to test?
2. Is the chosen numerical method the right method to determine that parameter or to test that hypothesis? Maybe there are other methods (analytical, experimental) that might be better suited, easier to perform, or even faster.

Potential parameters of interest in a bone-implant construct that could be computed by FEA are as follows:

• Interfragmentary movements in a fracture fixation construct
• Micromotions between bone and internal prosthesis
• Strain or stress distribution in an implant with respect to strength
• Strain or stress distribution in a bone with respect to strength or stress-shielding
• Strength and stiffness of bone-implant contacts

When a parameter of interest is identified, the whole simulation study and the process of modeling and simulation should be oriented toward this parameter.

23.2 Modeling and Simulation

The process of modeling and simulation usually starts with a system analysis of the aspect of reality that is of interest. The goal of that analysis is to formulate a conceptual model, which is a simplified representation of reality with respect to the parameter that has to be computed (▶ Fig. 23.1). The formulation of the conceptual model is probably the most important aspect of a simulation study. The following key issues have to be addressed for the modeling of a conceptual model of a bone-implant construct:

• Which components or details of the in vivo situation need to be considered when a bone-implant construct is investigated (e.g., do I need to consider muscles, cartilage, or soft tissue?)?
• Which components or details can be omitted with respect to the computed results? Do I need the lower leg with all muscles, tendons, and ligaments when my goal is to compute the interfragmentary motions in a femoral neck fracture?
• What are the relations between the different components of the system? Is the implant bonded to the bone, or does it slide over the bone with a specific coefficient of friction?

- What are the boundary and loading conditions? What are the joint kinematics, and how and where are forces applied?
- How can components, relations, and boundary and loading conditions be simplified? Do I need a bone model with inhomogeneous and anisotropic material properties when my goal is to compute the stress distribution in an intramedullary device?
- Where has nonlinearity to be considered or might be avoided? There are three sources of nonlinearity in an FEA:
  - Geometrical nonlinearity due to large displacements
  - Material nonlinearity (e.g., plastic behavior)
  - Nonlinear numerical contacts (e.g., friction contacts)

When the conceptual model is finally formulated, it has to be implemented in a computational model to be computable (▶ Fig. 23.1). The two-stage implementation of the conceptual model into a mathematical model and then into a computational model is usually accomplished within the preprocessor of FE software packages. The preprocessing generally involves the following steps when developing an FE model of a bone-implant construct:

1. Building of the geometry. This is usually performed within computer-aided design (CAD)-like software packages. Surgical procedures like drilling, filing, cutting, or milling can be simulated by Boolean operations.
2. Discretization of the geometry by a meshing algorithm. Appropriate types of elements (e.g., shells, solids) have to be chosen and the necessary degree of discretization has to be determined by mesh-convergence analysis

(see the following section titled "Verification and Validation").[3]

3. Application of material properties by constitutive laws (see Chapter 20).[4] If the inhomogeneous elasticity distribution of bone tissue has to be modeled, material mapping algorithms are employed that convert the bone density from q-computed tomography scans into elastic properties.[4] However, not every research question within the topic of bone-implant constructs has to be addressed with such sophisticated approaches.
4. Application of boundary and loading conditions. For validation purposes, the boundary and loading conditions have to be analogous to the validation experiment. For experimentation, more sophisticated boundary and loading conditions might be applied. Muscle forces, for example, can be derived from musculoskeletal multibody models (see Chapter 19).
5. Definition of numerical contacts. This is maybe the most crucial part of modeling in FEA of bone-implant constructs. Contacts between implants and bone tissue generally involve friction unless the bone has grown around the implant until bone and implant are bonded. Therefore, the interaction between implants and bone has to be modeled with friction contacts. However, friction contacts are nonlinear and computationally expensive. Thus, it often makes sense to simplify contacts by bonding implant and bone together. A good example for such an approach is the bonding of the threaded part of a screw to the bone tissue (▶ Fig. 23.2).

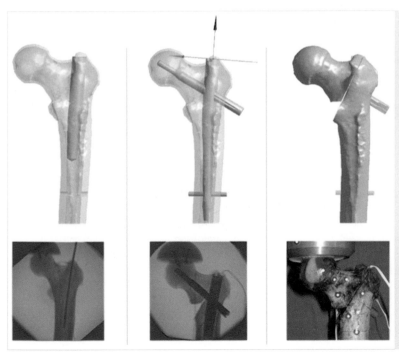

Fig. 23.2 Virtual surgery on a subject-specific bone model (*upper row*). The drilling was accomplished by a Boolean operation (*top left*). Then a short intramedullary nail was inserted (*top middle*), and a trochanteric fracture was set by virtual osteotomy (*top right*). The virtual operations simulated the surgical doing on an in vitro specimen (*lower row*).

23.3 Verification and Validation

The practice of verification is essential for the whole modeling process. Each step within the modeling procedure has to be verified, to assure that the "model is build right." Two important aspects of verification are code verification and calculation verification (▶ Fig. 23.1). While the code of commercial FE software is usually verified by the manufacturer, custom written code should be verified by benchmark problems. This applies, for example, to algorithms that are used to assign inhomogeneous material properties to bone tissue.[5] The numerical error of an FE model due to the nature of discretization has to be verified by mesh convergence analysis.[3] In h-method FE models, the degree of discretization has to be increased until the computed results converge (▶ Fig. 23.3). In p-method FE models, the polynomial degree of the elements has to be increased until the computed results converge.[6] In addition, global measures like the error in energy norm should be considered to check the overall mesh quality.

A further important aspect in computational models of bone-implant constructs is the accuracy of the geometry. The dimensions of bone and implant determine to some extent their stiffness and contact behavior. Particularly in subject-specific models of bones, where the bone geometry is derived from segmented q-computed tomography data, a verification of the dimensional accuracy is inevitable (▶ Fig. 23.4).[7]

When a computational model is verified, its underlying conceptual model has to be validated (▶ Fig. 23.1). All assumptions and simplifications that were made during the modeling of the conceptual model are checked by the validation procedure. Therefore, the physical model and the experimental design have to be based on the same conceptual model as the computational model (▶ Fig. 23.1). The experimental validation of a computational model and its underlying conceptual model is generally planned in three steps:

1. A physical model has to be established that represents the conceptual model. Furthermore, an experimental design has to be determined, which means that boundary and loading conditions, and location and type of validation measurements have to be defined. Preliminary computations can be used to help in designing the validation experiments (▶ Fig. 23.1).
2. An appropriate validation metric has to be set up that gives a measure of the deviation between computational model and experiment. The current "gold standard" in computational biomechanics is the Bland-Altman plot, which gives a measure of the mean deviation and the 95% confidence interval of the predictive errors of a computational model.[6]
3. A validation goal has to be set up—how accurate shall the model be? When using Bland-Altman plots, a range for the mean error and a maximum confidence interval could be used as validation goals. Based on the validation goal, it has to be decided whether the agreement between computed and measured values is acceptable. If the validation goal has not been achieved, the conceptual model has to be revised (▶ Fig. 23.1 and ▶ Fig. 23.5).

23.4 Experimentation

Once the simulation model is verified and validated, and the computed results are checked for plausibility, it can

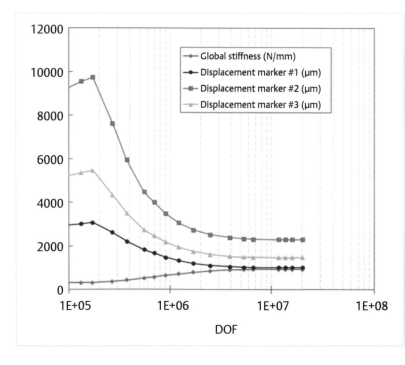

Fig. 23.3 Convergence behavior of computed results over an increasing number of degrees of freedom (*DOF*). In this case, the global axial stiffness and local displacements were computed. It is quite obvious that a too low degree of discretization would have caused a very large error in the computed results.

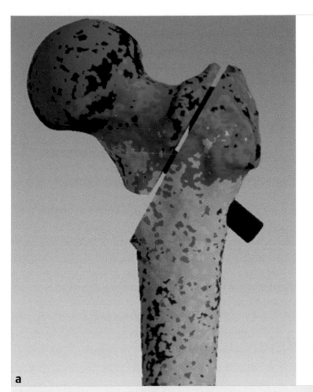
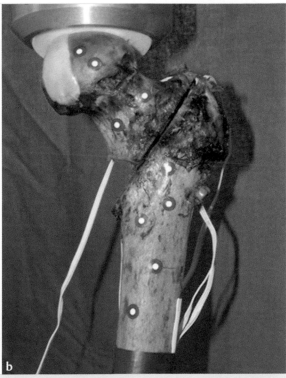

Fig. 23.4 (a) Subject-specific finite element model of the specimen. The contour plot shows the inhomogeneous distribution of elastic modulus values in the bone tissue. The finite element model was used to compute interfragmentary motions. **(b)** Human femur specimen with an artificial trochanteric fracture that was fixated with an intramedullary nail. Optical markers were glued to the bone surface to track local displacements. The experimentally determined displacements were used to validate the interfragmentary motions of the computational model.

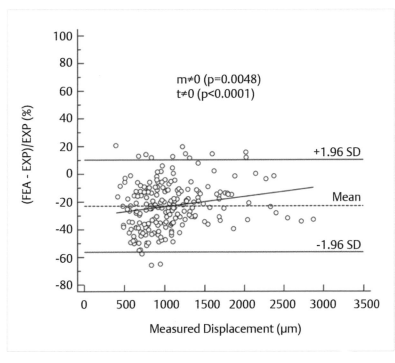

Fig. 23.5 Modified Bland-Altman plot of the predictive errors against the measured values. The *red dotted line* depicts the mean of all predictive errors, whereas the *red solid lines* show the 95% confidence interval of all predictive errors. The line of regression (*black*) of all values has a slope (*m*) and an offset (*t*) that is significantly different from zero. This means that the measured displacements were systematically underestimated by the finite element analysis, and that the predictive errors systematically depended on the magnitude of the measurements.[8]

be used to address the initial research question or to test the stated hypothesis. This virtual experimentation is very comparable to performing a series of mechanical experiments: for example, two implants are compared or different types of fractures and their effect on the implant are computed. However, the results of a single model are just deterministic results for the specific combination of input variables of that model. For that reason, it makes sense to vary the input variables in a plausible range to verify the sensitivity of the computed results to these variations. With such a sensitivity study, the significance of a model can be enhanced drastically (e.g., when implant A shows lower maximum stresses than implant B although the load vector is varied in its direction and amplitude, implant A might be really the better one in terms of strength). This extended validity of the results is termed robustness.

The robustness of results can be further increased when the probabilistic distribution (uncertainty) of input variables is known. With the known uncertainty of an input variable, the probabilistic distribution of a result can be computed. Uncertainties that might influence the computed results of bone-implant constructs could be:

- The probabilistic distribution of the mechanical properties of bone.
- The probabilistic distribution of loading conditions.
- The probabilistic distribution of implant dimensions due to manufacturing processes.
- The probabilistic distribution of contact properties between implant and bone.
- The probabilistic distribution of the implant position in the bone due to surgical procedures.

23.5 Results Interpretation

An often overlooked part of numerical simulation studies is the interpretation of the computed results. This is where the expertise of a computational engineer and/or biomechanical researcher comes into play. First, it has to be evaluated how reliable the results are based on the model validation. Second, the results have to be interpreted in terms of biomechanical or clinical relevance with the accuracy of the computations in mind.

23.6 Conclusion

Numerical simulation methods have an enormous potential in the field of biomechanical research. Particularly, hypotheses regarding the structural mechanics of bone-implant constructs are well suited to be addressed by numerical simulation methods like FEA. However, the prerequisite for numerical simulation studies in biomechanical research on bone-implant constructs is the valid application of the underlying methods. Finally, numerical simulation studies have to be applied as any other scientific method. It all starts with a good research question or

hypothesis. Then, the method needs to be qualified for that question or hypothesis.

Modeling and simplification of three major subjects have to be addressed when modeling and computing bone-implant constructs:
1. The contact between implant and bone
2. The material properties of bone
3. The in vivo boundary and loading conditions

Assumptions and simplifications in these three areas are particularly important when simulating bone-implant constructs and need to be well validated. Furthermore, the sensitivity of the computed results should be determined with respect to these three subjects. The topic of sensitivity is maybe the most important advantage of numerical simulation studies. The influence on the computed results by variation of single input variables can be determined. By incorporating the uncertainty of input variables, the significance of numerical models can be increased even further.

References

[1] Anderson AE, Ellis BJ, Weiss JA. Verification, validation and sensitivity studies in computational biomechanics. Comput Methods Biomech Biomed Engin 2007; 10: 171–184

[2] Oberkampf WL, Trucano TG, Hirsch C. Verification, validation, and predictive capability in computational engineering and physics. Appl Mech Rev 2004; 57: 345–384

[3] Schmidt H, Alber T, Wehner T, Blakytny R, Wilke H-J. Discretization error when using finite element models: analysis and evaluation of an underestimated problem. J Biomech 2009; 42: 1926–1934

[4] Eberle S, Göttlinger M, Augat P. An investigation to determine if a single validated density-elasticity relationship can be used for subject specific finite element analyses of human long bones. Med Eng Phys 2013; 35: 875–883

[5] Laz PJ, Browne M. A review of probabilistic analysis in orthopaedic biomechanics. Proc Inst Mech Eng H 2010; 224: 927–943

[6] Yosibash Z, Padan R, Joskowicz L, Milgrom C. A CT-based high-order finite element analysis of the human proximal femur compared to in-vitro experiments. J Biomech Eng 2007; 129: 297–309

[7] Trabelsi N, Yosibash Z, Wutte C, Augat P, Eberle S. Patient-specific finite element analysis of the human femur—a double-blinded biomechanical validation. J Biomech 2011; 44: 1666–1672

[8] Henninger HB, Reese SP, Anderson AE, Weiss JA. Validation of computational models in biomechanics. Proc Inst Mech Eng H 2010; 224: 801–812

Further Reading

Eberle S, Gerber C, von Oldenburg G, Hungerer S, Augat P. Type of hip fracture determines load share in intramedullary osteosynthesis. Clin Orthop Relat Res 2009; 467: 1972–1980

Oberkampf WL, Trucano TG, Hirsch C. Verification, validation, and predictive capability in computational engineering and physics. Appl Mech Rev 2004; 57: 345–384

Rathnayaka K, Sahama T, Schuetz MA, Schmutz B. Effects of CT image segmentation methods on the accuracy of long bone 3D reconstructions. Med Eng Phys 2011; 33: 226–233

Speirs AD, Heller MO, Duda GN, Taylor WR. Physiologically based boundary conditions in finite element modelling. J Biomech 2007; 40: 2318–2323

24 Numerical Simulation of Fracture Healing and Bone Remodeling

Ulrich Simon and Frank Niemeyer

Besides biological factors, the local mechanical environment is known to play a crucial role in directing the fracture healing process. The remarkably strong dependency of osteogenesis on mechanical factors is likely to be the reason why engineering methods and computer models found their way into this specific field of orthopedic research rather early on. Within the last 20 years, different research groups have developed dynamic models in order to predict the time-dependent fracture healing processes. While early models mainly served to test the plausibility of existing tissue differentiation hypotheses, more complex and more thoroughly validated models have since been used more frequently to generate clinically relevant predictions and recommendations.

In any case, computer models are very helpful in advancing our understanding of complex systems, especially if such numerical models are tightly coupled with experimental research methods.

24.1 Understanding and Creating Computer Models of Biological Processes

Let us now address some basic simulation concepts one has to understand first, in order to be able to classify existing numerical models. Anyone building a model of any biological process has to answer the following fundamental questions first.

24.1.1 First Question: What Are the Main Players, the State Variables?

First, you should think about the main players that participate in your "game," the so-called *state variables* or *dependent variables*. They describe the (changing) state of your system. They are the unknowns in your research question, the quantities you would like to measure, even if that is impossible experimentally. Start with one or only a few state variables and avoid unnecessary initial complexity; at first, include only the most important effects. It is your decision: You are the director; you can hire further players later on.

Examples of state variables:
- Local osteoblast concentration in a fracture callus
- Bone tissue distribution in a fracture callus
- Bone mineral density distribution around a hip stem

24.1.2 Second Question: Do You Like to Get a Single Picture or a Movie? What Are the Independent Variables?

Next, you need to choose the *independent variables* (i.e., time and spatial coordinates). They awaken your players and provide them with room to live in; otherwise, they would just be constants.

Examples of independent variables:
- Choose one, two, or three spatial coordinates (e.g., x, y, or z) in order to define the state variables as fields in a one-, two-, or three-dimensional space.
- Add a time coordinate t if your problem is time-dependent and if you are interested in that time dependency. Introducing time means switching from a static to a dynamic approach.

By choosing the independent coordinates, you implicitly define the mathematical type of your problem and thereby the numerical method, the algorithm(s)—and thus, the kind of software—suitable for solving the model (see remarks in the next section).

24.1.3 Third Question: What Is the Story About? Name Effects and Processes

Now that you have your players listed, you are able to write down the interactions between them. Most dynamical models, especially those of biological processes, use the following quite general form of equations, which is much easier to read and to construct than you might think at first. Such a mathematical formalism likely fits your problem as well. For each of your previously chosen state variables, you need to devise an equation that describes how the state variable changes over time. This results in a system of equations of the following form:

Rate of change of variable 1 = Effect A + Effect B + …
Rate of change of variable 2 = Effect C + Effect D + …

This system describes how the state variables (left side) change over time depending on several effects (right side). The effects can increase or decrease the rate of change. They can depend on any of the state variables, even the one that can be found on the left side of the same equation, as well as on any of the independent variables, explicitly. Mathematically speaking, we are dealing with a (potentially coupled) set of (linear or nonlinear) first-order ordinary differential equations.

Example: Rate of change of bone mineral density = bone matrix production rate – bone absorption rate

The bone matrix production itself might be modeled as a function depending on the local osteoblast concentration. It would therefore be nice to have that osteoblast concentration as a further state variable available. To describe more complex effects, we need to also include derivatives of state variables with respect to the spatial coordinates, leading to partial differential equations.

24.2 Biological Processes of Fracture Healing

In order to be able to capture the underlying biological processes of fracture healing in a mathematical model, we first need to understand them in detail. Please refer to Chapter 9, "Biomechanics of Trabecular and Cortical Bone," and Chapter 10, "Biomechanics of Fracture Fixation" for a detailed overview of the biological aspects of fracture healing and bone formation processes. In the context of this chapter, we only want to repeat briefly the most important aspects of the involved processes.

24.2.1 Processes of Fracture Healing

The natural form of fracture healing occurring in long bones is indirect or callus healing where the fragments, with or without artificial fixation, display a certain amount of so-called interfragmentary movement (IFM; i. e., relative movement toward each other).

The healing process (▶ Fig. 24.1) starts with the phase of acute inflammation within the blood clot. All cells enclosed in the hematoma die within days after the trauma due to acute hypoxia. Leukocytes invade the area; granulocytes, histiocytes, and mastocytes start clearing the site of debris tissue. Then trauma and inflammatory reactions trigger the primary callus response: Underneath the periosteum, at some distance from the gap, intramembranous ossification starts and produces large

amounts of woven bone. This primary response lasts for about 2 weeks.

In the meantime, revascularization of the hematoma begins and mesenchymal stem cells and fibroblasts invade the fracture site. The fibroblasts proliferate, produce collagen fibers, and replace the hematoma with well-vascularized granulation tissue. Within weeks, the initial granulation tissue is replaced by a cuff of fibrous connective tissue that encloses and connects both fracture fragments, forming a soft callus.

Near the fracture gap, where high strains predominate and prohibit both revascularization and intramembranous ossification, mesenchymal stem cells differentiate into chondroblasts that produce cartilage matrix. The produced cartilage further stabilizes the fracture site and provides the framework for the following ossification process.

Gradually, the fibrocartilage tissue mixture gets transformed into woven bone via endochondral ossification: Starting from the already existing woven bone that formed underneath the periosteum at some distance from the fracture gap, the ossification fronts of the two callus halves grow toward each other. While they approach, they increase their width as the mechanical strains in the vicinity of the fracture gap are far too high for the ossification process. This also increases the cross-sectional area and in turn the bending stiffness. Bony bridging through unification of the two callus wedges occurs typically in the periphery of the callus. When this happens, the fracture is considered to be "healed." Besides the periosteal response, there is also an endosteal reaction, which is however less pronounced due to the delayed medullary "vascular response."

24.2.2 Remodeling

Remodeling is a constantly ongoing process of resorption of old and formation of new bone to adapt the bone to new mechanical requirements, to repair microdamage, to regulate calcium homeostasis, to form the overall shape of the bone, or to transform woven into lamellar bone. Osteoclasts together with osteoblasts form a remodeling unit, where

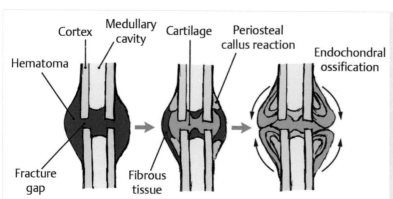

Fig. 24.1 Stages of callus healing: inflammation, primary callus response, and ossification.

the preceding osteoclasts resorb bone via phagocytosis by secreting enzymes that break up the existing bone tissue. The following osteoblasts produce the extracellular matrix called osteoid that becomes mineralized, resulting in the formation of new bone tissue. This process is strongly controlled by the local mechanical stimuli.

24.2.3 Tissue Differentiation and Mechanoregulation Hypotheses

The discovery of the functional adaptation of living tissues to their daily mechanical loading goes back to the 19th century. Julius Wolff observed that the trabeculae in the femoral head apparently are aligned along the trajectories of principal mechanical stresses. He deduced in 1892 that local mechanical stimuli determine local tissue formation.[1] Wilhelm Roux further hypothesized that the development of specific tissues is associated with specific types of mechanical stresses.[2] Friedrich Pauwels improved this concept and hypothesized that formation of either cartilage or fibrous tissue would be stimulated by shape changing or volume changing strain states, respectively.[3] A further differentiation into bone tissue, however, requires a stable situation with only very low strains but no preference for a specific deformation type. Pauwels therefore concluded that the primary goal of a fracture treatment must be the stabilization of the fracture site such that bone tissue can form.

Beginning in the 1960s, Harold Frost explored the relations between mechanical loading and the remodeling process of bone tissue, but also other potentially mechanosensitive tissues over the course of more than four decades.[4] He suggested that the skeletal physiology—its local strength and architecture—is controlled by biological factors and mechanical influences in such a way that the mechanical strains always fall within a certain acceptable range (Utah paradigm of skeletal physiology). If the mechanical load exceeded an upper threshold, the tissue's functional units would increase the strength of the tissue at that particular location. Respectively, if the stimulus dropped below a certain threshold, tissue would be resorbed until the local stimuli are again within the adapted window (▶ Fig. 24.2).

This negative feedback loop ("mechanostat") tends to plateau at equilibrium. Nearly all numerical remodeling simulations are based on this concept.

> ### Jargon Simplified: Invariant
>
> An invariant of the strain tensor (which can be represented by a matrix containing the strain components) is a value derived from the strain tensor's components and that is independent from the choice of a particular coordinate system. Using strain invariants as mechanical stimuli is plausible, as the cells' behavior should not depend on the arbitrary choice of a frame of reference.

Based on Pauwels ideas, Claes and Heigele[5] developed a first quantitative tissue differentiation function. Simon et al[6] enhanced that function and thermodynamically more consistently used only strain invariants as stimuli. Bone formation according to this function is possible only on existing bony surfaces with adequate blood supply and both strain stimuli lying within a certain range, called "medium" (▶ Fig. 24.3).

Prendergast et al[7] used a more complex biphasic (poroelastic) material model to describe the biological tissues and introduced a tissue differentiation algorithm dependent on shear strain (distortional strain γ) in the solid phase and the fluid flow velocity in the interstitial fluid phase (▶ Fig. 24.4). This function predicted bone formation for lower but not too low strains and fluid flows.

Though both hypotheses appear quite different at first sight, they both are able to explain the subsequent

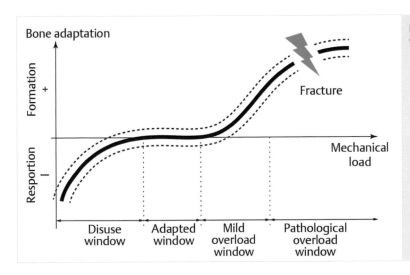

Fig. 24.2 Frost's concept of the bone adaptation mechanism, after Frost, H.[4]

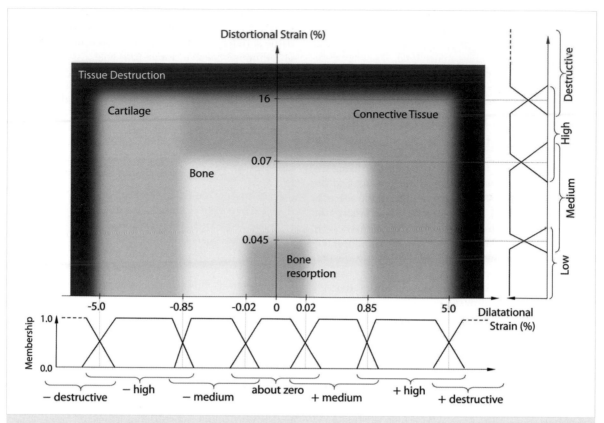

Fig. 24.3 The "New Ulm Differentiation Function" developed by Simon et al[6] based on the tissue differentiation hypothesis by Claes and Heigele.[5]

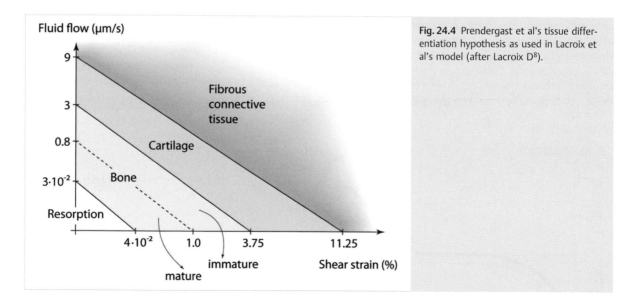

Fig. 24.4 Prendergast et al's tissue differentiation hypothesis as used in Lacroix et al's model (after Lacroix D[8]).

occurrence of fibrous soft tissue, cartilage, and bone, as both hypotheses associate tissue types with the magnitude of mechanical stimulation in an analogous order: Fibrous tissue can withstand high (in particular tensile) strains; chondrogenesis is the response to medium to high compressive and/or shear strains; and bone growth requires small but nonzero mechanical stimulation.

24.3 Numerical Models of Fracture Healing

24.3.1 Static Models

The goal of early numerical models of fracture healing was to compute the mechanical stimuli acting inside the callus, something that cannot be measured in vivo. The idea was that this could allow the verification of existing differentiation hypotheses by comparing the computed stimuli with the healing patterns found in vivo.

DiGioia et al[9] as well as Cheal et al[10] created geometrically simple static finite element models of the osteotomy gap of experimental healing cases and analyzed the strain distribution. Both groups concluded that the concept of axial interfragmentary strain (IFS) controlling the local tissue differentiation (Perren's hypothesis[11]) is probably too simple to account for the complex strain field. DiGioia et al[9] stated that possibly the hydrostatic stress together with the octahedral shear stress could be better indicators for tissue differentiation processes.

Following the ideas of Pauwels and DiGioia, Carter et al[12] chose two stress tensor invariants—hydrostatic stress and octahedral shear stress—and combined them in the "osteogenic index" as a stimulus for the bone forming process. The authors created two-dimensional finite element models (plane-stress assumption) of idealized femoral osteotomies in the initial healing phase. They computed the stress distribution inside the callus region for different load histories consisting of axial loading, bending, or a combination thereof. They found that hydrostatic pressure seems to be more important to ossification in the initial healing phase than octahedral shear stress, because high hydrostatic pressure could hinder the ingrowth of blood vessels.

Claes and Heigele[5] published a simple, axisymmetric finite element model of a transverse osteotomy of the right metatarsus in sheep. They compared the calculated stress and strain distributions in the callus with histological findings from three different healing stages. From this, they developed a new quantitative differentiation hypothesis, where tissue differentiation depends on the local hydrostatic stress and the local strain state, and bone formation happens on existing bony surfaces only, if stresses and strains are within a certain stimulating range. This hypothesis served as a basis for the new "Ulm Differentiation Function,"[6] which refers to strain invariants only (▶ Fig. 24.3).`

24.3.2 Dynamic Models

With the advent of more powerful computing hardware, researchers started to implement dynamic models of fracture healing. Dynamic in this context means that the models solve an initial value problem, usually in an iterative manner (compare to ▶ Fig. 24.5, *right part*): Starting with an initial distribution of tissue types and/or material properties, the mechanical stimuli for this configuration are computed, in the majority of cases by using the finite element method. Equipped with those stimuli, a tissue differentiation procedure modifies the tissue distribution and/or cell type concentrations and/or material properties according to some differentiation hypothesis. In the next iteration, this change of material properties in turn leads to slightly altered mechanical stimuli, which again promote an adaptation of the tissue distribution. This loop continues until some termination criterion is met (e. g., reaching a homeostatic state).

A first dynamic fracture healing model was presented in 1994 at the ISFR conference in Kobe by Ament and the group around Claes and Hofer.[13] They introduced the usage of fuzzy logic to model tissue differentiation processes that depend on the strain energy density as a mechanical stimulus. With this approach, they were able to simulate the callus healing of geometrically and constitutionally idealized cases.

The group around Prendergast, Lacroix, and Huiskes started to describe the mechanical behavior of biological tissues involved in the fracture healing process using more complex biphasic (poroelastic) material models. They also introduced the idea that tissue differentiation could be regulated by the fluid flow in the interstitial fluid phase beside the shear strain in the solid phase. Huiskes et al implemented an iterative, time-dependent model of mechano-regulated tissue differentiation around implants.[14] Lacroix et al additionally considered the migration of mesenchymal stem cells in their fracture healing model by a diffusion model. They were able to simulate first an idealized 2D callus[15] and later a 3D callus geometry.[16]

Pérez and Prendergast[17] and Checa and Prendergast[18] further improved the existing model by sub-finite processes to describe cell migration and capillary network formation using a lattice-based approach.

Bailón-Plaza and van der Meulen[19] in 2001 mainly modeled the influences of growth factors on the fracture healing process, first without considering any mechanical stimuli and later in 2003 with limited support for mechanostimulated tissue differentiation in a revised model.[20] They were able to predict the spatial distribution of cell densities (mesenchymal, bone, cartilage), matrix densities (combined connective tissue/cartilage matrix, bone matrix), and growth factor concentrations over time.

The Saragossa Group developed and improved numerical fracture healing models based on an approach from Kuiper et al.[21] What sets their models apart from other approaches is the inclusion of volumetric growth of the callus due to cell proliferation and chondrogenesis. Their model is able to describe how the callus changes its size and shape over time.[22,23]

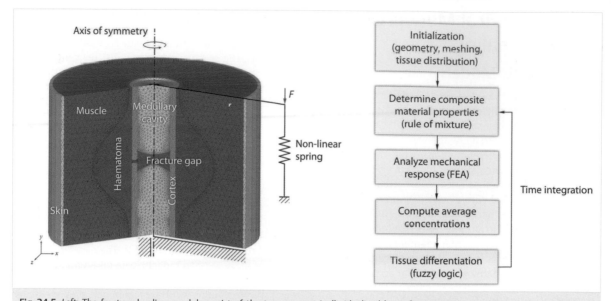

Fig. 24.5 *Left*: The fracture healing model consist of the two geometrically idealized bone fragments (cortical bone) separated by a fracture gap, enclosed by an initially avascular hematoma region; revascularization can commence from within the intramedullary canal as well as the surrounding soft tissue (muscle). The nonlinear spring represents the external fixator.
Right: After the initialization step, the simulation procedure follows an iterative scheme to compute how the tissue distribution evolves over time. For each iteration, it is necessary to determine the composite material properties based on the relative tissue concentrations for each finite element so that it is possible to determine the mechanical stimuli by solving the mechanical boundary value problem using the finite element method. Given the current mechanical stimulation as well as the biological stimuli (vascularity, local tissue concentration, distance-weighted average concentrations in finite neighborhood), the fuzzy logic controller determines the relative tissue changes for each element. (Source: Niemeyer, F.[29])

After extensive screening of different existing tissue differentiation models,[24] Isaksson et al[25] came up with a model that incorporated properties from both the "Prendergast family" of models and the bioregulatory approach of Bailón-Plaza and van der Meulen. The implementation consists of two finite element models: one poroelastic for the computation of the mechanical stimuli and one using a custom element type to solve the partial differential equations describing the cellular processes. A discrete, scalar function derived from the two continuous mechanical stimuli shear strain and fluid flow switches proliferation, differentiation, and apoptosis on and off, but does not influence the rate at which these processes take place. Cells also produce or break down matrix (fibrous tissue, cartilage, or bone) at a rate depending on the local cell concentration, but not on the mechanical stimulus as this, again, only acts as an on/off switch.

Geris et al first experimented mainly with Prendergast et al's approach[26] before turning towards models with a heavier emphasis on the bioregulatory side,[27] certainly inspired by the work of Bailón-Plaza and van der Meulen. Their contemporary model[28] combines both attempts and additionally accounts for the importance of the revascularization process (angiogenesis). These extensions required the addition of several state variables: vascular cell density, vascular matrix density, a generic angiogenic growth factor, fibroblasts, and a corresponding matrix type. The mechanical stimuli, hydrostatic pressure and fluid flow, influence the cellular processes in so far as the parameters of the bioregulatory model are modified depending on whether the stimulus is considered to be stimulating or inhibiting. Concerning the numerical implementation, Geris et al[28] used a poroelastic finite element model to determine the "stimulus of the day" (one load step per day), which then serves as input to the bioregulatory model. The custom finite volume method code used to solve the system of partial differential equations is so far restricted to rectangular geometries.

Jargon Simplified: Fuzzy Logic

"Fuzzy" in the context of fuzzy logic means "not sharp" (cf. fuzzy sets introduced by Lotfi Zadeh 1965 at the University of California, Berkeley). Fuzzy logic therefore is a "non-sharp logic" in that it not only operates on completely true (= 1) or false (= 0) truth values, but also on values in between (0 … 1). Evaluating fuzzy if-then expressions can therefore model smooth transitions between two states, in contrast to "classical" (sharp) logic, which can only model binary switching behavior.

24.3.3 The Ulm Fracture Healing Model

In the late 1990s, Simon et al[6] began building a more advanced, dynamic model of secondary fracture healing based on both Claes' and Heigele's work on finite element models and tissue differentiation functions and the fuzzy logic approach first introduced by Ament et al.[13] The first implementation of this model was a two-dimensional, yet axisymmetric finite element model[6] describing a fractured ovine metatarsus with a transverse osteotomy. The external fixator used in this experiment[30] featured a very high axial stiffness while still allowing a customizable amount of IFM. Simon et al[6] investigated two groups that differed in the amount of allowed IFM of either 0.25 mm or 1.25 mm. Comparisons with the experimental results showed that the model correctly predicts delayed healing for the less stable case.

Using an additional spatiotemporal state variable, Simon et al[2] added the local blood perfusion ("vascularity") as one of the most important biological factors besides the mechanical stimuli to the model. Processes to increase or decrease the blood perfusion, revascularization (angiogenesis), or tissue destruction, respectively, were also modeled dependent on the local mechanical and biological stimuli. The authors developed the "New Ulm Differentiation Function" (▶ Fig. 24.3) to describe these processes together with chondrogenesis, intramembraneous and endochondral ossification, and tissue destruction due to overloading. Strain invariants (pure dilatational and pure distortional strain) replace the stress-strain mixture used in the older Claes and Heigele differentiation function.

The Ulm model[31] has further been used and extended to simulate more realistic fracture geometries,[32] fracture healing in trabecular bone,[33] or complex load cases.[34] Niemeyer[29] made many important improvements and developed the currently most universal model that is able to successfully simulate many different cases of callus healing (see the example below) as well as distraction osteogenesis.

24.3.4 Simulating Distraction Osteogenesis

A few fracture healing models were further enhanced to simulate the more complex process of distraction osteogenesis. Isaksson et al[35] reported a dynamic model for distraction osteogenesis based on experimental work on bone segment transport using an intramedullary nail. Reina-Romo et al[36] enhanced the models from Gómez-Benito et al[23] and adapted it to different clinical applications of distraction osteogenesis. Also, the Ulm model was further advanced to also simulate experimental cases of both lateral bone distraction and callus distraction in sheep (see the following example).

Example of a Fracture Healing Model

Let us now investigate a sample healing simulation: Our goal shall be to simulate the different cases of ovine fracture healing described by Claes et al[30] with sufficient accuracy. Claes et al[30] investigated how different fracture gap sizes (1 mm, 2 mm, or 6 mm) and different fixator stiffnesses, resulting in low (7%) or high (30%) initial IFS, influence fracture healing in sheep. The following methods and results are based on the model presented by Niemeyer.[29]

Like the model by Simon et al,[6] this simulation employs two core numerical techniques to simulate the evolution of tissue distribution over time: Because bone healing is largely driven by mechanical stimulation, we need to determine the strain field inside the healing region. This elasticity problem can be solved using a conventional (static) finite element analysis, yielding the mechanical stimuli at a specific point in time. Depending on these mechanical stimuli, we then need to decide how the existing tissue reacts to these stimuli; in this model, we use a fuzzy logic controller to determine the rate of change for each tissue component (woven bone, lamellar bone, cartilage, soft/connective tissue, vascularity), which we then integrate (explicitly) over time.

Aside from these core ideas (relative tissue concentrations, finite element method, fuzzy logic–controlled tissue differentiation), Niemeyer[29] extended the original model by Simon et al[6] by the following features:

- Resorption: Understimulated and thus superfluous bone tissue is degraded and gradually resorbed over time.
- Remodeling: Lamellar bone slowly replaces the mechanically weaker woven bone. This leads to understimulation and hence resorption in large regions of the bony callus, eventually restoring the original shape of the bone.
- Delayed calcification: In reality, there is a finite delay between the occurrence of osteogenic stimuli and observable calcified bone tissue, as a number of biological processes have to take place first. Bone formation in the model therefore depends on a delayed version of the mechanical signal.
- Stimuli memory: In addition to the previous point, osteogenesis not only depends on instantaneous (delayed or not) mechanical stimuli, but also on stimuli it experienced in the past. The model captures this effect by maintaining a stimuli history for each element and for which it distills "effective stimuli" for the fuzzy logic controller.
- Viscoplastic material properties: Biological material display time-dependent behavior. The model therefore

uses viscoplastic material models, requiring transient finite element analyses.

- Decoupled spatial and temporal discretization: Osteogenesis and angiogenesis are surface processes (i.e., local bone increase/vessel growth requires a sufficient amount of bone and/or vascularity within a finite vicinity). In contrast to the original model, this requirement is formulated in terms of mesh-independent distance-weighted averaged concentrations, allowing the predicted evolution of tissue distribution to converge when increasing the mesh resolution.
- Remeshing: Because the model should be able to model distraction osteogenesis as well, where immense plastic straining occurs regularly, we also included a remeshing and mesh-to-mesh state mapping procedure.

Using this model (▶ Fig. 24.5) to simulate two of the six in vivo cases (2 mm gap, 7% versus 30% initial IFS) shows that the version with the less stiff fixator and thus higher IFS takes considerably longer to bridge the fracture gap, resulting in overall delayed healing (▶ Fig. 24.6). In fact, at day 56, the end of the in vivo study, according to the simulation there is still a gap of approximately 2 mm between the distal and proximal callus segments. The overall reduction in IFM is only due to an increased cross-sectional area combined with large amounts of cartilage that forms inside the fracture gap. The low-IFS case, on the other hand, heals rapidly and displays bony bridging as soon as day 35, although we can also discover some amount of bone resorption during the initial 2 weeks due to partial stress shielding, caused by the relatively stiff fixator.

All in all, these results fit comparatively well to the in vivo results, although the high-IFS case seems to have healed a bit better in the experiments than the model predicts. Yet, the scatter in the experimental results is significant, and the deviation from the exact mean values should probably not be overrated. What we can undoubtedly conclude is that the experiment and the numerical model based on its underlying tissue differentiation hypothesis agree that too flexible fixation can lead to delayed bony union.

24.4 Conclusion

Numerical models of fracture healing and bone remodeling processes let us look much deeper into the complexity of the involved biological systems. Numerical modeling is an excellent tool to develop, proof, and improve theories and hypotheses. While early models mainly served to test the plausibility of existing tissue differentiation hypotheses, more complex and more thoroughly validated models have since been used more and more frequently to generate clinically relevant predictions and recommendations. Yet, simulations should always be used in tight conjunction with experimental methods and can help to optimize clinical devices and treatments. We are still only at the beginning of a flourishing development and a lot of progress is still to be made; future, more advanced models will likely include more biological processes in a more mechanistic manner and on different scales.

24.5 Acknowledgments

The simulation example and much of the other material presented in this chapter was adapted from the recently published PhD thesis by the coauthor Frank Niemeyer.[29] This dissertation project was supervised by Prof. Lutz Claes at the Institute of Orthopaedic Research and Biomechanics at the University of Ulm and was funded by a research grant of the German Research Foundation (DFG CL77/14).

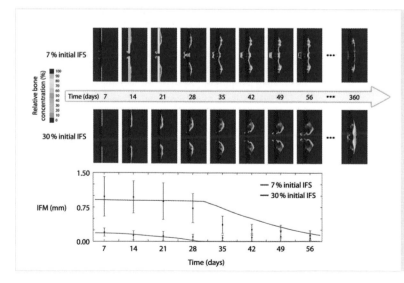

Fig. 24.6 Experimental versus numerical results. The simulations of two of the cases investigated by Claes et al[30] with a gap size of 2 mm and 7% or 30% initial interfragmentary strain (IFS), respectively, agree well with the reported experimental results (*corresponding bars*): The interfragmentary movement drops considerably faster for the stiffer case (*bottom, blue line*). These results are not very surprising, given that the low-IFS case is already bridged at day 35 whereas the high-IFS case is still not healed at day 56 (*top*). Simulating the evolution of bone tissue beyond the time frame of the experiment predicts slow but steady remodeling of the now dispensable callus as the newly formed bone matures over time.

References

[1] Wolff J. Das Gesetz der Transformation der Knochen. Berlin: Hirsch-wald; 1892

[2] Roux W. Der züchtende Kampf der Theile oder die Theilauslese im Or-ganismus. Zugleich eine Theorie der functionellen Anpassung. Ein Bei-trag zur Vervollständigung der Lehre von der mechanischen Entste-hung des sogenannten Zweckmäßigen. In: Gesammelte Abhandlungen über Entwicklungsmechanik der Organismen. Vol. 1. 1881, 135–442

[3] Pauwels F. Eine neue Theorie über den Einfluss mechanischer Reize auf die Differenzierung der Stützgewebe. Anatomy and Embryology 1960;6:478–515

[4] Frost HM. The Utah paradigm of skeletal physiology: an overview of its insights for bone, cartilage and collagenous tissue organs. J Bone and Mineral Metabolism 2000;18(6): 305–316

[5] Claes LE, Heigele CA. Magnitudes of local stress and strain along bony surfaces predict the course and type of fracture healing. J Biomech 1999;32(3):255–266

[6] Simon U, Augat P, Utz M, Claes L. A numerical model of the fracture healing process that describes tissue development and revascularisa-tion. Comput Methods Biomech Biomed Engin 2011;14(1):79–93

[7] Prendergast PJ, Huiskes R, Søballe K. Biophysical stimuli on cells dur-ing tissue differentiation at implant interfaces. J Biomech 1997:30 (6):539–548

[8] Lacroix D, Prendergast PJ, Li G, Marsh D. Biomechanical model to sim-ulate tissue differentiation and bone regeneration: application to fracture healing. Med Biol Eng Comput 2002; 40: 14–21

[9] DiGioia AM III, Cheal EJ, Hayes WC. Three-dimensional strain fields in a uniform osteotomy gap. J Biomech Eng 1986; 108: 273–280

[10] Cheal EJ, Mansmann KA, Digioia AM, Hayes WC, Perren SM. Role of interfragmentary strain in fracture healing: Ovine model of a healing osteotomy. J Orthop Res 1991;9(1):131–142

[11] Perren SM, Cordey J. The concept of interfragmentary strain. Current concepts of internal fixation of fractures 1980:63–77

[12] Carter DR, Blenman PR, Beaupré GS. Correlations between mechani-cal stress history and tissue differentiation in initial fracture healing. J Orthop Res 1988; 6: 736–748

[13] Ament C, Hofer EP. A fuzzy logic model of fracture healing. J Biomech 2000;33(8):961–968

[14] Huiskes R, Van Driel WD, Prendergast PJ, Søballe K. A biomechanical regulatory model for periprosthetic fibrous-tissue differentiation. J Materials Science 1997;8(12):785–788

[15] Lacroix D, Prendergast PJ. A mechano-regulation model for tissue dif-ferentiation during fracture healing: analysis of gap size and loading. J Biomech 2002;35(9):1163–1171

[16] Lacroix D, Prendergast PJ. Three-dimensional simulation of fracture repair in the human tibia. Comput Methods Biomech Biomed Engin 2002;5(5):369–376

[17] Pérez M, Prendergast PJ. Random-walk models of cell dispersal in-cluded in mechanobiological simulations of tissue differentiation. J Biomech 2007;40(10):2244–2253

[18] Checa S, Prendergast PJ. Effect of cell seeding and mechanical loading on vascularization and tissue formation inside a scaffold: A mechano-biological model using a lattice approach to simulate cell activity. J Biomech 2010;43(5):961–968

[19] Bailón-Plaza A, van der Meulen MCH. A Mathematical Framework to Study the Effects of Growth Factor Influences on Fracture Healing. J Theoretical Biol 2001;212(2):191–209

[20] Bailón-Plaza A, van der Meulen MCH. Beneficial effects of moderate, early loading and adverse effects of delayed or excessive loading on bone healing. J Biomech 2003;36(8):1069–1077

[21] Kuiper et al. ESB, 2000, Dublin

[22] García-Aznar JM, Kuiper JH, Gómez-Benito MJ, Doblaré M, Richardson JB. Computational simulation of fracture healing: influence of inter-fragmentary movement on the callus growth. J Biomech 2007;40 (7):1467–1476

[23] Gómez-Benito M, García-Aznar J, Kuiper J, Doblaré M. Influence of fracture gap size on the pattern of long bone healing: a computation-al study. J Theor Biol 2005;235(1):105–119

[24] Isaksson H, Wilson W, van Donkelaar CC, Huiskes R, Ito K. Com-parison of biophysical stimuli for mechano-regulation of tissue differentiation during fracture healing. J Biomech 2006;39 (8):1507–1516

[25] Isaksson H, van Donkelaar CC, Huiskes R, Ito K. A mechanoregulatory bone-healing model incorporating cell-phenotype specific activity. J Theor Biol 2008;252(2):230–246

[26] Geris L, Oosterwyck HV, Sloten JV, Duyck J, Naert I. Assessment of Mechanobiological Models for the Numerical Simulation of Tissue Differentiation around Immediately Loaded Implants. Comput Meth-ods Biomech Biomed Engin 2003;6(5):277

[27] Geris L, Gerisch A, Sloten JV, Weiner R, Oosterwyck HV. Angiogenesis in bone fracture healing: A bioregulatory model. J Theor Biol 2008;251(1):137–158

[28] Geris L, Sloten JV, Oosterwyck HV. Connecting biology and mechanics in fracture healing: an integrated mathematical modeling framework for the study of nonunions. Biomech Model Mechanobiol 2010;9 (6):713–724

[29] Niemeyer F. Simulation of fracture healing - applied to distraction os-teogenesis. PhD thesis, University of Ulm, Ulm, Germany 2013

[30] Claes L, Wilke H-J, Augat P, Rübenacker S, Margevicius K. Effect of dy-namization on gap healing of diaphyseal fractures under external fix-ation. Clin Biomech (Bristol, Avon) 1995;10(5):227–234

[31] Simon, U., Augat, P., and Claes, L. Dynamical Simulation of the Frac-ture Healing Process Including Vascularity. In: 13th Conference of the European Society of Biomechanics (ESB), Acta of Bioengineering and Biomechanics. Vol. 4. Wroclaw, Poland, 2002

[32] Wehner T, Claes L, Niemeyer F, Nolte D, Simon, U. Influence of the fixation stability on the healing time–a numerical study of a pa-tient-specific fracture healing process. Clin Biomech 2010;25 (6):606–612

[33] Shefelbine SJ, Augat P, Claes L, Simon U. Trabecular bone fracture healing simulation with Finite element analysis and fuzzy logic. J Bio-mech 2005;38(12):2440–2450

[34] Steiner M, Claes L, Ignatius A, Niemeyer F, Simon U, Wehner T. Predic-tion of fracture healing under axial loading, shear loading and bend-ing is possible using distortional and dilatational strains as determin-ing mechanical stimuli. Journal of the Royal Society, Interface / the Royal Society 2013;10(86):20130389

[35] Isaksson H, Comas O, van Donkelaar CC, et al. Bone regeneration dur-ing distraction osteogenesis: Mechano-regulation by shear strain and fluid velocity. J Biomech 2007;40(9):2002–2011

[36] Reina-Romo E, Gómez-Benito MJ, García-Aznar JM, Domínguez J, Doblaré M. Growth mixture model of distraction osteogenesis: ef-fect of pre-traction stresses. Biomech Model Mechanobiol 2009;9 (1):103–115

Part 5
Imaging

25 Micro-Computed Tomography Imaging of Bone Tissue

Timothy M. Jackman, Gabriel McDonald, and Elise F. Morgan

Since the introduction of micro-computed tomography (μCT) for imaging of trabecular bone approximately 25 years ago, this imaging modality has rapidly become the standard technique for assessment of bone micro- and macrostructure in laboratory research. Estimating bone mineral density from μCT images has also become commonplace. The purpose of this chapter is to provide an introduction and survey of the use of μCT in bone research. We begin with a brief overview of the basic operating principles of μCT systems and then proceed to summarize the capabilities of μCT as an imaging modality for assessing the microstructure, macrostructure, and mineralization of bone. The particular application of μCT to rodent bone is then discussed, along with applications that use μCT imaging to assess the biomechanical behavior of bone. We end the chapter with a summary of the recent trajectory of research in μCT imaging of bone.

25.1 Overview of Micro-Computed Tomography

Modern μCT systems are the evolutionary successors of X-ray technology, incorporating rapid digital image acquisition and high-performance computing to produce detailed, three-dimensional (3D) fields of data. All μCT scanners use the same basic operating scheme, which is to place the specimen in between an X-ray source and X-ray detector, and to rotate either the specimen or the

source-detector pair during the course of image acquisition (▶ Fig. 25.1). The X-ray source produces photons, which are attenuated as they pass through the specimen, prior to striking the detector. The detector is an X-ray–sensitive camera that records a two-dimensional (2D) radiographic projection of the specimen at the particular angular position. The angular position is then changed, and a new projection is gathered. The number of projections required depends on the nature of the specimen and the desired image resolution, but usually several hundred projections (e.g., one per degree of rotation) are necessary. The resulting set of 2D projections is then reconstructed to generate image data representing the full 3D volume. This 3D representation is simply a 3D array of *voxels* (volumetric pixels).

For the typical range of photon energies used in μCT (20 to 100 keV), photon attenuation occurs via photoelectric absorption and Compton scattering. Photoelectric absorption, whereby the attenuation scales with the atomic number of the material, is foremost for lower-energy photons (< 25 keV). Compton scattering, whereby the attenuation scales with the density of the material, is dominant for higher-energy photons. Owing to its high calcium content and high density, bone tissue attenuates the incident photons to a greater degree than do soft tissues. This differential attenuation produces sharp contrast between bone and surrounding soft tissues in μCT images, wherein the grayscale value of a given voxel represents the attenuation of the material present at that location in the specimen.

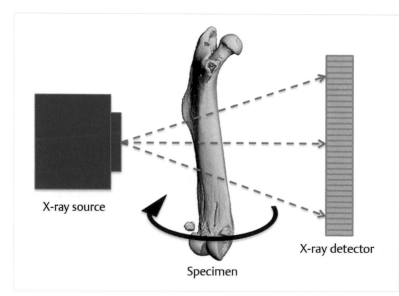

X-ray source

Specimen

X-ray detector

Fig. 25.1 Basic scheme of a micro-computed tomography scanner in which the specimen is placed on a stage that rotates relative to the X-ray source and detector.

Two different types of µCT scanners have been used extensively in bone research: X-ray tube µCT and synchrotron µCT. These two types of scanners differ in the nature of the C-ray source, availability, and imaging capabilities.

25.1.1 X-ray Tube Micro-Computed Tomography

X-ray tube µCT systems are so named because they use an X-ray tube to produce photons. They are generally known as "bench-top" µCT systems because of their comparatively small size. X-ray tubes are solid-state components and are based on mature, commercially available technology. This combination of size, reliability, and low maintenance makes X-ray tube µCT the most common µCT system for research applications. To a large extent, the performance of x-ray tube µCT scanners can be characterized with just a few parameters (▶ Table 25.1).

While X-ray tubes are compact and relatively inexpensive, one important drawback is that they produce only polychromatic X-rays. The emitted X-ray beam is thus subject to *beam hardening*, a phenomenon in which the photons of lower energy are preferentially absorbed as they pass through the specimen, resulting in a "harder" beam, or a beam of higher mean energy. Image artifacts created by beam hardening can confound measurements of mineral density and can also blur distinctions between high- and low-attenuating materials, thereby decreasing the effective spatial resolution. The negative effects of beam hardening can be reduced by placing an aluminum filter in front of the X-ray source to "preharden" the beam[1] and/or by applying a correction during image reconstruction based on empirically derived calibration data.[2]

X-ray tube µCT scanners specially designed for high-resolution imaging can achieve isotropic voxel sizes of side length ~2 µm, though most bench-top systems are limited to ~5 µm. The best achievable resolution, expressed in terms of voxel size, is typically in proportion to the specimen diameter. For medium- to high-attenuating materials such as bone, the signal-to-noise ratio is more than sufficient to discern the material from background noise. However, these systems cannot be used to distinguish among low attenuating materials, such as cartilage and many other soft tissues, without use of a contrast agent.

25.1.2 Synchrotron Micro-Computed Tomography

Synchrotron µCT systems produce photons from synchrotron particle accelerators, rather than X-ray tubes, and are thus not as widely available as X-ray tube systems. Synchrotron radiation has several advantages over radiation produced by an X-ray tube. First, the beam is monochromatic and is not subject to beam hardening. Second, the narrower spread of photon energy makes for improved signal-to-noise ratios, especially when imaging lower-attenuating materials. Third, the synchrotron can generate a parallel photon beam (whereas X-ray tube sources generate fan- or cone-shaped beams), which enables greater magnification and improved spatial resolution.

Synchrotron µCT systems can achieve submicron resolution. As with µCT systems using X-ray tubes, the best achievable resolution expressed in voxel size is proportional to specimen diameter. Further, the absence of beam-hardening artifacts allows accurate measurement of mineral density in bone tissue.[3]

25.2 Micro-Computed Tomography Imaging of Trabecular Bone

The first published reports of the use of µCT in bone research were studies of trabecular bone.[4,5] Prior to these reports, the gold standard for quantifying the microstructure of trabecular bone was to cut thin, serial sections of a specimen and to perform histomorphometric analyses of each section. µCT provided an alternative that is nondestructive, 3D, and, with the continued improvements in computing power, increasingly more time-efficient and less labor-intensive.

Critical to the validity of µCT analyses of trabecular microstructure are choices of several parameters involved in scanning and image processing. For scanning, the

Table 25.1 Parameters that Characterize the Performance of X-ray Tube Micro-Computed Tomography Scanners

Parameter	Description	Typical units
Tube (peak) voltage	The applied electrical potential across the X-ray tube. Tube voltage largely determines the mean energy of the photons created.	Kilovolts, kVp (where "p" stands for peak)
Tube current	The electrical current flowing through the X-ray tube. Tube current controls the quantity of photons generated.	Milliamps, mA
Exposure time	The amount of time the tube and detector are actively generating and collecting photons	Milliseconds, ms

parameters are the nominal resolution of the scan or, equivalently, the voxel size in the resulting image; the tube voltage and current; the integration time (the amount of time the detector is active for each projection); and the frame averaging (the number of times each projection is repeated). The chosen resolution should balance the need for accurate measurement of small features within the specimen with eight-fold increase in dataset size caused by doubling the resolution. For a feature such as a trabecula to be detected, the voxel size must be no greater than one half the thickness of the feature; however, in practice, the voxel size should be smaller, particularly for the purposes of quantitative analyses of microstructure and density. The appropriate tube voltage for bone specimens is typically toward the high end of the voltage range offered by bench-top µCT systems (20 to 100 kVp), because specimens of higher density and/or larger diameter require higher beam energies. The tube current, integration time, and frame averaging collectively determine the number of photons collected by the detector, which is generally proportional to the signal-to-noise ratio for the scan.

Regarding image processing, the key parameters are those that control the noise filtering and the threshold. Filtering is essential for noise reduction prior to calculation of the microstructural parameters. Filtering involves smoothing the spatial variation of grayvalues within a small neighborhood of voxels. A Gaussian filter is most commonly used. Selecting a correct threshold is crucial, because the threshold defines which voxels are considered to contain bone tissue (▶ Fig. 25.2). For trabecular bone, routine algorithms exist to identify an appropriate threshold for segmenting bone voxels from those containing marrow, other soft tissues, and background medium.[6,7] However, the binary images resulting from applying the threshold should always be examined in conjunction with the original, grayscale images to check on the suitability of the threshold. The aforementioned algorithms may not produce good segmentation of the microstructure for a given combination of voxel size and other scanning parameters. Moreover, use of a single value for the threshold (a global threshold) for the entire image and for every experimental group may not be feasible for a given study.

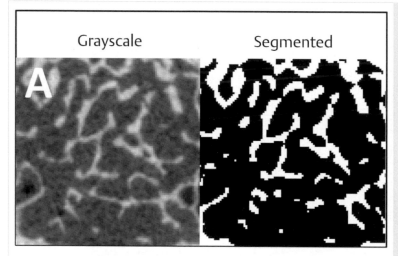

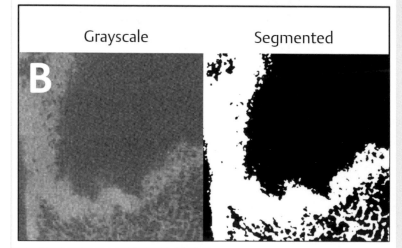

Fig. 25.2 Representative results of applying a global threshold to a micro-computed tomography image of (a) rabbit trabecular bone and (b) human vertebral end plate. In each case, a region of a two-dimensional cross-section of the three-dimensional grayscale micro-computed tomography image is shown on the *left*, and the binary image that results from applying the global threshold to segment bone tissue from marrow is shown on the *right*.

25.2.1 Trabecular Microstructure

A slate of common metrics describing the microstructure of trabecular bone now exits (▶ Table 25.2). *Bone volume* (BV) is defined as only the volume of the specimen (or the region of interest [ROI] within the specimen) that is occupied by bone. Commonly, BV is more meaningful when it is normalized by the *total volume* of the specimen (or ROI); the resulting metric, BV/total volume, is known as the *bone volume fraction*. The remaining metrics quantify the *trabecular architecture*, or the arrangement of BV in space. *Trabecular thickness* (Tb.Th*: The measures of trabecular thickness, separation, and number that are appended with an asterisk are determined directly from the 3D images of the trabecular structure without making any assumption about the type of structure. Traditional histomorphometric measurements [e.g., Tb.Th] assume a type of structure, such as rod-shaped or plate-shaped trabeculae, in order to calculate these architectural metrics.[9]) is the mean thickness of the individual trabeculae, while *trabecular separation* (Tb.Sp*) is the mean distance between trabeculae. *Trabecular number* (Tb.N*) is the average number of trabeculae per unit length for an arbitrary line through the volume. The *structure model index* (SMI) is a quantitative measure of how "rod-like" or "plate-like" the trabeculae are. The structure model index values typically range from 0 (plate-like) to 3 (rod-like) but can also include 4 (sphere-like) and negative values (trabeculae with concave surfaces that nearly enclose marrow pores).[10] *Connectivity density* is defined as the number of connections between trabeculae per unit volume. *Degree of anisotropy* (DA) describes the extent of preferential alignment of the trabeculae. A DA value greater than 1 indicates that a preferential alignment, or anisotropy, exists (consider, e.g., the primary compressive group in the femoral head). The minimum value of DA, 1, indicates no preferential orientation (i.e., isotropy). Importantly, DA quantifies the extent of the preferential alignment, not the direction of that alignment. However, the same calculations used to determine DA also identify the direction.

25.2.2 Tissue Mineral Density

In the absence of beam hardening, or at least with sufficient correction for beam-hardening artifacts, the grayvalues or values of linear attenuation contained in µCT images can be converted into values of mineral density. This conversion requires a standard curve that can be obtained from a scan of a calibration phantom—a set of standardized specimens of known mineral density. It is important to note that the resulting values of mineral density are not true density measures but rather estimates of the partial density (mass concentration) of a mineral solution that would have the same linear attenuation as the region of tissue imaged. For example, if the calibration phantom contains varying concentrations of hydroxyapatite, then the mineral densities obtained from conversion of the voxel grayvalues are in units of mass of hydroxyapatite per volume (e.g., mg hydroxyapatite/

Table 25.2 Parameters Used to Describe Trabecular Microstructure in Three Dimensions

Symbol	Variable	Description	Standard units
BV	Bone volume	Volume of region of interest above threshold	mm^3
TV	Total volume	Volume of entire region of interest	mm^3
BV/TV	Volume fraction	Ratio of segmented bone to total volume	-
Tb.Th*	Trabecular thickness	Mean thickness of trabeculae	mm
Tb.Sp*	Trabecular separation	Mean separation between trabeculae	mm
Tb.N*[1]	Trabecular number	Average number of trabeculae per unit length	mm^{-1}
SMI	Structure model index	Indicator of structure of trabeculae (rod-like or plate-like)	-
ConnD	Connectivity density	Connections in trabecular network per unit volume	mm^{-3}
DA	Degree of anisotropy	Measure of the extent of preferential alignment of trabeculae	-

[1] Tb.N* is coupled to Tb.Sp* in that Tb.N* is the inverse of the mean distance between trabeculae (Tb.Sp*), as determined by the sphere-fitting technique.[8]

cm^3). This conversion can be done for any collection of voxels in the image; however, a standard approach is to report the average mineral density for all voxels whose grayvalue exceeds the specified threshold. This average value is known as the *tissue mineral density* (TMD).

Values of TMD are sensitive to *partial-volume effects.* These effects arise from the discrete nature of the image data: Voxels at the surface of a trabecula, or any boundary between materials with different attenuation, are only partially filled with the higher attenuating material and therefore have a lower grayvalue than would be commensurate with the higher-attenuating material alone. A coarse image resolution will exacerbate partial-volume effects; however, these effects will always be present to some degree. Moreover, while partial-volume effects can degrade the accuracy of all measures of trabecular microstructure, they are more damaging to measurement of TMD. Many techniques used to measure TMD will account for partial-volume effects by "peeling" a set number of voxels away at any interface identified during segmentation. For trabecular bone, users should exercise caution, because if the image resolution is not sufficiently high, this peeling may leave too few trabeculae with meaningful volume left for calculation of TMD.

25.3 Micro-Computed Tomography Imaging of Cortex

In a manner similar to the analyses of trabecular architecture, µCT images can be used to measure the morphometry of the cortex in a region of the bone of interest. *Cortical volume* (Ct.V) and *cortical thickness* (Ct.Th) give the total volume and mean thickness, respectively, of the cortex (▶ Table 25.3). Area measurements include *total cross sectional area* (Tt.Ar), *marrow area* (Ma.Ar), and *cortical bone area* (Ct.Ar). The *moment of inertia* (I) of the cortex is a geometrical property that describes the structural resistance of the cortex to flexion about a given axis. The value of I depends on the axis—whether the anteroposterior, mediolateral, or other axis—so an efficient set of values to report consists of the maximum and minimum values along with the orientation of the axes that correspond to these values. The *polar moment of inertia* (J) is a geometric property that describes the structural resistance of the cortex to twisting.

25.4 Micro-Computed Tomography Imaging of Trabecular and Cortical Tissue

As discussed earlier, synchrotron µCT has the distinct advantage of providing accurate measurement of TMD, without any correction for beam hardening. This advantage, combined with the higher resolution that

synchrotron µCT typically affords as compared to bench-top µCT systems, enables detailed measurement of spatial variations in mineralization within small regions of cortical tissue and trabecular tissue.

Current synchrotron µCT systems and the most recent X-ray tube µCT systems also provide sufficient image resolution to quantify porosity in cortical and trabecular tissue, offering an alternative to 2D histomorphometric assessments of this parameter. From these analyses of porosity, values of *pore volume* (Po.V), *pore number* (Po.N), *cortical porosity* (Ct.Po, defined as Po.V/Ct.V), and *pore density* (Po.Dn, defined as Po.N/Ct.V) can all be obtained (▶ Table 25.3). Depending on the image resolution, one may be able to resolve haversian canals and, separately, Volkmann canals, resorption cavities, and lacunae (▶ Fig. 25.3).[11,12,13] For analyses of the haversian and Volkman canals, which together describe the morphology of the vascular system in bone, parameters such as *canal volume* (Ca.V), *canal volume fraction* (Ca.V/Ct.V), mean *canal diameter* (Ca.Dm), mean *canal separation* (Ca.Sp), and *canal number* (N.Ca) can be obtained in much the same manner as the measures of trabecular architecture.[13] Calculations of *degree of anisotropy* can be used to describe the preferential alignment of Volkmann and, predominantly, haversian canals.[14] These measurements may provide new insight into disease-related changes in bone tissue. For example, measures of intracortical canal network, including measures of the intraspecimen variation in parameters such as canal length, were recently found to aid in predictions of the flexural strength of the murine diaphysis.[13] Further, microcracks within cortical and trabecular tissue can be assessed via µCT scans at resolutions approaching 1 µm/voxel,[15,16] potentially providing greater statistical power in examining relationships among mechanical loading, damage, failure, and remodeling.

25.5 Micro-Computed Tomography Imaging to Assess the Phenotype of Murine Bones

A common application of the techniques previously described for trabecular and cortical bone is to identify the bone phenotype associated with a particular mutant mouse or a particular treatment in mice. A complete assessment of bone phenotype would include analyses of trabecular bone and cortical bone, each in both the axial and appendicular skeleton. The sites most commonly chosen for these analyses are the distal femoral metaphysis (trabecular), the femoral midshaft (cortical), and a lumbar vertebra (trabecular and cortical) (▶ Fig. 25.4).

At each of these sites, care must be taken to define a suitable and consistent ROI. In the case of long bones, the ROI should be chosen based on landmarks that are readily identifiable in all specimens in the study. For example, a suitable ROI in a vertebral body may span the distance, or

Table 25.3 Parameters Used to Describe Cortical Morphometry and Microstructure in Three Dimensions

Symbol	Variable	Description	Standard units
Ct.V	Cortical volume	Volume of cortical region of interest above threshold	mm³
Ct.Th	Cortical thickness	Mean thickness of cortical bone	mm
Po.V	Pore volume	Total volume of pores in cortical bone	mm³
Po.N	Pore number	Total number of pores in cortical bone	-
Ct.Po	Cortical porosity	Ratio of pore volume to total volume of cortical region	-
Po.Dn	Pore density	Ration of pore number to total volume of cortical region	mm³
I_{max}	Maximum moment of inertia	Maximum structural resistance of the cortex to flexion, considering all possible axes of flexion	mm⁴
I_{min}	Minimum moment of inertia	Minimum structural resistance of the cortex to flexion, considering all possible axes of flexion	mm⁴
I_{ap}	Anteroposterior moment of inertia	Structural resistance of the cortex to flexion about the anteroposterior axis	mm⁴
I_{mL}	Mediolateral moment of inertia	Structural resistance of the cortex to flexion about the mediolateral axis	mm⁴
J	Polar moment of inertia	Structural resistance of the cortex to twisting	mm⁴
Tt.Ar	Total cross-sectional area	Total cross-sectional area inside periosteal perimeter	mm²
Ma.Ar	Marrow area	Cross-sectional area inside periosteal perimeter below bone threshold	mm²
Ct.Ar	Cortical bone area	Cross-sectional area inside periosteal perimeter above bone threshold	mm²

a fraction of the distance, between physes or end plates. In the appendicular skeleton, a commonly chosen ROI begins at a small, fixed distance from the hypertrophic zone of the growth plate and traverses some fixed distance toward the metaphyseal-diaphyseal boundary. In cases where the bone length varies among groups, the length of the ROI for each group should be scaled to the median bone length of that group, to ensure that regions being analyzed are comparable anatomically and biomechanically. If scaling is not performed to compensate for differences in bone lengths, the ROIs will likely include a disproportionately large amount of bone for the smaller group.[17] Other methods exist to determine the ROI when analyzing trabecular architecture in other bones, such as the mandible.[18]

For analysis of trabecular bone in the metaphysis, the surrounding cortex must be excluded from the ROI. Similarly, for analysis of metaphyseal cortical bone, the trabecular compartment must be excluded. Both of these tasks can be carried out by defining the endocortical boundary, either manually or using automated techniques[20] (► Fig. 25.5).

One recent extension of the phenotypic assessment just described is to consider the overall shape of and variations in density and microstructure throughout the entire bone, rather than only the density and microstructure of individual regions. A challenge that arises immediately is the large increase in the number of parameters contained in the data set. Statistical shape modeling is a method of analyzing these large sets of data so as to allow

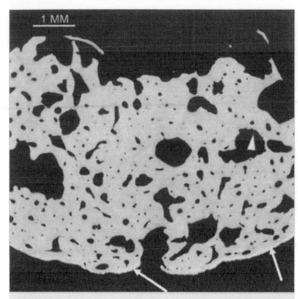

Fig. 25.3 Transverse cross-section of a micro-computed tomography image of cortical bone in the human femoral neck. Resorption cavities (*arrow*) and haversian canals are evident.[19]

quantitative description of complex shapes and property distributions with a reduced number of parameters. Statistical shape modeling analyses of human bones have been performed with several imaging modalities such as radiographs and magnetic resonance imaging that have lower resolution than μCT. Recently, statistical shape modeling using μCT images was demonstrated for describing developmental changes in bone shape in mice.[21]

25.6 In Vivo Micro-Computed Tomography Imaging

With the capacity to move beyond nondestructive imaging to noninvasive imaging, in vivo μCT systems offer unprecedented opportunities to examine longitudinal changes in bone density, bone microstructure, and bone shape. However, to reap the benefits of in vivo μCT, the investigator must consider some important limitations and challenges of this imaging method.

The first limitation is that the ionizing radiation delivered to the animal during the scan may confound the effects one is seeking to measure. Many biological functions, including those associated with bone development, homeostasis, and healing, are affected by radiation exposure. Moreover, the scan settings that are most desirable with respect to achieving high-quality μCT images of bone—high voltage and current, small voxel size, long integration times, and use of scan averaging—are also those that increase radiation exposure.

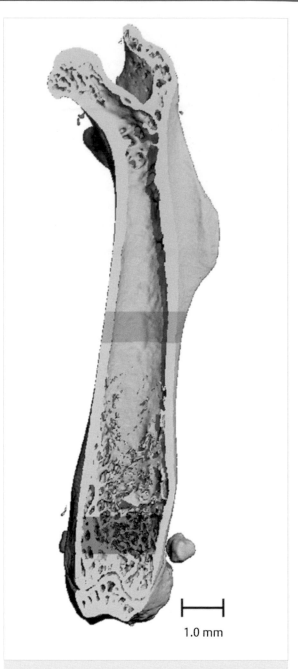

Fig. 25.4 Coronal, cut-away view of a micro-computed tomography rendering of a murine femur, showing two regions of interest commonly used for analyzing the bone phenotype. Shown in *green* is the segment of the middiaphysis used to examine the cortical phenotype; shown in *purple* is the segment of the trabecular compartment of the distal femoral metaphysis, which is commonly used to examine the trabecular phenotype.

The CT dose index and the multiple scan average dose are measures of the radiation absorption by the animal during a CT scan. Estimates of CT dose index and multiple

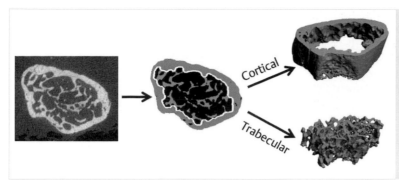

Fig. 25.5 Schematic of the process of separating the cortical shell from the trabecular compartment, for the purpose of analyzing these two regions separately. In a given transverse cross-section of the three-dimensional image, the endocortical boundary is defined. The region outside this boundary is analyzed as the cortical shell, whereas the region inside the boundary is analyzed as the trabecular compartment.

scan average dose are provided by the system manufacturers and are based on the energy and quantity of photons absorbed, as well as the geometry of the object being scanned.[22] Different organs and regions of the body have different sensitivities to radiation exposure. The extremities such as the tail and hind legs, for example, can safely absorb more radiation than the heart and brain. The precise effects of a given radiation dose on bone density and morphometry are often difficult to predict.

Given this uncertainty, early studies on use of in vivo µCT made major contributions by comparing changes in bone microstructure between limbs scanned repeatedly and contralateral limbs. These studies generally agreed that a small number (approximately four to seven) of weekly scans does not produce detectable, artifactual changes in bone mass or architecture.[23,24,25] However, given that deleterious effects on osteoblastic cells have been observed[26] at a radiation dose (4 Gy) that is approximately 5- to 10-fold higher than the dose per scan (~0.4 to 0.8 Gy[23,24,27]), continued consideration of the potential problems caused by radiation exposure in a given study design is warranted.

A second limitation of in vivo µCT scanning is the susceptibility of the images to movement-induced artifacts. The motions associated with heart rate and respiration will cause blurring and degrade final image quality, especially in the axial skeleton, and care must be taken to use a restraint system that minimizes movement of the regions to be scanned. Shortening the scan time can reduce the presence of movement artifacts; however, shorter scan times can compromise image resolution and overall image quality.

With respect to image analysis, a primary challenge for in vivo µCT scanning is ensuring comparisons across scans are performed on the same ROI. Even if the ROI is rigorously defined based on clearly identifiable landmarks, a misalignment of only several degrees between the position of the bone in one scan compared to another in the series can affect conclusions regarding temporal changes in microarchitecture or morphometry. This misalignment can be removed, or at least greatly reduced, by aligning, or registering, the 3D image sets with one another.

25.7 Biomechanical Analyses Using Micro-Computed Tomography

For many of the types of analyses presented previously, the information on bone density and microstructure gathered by µCT imaging can be used to develop hypotheses regarding the effects of the experimental conditions on biomechanical properties of the bones under study. For example, a loss of BV/total volume and decrease in Tb.Th* in a region of trabecular bone would suggest decreased stiffness and strength. Although testing such hypotheses is not possible with the µCT images alone, two methods that rely on µCT images, micro-finite element modeling (µFE) and image-guided failure analysis, can provide more direct biomechanical assessments.

25.7.1 Micro-Finite Element Modeling

Finite element analysis is a standard, widely used engineering method that estimates how a structure (such as a region of trabecular bone) behaves when it is subjected to external loads. An essential step in the finite element method is representing the object as a collection of a finite number of building blocks, or elements. Recognizing that CT images contain exactly this type of discretization, investigators began to create finite element models directly from quantitative CT images[28] and, subsequently, µCT images.[29] The latter models, µFE models, can represent the trabecular structure in fine detail and have been used extensively to estimate the stiffness and strength of regions of trabecular bone and whole bones, to estimate strains induced within trabecular tissue by applied loads (▶ Fig. 25.6), and to simulate bone remodeling in response to mechanical stimuli. Although µFE analyses of whole bones (e.g., vertebra, proximal femur) require high-end computational resources and custom software, µFE analyses of regions of trabecular bone or of small sections of whole bones, are very manageable for off-the-shelf, modern desktop computers and commercially available software.

However, there are some important limitations to µFE modeling. As with any finite element model, the accuracy and physiological relevance of the results depends strongly on the quality of the input. Errors resulting from discretization of the bone structure into elements, and the impact of decisions regarding the type of element, are inherent in any finite element analysis. These errors can be moderated by using higher-resolution scans and by preserving this high resolution when converting the voxels to finite elements; however, these steps will increase the complexity and computation time of the analysis. Also of concern is the accuracy of the material properties assigned to the elements and the accuracy of the loading that is applied in the analyses. The stiffness of the tissue represented by each element in the model is commonly assigned based on values in the literature, the local grayvalue, or measurements obtained from nanoindentation. Fewer data are available to use to assign values of strength and other postyield tissue properties to the elements, thus making µFE estimates of bone failure less standard and less well validated. Similarly, quantifying the accuracy of the applied loading is difficult, because of biological variation and other challenges associated with measuring joint contact forces and muscle forces in vivo.

25.7.2 Image-Guided Failure Analysis

Experimental approaches to studying the process of bone failure have been developed that use a series of µCT scans performed during the course of mechanical loading. These approaches grew out of a 2D technique that used contact radiography to image deformations of the microstructure of thin sections of trabecular bone as the sections were loaded.[31] The early 3D studies using µCT were in one of two categories. The first consisted of qualitative inspection of the time-lapsed series of µCT images to identify the region in which failure is first observable and to determine whether regional measures of the BV fraction and/or trabecular architecture can predict the regions of failure initiation (▶ Fig. 25.7).[16,30,32]

The second category of early studies in image-guided failure analysis focused on development of a quantitative method for analyzing the image series. This method is a 3D extension of digital image correlation, a standard, 2D method in experimental mechanics for quantifying local deformations on the surface of a specimen subjected to mechanical loading.[34] Briefly, this method can measure surface strains by tracking, via sequential digital images, the movement of surface features—such as paint speckles applied to the specimen surface—in response to the

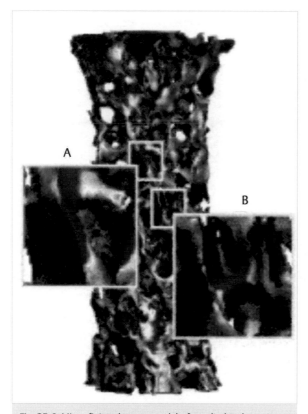

Fig. 25.6 Micro-finite element model of a cylindrical specimen trabecular bone, showing the estimated distribution of Von Mises stress developed under axial compressive loading of the specimen. High estimated Von Mises stress is observed in a longitudinal trabecula (*inset A*) and transverse trabecula (*inset B*).[30]

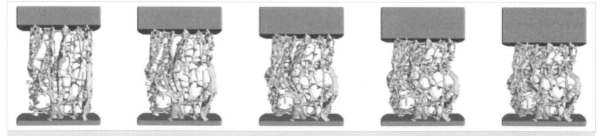

Fig. 25.7 Image-guided failure assessment of a small cylinder of human trabecular bone.[32] The series of time-lapsed micro-computed tomography images were captured at applied compressive strains of 0%, 4%, 8%, 12%, and 16% (*left to right*). Each rendering depicts the back half of the cylindrical specimen (i.e., the cut plane is the longitudinal midplane of the cylinder).

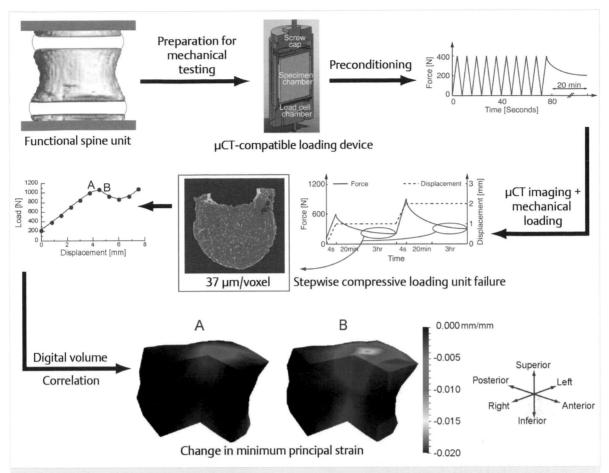

Fig. 25.8 Quantitative image-guided failure analysis of the human lumbar vertebra. Shown in this schematic is the experimental procedure for acquiring the series of micro-computed tomography (μCT) images during stepwise compressive loading of a functional spine unit, as well as a sampling of the results of digital volume correlation analyses applied to the image series (adapted from Hussein et al[33]). The contour plots shown of the digital volume correlation results (*bottom row*) represent the measured values of the change in minimum compressive strain during the increments labeled *A* and *B* on the load-displacement curve (*middle row, far left*). In these contour plots, the anterior-right quadrant of the vertebral body is removed to reveal strains measured in the interior of the vertebral body.

applied loading. For trabecular bone, the spatially heterogeneous microstructure naturally provides features to track, and μCT provides the images with which this tracking can be performed in 3D. The 3D method, known as digital volume correlation (DVC) or volumetric digital image correlation, has been applied to compression tests of cylindrical specimens of trabecular bone[31,35] and, more recently, entire vertebrae[33,36] (▶ Fig. 25.8).

As a purely experimental approach, DVC can provide an important complement to CT-based finite element models of bone. The DVC data on deformations created in regions of trabecular tissue or trabecular bone by the applied loads can be compared against the deformations predicted by μFE models or quantitative CT–based finite element models, respectively, to assess in great detail the accuracy of the models.

With many of the current μCT systems, DVC analyses of bone may be restricted to measurement of strains just prior to and following the yield point, because the strains in the preyield regime are not sufficiently large enough to be distinguished from measurement error.[31,37] It remains to be seen whether this restriction will be relaxed as a result of the higher image resolution afforded by newer-generation μCT systems.

25.8 Conclusion

In the present day, μCT imaging of bone is both a routine enterprise and an ever-evolving, applied technology. The main routine application is quantification of trabecular microstructure and cortical morphometry in specimens of human tissue and in animal models. Newer approaches that are pushing the envelope of image resolution and image processing are those that seek to quantify increasingly smaller-scale features of the microstructure and mineralization of cortical and trabecular tissue. However, even for the routine applications, µCT imaging of bone is not fully turn-key: Choices of parameters used for scanning and image processing can have major effects on the suitability of the results for addressing the research question at hand.

As a nondestructive, 3D imaging modality, µCT has a strong foothold in bone research with respect to the ability to allow integration of microstructural and anatomical assessments with assays of biological function and evaluations of mechanical behavior. For example, in vivo µCT imaging is a powerful technique for the study of bone adaptation, bone loss, and anabolic effects of pharmacological agents. Use of µCT to characterize the morphology of the vascular system and microcracks, particularly with respect to the spatial distributions of osteocyte lacunae and resorption cavities, can provide insights into bone-vascular interactions and bone remodeling. Finally, µFE modeling and image-guided failure analysis are clear illustrations of µCT-based approaches that move beyond mere morphological assessment to more direct evaluations of mechanical competence and mechanisms of failure. The diversity of uses of µCT in bone research is a testament to the utility of this imaging modality and an indicator that the spectrum of µCT-based approaches to studying bone will continue to grow.

25.9 Acknowledgments

Funding provided by National Institutes of Health (AR054620). The authors acknowledge the technical contributions of Benjamin Pritz.

References

[1] Meganck JA, Kozloff KM, Thornton MM, Broski SM, Goldstein SA. Beam hardening artifacts in micro-computed tomography scanning can be reduced by X-ray beam filtration and the resulting images can be used to accurately measure BMD. Bone 2009; 45: 1104–1116

[2] Burghardt AJ, Kazakia GJ, Laib A, Majumdar S. Quantitative assessment of bone tissue mineralization with polychromatic micro-computed tomography. Calcif Tissue Int 2008; 83: 129–138

[3] Nuzzo S, Peyrin F, Cloetens P, Baruchel J, Boivin G. Quantification of the degree of mineralization of bone in three dimensions using synchrotron radiation microtomography. Med Phys 2002; 29: 2672–2681

[4] Feldkamp LA, Goldstein SA, Parfitt AM, Jesion G, Kleerekoper M. The direct examination of three-dimensional bone architecture in vitro by computed tomography. J Bone Miner Res 1989; 4: 3–11

[5] Layton MW, Goldstein SA, Goulet RW, Feldkamp LA, Kubinski DJ, Bole GG. Examination of subchondral bone architecture in experimental osteoarthritis by microscopic computed axial tomography. Arthritis Rheum 1988; 31: 1400–1405

[6] Otsu N. A threshold selection method from gray-level histograms. Automatica 1975; 11: 23–27

[7] Ridler TW, Calvard S. Picture thresholding using an iterative selection method. IEEE Trans Syst Man Cybern 1978; 8: 630–632

[8] Hildebrand T, Rüegsegger P. A new method for the model-independent assessment of thickness in three-dimensional images. Journal of Microscopy 1997,185.67-75

[9] Hildebrand T, Laib A, Müller R, Dequeker J, Rüegsegger P. Direct three-dimensional morphometric analysis of human cancellous bone: microstructural data from spine, femur, iliac crest, and calcaneus. J Bone Miner Res 1999; 14: 1167–1174

[10] Hildebrand T, Rüegsegger P. Quantification of bone microarchitecture with the Structure Model Index. Comput Methods Biomech Biomed Engin 1997; 1: 15–23

[11] Cooper DM, Turinsky AL, Sensen CW, Hallgrímsson B. Quantitative 3D analysis of the canal network in cortical bone by micro-computed tomography. Anat Rec B New Anat 2003; 274: 169–179

[12] Hannah KM, Thomas CD, Clement JG, De Carlo F, Peele AG. Bimodal distribution of osteocyte lacunar size in the human femoral cortex as revealed by micro-CT. Bone 2010; 47: 866–871

[13] Schneider P, Voide R, Stampanoni M, Donahue LR, Müller R. The importance of the intracortical canal network for murine bone mechanics. Bone 2013; 53: 120–128

[14] Basillais A, Bensamoun S, Chappard C et al. Three-dimensional characterization of cortical bone microstructure by microcomputed tomography: validation with ultrasonic and microscopic measurements. J Orthop Sci 2007; 12: 141–148

[15] Larrue A, Rattner A, Peter ZA et al. Synchrotron radiation micro-CT at the micrometer scale for the analysis of the three-dimensional morphology of microcracks in human trabecular bone. PLoS ONE 2011; 6: e21297

[16] Voide R, Schneider P, Stauber M et al. Time-lapsed assessment of microcrack initiation and propagation in murine cortical bone at submicrometer resolution. Bone 2009; 45: 164–173

[17] Fajardo RJ, Müller R. Three-dimensional analysis of nonhuman primate trabecular architecture using micro-computed tomography. Am J Phys Anthropol 2001; 115: 327–336

[18] Moon HS, Won YY, Kim KD et al. The three-dimensional microstructure of the trabecular bone in the mandible. Surg Radiol Anat 2004; 26: 466–473

[19] Bousson V, Peyrin F, Bergot C, Hausard M, Sautet A, Laredo JD. Cortical bone in the human femoral neck: three-dimensional appearance and porosity using synchrotron radiation. J Bone Miner Res 2004; 19: 794–801

[20] Buie HR, Campbell GM, Klinck RJ, MacNeil JA, Boyd SK. Automatic segmentation of cortical and trabecular compartments based on a dual threshold technique for in vivo micro-CT bone analysis. Bone 2007; 41: 505–515

[21] Chan EF, Harjanto R, Asahara H et al. Structural and functional maturation of distal femoral cartilage and bone during postnatal development and growth in humans and mice. Orthop Clin North Am 2012; 43: 173–185, vv.

[22] Goldman LW. Principles of CT: radiation dose and image quality. J Nucl Med Technol 2007; 35: 213–225, quiz 226–228

[23] Brouwers JE, van Rietbergen B, Huiskes R. No effects of in vivo micro-CT radiation on structural parameters and bone marrow cells in proximal tibia of wistar rats detected after eight weekly scans. J Orthop Res 2007; 25: 1325–1332

[24] Klinck RJ, Campbell GM, Boyd SK. Radiation effects on bone architecture in mice and rats resulting from in vivo micro-computed tomography scanning. Med Eng Phys 2008; 30: 888–895

[25] Laperre K, Depypere M, van Gastel N et al. Development of micro-CT protocols for in vivo follow-up of mouse bone architecture without major radiation side effects. Bone 2011; 49: 613–622

[26] Dare A, Hachisu R, Yamaguchi A, Yokose S, Yoshiki S, Okano T. Effects of ionizing radiation on proliferation and differentiation of osteoblast-like cells. J Dent Res 1997; 76: 658–664

[27] Waarsing JH, Day JS, van der Linden JC et al. Detecting and tracking local changes in the tibiae of individual rats: a novel method to analyse longitudinal in vivo micro-CT data. Bone 2004; 34: 163–169

[28] Faulkner KG, Cann CE, Hasegawa BH. Effect of bone distribution on vertebral strength: assessment with patient-specific nonlinear finite element analysis. Radiology 1991; 179: 669–674

[29] van Rietbergen B, Weinans H, Huiskes R, Odgaard A. A new method to determine trabecular bone elastic properties and loading using micromechanical finite-element models. J Biomech 1995; 28: 69–81

[30] Nagaraja S, Couse TL, Guldberg RE. Trabecular bone microdamage and microstructural stresses under uniaxial compression. J Biomech 2005; 38: 707–716

[31] Bay BK. Texture correlation: a method for the measurement of detailed strain distributions within trabecular bone. J Orthop Res 1995; 13: 258–267

[32] Nazarian A, Müller R. Time-lapsed microstructural imaging of bone failure behavior. J Biomech 2004; 37: 55–65

[33] Hussein AI, Barbone PE, Morgan EF. Digital Volume Correlation for Study of the Mechanics of Whole Bones. Procedia IUTAM 2012; 4: 116–125

[34] Sutton MA, Wolters WJ, Peters WH, Ranson WF, McNeill SR. Determination of displacements using an improved digital correlation method. Image and Vision Computing 1983;3(1): 133–139

[35] Zauel R, Yeni YN, Bay BK, Dong XN, Fyhrie DP. Comparison of the linear finite element prediction of deformation and strain of human cancellous bone to 3D digital volume correlation measurements. J Biomech Eng 2006; 128: 1–6

[36] Hardisty MR, Whyne CM. Whole bone strain quantification by image registration: a validation study. J Biomech Eng 2009; 131: 064502

[37] Liu L, Morgan EF. Accuracy and precision of digital volume correlation in quantifying displacements and strains in trabecular bone. J Biomech 2007; 40: 3516–3520

Further Reading

Barrett JF, Keat N. Artifacts in CT: recognition and avoidance. Radiographics 2004; 24: 1679–1691

Bouxsein ML, Boyd SK, Christiansen BA, Guldberg RE, Jepsen KJ, Müller R. Guidelines for assessment of bone microstructure in rodents using micro-computed tomography. J Bone Miner Res 2010; 25: 1468–1486

Ritman EL. Micro-computed tomography-current status and developments. Annu Rev Biomed Eng 2004; 6: 185–208

26 Imaging Bone

Spencer Behr, Jeffrey Meier, and Thomas M. Link

Standard techniques for quantitative imaging of bone are dual energy X-ray absorptiometry (DXA) and quantitative computed tomography (QCT), these methods provide information on bone mineral density. Nuclear medicine techniques do not simply provide density information of bone but characterize bone metabolism; among these, positron emission tomography (PET) is a more novel technique. These technologies are currently used for both research and clinical applications.

26.1 Bone Densitometry

Bone densitometry can be used (1) to assess fracture risk based on the absolute or relative density of bone, (2) to provide recommendations on potential therapy, and (3) to monitor therapy. The most frequently measured sites include the proximal femur, the lumbar spine, and the distal radius, all sites that are also at risk for fragility fractures. Bone mineral density (BMD) is the single most important determinant of fracture, accounting for approximately 70% of bone strength. The lower the peak bone density at a young age, the higher the risk of fracture in later life. In addition to these indications, methods of measuring BMD are also relevant to the study of skeletal development and to diagnose osteopenia and osteoporosis. Most BMD measurement techniques are accurate, reproducible, and sensitive to small changes with time and to differences in patient

groups with high and low fracture risk; they are also inexpensive and involve minimal exposure to ionizing radiation.

26.1.1 Dual Energy X-Ray Absorptiometry

DXA measurements of BMD have been universally adopted as a standard to define osteoporosis and osteopenia. DXA uses two X-ray beams with differing kVp (30 to 50 keV and > 70 keV), which enables subtraction of the soft tissue component. DXA measures "areal" BMD (g/cm^2) typically of the lumbar spine (L1–L4), proximal femur (femoral neck and total), and distal radius (▸ Fig. 26.1). The accuracy of DXA is between 3% and 8%, with a precision better than 1% (coefficient of variation in percent) at the anterior-posterior spine and the total femur, and 1 to 2% at the femoral neck. Also radiation dose is low (1 to 6 micro Sievert (Sv) for BMD and up to 50 microSv if performed with vertebral fracture assessment).[1] In addition to areal density values in g/cm^2, DXA provides T-scores and Z-scores. Z-scores are standard deviations (SD) compared to an age-matched reference population, whereas T-scores are SD compared to a young adult, healthy reference population, matched for gender and ethnicity. In 1994, the World Health Organization (WHO)[2] established T-scores at the proximal femur, the lumbar spine, and the distal radius to classify and define

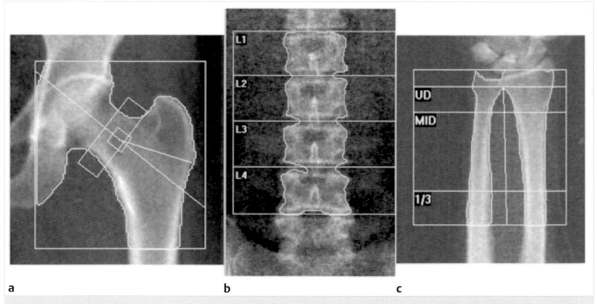

Fig. 26.1 Dual energy X-ray absorptiometry images of the proximal femur (**a**), lumbar spine (**b**), and distal radius (**c**) with regions of interest.

BMD measurements. According to the WHO, normal, osteopenic, and osteoporotic BMD are differentiated.

Normal: BMD above (≥) – 1 SD of the young adult reference mean (peak bone mass).

Osteopenia: BMD between (<) –1 and (>) –2.5 SD below that of the young adult reference mean.

Osteoporosis: BMD more than (≤) –2.5 SD below the young adult reference mean.

The WHO definition is *not applicable* to other bone densitometry techniques (QCT, quantitative ultrasound) or other anatomical sites (e.g., calcaneus). Whole-body DXA with regional analysis gives information not only on total and regional BMD but also on body composition (lean muscle mass and fat mass).

DXA has some limitations: (1) it measures density/area (in g/cm^2) of integral (cortical and trabecular) bone and not the volumetric density (in mg/cm^3) as is provided by QCT. That means areal BMD is dependent on bone size and will thus overestimate fracture risk in short individuals with small bones, who will have lower areal BMD than normal-sized individuals. (2) Spine and hip DXA are also sensitive to artifacts caused by degenerative changes, and individuals with significant degenerative disease will have falsely increased areal BMD, which will indicate a lower fracture risk than is actually present. Also all structures overlying the spine such as aortic calcifications, or morphological abnormalities of the vertebrae such as fractures (false elevation of BMD) or laminectomy (false reduction) will affect DXA BMD measurements.

26.1.2 Quantitative Computed Tomography

QCT provides a true volumetric density in mg/cm^3, rather than the "areal" density (mg/cm^2) of DXA. Using a calibration phantom, density values, measured in Hounsfield units, are transformed into BMD measured in mg hydroxyapatite/cm^3. Typically, the L1–L3 vertebral bodies are measured (▶ Fig. 26.2). In addition to the true volumetric measurements provided by QCT, the technique has several other important advantages over DXA. QCT can provide separate measures of cortical and trabecular BMD. Trabecular BMD is more sensitive to monitoring changes with disease and therapy, as trabecular bone is more metabolically active than cortical bone.[3] Cross-sectional studies have shown that QCT BMD of the spine allows better discrimination of individuals with and without vertebral fractures.[4,5] QCT is also better suited to examining obese patients as DXA makes assumptions about body composition and so has limitations in measuring BMD in patients with a body mass index over 25 kg/m^2.

Limitations of QCT are a higher radiation dose (0.06 to 2.9 mSv depending on whether lumbar spine or hip are scanned and whether single-slice or volumetric techniques are used)[1] and that the WHO T-score of −2.5 defining osteoporosis is not applicable to QCT. Currently, volumetric QCT techniques are preferred over single-slice techniques,[6,7,8,9] and in clinical practice absolute measurements of BMD have been defined to characterize

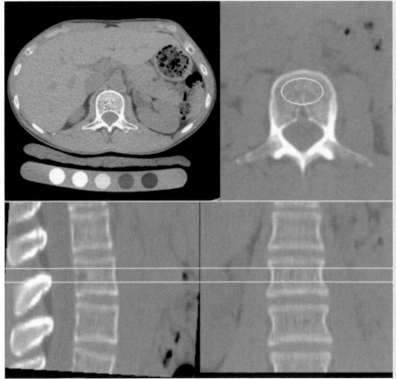

Fig. 26.2 Volumetric quantitative computed tomography of the L2 vertebral body with region of interest in the axial, coronal, and sagittal plane.

fracture risk: below 50 mg/cm³ = severe increase in fracture risk, 50 to 80 mg/cm³ = moderate increase in fracture risk, and 80 to 110 mg/cm³ = mild increase in fracture risk. According to the American College of Radiology Guidelines for QCT, a BMD range of 80 to 120 mg/cm³ is defined as osteopenic and values below 80 mg/cm³ as osteoporotic (*ACR Practice Guideline for the Performance of Quantitative Computed Tomography*, 2008).

26.1.3 Other Techniques

Other technologies available to quantitatively assess bone provide information on bone architecture such as high-resolution peripheral QCT (HR-pCT) and quantitative ultrasound. Recent meta-analyses confirmed that both DXA and calcaneal quantitative ultrasonography predict fractures in an older patient population but that the correlation between the two techniques is low.[10] The propagation of ultrasound waves through the bone is characterized by the velocity of transmission and the amplitude of the ultrasound signal.

Compared to multidetector-CT (MD-CT) and magnetic resonance imaging, HR-pCT has the advantage of significantly higher signal-to-noise ratio and spatial resolution (nominal isotropic voxel dimension of 82 μm)[11] (▶ Fig. 26.3). MD-CT has a maximum in plane spatial resolution of 250 to 300 μm and magnetic resonance imaging of 150 to 200 μm with slice thicknesses of 0.5 to 0.7 mm and 0.3 to 0.5 mm, respectively. Furthermore, the effective radiation dose for HR-pCT is substantially lower compared to whole-body MD-CT, and primarily does not

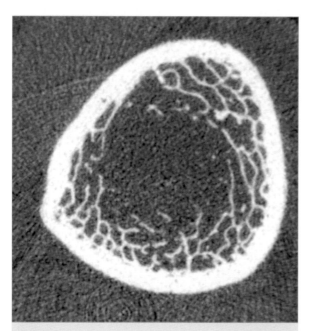

Fig. 26.3 High-resolution peripheral quantitative computed tomography image of the distal radius depicting trabecular and cortical bone structure.

involve critical, radiosensitive organs (effective dose < 3 microSv). The scan time for HR-pCT is long at approximately 3 minutes for each scan of the tibia and radius, so motion artifacts can be problematic. The disadvantage of HR-pCT is its limitation to peripheral skeletal sites thus not being able to provide direct insights into bone quality in the lumbar spine or proximal femur, which are common sites for osteoporotic insufficiency fractures.[11]

26.2 Nuclear Medicine Techniques

Historically, the imaging of bone with nuclear medicine has typically been reserved for the assessment of focal osseous abnormalities such as stress fractures, skeletal infections, and primary and secondary bone tumors, as well as to evaluate for response of these abnormalities to therapy. Several conventional nuclear medicine radiopharmaceuticals are available for such imaging bone, including technetium-99 m (99mTc)-labeled agents like diphosphonates (e.g., methylene diphosphonate), colloids, and sestamibi, gallium-67 citrate, thallium-201, and indium-111 oxine- or 99mTc hexamethlypropylene-amine oxime–labeled leukocytes, monoclonal antibodies, and polyclonal antibodies. With the expanding utilization of PET and PET/CT, radiotracers such as 18-fluorodeoxyglucose, which is taken up like glucose by cells and so demonstrates areas of increased metabolic activity, and fluorine-18 (18F)-fluoride, which binds to newly mineralizing bone and so reflects osteoblastic activity, are increasingly used to evaluate for the presence and response to therapy of primary and secondary bone tumors. This increased use of PET agents is due in part to the higher first pass extraction and greater bone uptake of 18F-fluoride relative to 99mTc–methylene diphosphonate (▶ Fig. 26.4) and the associated improved accuracy of 18-fluorodeoxyglucose and 18F-fluoride relative to conventional imaging.[12,13,14]

Imaging of osteoporosis represents a developing field of imaging within nuclear medicine. Hawkins et al[14] demonstrated that dynamic PET, using 18F-fluoride, can be used to determine bone plasma flow and plasma clearance, reflections of bone metabolism, and osteoblast activity.[15] Building on this work, recent studies have begun evaluating the use of 18F-fluoride in assessing for osteopenia and osteoporosis and bone formation in the treatment of osteoporosis. For example, studies using a nude rat model showed increased plasma clearance and movement of 18F-fluoride into bound bone in osteoporotic bone in rats with diets poor in calcium and vitamin D versus normal bone in control animals.[16] Another study using the same nude rat model demonstrated significantly reduced movement of 18F-fluoride into bound bone in rats with osteoporosis and receiving corticosteroids.[17] In humans, net uptake of 18F-fluoride into the

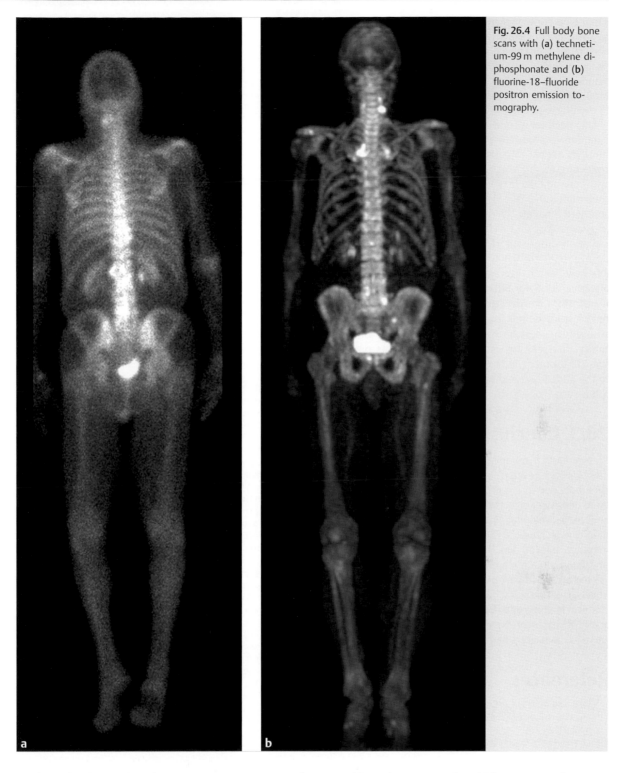

Fig. 26.4 Full body bone scans with (**a**) technetium-99 m methylene diphosphonate and (**b**) fluorine-18–fluoride positron emission tomography.

a

b

lumbar spine bone mineral compartment, a measure of bone formation, was found to be significantly lower in patients with osteoporosis than in normal controls and osteopenic patients.[18] Furthermore, plasma clearance of 18F-fluoride has been found to increase significantly in the bones of patients treated with teriparatide, a recombinant human parathyroid hormone used to treat osteoporosis, compared with patients not receiving that therapy.[19] Of note, another study evaluating changes in 18F-fluoride and 99mTc–methylene diphosphonate bone uptake and plasma clearance with teriparatide therapy showed that although plasma clearance (measured using serial blood draws) increases following teriparatide therapy, this did not translate into significantly changed lumbar spine standardized uptake values for 18F-fluoride.[20] As such, blood sampling—and not simply noninvasive standardized uptake value measurement—may be required to accurately assess for response of osteoporosis to therapy with 18F-fluoride.

This need for a somewhat invasive procedure to evaluate for response to therapy using 18F-fluoride may limit its appeal to patients, much as the complexity of collecting the information to calculate plasma clearance and bone uptake may limit its appeal to clinicians. Further limitations of 18F-fluoride relative to the current standard imaging for osteoporosis (i.e., DXA) include increased cost of 18F-fluoride PET and PET/CT, higher radiation dose with 18F-fluoride PET (i.e., an effective dose of 0.001 to 0.006 mSv for an average DXA versus 8.9 mSv for an average 18F-fluoride PET and higher effective doses for PET/CT), and more limited availability of 18F-fluoride PET than DXA.[21] What is more, a recent study demonstrated that abdominal CTs can also be used to assess for osteoporosis, providing an opportunity to screen for osteoporosis in patients obtaining the CTs for other indications without exposing patients to the added cost and radiation of a 18F-fluoride PET or other such study.[22]

26.3 Conclusion

In summary, a number of quantitative imaging techniques for bone research applications are available that can be subdivided into morphological technologies assessing bone density or structure such as DXA, QCT, and HR-pCT, and those studying bone metabolism such as nuclear medicine techniques. These technologies provide complementary information on normal and abnormal bone physiology. In a research environment, they may be used (1) to test the impact of new therapies on bone, such as novel drug therapies; (2) to study the effects of biomechanical loading; and (3) to analyze the evolution of metabolic diseases of bone and bone marrow. They may serve as biomarkers for bone strength and viability.

References

[1] Damilakis J, Adams JE, Guglielmi G, Link TM. Radiation exposure in X-ray-based imaging techniques used in osteoporosis. Eur Radiol 2010; 20: 2707–2714
[2] World Health Organization. Technical report: assessment of fracture risk and its application to screening for postmenopausal osteoporosis: a report of a WHO study group. Paper presented at: World Health Organization, Geneva, Switzerland,1994
[3] Black DM, Greenspan SL, Ensrud KE et al. PaTH Study Investigators.. The effects of parathyroid hormone and alendronate alone or in combination in postmenopausal osteoporosis. N Engl J Med 2003; 349: 1207–1215
[4] Bergot C, Laval-Jeantet AM, Hutchinson K, Dautraix I, Caulin F, Genant HK. A comparison of spinal quantitative computed tomography with dual energy X-ray absorptiometry in European women with vertebral and nonvertebral fractures. Calcif Tissue Int 2001; 68: 74–82
[5] Yu W, Glüer CC, Grampp S et al. Spinal bone mineral assessment in postmenopausal women: a comparison between dual X-ray absorptiometry and quantitative computed tomography. Osteoporos Int 1995; 5: 433–439
[6] Bousson V, Le Bras A, Roqueplan F et al. Volumetric quantitative computed tomography of the proximal femur: relationships linking geometric and densitometric variables to bone strength. Role for compact bone. Osteoporos Int 2006; 17: 855–864
[7] Farhat GN, Cauley JA, Matthews KA et al. Volumetric BMD and vascular calcification in middle-aged women: the Study of Women's Health Across the Nation. J Bone Miner Res 2006; 21: 1839–1846
[8] Farhat GN, Strotmeyer ES, Newman AB et al. Volumetric and areal bone mineral density measures are associated with cardiovascular disease in older men and women: the health, aging, and body composition study. Calcif Tissue Int 2006; 79: 102–111
[9] Lang TF, Li J, Harris ST, Genant HK. Assessment of vertebral bone mineral density using volumetric quantitative CT. J Comput Assist Tomogr 1999; 23: 130–137
[10] Nelson HD, Haney EM, Dana T, Bougatsos C, Chou R. Screening for osteoporosis: an update for the U.S. Preventive Services Task Force. Ann Intern Med 2010; 153: 99–111
[11] Krug R, Burghardt AJ, Majumdar S, Link TM. High-resolution imaging techniques for the assessment of osteoporosis. Radiol Clin North Am 2010; 48: 601–621
[12] Schirrmeister H, Glatting G, Hetzel J et al. Prospective evaluation of the clinical value of planar bone scans, SPECT, and (18)F-labeled NaF PET in newly diagnosed lung cancer. J Nucl Med 2001; 42: 1800–1804
[13] Yen RF, Chen CY, Cheng MF et al. The diagnostic and prognostic effectiveness of F-18 sodium fluoride PET-CT in detecting bone metastases for hepatocellular carcinoma patients. Nucl Med Commun 2010; 31: 637–645
[14] Hawkins RA, Choi Y, Huang SC et al. Evaluation of the skeletal kinetics of fluorine-18-fluoride ion with PET. J Nucl Med 1992; 33: 633–642
[15] Reeve J, Arlot M, Wootton R et al. Skeletal blood flow, iliac histomorphometry, and strontium kinetics in osteoporosis: a relationship between blood flow and corrected apposition rate. J Clin Endocrinol Metab 1988; 66: 1124–1131
[16] Cheng C, Alt V, Dimitrakopoulou-Strauss A et al. Evaluation of new bone formation in normal and osteoporotic rats with a 3-mm femur defect: functional assessment with dynamic PET-CT (dPET-CT) using 2-deoxy-2-[(18)F]fluoro-D-glucose (18)F-FDG) and (18)F-fluoride. Mol Imaging Biol 2013; 15: 336–344
[17] Cheng C, Heiss C, Dimitrakopoulou-Strauss A et al. Evaluation of bone remodeling with (18)F-fluoride and correlation with the glucose metabolism measured by (18)F-FDG in lumbar spine with time in an experimental nude rat model with osteoporosis using dynamic PET-CT. Am J Nucl Med Mol Imaging 2013; 3: 118–128
[18] Frost ML, Fogelman I, Blake GM, Marsden PK, Cook G Jr. Dissociation between global markers of bone formation and direct measurement of spinal bone formation in osteoporosis. J Bone Miner Res 2004; 19: 1797–1804
[19] Frost ML, Moore AE, Siddique M et al. 18F-fluoride PET as a noninvasive imaging biomarker for determining treatment efficacy of bone active agents at the hip: a prospective, randomized, controlled clinical study. J Bone Miner Res 2013; 28: 1337–1347
[20] Blake GM, Siddique M, Frost ML, Moore AE, Fogelman I. Radionuclide studies of bone metabolism: do bone uptake and bone plasma clearance provide equivalent measurements of bone turnover? Bone 2011; 49: 537–542
[21] Segall G, Delbeke D, Stabin MG et al.. SNM practice guideline for sodium 18F-fluoride PET/CT bone scans 1.0. J Nucl Med 2010; 51: 1813–1820
[22] Pickhardt PJ, Pooler BD, Lauder T, del Rio AM, Bruce RJ, Binkley N. Opportunistic screening for osteoporosis using abdominal computed tomography scans obtained for other indications. Ann Intern Med 2013; 158: 588–595

27 Ultrasound Techniques for Imaging Bone

Thomas J. MacGillivray and Erin Ross

Fracture recovery is currently assessed using a combination of physical assessment and X-ray.[1] The limitations of this approach are a long-held concern by clinicians because both methods are subject to interobserver variability.[2,3] In addition, signs of fracture healing are not normally visible on radiographs until after 6 to 8 weeks, when the forming fracture callus has become sufficiently dense with calcium to be visible.[4] Earlier signs of the healing process cannot be detected by X-ray, which means if complications occur in the healing process, these may go undetected for weeks or months. This prolongs rehabilitation times, causes further distress to the patient, and is ultimately costly. Furthermore, the amount of callus observed using this traditional imaging modality does not correlate well with the true state of healing or the clinical assessment of bony union.[5] As a final point, X-ray yields a two-dimensional (2D) projection image and so three-dimensional (3D) information regarding surface, volume, and depth is inherently difficult to perceive.

27.1 Overview of Three-Dimensional Freehand Ultrasound

Ultrasound as an imaging modality for monitoring fracture healing and repair can reveal details about the initial stages of healing from 1 to 2 weeks postfracture and enable earlier detection of complications.[6] Soft tissue and bone are imaged simultaneously, which allows surrounding tissue damage to be examined along with the hematoma that forms at the first stage of fracture repair.[7]

3D ultrasound is yet more advantageous than conventional 2D ultrasound because it can provide effective 3D views of the anatomy that enhance interpretation and aid diagnosis. This is of particular relevance to monitoring fracture healing and bone repair where 3D details of callus formation are of considerable interest. The last 15 years have seen the emergence of 3D freehand ultrasound as a viable technique for medical imaging,[8,9,10] though its potential for monitoring fracture healing remains largely undiscovered.[11]

A six-degree-of-freedom position sensing device is easily attached to the transducer of a conventional diagnostic ultrasound machine.[8] As the probe is moved over the object of interest, its position and orientation in space are then recorded along with the 2D ultrasound images (B-scans) to form an irregularly sampled 3D dataset describing the scan volume. Slices through this scan volume can be extracted, yielding views that would be inaccessible with conventional 2D ultrasound.

From these irregularly distributed B-scans and their positions, a regular 3D lattice volume can be reconstructed, similar to computed tomography (CT) and magnetic resonance (MR) imaging. This allows the application of 3D image postprocessing algorithms such as object segmentation, surface rendering, and volumetric registration. Further quantitative analysis of object parameters such as length, area, perimeter, and volume is also possible.

27.1.1 Position Sensing

Two types of tracking system are commonly used: electromagnetic and optical. Electromagnetic tracking comprises a transmitter that generates a magnetic field and a sensor that is attached to the probe.[12] There are two technologies for electromagnetic tracking; direct current systems use pulsed direct current to build up electromagnetic fields, whereas alternating current systems are based on alternating magnetic fields. Electromagnetic position sensors can achieve an accuracy of up to ± 0.5 mm in location and ± 0.7 degrees in orientation for the position sensor alone. However, direct current systems are sensitive to the close proximity of ferromagnetic

Table 27.1 Time from Fracture to the First Signs of Callus Formation Imaged by Three-Dimensional Freehand Ultrasound and by X-ray. Also Shown is a Description of the Nature of Bone Repair and the Time from Fracture to First Three-Dimensional Ultrasound Scan

Patient	Age (years)	Bone repair	First three-dimensional ultrasound scan (weeks)	Callus first visible	
				Three-dimensional ultrasound (weeks)	X-ray (weeks)
1	30	Tibial fracture	6	6	19
2	17	Tibial fracture	2	2	7
3	26	Tibial fracture	3	3	8
4	38	Femoral fracture	8	8	8
5	33	Lengthening	4	4	4

materials, whereas alternating current systems are affected by metal because of the induced current within. In addition, attaching a position sensor to an ultrasound probe will also introduce interference and increase susceptibility to error.[13]

As an alternative, optical tracking is not only immune to distortions caused by ferromagnetic or metal objects and interference, it has a greater accuracy and precision than electromagnetic tracking devices (± 0.2 mm for the position sensor alone).[9] Optical tracking consists of an infrared position sensor mounted on a tripod and a tracking tool attached to the ultrasound probe. The position sensor detects infrared light emitted from several light-emitting diode markers on the tracking tool and calculates the position and orientation based on the information received from those markers, though only when there is a clear line-of-sight between the tracking tool and the position sensor.

Regardless of the tracking implemented, freehand scanning works by combining 2D B-scan images from the ultrasound machine with transducer positional information from the tracking system using dedicated software (STRADWIN, Cambridge University, Cambridge, UK) on an additional computer to compute 3D ultrasound images in near real-time.

27.1.2 Image Data Transfer

Image data transfer takes place by recording radiofrequency ultrasound signals live from the ultrasound scanner. For example, using a Gage Compuscope 14200 14-bit digitizer (Cambridgeshire, UK), the analogue radiofrequency signals can be digitized after receive-focusing and time-gain compensation but before log-compression and envelope detection. Whole frames are then stored in on-board Gage memory before transferring to computer memory at 200 MB/s. Such an arrangement can operate in real-time with acquisition rates of approximately 30 frames per second and sampling at 66.67 MHz synchronous with the ultrasound machine's internal clock. The STRADWIN software can convert the radiofrequency data to a displayable B-scan format.

27.1.3 Calibration

A 3D freehand system must be calibrated prior to use, and this is a two-step process.[10] Firstly, the delay between acquired B-mode scans from the ultrasound machine and incoming positions from the optical tracking system must be calculated. Secondly, the coordinate transformation from the ultrasound scan plane to the infrared camera of the tracking system should be determined. After calibration, pixel coordinates in any recorded B-scan image are transformed into 3D space with typical error of less than ± 0.25 mm.

27.1.4 Three-Dimensional Image Interpretation

A single 3D freehand ultrasound scan can contain anywhere between 200 and 500 2D images. Views of a fracture not achievable with conventional 2D ultrasound can be obtained by "re-slicing" the 3D dataset (in a manner similar to MR or CT imaging) and examining for signs of healing such as hematoma and callus formation. 3D computer models of the fracture site are constructed by manually segmenting different soft tissues, callus deposits, bone fragments, and sections of healthy bone. Information on the progression of fracture healing from 3D ultrasound is attained by repeating the process temporally.

27.2 Imaging Fracture and Bone Repair

3D freehand scanning retains all the flexibility and freedom of movement associated with conventional ultrasound scanning but with the added ability to reconstruct 3D datasets of the volume of interest. The modality is well suited to monitoring fracture healing and bone repair, particularly in closed fracture to one of the long bones of the lower limb and in limb lengthening. Patients treated conservatively using a plaster cast have to be excluded as this would entail a "window" being cut in the cast to allow ultrasound scanning.

27.2.1 Three-Dimensional Freehand Scanning

3D freehand ultrasound scanning is, in our experience,[11] tolerated well by patients despite some initial reservations that the contact pressure exerted by the probe on the skin surface over the fracture site might cause discomfort. It takes on average 15 minutes to position a patient and complete freehand ultrasound scanning. Time required to interpret 3D ultrasound image data is largely dependent on the ease of identification of different soft tissues, callus, and bone, and typically requires about 60 minutes to complete per scan.

Time spent segmenting scans to create 3D computer models is a restricting factor of 3D freehand ultrasound. However, recent developments in computational postprocessing techniques, such as the automatic detection of bone surfaces,[14] speed up analysis by allowing the operator to concentrate on segmenting callus material and soft tissue damage. This in turn increases the viability of 3D freehand ultrasound as a clinically useful tool.

One of the key advantages of freehand ultrasound is that the position-sensing equipment can be transferred between scanners and probes, and so existing ultrasound machines could easily be upgraded to 3D and utilized more comprehensively for musculoskeletal examinations.

In addition, multiple freehand sweeps, stitched together in postprocessing, allow the imaging of complex fracture sites. 3D freehand ultrasound is a flexible and portable imaging tool that can be brought to the bedside, clinic, or theater, and is well suited to scanning elderly people as well as frail patients and children. It is also important to note that there are no restrictions for people with pacemakers or metal implants/fixators, and frequent repeat scanning is possible as there is no dose of ionizing radiation.

27.2.2 Comparing to X-ray

Two X-ray views are routinely required (anteroposterior and lateral) to image a fracture sufficiently when a patient attends the clinic. The clinician interprets the X-rays for the appearance of the fracture line and the amount and location of callus. However, even with these two orthogonal views, the shape and appearance of the fracture is subject to interobserver variability.[3] The projection nature of X-ray means that 3D surface and depth detail such as the shape of the fracture line and the location of bone fragments are difficult to perceive with this traditional modality.

3D freehand ultrasound images both the nature of the fracture pattern and the location of callus in 3D. Fibrous material forming within the gap to stabilize the fracture is identifiable along with developing periosteal callus. Such material is not visible on X-ray. Also, 3D computer models constructed from 3D ultrasound provide a means of visualizing and monitoring the progression of healing temporally.

To assess the performance of 3D freehand ultrasound, we compared information on the progression of fracture healing obtained with this modality to the clinical interpretation of X-rays (see Table 27.1). We followed a small group of patients ($n = 6$) from their first attendance at the outpatients fracture clinic at the Royal Infirmary of Edinburgh up until their consultant deemed that their fracture had united or until the occurrence of any complications had been identified. Three patients had sustained tibial fractures that were stabilized using an intramedullary nail, one had a fractured femur that was stabilized using a unilateral external fixation device, and the remaining two were undergoing tibial lengthening (one through the use of an Ilizarov frame and the other with an internal lengthening nail).

It is important to note that X-rays were not used as an aid to interpreting 3D ultrasound but were compared to the results of ultrasound scanning once the 3D data had been analyzed. The time at which the first signs of callus formation became visible was noted for each modality. Images acquired via both modalities were also assessed in a qualitative manner with particular focus given to the presence, location, and progression of healing.

27.3 Tibial Fracture

In three patients with tibial fractures, callus formation was detectable with 3D freehand ultrasound 5 to 13 weeks before X-ray. The fibrous deposits, which are the initial foundations for the callus, are observable forming between the ends of the broken bone with 3D ultrasound but not with X-ray. ▶ Fig. 27.1 shows a "re-sliced" view of the fracture site at 2 weeks postfracture from one of the patients. This view reveals a faint outline in the

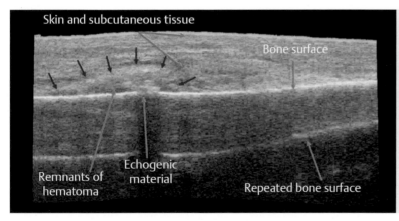

Fig. 27.1 View obtained by "re-slicing" a three-dimensional ultrasound scan of patient 2 at 2 weeks postfracture. The *red arrows* indicate the location of the hematoma before it was reabsorbed. The "repeated bone surface" artifact appears under normal, healthy bone and is caused by this hard reflecting surface. It does not appear under the fracture site as the lower density of the forming callus allows for some transmission of ultrasound.

surrounding soft tissues that indicates the location of the hematoma that had formed after fracture and before it was reabsorbed. Such soft tissue detail is unobtainable under X-ray.

For another patient, the 3D computer models constructed from freehand ultrasound scans (see ► Fig. 27.2) show the spiral nature of the fracture far more clearly than X-ray (see ► Fig. 27.3). The series of 3D computer models constructed for the third patient and shown in ► Fig. 27.4 chart the growth and progression of the fracture callus. At 17 weeks, the fracture callus as viewed on 3D ultrasound completely bridges the break, whereas on the corresponding X-rays (see ► Fig. 27.5) the fracture gap is still clearly visible with only a small region of bridging callus present on the medial side.

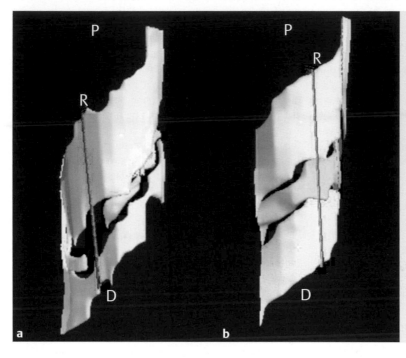

Fig. 27.2 Three-dimensional models of a tibial fracture at (a) 6 weeks and (b) 19 weeks postfracture reconstructed from three-dimensional ultrasound scans of patient 1. The spiral nature of the break can clearly be seen, and the increase in clearly identifiable forming callus (*yellow*) is also notable. D, distal; P, proximal.

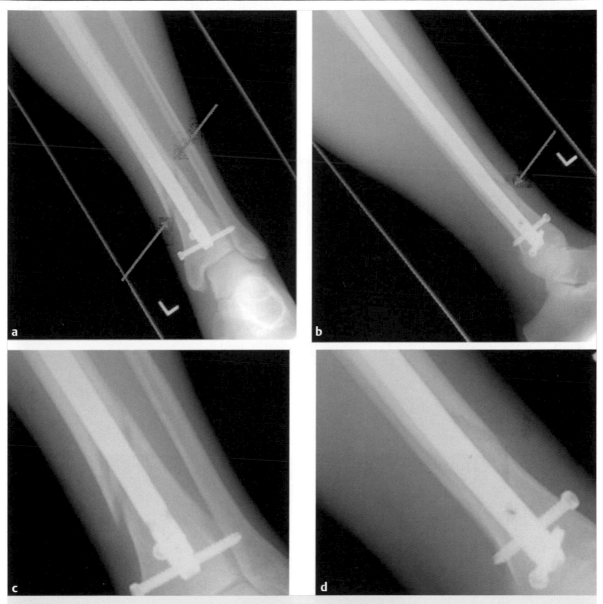

Fig. 27.3 (a–d) Lateral and anteroposterior X-rays of the tibial fracture experienced by patient 1 and taken at 2 weeks postfracture. The location of the fracture is indicated by the arrows.

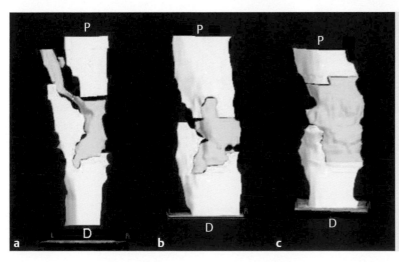

Fig. 27.4 Three-dimensional computer models for patient 3 constructed from three-dimensional ultrasound scans at (a) 3 weeks, (b) 8 weeks, and (c) 17 weeks postfracture. D, distal; P, proximal. Healthy, normal bone (*white*) and regions of clearly identifiable callus (*yellow*) have also been included in the models.

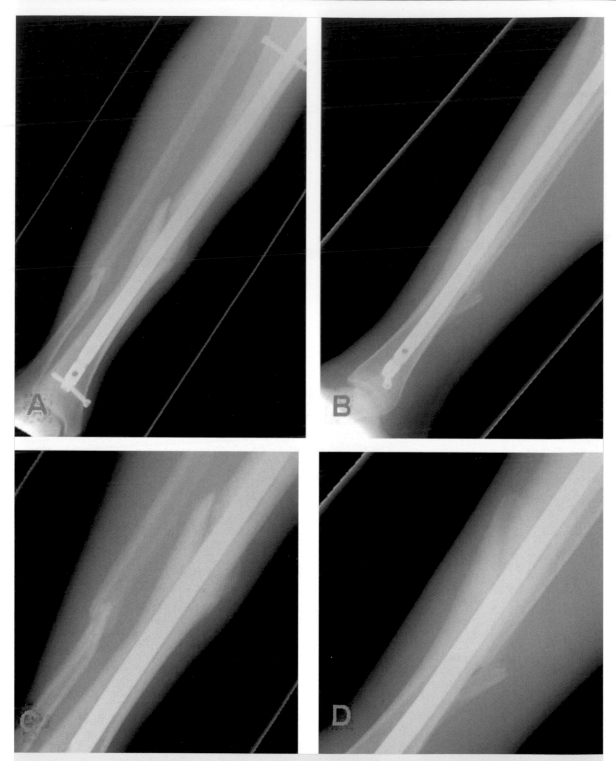

Fig. 27.5 (a–d) Lateral and anteroposterior X-rays at 17 weeks postfracture for patient 3. The fracture line remains well defined, and only small regions of callus are visible.

27.4 Femoral Fracture Case

The healing process was well under way for our femoral fracture patient when the first 3D ultrasound scans were obtained. Thus callus was detectable on both imaging modalities at the same time. However, the amount of callus visible with freehand 3D ultrasound is more substantial than with X-ray. 3D ultrasound also allows changes in the appearance of callus to be monitored as healing progresses. Comparing the 3D ultrasound scans temporally revealed that callus appeared more extensive at 44 weeks and had greater grayscale intensity than at 28 weeks. This is illustrated in ▶ Fig. 27.6.

27.5 Limb Lengthening Cases

For a patient who was undergoing lengthening using an Ilizarov frame, 3D freehand ultrasound allowed callus formation to be monitored in relation to the rate of lengthening. We observed a lag between the amounts of callus visible on X-ray compared to 3D ultrasound. Although, as periosteal callus forming on the bone ends matured, it became difficult to accurately determine the location of the original bone ends using 3D ultrasound and between which the amount of length gained was measured.

Complications were identified by 3D ultrasound for a patient who was undergoing tibial lengthening using an

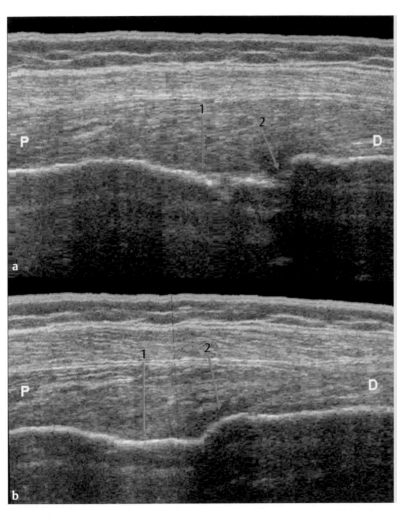

Fig. 27.6 Views obtained by "re-slicing" three-dimensional ultrasound scans of patient 4 at (a) 28 weeks and (b) 44 weeks postfracture. Each "slice" is through the middle of the anterior face of the femur. There is a clear change in appearance of the callus, particularly at regions 1 and 2 as indicated on both images. D, distal; P, proximal.

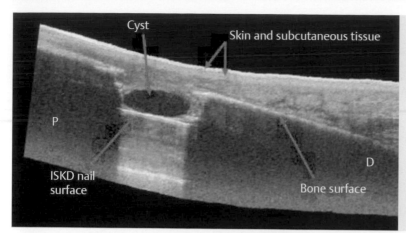

Fig. 27.7 View obtained by "re-slicing" three-dimensional ultrasound scan of patient 6 that shows the location of the cyst within the lengthening gap. D, distal; ISKD, intramedullary skeletal kinetic distractor; P, proximal.

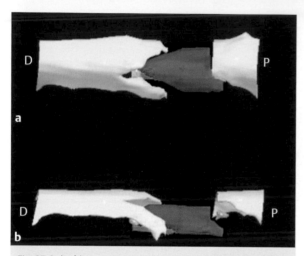

Fig. 27.8 (a, b) Two views of the three-dimensional computer model constructed from the ultrasound scans of patient 6. The cyst (*red*) and small areas of callus (*yellow*) have been identified along with the surface of the lengthening nail (*blue*). D, distal; P, proximal.

internal nail device. ▶ Fig. 27.7 shows an image obtained by "re-slicing" through the 3D ultrasound scan, and this reveals a cyst that can be seen within the lengthening gap and residing on the surface of the nail. The full extent of the cyst (shown in *red* in ▶ Fig. 27.8) can be seen from two views of the corresponding 3D computer model. A volume of 1.05 mL for the cyst was measured using 3D ultrasound. Small areas of callus growth are detected at the edges of the lengthening gap (*yellow*), and the patient's normal, healthy bone is also marked (*white*). Further, it is also possible to identify the surface of the nail beneath the cyst (*blue*). On the corresponding X-ray, there were no obvious signs of complications; however, new bone growth was noted to be occurring slower than expected. The identification of the cyst by 3D ultrasound led to interventional treatment by the consultant. Without 3D ultrasound, it would have been several more weeks before this patient was sent for a conventional 2D ultrasound scan to check for cysts or other complications.

27.6 Conclusion

3D freehand ultrasound is an effective imaging technique for monitoring fracture healing. Such a system typically consists of a standard clinical ultrasound machine and an optical tracking device, both of which are relatively inexpensive compared to the cost of other medical imaging devices. 3D ultrasound scans can be "re-sliced" to provide unique views of the anatomy not offered by conventional 2D ultrasound or X-ray, and segmented to produce 3D computer models for clinical evaluation. 3D freehand ultrasound has the potential to provide extra information compared to X-ray by revealing more detail about the progression of healing and allow earlier detection of complications. A role exists for 3D freehand ultrasound alongside X-ray for monitoring the bone repair process and identifying problematic healing. Finally, the technique has additional applications such as monitoring joint swelling and tumor size.

References

[1] McRae R. Pocket book of orthopaedics & fracture. 2 e. Edinburgh: Churchill Livingstone; 2006

[2] Bhandari M, Guyatt GH, Swiontkowski MF, Tornetta P III Sprague S, Schemitsch EH. A lack of consensus in the assessment of fracture healing among orthopaedic surgeons. J Orthop Trauma 2002; 16: 562–566

[3] Whelan DB, Bhandari M, McKee MD et al. Interobserver and intraobserver variation in the assessment of the healing of tibial fractures after intramedullary fixation. J Bone Joint Surg Br 2002; 84: 15–18

[4] Hamblen D, Simpson A. Outline of fractures. 12 e. Edinburgh: Churchill Livingstone; 2007

[5] Siegel IM, Anast GT, Fields T. The determination of fracture healing by measurement of sound velocity across the fracture site. Surg Gynecol Obstet 1958; 107: 327–332

[6] Young JW, Kostrubiak IS, Resnik CS, Paley D. Sonographic evaluation of bone production at the distraction site in Ilizarov limb-lengthening procedures. AJR Am J Roentgenol 1990; 154: 125–128

[7] Craig JG, Jacobson JA, Moed BR. Ultrasound of fracture and bone healing. Radiol Clin North Am 1999; 37: 737–751, ix

[8] Prager R, Gee A, Berman L. Stradx: Real-time acquisition and visualisation of freehand 3D ultrasound. Cambridge University Engineering Department Technical Report. 1998

[9] Treece GM, Gee AH, Prager RW, Cash CJC, Berman LH. High-definition freehand 3-D ultrasound. Ultrasound Med Biol 2003; 29: 529–546

[10] Hsu PW, Prager RW, Gee AH, Treece GM. Rapid, easy and reliable calibration for freehand 3D ultrasound. Ultrasound Med Biol 2006; 32: 823–835

[11] Ross E. Freehand 3D Ultrasound for imaging components of the musculoskeletal system. PhD thesis, University of Edinburgh, 2009

[12] Weller R, Pfau T, Ferrari M, Griffith R, Bradford T, Wilson A. The determination of muscle volume with a freehand 3D ultrasonography system. Ultrasound Med Biol 2007; 33: 402–407

[13] Hastenteufel M, Vetter M, Meinzer HP, Wolf I. Effect of 3D ultrasound probes on the accuracy of electromagnetic tracking systems. Ultrasound Med Biol 2006; 32: 1359–1368

[14] Hacihaliloglu I, Abugharbieh R, Hodgson AJ, Rohling RN, Guy P. Automatic bone localization and fracture detection from volumetric ultrasound images using 3-D local phase features. Ultrasound Med Biol 2012; 38: 128–144

Further Reading

Fenster A, Downey DB, Cardinal HN. Three-dimensional ultrasound imaging. Phys Med Biol 2001; 46: R67–R99

Hoskins P, MacGillivray T. 3D ultrasound. In Diagnostic ultrasound: physics and equipment. 2 e. Cambridge: Cambridge University Press; 2010: 171-181

MacGillivray TJ, Ross E, Simpson HA, Greig CA. 3D freehand ultrasound for in vivo determination of human skeletal muscle volume. Ultrasound Med Biol 2009; 35: 928–935

28 In Vivo Scanning

Scott Ian Kay Semple

Magnetic resonance imaging (MRI) is an ideal tool for investigation of the musculoskeletal system and of cartilage in particular. Since MRI was introduced into the clinical environment 30 years ago, constant advances have been made to continually improve hardware and software relating to both acquisition and analysis of MRI data.

MRI is an exceptionally versatile tool for clinical imaging. Through selection and manipulation of the various acquisition parameters available, the MRI user is able to obtain a range of different soft tissue contrast data noninvasively and investigate a range of physiological processes influenced by the biochemical structure of tissues. Although MRI may be used as a whole-body imaging modality, individual purpose built "coils" are used to focus data acquisition on individual body areas. A range of coils is available for most clinical imaging systems (head coil, spine coil, knee coil, cardiac coil). Each of these is designed both in shape and function for use on a particular body area.

The fundamental principle of MRI is that when a proton is placed in a strong magnetic field and then "excited" through the application of an applied radiofrequency pulse, the proton will oscillate at a resonant frequency proportional to the type of proton and the magnetic field strength. MRI soft tissue contrast relies on intrinsic magnetic relaxation properties of each tissue type (such as the nuclear relaxation times T1, T2, T2*, etc.) to generate image contrast between tissues within the MRI. By varying the MRI acquisition parameters, different intrinsic tissue processes can be made to form the dominant contrast within the resulting image (see ▶ Fig. 28.1a,b). It is also possible to directly measure several of these intrinsic

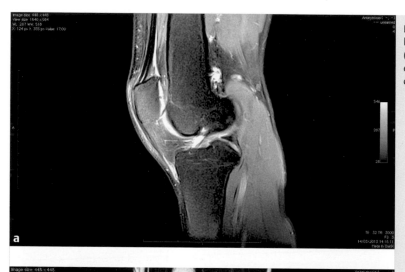

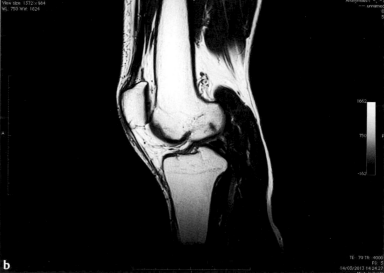

Fig. 28.1 (a) Proton density–weighted turbo spin echo sagittal acquisition of the knee (acquired at 3T). (b) T2-weighted turbo spin echo sagittal acquisition of the knee (acquired at 3T).

magnetic tissue properties through specific MRI acquisition analysis. Calculation and mapping of these properties allows quantitative diagnostic and intervention/therapy response measurements to be made.

This chapter attempts to summarize some of the current research MRI tools that are available for assessment of cartilage in vivo.

28.1 Magnetic Relaxation Times

Magnetic relaxation times (T1, T2, etc.) govern the processes that dictate the decay of MRI signal amplitude during an MRI acquisition and can be exploited to manipulate the tissue contrast in the resulting image.

T2: The spin-spin or transverse relaxation time T2 refers to the rate of the decay of the MRI signal over time resulting from the loss of phase coherence from neighboring nuclear magnetic moments after excitation has occurred, hence the term "spin-spin relaxation." When the magnetic moments have phase coherence immediately after they have been excited by a radiofrequency pulse, they create a detectable net magnetization vector (the MRI signal). As the individual magnetic dipole moments influence one another, they lose phase coherence and no longer contribute toward the MRI signal (the signal strength decays to zero over time). This process is quite rapid, with soft tissue T2 times typically ranging from 40 ms and greater. Images that are obtained in order to primarily focus on this process are said to be "T2-weighted."

T2*: In practice, localized inhomogeneities of the main magnetic field also contribute toward the rate of loss of phase coherence from neighboring spins. Combining this effect with the spin-spin dephasing governed by T2 relaxation gives a combined dephasing rate T2*. Images may specifically be acquired to be either T2- or "T2*-weighted."

T1: The spin-lattice or longitudinal relaxation time T1 refers to the rate at which excited magnetic moments realign back to their unexcited equilibrium orientation over time. The term "spin-lattice relaxation" refers to the fact that this relaxation process is the loss of energy from the excited magnetic moments to their surroundings (typically large macromolecules). Due to the energy exchange nature of this process, T1 is typically an order of magnitude longer than T2 for most tissues, and it increases with magnetic field strength. Images that are obtained in order to primarily focus on this process are said to be "T1-weighted."

T1ρ: Through the application of a continuous radiofrequency pulse to lock the spins in a single orientation, loss of phase coherence can be prevented and instead the rate of decay of the MRI signal can be made proportional to the low-frequency thermal interactions between the excited hydrogen molecules and local macromolecules. This process

is governed by the relaxation time T1ρ. Through application of specific acquisition sequences that involve longer applications of continuous radiofrequency pulses, images may be acquired that are strongly "T1ρ-weighted."

The number of protons available within a unit volume of tissue will also affect the amount of signal that tissue can contribute to MRI. If acquisition parameters are chosen such that there is no notable contrast in the image from either T1 or T2 decay, the image is said to be "proton density (or spin density) weighted."

There are an incredible variety of additional types of MRI contrast available, as well as the ability to mix contributions of contrast in order to optimally focus on tissue and biological processes with MRI.

MRI may be acquired in either two or three dimensions in any orientation, with the static nature of most joints making them ideal targets for high-resolution three-dimensional imaging, which tends to require longer acquisition times. Three-dimensional MRI also benefits from the ability to reconstruct the data in multiple planes to observe a variety of structures within a joint. MRI is now widely held as a clinical gold standard for assessment of cartilage and joints.[1,2]

28.2 Imaging Coils

Most clinical MRI systems are whole-body imaging systems with a range of radiofrequency coils used to acquire images of specific body areas. Knee imaging, for example, is commonly acquired using a dedicated knee coil (see ▶ Fig. 28.2), although dedicated extremity systems are

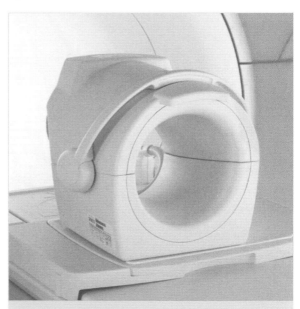

Fig. 28.2 Typical magnetic resonance imaging dedicated extremity (knee) coil. The rigid design allows reproducible positioning for longitudinal assessment of patients and also to assess knee alignment. (Image courtesy of Siemens Medical.)

also available for rapid throughput of extremity imaging (see ▶ Fig. 28.3).

Extremity coils (such as knee coils) tend to have multiple receiver elements and benefit from a broadly cylindrical design to give excellent signal-to-noise ratio (SNR) and homogeneity of transmit field (B_1). Image quality and spatial resolution on these coils therefore tend to be some of the best available on clinical imaging systems. The majority of quantitative MRI cartilage research is therefore performed on whole-body MRI systems with dedicated body area–specific coils.

Dedicated extremity coils also benefit from a more reproducible placement of the body part than flexible, general purpose coils. Dedicated extremity coils are generally of solid construction and therefore fixate the volume of interest more reproducibly than flexible coils. When imaging subjects longitudinally (before and after surgical repair, for example), reproducibility of patient positioning within the imaging system is essential to assess subtle changes in joint morphology or geometry. A reproducible and rapid patient positioning protocol is also essential for studies involving large populations.

Due to their rigid construction, dedicated extremity coils do, however, have a finite bore size, so larger subjects may need to be scanned using flexible coils.

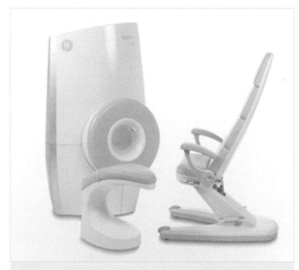

Fig. 28.3 Dedicated 1.5 T extremity magnetic resonance imaging system. (Image courtesy of GE Healthcare.)

28.3 Multinuclear Coils

Hydrogen is the nucleus most commonly used in MRI due to the natural abundance of ^{1}II in the body as well as the high nuclear magnetic resonance sensitivity of ^{1}H. Most clinical imaging systems therefore use imaging coils tuned to the resonant frequency of ^{1}H. To obtain data from other nuclei such as in applications using ^{31}P magnetic resonance spectroscopy (MRS) or ^{23}Na imaging, for example, coils must be used that are tuned to the specific resonant frequency of those nuclei. Multinuclear coils may be purchase or constructed that are either tuned to one specific frequency, or are switchable between frequencies (known as "dual-tuned"). For example, a ^{31}P coil may be used that is "dual-tuned" to allow acquisition of ^{1}H data as well as ^{31}P data. The much lower relative nuclear magnetic resonance sensitivity of non-^{1}H nuclei means that SNR of this type of data is much lower and that acquisition times may often therefore be much longer and data acquisition more challenging (see ▶ Table 28.1).

28.4 Magnet Field Strength

MRI systems are available in a range of magnetic field strengths, with most clinical imaging systems currently either 1.5 T or 3 T. There is a fundamental relationship between the amount of signal available within a unit volume of tissue and the field strength of the MRI system. The amount of signal available increases with increasing field strength.

Due to magnetic susceptibility effects and a nonlinear dependence of noise at field strengths greater than 1 T, the gain in SNR from 1.5 T to 3 T is approximately 30 to 60%, the exact gain being highly dependent on the body area being imaged and the type of imaging coil used. This increase in SNR may be used to either acquire faster MRI, or to increase the spatial resolution or image quality of the images being obtained.

Increasing field strength above 3 T can help to further increase SNR and can be very useful when multinuclear MRS or imaging is being undertaken. As of 2013, there are approximately 50 7 T clinical MRI systems installed worldwide. While the majority of MRI performed at 7 T is neuroradiological, some whole-body 7 T systems are now available for musculoskeletal imaging. ^{1}H imaging at 7 T does pose some safety concerns with the specific absorption rate (a measure of transmitted power into the body) being >

Table 28.1 Nuclear Magnetic Resonance Properties of Common Nuclei Used in Biomedical Research

Nucleus	Resonant frequency (MHz T^{-1})	Natural abundance	Typical concentration in vivo (mM)	Relative nuclear magnetic resonance sensitivity
^{1}H	42.57	100	10^5	1.0
^{31}P	17.23	100	10	6.6×10^{-2}
^{13}C	10.71	1.108	10	1.8×10^{-4}
^{23}Na	11.26	100	80	9.3×10^{-2}

20 times higher at 7 T than at 3 T. However, with the increase in SNR, non-^{1}H MRI becomes significantly more achievable at 7 T than at lower field strengths. A good example of this has been the development of ^{23}Na at high field strengths with applications in cartilage imaging.

^{23}Na MRI signal has been demonstrated to be directly proportional to glycosaminoglycan (GAG) content in articular cartilage[3] and may have a role to play in very early detection of degenerative changes in cartilage. Even at 7 T, ^{23}Na remains challenging. The very short T2 relaxation time for ^{23}Na (1 ms for the short component representing 60% of the available sodium signal and approximately 10 ms for the longer T2 component of the remainder of the sodium signal) means that even with the increased SNR available at 7 T, specially customized acquisition techniques employing rapid radial data acquisition, fluid suppression, and ultrashort echo times are currently being investigated in order to make in vivo ^{23}Na cartilage imaging achievable, as shown in ▶ Fig. 28.4.[4]

^{31}P MRS is more suited to assessment of muscle metabolism than cartilage.[5] MRS also benefits from the higher SNR available at higher field strengths.[6] For MRS applications, the higher SNR results in more easily discernible spectral peaks, meaning that shorter acquisition times can be used in vivo. The reduction in ^{31}P longitudinal (or spin-lattice) relaxation time T1 also means that shorter acquisition times can be used at 7 T, bringing in vivo acquisition times down to several minutes,[6] whereas the higher field strength also increases chemical shift and results in better peak separation (see ▶ Fig. 28.5). All of these factors combine to improve ^{31}P data quality obtained at 7 T.

28.5 Magnetic Resonance Imaging Contrast Agents

By careful selection of MRI acquisition parameters, it is possible to calculate the intrinsic relaxation properties of tissue. Calculation of MRI relaxation parameters on a voxel-by-voxel basis allows "mapping" of biochemical properties of tissues. T1 (or spin-lattice) relaxation mapping is now commonly exploited in assessment of cartilage combined with the application of an MRI contrast agent.

Native tissue relaxation times may be altered with the administration of exogenous contrast agents.

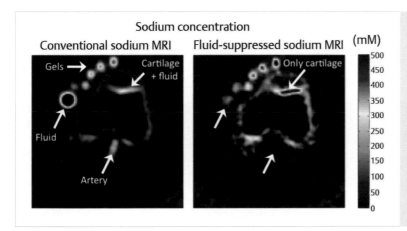

Fig. 28.4 In-vivo ^{23}Na knee cartilage image obtained at 7 T demonstrating ^{23}Na signal obtained in cartilage with and without the presence of fluid suppression. Image contains sodium- and fluid-filled gels to confirm fluid suppression sodium signal detection. (Image courtesy of Prof. G. Madelin, New York University Medical Center.)

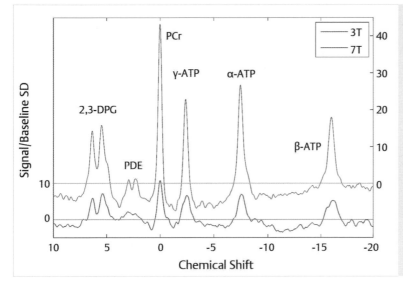

Fig. 28.5 ^{31}P magnetic resonance spectroscopy spectra comparison of 3 T and 7 T taken from an interventricular septum in a typical subject. Note the significant increase in signal-to-noise ratio obtained at increased field strength as demonstrated by increased peak height. ATP, adenosine triphosphate; DPG, 2,3-diphosphoglycerate; PCr, phosphocreatine; PDE, phosphodiester. (Image provided by Dr. Chris Rodgers, Oxford Centre for Clinical Magnetic Resonance Research, University of Oxford.)

28.5.1 Gadolinium and T1 Mapping

The most commonly used MRI contrast agents in human imaging are small-molecular-weight compounds containing gadolinium. Due to the paramagnetic nature of gadolinium, these contrast agents significantly shorten T1 relaxation times in tissues in which they accumulate, such that tissues containing the contrast agent will appear "brighter" in images. Gadolinium is toxic and therefore commonly administered in chelated form to diethylenetriaminepentaacetic acid. The use of gadolinium-diethylenetriaminepentaacetic contrast agents has been linked to cases of nephrogenic systemic fibrosis in patients with severe kidney failure and is therefore contraindicated in these patients.

As gadolinium-based contrast agents are negatively charged, they are repelled by the similarly negative charged GAG in healthy cartilage. Distribution of contrast agent within cartilage is therefore inversely proportional to presence of GAG and can be a sensitive indicator of early cartilage breakdown and repair.[7]

28.5.2 Delayed Gadolinium-Enhanced Magnetic Resonance Imaging of the Cartilage

Delayed gadolinium-enhanced MRI of the cartilage (dGEMRIC) continues to be the subject of ongoing research in a range of cartilage pathology and repair applications.

Once gadolinium has been intravenously administered and allowed an appropriate time to circulate (commonly 30 to 60 minutes postinfusion), the measured T1 value postinfusion (T1Gd) due to contrast accumulation within cartilage (also known as the dGEMRIC index) has been shown to directly reflect localized GAG content.[8]

High T1Gd reflects healthy cartilage due to lack of contrast accumulation, whereas lower T1Gd values reflect degenerated cartilage. The sensitivity of spatial distribution of GAG content is therefore only limited by the spatial resolution of the dGEMRIC acquisition.

Due to potential variability of native T1 values of cartilage precontrast infusion, or any other potential confounding acquisition or MRI scanner-related factors, native T1 precontrast *must* be measured to accurately assess T1Gd. This allows calculation of ΔR_1 (where $R_1 = 1/T1$). Calculation of native T1 is particularly important when T1 is being calculated using the variable flip angle method, where any inhomogeneity in the transmit field may cause systematic errors in calculated T1 values, and must be corrected for. An example native T1 map is shown in ▶ Fig. 28.6a. These errors become more notable at increasingly higher field strengths, where body loading effects at 3 T and above can contribute to a higher degree of B_1 inhomogeneity and therefore flip angle errors. Various scanner vendors have increasingly implemented hardware modifications on modern high field systems

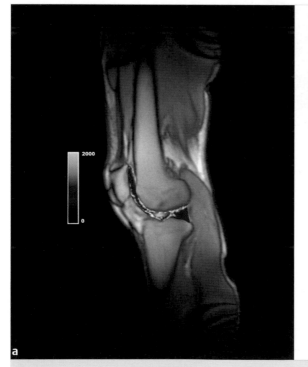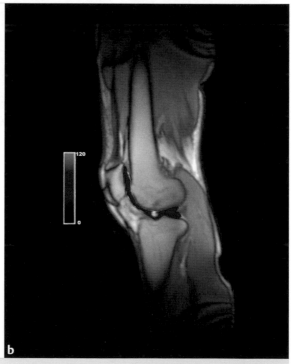

Fig. 28.6 (a) T1 map of cartilage of the knee in sagittal plane. T1 scale shown in ms. (b) T2 map of cartilage of the knee in sagittal plane. T2 scale shown in ms.

(such as dual transmit fields) in order to mitigate these errors.

As with all quantitative analysis of research data, it is vital to ensure that the MRI system is capable of accurately measuring known relaxation times. Therefore, if any research studies involving dGEMRIC are being undertaken, a robust quality assurance (QA) program is vital to ensure confidence in the accuracy of the MRI system. Various commercial test objects (known as phantoms) with known and stable relaxation times are available, and regular measurements of these objects should be made, with measured relaxation time values logged over time. Appropriate test objects should be selected that mimic the typical range of relaxation times observed in vivo. These will commonly consist of saline water, agar gel, or oil, doped with various paramagnetic salts ($CuSO_4$, $MnCl_2$, $GdCl_2$, $NiCl_2$, for example). Care should also be taken to appropriately mimic in vivo conditions by adequately "loading" the MRI coil during QA. Inadequate "loading" of the coil due to an inappropriate test object being imaged rather than the body area the coil was designed for may result in QA values being an inadequate control for research studies (see ▶ Fig. 28.7).

Regular QA will enable detection of any potential scanner "drift" or systematic error over time, and highlight any relevant problems (such as errors in the transmit field causing B_1 inhomogeneity). This type of regular QA is particularly important in ongoing research trials where longitudinal data are being obtained (such as in cartilage repair studies) or when large cohorts are being imaged with a reproducible protocol.

dGEMRIC is now regularly being performed in research trials at both 1.5 T and 3 T, demonstrating excellent reproducibility at these field strengths.

28.5.3 Ultrasmall Superparamagnetic Particles of Iron Oxide and T2* Mapping

An alternative type of MRI contrast agent is ultra-small superparamagnetic particles of iron oxide (USPIO). Because of their size (commonly 10 to 30 nm in diameter), these particles escape immediate detection by the reticuloendothelial system and persist for long enough in the bloodstream to undergo macrophage phagocytosis and can be used to assess accumulation within vascular and lymphatic tissues. These particles have been widely used to investigate joint inflammation or infection.

Due to the superparamagnetic nature of these particles, they have an extremely strong effect on the local magnetic field homogeneity. On T2*-weighted scans, this results in localized signal reduction. Darker areas are seen around areas of USPIO accumulation. Similarly to the requirement to calculate native T1 values in the application of gadolinium-based agents, it is important to image the tissue of interest before and after administration of USPIO. This is important to discount signal reduction post-USPIO being due to some other factor. The optimal time for detection of macrophage-USPIO uptake is approximately 36 hours postinfusion, and as such, two imaging sessions will be needed. Spatial registration of pre- and post-USPIO infusion data is therefore also important to appropriately quantify USPIO uptake. Much of the work in inflammatory cartilage has been performed in animal models due to the unavailability of USPIO agents suitable for human application. However, recent applications have been performed in human cardiovascular disease with newly marketed human USPIO applications. Some research has been published in USPIO imaging of the knee of asymptomatic volunteers,[9] and in vivo human USPIO inflammatory imaging of joints is ripe for exploration.

T2 and T2* mapping may be performed without the application of USPIO. Native T2 and T2* mapping of cartilage has been shown to reflect the collagen component of cartilage[10] (see ▶ Fig. 28.6b). As with T1 mapping in dGEMRIC, T2 and T2* mapping can provide zonal distribution information within the cartilage according to the spatial resolution of the image acquired. Higher SNR dedicated coils and higher MRI field strengths therefore result in better differentiation of spatial distribution of collagen within the cartilage.

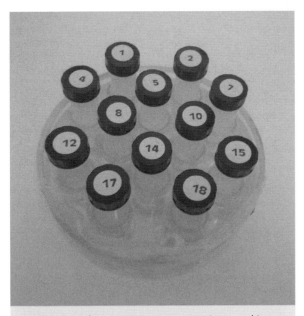

Fig. 28.7 Example magnetic resonance imaging test objects (phantoms) used to perform regular quality assurance so that the system is able to reliably calculate known relaxation times. Each numbered test tube contains an agar solution doped with paramagnetic salts with known relaxation times (T1, T2). Tubes are placed in a loading annulus filled with doped water in order to adequately "load" the imaging coil used. (Image provided by Dr. Dan Wilson, Department of Medical Physics, Leeds Teaching Hospitals NHS Trust.)

28.6 Other Magnetic Resonance Imaging Contrast Mechanisms in Cartilage Imaging

28.6.1 T1ρ Imaging

T1ρ values in T1ρ-mapped MRI of the cartilage have been shown to correlate with proteoglycan content in bovine and clinical osteoarthritic specimens.[10] There are indications that T1ρ mapping may be more sensitive to early changes in cartilage extracellular matrix than T2 mapping.

Due to the longer radiofrequency applications required to weight MRI contrast toward T1ρ processes, application of T1ρ mapping at higher field strength can be challenging, where in vivo specific absorption rate limits (a measure of the transmitted power into the body) can limit the application of the required T1ρ "locking" radiofrequency pulse.

28.6.2 Diffusion-Weighted Magnetic Resonance Imaging

Diffusion-weighted MRI (DWI) is an MRI technique that uses the repeated application of two balanced magnetic field gradients to sensitize the MRI acquisition to the three-dimensional Brownian motion of water molecules. This technique has mostly been developed to "map" brain white matter structure and connectivity.[11] Quantitative measures reflective of this motion can be made to calculate the apparent diffusion coefficient, which is reflective of the overall motion of water molecules. Another useful characteristic is the fractional anisotropy that is indicative of the directional coherence of the water molecule diffusion. Both apparent diffusion coefficient and fractional anisotropy have been shown to be sensitive to collagen degeneration in cartilage,[12] and DWI is a promising technique for investigation of cartilage. Again, due to the otherwise static nature of most joints, cartilage assessment is particularly well suited to DWI investigation (because DWI is inherently very sensitive to macroscopic motion and therefore prone to motion-related image artifacts).

28.7 Conclusion

In conclusion, MRI offers a wide range of research applications shown to demonstrate merit in the investigation of degenerative cartilage and cartilage repair. Most of these techniques are under current research and are being further developed and refined, both in their technical application and in clinical use. With the advent of increasingly high field MRI systems, dedicated coils with multiple receiver elements capable of parallel imaging to speed up acquisitions and obtain higher spatial resolution, MRI will continue to develop in the application of musculoskeletal imaging and noninvasive assessment of cartilage pathology, in particular.

References

[1] Binks DA, Hodgson RJ, Ries ME et al. Quantitative parametric MRI of articular cartilage: a review of progress and open challenges. Br J Radiol 2013; 86: 20120163

[2] Trattnig S, Domayer S, Welsch GW, Mosher T, Eckstein F. MR imaging of cartilage and its repair in the knee—a review. Eur Radiol 2009; 19: 1582–1594

[3] Wheaton AJ, Borthakur A, Shapiro EM et al. Proteoglycan loss in human knee cartilage: quantitation with sodium MR imaging—feasibility study. Radiology 2004; 231: 900–905

[4] Madelin G, Babb J, Xia D et al. Articular cartilage: evaluation with fluid-suppressed 7.0-T sodium MR imaging in subjects with and subjects without osteoarthritis. Radiology 2013; 268: 481–491

[5] Lindquist D. What can 31 P MR spectroscopy tell us about muscle disease? Radiology 2008; 247: 1–2

[6] Bogner W, Chmelik M, Andronesi OC, Sorensen AG, Trattnig S, Gruber S. In vivo 31 P spectroscopy by fully adiabatic extended image selected in vivo spectroscopy: a comparison between 3 T and 7 T. Magn Reson Med 2011; 66: 923–930

[7] Bittersohl B, Zilkens C, Kim YJ et al. Delayed gadolinium-enhanced magnetic resonance imaging of hip joint cartilage: pearls and pitfalls. Orthop Rev (Pavia) 2011; 3: e11

[8] Burstein D, Velyvis J, Scott KT et al. Protocol issues for delayed Gd (DTPA)(2-)-enhanced MRI (dGEMRIC) for clinical evaluation of articular cartilage. Magn Reson Med 2001; 45: 36–41

[9] Reiner CS, Lutz AM, Tschirch F et al. USPIO-enhanced magnetic resonance imaging of the knee in asymptomatic volunteers. Eur Radiol 2009; 19: 1715–1722

[10] Jazrawi LM, Alaia MJ, Chang G, Fitzgerald EF, Recht MP. Advances in magnetic resonance imaging of articular cartilage. J Am Acad Orthop Surg 2011; 19: 420–429

[11] Le Bihan D, Mangin JF, Poupon C et al. Diffusion tensor imaging: concepts and applications. J Magn Reson Imaging 2001; 13: 534–546

[12] Deng X, Farley M, Nieminen MT, Gray M, Burstein D. Diffusion tensor imaging of native and degenerated human articular cartilage. Magn Reson Imaging 2007; 25: 168–171

29 Imaging of Cartilage Function

Gabby B. Joseph and Thomas M. Link

Osteoarthritis (OA) is a degenerative joint disease affecting more than 27 million people in the United States alone.[1] OA is characterized by biochemical and morphological degradation of joint tissues, including the articular cartilage. Despite the high prevalence of OA worldwide, diagnosis in the early stages of disease is difficult, because many asymptomatic subjects have morphological cartilage degeneration. The traditional method for imaging OA is radiography, which assesses osseous changes. Although magnetic resonance imaging (MRI) is widely used for the clinical diagnosis of OA, conventional imaging protocols assess degeneration primarily based on morphological changes (late stage in the disease process). Quantitative MRI methods for measuring the relaxation properties in cartilage may aid in the diagnosis of early OA prior to irreversible morphological changes. Such methods, which characterize changes in the molecular composition of the extracellular matrix (ECM), include T2 relaxometry, T1rho relaxometry, T1Gd relaxometry (delayed gadolinium-enhanced MRI contrast [dGEMRIC]) and sodium imaging. This chapter will review the T1rho relaxometry, T2 relaxometry, T1Gd relaxometry (dGEMRIC), and sodium MRI quantification techniques for cartilage assessment and their applications in OA imaging.

29.1 Osteoarthritis and Cartilage

OA is a heterogeneous and multifactorial disease characterized by the progressive loss of hyaline articular cartilage and the development of altered joint congruency, subchondral sclerosis, intraosseous cysts, and osteophytes. It affects approximately 14% of the adult population[2] and is the second most common cause of permanent disability among people over the age of 50[3]; knee OA is the most common form of OA followed by hip OA. The initiation and pathogenesis of OA can be affected by many factors including altered mechanical loading and previous knee injury.

Hyaline cartilage lines the articular surfaces of the joints; at the knee, it covers the distal femur, proximal tibia, and patella. The primary function of cartilage is to minimize the contact stresses that occur during the joint loading,[4] thus acting as a cushion in the joint. Cartilage is composed of an ECM, which contains chondrocytes, collagen, proteoglycan (PG), and water molecules. Chondrocytes are cartilage cells that regulate the production and maintenance of the ECM. In healthy tissue, the water constitutes about 65 to 80% of the dry tissue weight. The collagen constitutes approximately 75% of the dry weight of tissue and is responsible for the tensile strength.[4] Proteoglycans are negatively charged macromolecules that constitute approximately 20 to 30% of the dry tissue weight. The strong negative charge is neutralized by positive ions in the surrounding fluid, therefore creating a swelling pressure. The PG is responsible for the compressive strength in the cartilage. It is made up of a protein core with glycosaminoglycan (GAG) sidechains (chondroitin sulfate and keratin sulfate).

The initial stages of OA include PG loss, increased water content, and disorganization of the collagen network. With further degeneration, cartilage tissue becomes ulcerated causing PGs to diffuse into the synovial fluid, thus decreasing water content in cartilage. The intermediate stages of OA include cartilage thinning, fibrillation, and decreased PG and water content. In the late stages of OA, collagen, PG, and water content is further reduced, and the collagen network is severely disrupted. Because the cascade of events leading to cartilage loss is initiated by a disruption in the biochemical composition of the ECM, the noninvasive detection of early changes in the ECM would be key for understanding the natural history of OA. MRI T2 relaxometry, T1rho relaxometry, and T1Gd relaxometry (dGEMRIC), and sodium imaging are recently developed MRI techniques that can assess early stages of cartilage degeneration; implementation of such techniques in clinical practice may improve diagnostic capabilities and may enable preventive and therapeutic measures to be taken at the early stages of the disease.

29.2 Diagnostic Techniques for in Vivo Imaging of the Cartilage Matrix

29.2.1 T2 Mapping

Quantitative T2 relaxation time is a noninvasive marker of cartilage degeneration as it is sensitive to tissue hydration and biochemical composition. Immobilization of water protons in cartilage by the collagen-PG matrix promotes T2 decay. Increases in the mobility of water in the cartilage ECM occur as a result of degeneration, and thus increase cartilage T2 relaxation time. Because alterations of the collagen network and changes in hydration are characteristics of early cartilage degeneration, T2 mapping is a viable technique for the noninvasive evaluation of OA. The following sections describe (1) the methodology for T2 measurement and (2) in vivo research studies relating to OA.

T2 Mapping: Methodology

T2 relaxation time in in vivo imaging is generally performed using 1.5 T or 3 T MRI scanners. Various MRI sequences can be used for acquisition including spin echo, multislice multiecho (MSME), fast spin echo, and three-dimensional spoiled gradient recalled. A comparison of these sequences for T2 measurement has been previously performed, demonstrating various differences in quantified T2 values between sequences. Thus, the direct comparison of T2 values between sequences is not recommended.

In addition to the type of MRI sequence used for quantification, an imaging parameter called "echo time" must also be optimized for T2 quantification. In general, the greater the number of echo times, the more accurate the quantification. Many studies have used four echo times, while others including the Osteoarthritis Initiative (OAI) study have used seven (echo times = 10, 20, 30, 40, 50, 60, and 70 ms). While it would be ideal to use the greatest number of echo times with the least time separation between them, these values are optimized based on limitations of the MRI hardware and as well as scan time—the greater the number of echoes, the longer the scan time.

The scan time is an important factor to consider when designing an MRI sequence for T2 measurement. The scan time is ideally as short as possible, in order to ensure feasibility of T2 relaxation time measurements in clinical practice. Compared to single-echo spin echo and single-slice multiecho spin echo sequences, the application of an MSME spin echo sequence considerably reduces the acquisition time. However, potential sources of error are introduced by using an MSME spin echo sequence.

Watanabe et al[5] reported that the average T2 value measured with multislice acquisition was shorter than that measured with single-slice acquisition. However, they found only a relatively small decrease in T2 and observed no obvious inter-slice variation in T2 values when multislice acquisition was used. They concluded that multislice acquisitions for T2 measurements are clinically applicable. Thus, large clinical trials such as the OAI are using MSME acquisition.

Cartilage T2 maps are created using the following process: Typically, T2-weighted multiecho, spin echo images with varying echo times and identical repetition times are acquired. Second, T2 maps are computed assuming exponential signal decay. The T2 relaxation time value for each pixel in an image is calculated by fitting the measured signal intensity S at each echo times to a mono-exponential decay function:

$$S(TE_i) = S_0 \cdot e^{\left(\frac{-TE_i}{T2}\right)}$$

where S_0 is the signal intensity at zero echo times. The last step of image processing is the creation of T2 maps containing the calculated T2 values of each pixel. A T2 map can be visualized by creating a color-coded representation of the T2 values where high values signify cartilage degeneration (▶ Fig. 29.1). Such maps can be used to localize areas of cartilage degeneration, which may be helpful in surgical planning.

Because many factors—such as previous injury, knee alignment, and altered mechanical loading patterns—may contribute to OA, the disease is heterogeneous and may develop in different areas of the knee. Thus, cartilage T2

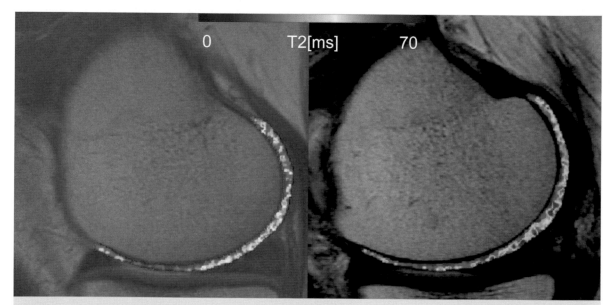

Fig. 29.1 Representative T2 maps from a normal control subject (*left*) and a subject with risk factors for osteoarthritis (*right*). Both subjects have no cartilage abnormalities and no pain; however, the subject with risk factors has elevated mean T2, gray-level co-occurrence matrix (GLCM) variance, GLCM contrast, and GLCM entropy.

is often assessed on a knee level as well as in a localized manner in order to capture the heterogeneous nature of OA degeneration. Generally, T2 is quantified as the mean T2 value in a region of interest (ROI). Research studies often report mean T2 values in various regions of the knee cartilage including the patella, medial femur, lateral femur, medial tibia, lateral tibia, and trochlea. Further subdivision of ROIs into weight-bearing and nonweight-bearing regions has been performed in order to assess the effects of mechanical loading on the pathogenesis of OA. Thus, subdividing the analysis into subregions facilitates the assessment of different areas of the joint that may behave uniquely due to varied mechanical load patterns and weight-bearing properties.

In addition to this subregional analysis, recent studies have developed novel image-processing tools to assess the cartilage layers. Cartilage is composed of three primary layers: The "superficial layer" is closest to the cartilage surface and contains collagen fibers that are oriented parallel to the surface. The "transitional layer" is the largest zone that is adjacent to the "superficial layer" and has collagen fibers that are randomly oriented. The "deep layer" contains collagen fibers that are oriented perpendicular to the joint surface. MRI laminar analysis is a method that partitions the regions of interest into cartilage layers; studies have demonstrated elevated T2 values in the superficial layer compared to the deep layer. Thus, in addition to mean subregional values, laminar analysis may provide additional insight on the pathogenesis of cartilage degeneration.

Another technique that captures localized changes to cartilage is gray-level co-occurrence matrix (GLCM) texture analysis, a method developed by Haralick et al.[6] This technique has been used to assess the spatial distribution of cartilage T2. The GLCM determines the frequency that neighboring gray-level values occur in an image. Various GLCM texture parameters including contrast, variance, and entropy can be calculated in each region. Each texture parameter provides unique information on the spatial distribution of T2 values in the cartilage. Preliminary studies have shown that subjects with OA have a more heterogeneous distribution of T2 values than controls[7,8,9] (as reflected by higher values of GLCM contrast, entropy, and variance), demonstrating that the mean and heterogeneity of cartilage T2 pixels may be indicative of early cartilage matrix degeneration. ► Fig. 29.1 illustrates two representative T2 maps from a control and a subject at risk for OA, respectively. While both subjects do not have cartilage abnormalities, the subject from the incidence cohort has greater mean T2, GLCM contrast, GLCM variance, and GLCM entropy of cartilage T2.

T2 Mapping: In Vivo Research Studies

T2 mapping has been used to assess a multitude of research topics including pathogenesis of OA in various joints including the knee and hip, the efficacy of cartilage repair surgical procedures, and relationship with physical activity. This section will focus on research studies relating to knee cartilage.

Studies have utilized cartilage T2 to study OA in order to understand the role of cartilage biochemistry in the initiation and progression of disease. Cross-sectional studies have demonstrated elevated cartilage T2 values in subjects with OA as compared to controls, demonstrating alterations in cartilage biochemistry with disease. Another interesting characteristic of OA is the relationship between cartilage biochemistry and cartilage morphology. Studies have shown an inverse relationship between cartilage T2 and cartilage thickness, and that elevated T2 at baseline is associated with cartilage loss at 12 months. Other studies have assessed the relationship between cartilage degeneration and degeneration in other tissues of the knee including the bone marrow and the meniscus, and have demonstrated elevation in cartilage T2 in relation to bone marrow edema pattern and meniscus degeneration. These studies highlight the complexity of OA and that degenerative changes in one tissue may cause a cascade of degenerative changes in other neighboring regions of the knee.

Assessing the longitudinal changes in joint biochemistry, morphology, and symptoms has been a key focus in recent studies on OA. The OAI is a national and multicenter, ~5,000-patient natural history and prevalence database of OA images. This study aims to evaluate the pathogenesis of OA and to classify biomarkers that can predict the development and progression of the disease. The OAI is a cross-sectional and longitudinal dataset that includes both MRI and radiographic images of subjects scanned annually over 8 years. MRI for the assessment of cartilage morphology and cartilage T2 are available, and the longitudinal follow-up facilitates assessment of the progression of the disease. Recent studies have utilized the OAI database to assess whether cartilage T2 relaxation time can predict longitudinal changes in joint morphology—having an elevated T2 relaxation time at baseline was predictive of developing joint degeneration 3 years later. These results suggest that the initial changes to the cartilage matrix may be indicative of future joint degeneration and demonstrate the utility of the OAI dataset in the study of biomarkers for OA progression.

While a multitude of research studies have used T2 to assess cartilage degeneration during the pathogenesis of OA, recently T2 has been used to assess the outcomes of cartilage repair. Previous studies have measured T2 relaxation time following chondrocyte transplantation and microfracture surgical repair techniques, demonstrating changes in T2 following repair. These studies demonstrate that cartilage T2 measurements may supplement the standard MRI clinical protocol for the noninvasive assessment of treatment efficacy.

Overall, these studies demonstrate that T2 mapping may be a viable biomarker for early degenerative cartilage disease, and may be useful for the early detection of OA as well as for therapeutic assessment.

29.2.2 T1rho Mapping

In addition to T2 mapping, T1rho mapping is an imaging technique that can be used to noninvasively assess the early stages of cartilage degeneration in OA. In cartilage, the PG, which is largely responsible for the high elasticity and resilience of tissue, consists of a central protein core to which a large number of negatively charged GAG side-chains are covalently attached. The PG content of cartilage can be probed using spin lattice relaxation in the rotating frame (T1rho-weighted imaging).[10,11,12] Because the PG content is depleted during early stages of cartilage degeneration, T1rho mapping may be valuable tool for the noninvasive assessment of early OA.

T1rho: Methodology

Similar to T2 mapping, T1rho MRI is often performed at 1.5 T or 3 T. Various MRI sequences can be used to quantify the T1rho value in cartilage including two-dimensional spin echo, fast spin echo, spiral imaging, echo planar imaging, or three-dimensional gradient echo sequences. T1rho relaxation time describes the spin-lattice relaxation in the rotating frame and is sensitive to slow molecular motion. T1rho is measured by applying a spin lock pulse, which allows the magnetization to relax with a T1rho time constant. In the T1rho experiment, various spin lock times are implemented in the MRI sequence and the signal is measured at each spin lock time. Similar to T2, T1rho has exponential signal decay, and the T1rho time constant is measured on a pixel-by-pixel basis. The mean T1rho value in an ROI is often reported in research studies; however, subregional analysis, including subdivision of cartilage into weight-bearing and nonweight-bearing sections as well as laminar and texture analysis, have also been performed. In addition to the mean T1rho value, which provides an overall assessment of the cartilage biochemical composition, the subregional analysis provides insight on the spatial distribution of PG content in the cartilage.\

T1rho: In Vivo Research Studies

Because T1rho is sensitive to PG content, many research studies have used T1rho to investigate cartilage biochemistry in OA. Studies have demonstrated elevated T1rho values in subjects with cartilage degeneration and have shown correlations with the degree of knee joint degeneration, as assessed by radiography and clinical MRI sequences. More interestingly, previous studies have reported elevated T1rho values in cartilage regions that showed no obvious morphological changes in clinical MRI. These results suggest that T1rho can detect in vivo cartilage degeneration at very early stages and that the technique is more sensitive than current clinical imaging techniques. In addition, T1rho has been used to investigate the relationship between cartilage degeneration and other aspects of OA including bone marrow abnormalities and meniscal lesions. Interestingly, bone marrow abnormalities were related to cartilage degeneration, as evidenced by elevated T1rho values and clinical gradings. Furthermore, meniscal abnormalities were related to elevated cartilage T1rho values. These studies suggest that early signs of cartilage degeneration, as measured by T1rho, may not only be associated with cartilage thinning, but also with neighboring tissue degeneration, thus highlighting the interplay between cartilage and other joint tissues in the pathogenesis of OA.

Studies have compared the utility of both T1rho and T2 in the assessment of OA, and have demonstrated that both T1rho and T2 may provide complementary information on cartilage biochemistry. An in vivo study quantified the pixel-by-pixel correlation of T1rho and T2 values in patients with OA and healthy controls, demonstrating that the pixel-by-pixel correlation between T1rho and T2 showed a large range in both controls and patients with OA ($R = 0.522 \pm 0.183$, ranging from 0.221 to 0.763 in patients with OA, versus $R = 0.624 \pm 0.060$, ranging from 0.547 to 0.726 in controls,).[13] ▶ Fig. 29.2 shows T1rho and T2 maps from a control subject, a subject with mild OA, and a subject with severe OA, demonstrating differences in the spatial distribution of T1rho and T2 values. These results suggested that T1rho and T2 have different spatial distributions and may provide complementary information regarding cartilage degeneration in OA. Combining these two parameters may further improve our capability to diagnose early cartilage degeneration and injury.

T1rho has also been used to evaluate knee cartilage biochemistry following injury and after cartilage repair. Because injury is a risk factor for the future development of OA, it is important to understand the cascade of events following injury and leading to OA. Interestingly, T1rho is elevated in subjects with anterior cruciate ligament injuries, demonstrating compromised cartilage biochemical composition, which may lead into posttraumatic OA development in anterior cruciate ligament-injured joints. T1rho has also been used to study the biochemical response of cartilage following surgery. Methods for cartilage repair including microfracture, which relies on bone marrow stimulation, and osteochondral transfer, which relies on harvesting cartilage plugs from a different area of the joint, have been studied using T1rho. Cartilage T1rho values were elevated in subjects following each procedure, demonstrating a biochemical response in the cartilage ECM. Future studies utilizing T1rho to study the longitudinal changes in the cartilage biochemistry following surgical procedures may be useful in the assessment of treatment efficacy.

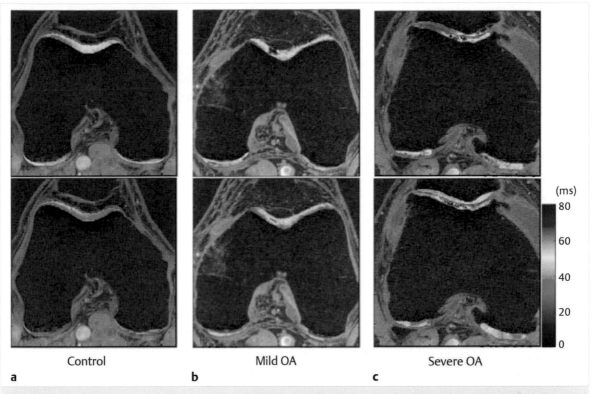

Fig. 29.2 T1rho maps (*top row*) and T2 maps (*bottom row*) for a healthy control (**a**), a patient with mild osteoarthritis (OA) (**b**), and a patient with severe OA (**c**). (**a**) Control: The average T1rho value was 40.1 ± 11.4 ms and T2 value was 33.3 ± 10.5 ms in cartilage. (**b**) A patient with early OA (male, 66 years old). The average T1rho value was 45.5 ± 14.5 ms and T2 value was 35.0 ± 10.9 ms in cartilage. (**c**) A patient with advanced OA (male, 46 years old). The average T1rho value was 55.4 ± 26.0 ms and T2 value was 43.8 ± 11.1 ms in cartilage. The maps illustrate the differences in T1rho and T2 between OA severity, and demonstrate potential different spatial distribution between T2 and T1rho elevation in osteoarthritic cartilage (patient C).

The impact of physical activity on cartilage structure and overall joint health is a critical area of research, because exercise is often advised for patients as a noninvasive treatment for OA, and the long-term effects of exercise on joint structure are unclear. Because the magnitude and types of exercise may have varied effects on the joint, it would be important to understand the immediate and long-term responses of joint biochemistry and morphology to exercise. Studies have used T1rho and T2 MRI to assess joint structure following marathon running and have demonstrated elevations in both T1rho and T2 immediately following exercise. While the T2 values recovered 3 months following the marathon, the T1rho values remained elevated. These elevated T1rho values are suggestive of a disrupted cartilage ECM, in particular, PG. The biochemistry of the meniscus following marathon running has also been assessed using T1rho and T2 imaging. Of interest, both the T1rho and T2 values in the meniscus following the marathon were elevated; however, 3 months later, the T2 values decreased and the T1rho values remained elevated. Overall, these results suggest that persisting changes in the ECM months following the completion of a marathon. These results demonstrate the utility of quantitative joint imaging to assess the impact of physical activity on the joint.

Overall, previous research studies have demonstrated that T1rho is sensitive to macromolecular changes in cartilage composition as a result of disease, injury, and mechanical loading, and thus may be useful to detect early signs of deterioration of the cartilage ECM.

29.3 Delayed Gadolinium-Enhanced Magnetic Resonance Imaging of Cartilage

dGEMRIC is an MRI technique that can detect changes in the fixed charged density of cartilage, and thus GAG concentration. Because changes in GAG concentration are one of the primary characteristics of early stage cartilage degeneration and are related to the mechanical properties of cartilage, dGMERIC has been widely investigated in the study of OA, cartilage repair, and physical activity.

29.3.1 Methodology

In the dGEMRIC imaging protocol, a negatively charged gadolinium diethylenetriaminepentaacetic (Gd-DTPA)$^{2-}$ contrast agent is injected intravenously, the subject exercises for approximately 10 minutes (in order for the contrast agent to penetrate the cartilage), and imaging is performed after about 1.5 hours for the knee.[14] It is also possible to inject the contrast agent intra-articularly; however, the penetration is more efficient when using the intravenous method. The negatively charged GAG in articular cartilage repels the negatively charged contrast agent. A low concentration of Gd-DTPA^{2-} will accumulate in areas of high GAG content and will have a slower T1 relaxation time as compared to areas of low GAG content. In diseased cartilage, the contrast agent is easily absorbed due to the lack of GAG. However, in healthy cartilage, the contrast agent is less likely to be absorbed due to the abundance of GAG.

Following contrast agent penetration, MRI T1 maps are acquired. The distribution of Gd-DTPA^{2-} is calculated based on the T1 relaxation time of the tissue. Three-dimensional dGEMRIC sequences have been implemented at 1.5 T and 3 T for use in clinical studies,[15] and research studies using a 7 T scanner have been performed. ▶ Fig. 29.3 illustrates sagittal images of the knee (identical window and level) that can be used to measure T1 relaxation time and determine the distribution of Gd-DTPA^{2-} in cartilage. Many factors can contribute to the sensitivity of dGEMRIC, including the amount of contrast agent absorbed into the cartilage and the body mass index of the subject. Such factors need to be considered when designing clinical studies in order to standardize the clinical protocol.

The spatial variation of the dGEMRIC values may be an important indicator of cartilage composition and integrity. Similar to T2 and T1rho, depth-wise variations in the dGEMRIC index have been demonstrated and suggest varied GAG concentrations throughout the depth of the cartilage. Thus, it is important to not only consider bulk dGEMRIC values, but also the spatial distribution of dGEMRIC values when assessing OA. Monitoring the changes in GAG content in the deep and superficial layers during disease progression may shed light on whether cartilage degeneration is initiated from the deep layers of cartilage or the superficial layer closest to the joint surface.

29.3.2 In Vivo Evaluation

In addition to T2 and T1rho, dGEMRIC is a valuable tool in the assessment of cartilage biochemical composition in OA, and studies have shown promise for dGEMRIC as an early indicator and predictor for future joint degeneration. A wide range of dGEMRIC values have been demonstrated in subjects without radiographic evidence of OA, suggesting that the GAG content in these patients may be varied despite having a healthy joint as evidenced by radiography. In addition, the dGEMRIC index has been associated with the severity of OA as assessed from radiography: subjects with joint space narrowing had higher dGEMRIC indices than subjects without joint space narrowing, demonstrating a relationship between morphological joint degeneration and cartilage biochemical changes. A recent longitudinal study reported that a low dGEMRIC index at baseline was associated with the development of radiographic OA at 6 years follow-up. At 6 years follow-up, 9 of the 16 knees studied developed radiographic OA—those 9 knees also had lower dGEMRIC indices at baseline than the remaining knees that did not develop radiographic evidence of OA.[16] This study demonstrates that the dGEMRIC index may be a biomarker for the longitudinal development of radiographic OA.

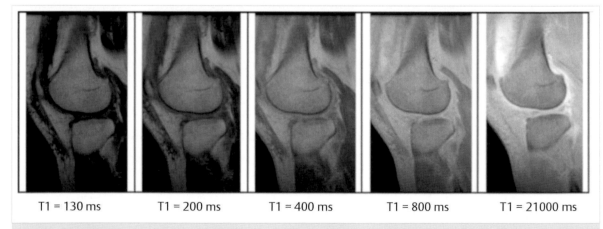

| T1 = 130 ms | T1 = 200 ms | T1 = 400 ms | T1 = 800 ms | T1 = 21000 ms |

Fig. 29.3 An example of sagittal images of the knee (identical window and level) used to measure T1 relaxation time and determine the distribution of Gd-DTPA^{2-} in cartilage. A fast gradient echo sequence is used with the following scanning parameters: TI1/TI2/TI3/TI4/TI5 = 130/200/400/800/2100 ms, repetition times = 6.2 ms, resolution = 0.625 × 0.625 × 3 mm^3, field of view = 16 cm. The images reflect an uptake of Gd-DTPA^{2-} as demonstrated by the increases in image signal intensity, particularly in the cartilage.

dGEMRIC has been used to study various aspects of OA including knee mechanical properties. Varus malalignment (bow legged) is associated with a lower dGEMRIC index on the medial side, whereas the opposite trend is evident in valgus malalignment, demonstrating that malalignment not only affects the joint morphology, but also cartilage biochemistry.

dGEMRIC is also a viable method for the study of postsurgical cartilage composition. Various animal models have been used to study cartilage biochemistry following repair procedures and have shown that a return of dGEMRIC values to "normal" after surgery. In a rabbit model of spontaneous repair of osteochondral defects, the dGEMRIC index approached "normal" values 6 months after injury, suggesting repair of the cartilage matrix. Studies have shown that dGEMRIC can be used to monitor GAG content in autologous chondrocyte transplantation, microfracture procedures, and following anterior cruciate ligament reconstruction. A study by Trattnig et al[17] performed dGEMRIC scans on patients who had undergone matrix-associated autologous chondrocyte transplantation ($n = 10$) and microfracture ($n = 10$). The study reported a higher cartilage GAG content, as measured by dGEMRIC, in the matrix-associated autologous chondrocyte transplantation group as compared to the microfracture group,[17] demonstrating varied response of cartilage following different types of surgeries. dGMERIC has also been used to study the efficacy of anterior cruciate ligament repair: The dGMERIC index was similar to that of surrounding cartilage approximately 1 year after anterior cruciate ligament reconstruction, suggesting the incorporation of a graft tissue. These studies demonstrate that dGEMRIC is not only useful for evaluating cartilage degeneration, but also valuable in the assessment of cartilage integrity following cartilage repair.

Overall, research studies have demonstrated that dGEMRIC may be a useful biomarker for OA, mechanical alignment, and postsurgical evaluation, demonstrating the utility of this technique for assessing the biochemical composition of cartilage.

29.4 Sodium Imaging

Sodium imaging is a novel method that has been developed to assess cartilage biochemical composition. The principals of sodium imaging rely on assessing the fixed charge density of cartilage, which decreases during cartilage degeneration. In healthy cartilage, the PGs impart a negative fixed charge density and attract positive ions into the tissue. This action provides a swelling pressure in cartilage, which contributes to its tensile and compressive mechanical properties. During cartilage degeneration in OA, PG loss occurs, thus leading to decreases in the fixed charge density of cartilage. Sodium MRI quantifies the fixed charge density using of the sodium concentration (^{23}Na) in cartilage. By quantifying fixed charge density, sodium imaging can be used to assess PG content in the cartilage.

Sodium imaging has been used to assess cartilage degeneration and has demonstrated that regions of PG loss exhibit lower signal. However, sodium imaging has several drawbacks including low signal-to-noise ratio (and thus resolution) and the requirement of specialized MRI coil hardware. To achieve adequate signal-to-noise ratio, relatively long imaging times are requires. Thus, sodium imaging for cartilage may benefit from higher magnetic fields as well as improvements in MRI coil technology.

29.5 Conclusion

This chapter discussed various MRI methods that probe early degenerative changes in cartilage biochemistry associated with OA. Quantitative MRI techniques including T2 mapping, T1rho mapping, dGEMRIC, and sodium imaging have been used to evaluate the ECM of cartilage noninvasively. Each of these techniques is unique in its inherent mechanism for cartilage assessment, and each offers a distinctive perspective in the assessment of various components to the ECM. Quantitative MRI that is sensitive to biochemical changes appears promising and may potentially provide information beyond morphological changes in articular cartilage, with regards to early cartilage degeneration and biochemistry.

References

[1] Lester G, McGowan J, Panagis J, et al. NIAMS Osteoarthritis Handout on Health. 2006. http://www.niams.nih.gov/Health_Info/Osteoarthritis/default.asp

[2] Forman MD, Malamet R, Kaplan D. A survey of osteoarthritis of the knee in the elderly. J Rheumatol 1983; 10: 282–287

[3] Peyron JG. The epidemiology of osteoathritis. In: Moskowitz R, ed. Osteoarthritis diagnosis and management. Philadelphia: W. B. Saunders; 1984:9–27

[4] Mow VC, Guo XE. Mechano-electrochemical properties of articular cartilage: their inhomogeneities and anisotropies. Annu Rev Biomed Eng 2002; 4: 175–209

[5] Watanabe A, Boesch C, Obata T, Anderson SE. Effect of multislice acquisition on T1 and T2 measurements of articular cartilage at 3T. J Magn Reson Imaging 2007; 26: 109–117

[6] Haralick RM, Shanmugam K, Dinstein I. Textural features for image classification. IEEE Trans Syst Man Cybern 1973; 3: 610–621

[7] Blumenkrantz G, Dunn TC, Carballido-Gamio J, Link TM, Majumdar S. Spatial heterogeneity of cartilage T2 in osteoarthritic patients. Paper presented at: OARSI2005; Boston, MA

[8] Carballido-Gamio J, Stahl R, Blumenkrantz G, Romero A, Majumdar S, Link TM. Spatial analysis of magnetic resonance T1rho and T2 relaxation times improves classification between subjects with and without osteoarthritis. Med Phys 2009; 36: 4059–4067

[9] Li X, Pai A, Blumenkrantz G et al. Spatial distribution and relationship of T1rho and T2 relaxation times in knee cartilage with osteoarthritis. Magn Reson Med 2009; 61: 1310–1318

[10] Duvvuri U, Reddy R, Patel SD, Kaufman JH, Kneeland JB, Leigh JS. T1rho-relaxation in articular cartilage: effects of enzymatic degradation. Magn Reson Med 1997; 38: 863–867

[11] Regatte RR, Akella SV, Borthakur A, Kneeland JB, Reddy R. In vivo proton MR three-dimensional T1rho mapping of human articular cartilage: initial experience. Radiology 2003; 229: 269–274

[12] Akella SV, Regatte RR, Gougoutas AJ et al. Proteoglycan-induced changes in T1rho-relaxation of articular cartilage at 4T. Magn Reson Med 2001; 46: 419–423

[13] Li X, Pai A, Blumenkrantz G et al. Spatial distribution and relationship of T1rho and T2 relaxation times in knee cartilage with osteoarthritis. Magn Reson Med 2009; 61: 1310–1318

[14] Burstein D, Velyvis J, Scott KT et al. Protocol issues for delayed Gd (DTPA)(2-)-enhanced MRI (dGEMRIC) for clinical evaluation of articular cartilage. Magn Reson Med 2001; 45: 36–41

[15] McKenzie CA, Williams A, Prasad PV, Burstein D. Three-dimensional delayed gadolinium-enhanced MRI of cartilage (dGEMRIC) at 1.5T and 3.0T. J Magn Reson Imaging 2006; 24: 928–933

[16] Owman H, Tiderius CJ, Neuman P, Nyquist F, Dahlberg LE. Association between findings on delayed gadolinium enhanced magnetic resonance imaging of cartilage and future knee osteoarthritis. Arthritis Rheum 2008; 58: 1727–1730

[17] Trattnig S, Mamisch TC, Pinker K et al. Differentiating normal hyaline cartilage from post-surgical repair tissue using fast gradient echo imaging in delayed gadolinium-enhanced MRI (dGEMRIC) at 3 Tesla. Eur Radiol 2008; 18: 1251–1259

30 Histochemistry Bone and Cartilage

Yan-Yiu Yu

Histological and histochemical analysis of bone are useful techniques for examining growth and development as well as diseases associated with bone. To obtain high-quality data, every step from the choice of fixative through mounting of slides can affect the final outcome of the stain quality. Unfortunately, all specimen-handling procedures may be suitable for one of the analyses but not for others. For example, the fixation and embedding step affects the histological appearance of morphological details in bone specimens, whereas it is the most problematic step for the detection of bone specimens in regard to immunohistochemistry. In this chapter, we will discuss the technical difficulties associated with different histological and histochemical stainings.

30.1 Tissue Fixation

After tissue collection, the first step of the procedure is tissue preservation for future investigation. The purpose of fixation is to stabilize the proteins in the tissues and preserve their microarchitecture for investigation. Fixatives also inhibit the growth of bacteria and molds that give rise to putrefactive changes. Currently, 10% buffered formalin, 2.5% gluteraldehyde, and alcohol fixatives are the most widely used fixatives for routine light microscopy and ultrastructural studies. However, every fixative has different capabilities for staining certain organelles and maintaining tissue integrity, and the choice of fixative should be based on the tissue being stained.

30.1.1 Fixatives

Formaldehyde (4% buffered formaldehyde, 10% buffered formalin)
- Widely used universal fixative for paraffin embedded sections
- Requires a relatively short fixation time but can also be used for long-term storage
- Produces no deleterious effects on tissue morphology with nuclear and cytoplasmic detail
- Slow penetration
- Requires fixation at temperatures of 1 to 4°C
- Fixed tissue specimen can be stored in buffer solution for many months

Alcoholic fixatives
- Include Clarke's fluid (ethanol and acetic acid, 3:1 by volume), Carnoy's fluid (ethanol, chloroform, and acetic acid, 60:30:10 by volume), and 70% ethanol diluted in acetic acid
- Better histological preservation and retain reactivity for labile lymphocyte membrane antigens

30.1.2 Factors that Affect Fixation

- Volume ratio: Ratio of the fixative volume to the tissue volume needs to be more than 10 times.
- Temperature: For standard histology, fixation can be carried out at room temperature; for electron microscopy and histochemical procedures, fixation should be done at 4°C.
- Size: Tissue blocks should either be small or thin. Recommended thickness is ≤ 3 mm.
- Time: 2 mm thick tissue blocks = 4 to 8 hours; large specimens = overnight.

30.2 Decalcification

Decalcification is usually carried out between the fixation and processing steps. The removal of calcium deposits in bone or other tissues that contain calcified areas is essential to improve sectioning and staining quality.

30.2.1 Decalcifying Agents

Mineral acids: dilute nitric or hydrochloric acid
- Fast decalcification, suitable for dense cortical bone
- Damage cellular morphology
- Not recommended for delicate tissues such as bone marrow

Organic acids: acetic acid, formic acid
- Not as harsh as mineral acid
- Damage cellular morphology if expose too long
- Suitable for bone marrow or other soft tissues
- Require longer decalcification time

Chelating agents: ethylenediaminetetraacetic acid
- Slow penetration and slow decalcification
- Take weeks for decalcification
- Better for histochemical methods

30.3 Histology and Histochemical Staining Methods

30.3.1 Hematoxylin and Eosin Stain

The hematoxylin and eosin (H&E) technique is widely used in the histopathology laboratory and is essential to demonstrate the general tissue structures, enabling recognition of malignant and nonmalignant cells as well as several intracellular and extracellular substances necessary for medical diagnosis. This staining has been used for a long time because it works well with a variety of fixatives and displays a broad range of cytoplasm, nuclear, and extracellular matrix features.

Hematoxylin is a natural dye, obtained from the heartwood of the logwood tree. It has no staining properties until it is oxidized to hematein, a compound that forms strongly colored complexes with metal ions such as iron. In H&E staining, hematoxylin stains the nuclei blue, enabling recognition of the nuclear features of different types of cells, such as malignant and nonmalignant cells. Hematoxylin can be used as a nuclear counterstain.

Eosin is a fluorescent red dye resulting from the action of bromine on fluorescein. Eosin Y is most often used as a counterstain to hematoxylin in H&E staining. It is typically used in concentration of 1 to 5% by weight volume dissolved in 1% acetic acid.

Before using a new batch of H&E solutions, a simple test should be performed for quality assurance. From that, we should be able to (1) determine the performance of each new container of stain, (2) decide suitable staining times, (3) find out how many slides can be stained satisfactorily by a given volume of each stain, (4) how many rinses should be changed, and (5) troubleshoot the cause of an observed staining problem. After staining times and stain and rinse change schedules have been determined, the use of control sections is not necessary for the remainder of the life of the particular stain that has been validated.

> ### Key Concepts: The Final Staining Pattern of Hematoxylin and Eosin
>
> - Cytoplasm: Pink to orange
> - Nuclei: Blue

Factors that Affect Hematoxylin and Eosin Stain

Rinses: The purposes of rinses include to remove paraffin, effect transition from organic solvents to aqueous solutions and vice versa, stop action of previous solution, differentially extract excess hematoxylin, convert hematoxylin from red to blue color, promote redistribution of dyes within tissues, dehydrate and clear, etc. By arbitrary means, the amount of stain that remains within cells represents the difference between what the staining solutions put in and the rinses take out.

To obtain a good H&E stain, sections must be effectively rinsed in the posteosin step. This means that there is maximum difference in concentration gradient between the dyes in the cells and the rinse. When stained tissue is immersed in clean alcohol, the dyes diffuse into the surrounding rinse. As the rinses become dye-laden, the concentration gradient is reduced and diffusion slows. When the concentration of dye in the tissue equals that in the rinse, no diffusion occurs and the benefits of rinsing are lost.

To promote effective rinsing:
- Keep the rinses deep for maximum dilution (not just simply covering the tops of the slides).
- Use a set of three.
- Dip racks at least 10 times in each.
- Change as needed. In general, once the third rinse becomes colored with carryover dye, discard the contents of the first dish, move rinses 2 and 3 back one step to become rinse 1 and 2, and refill the third dish with fresh rinse. The third dish in each series of three posteosin rinses should remain color-free. Maintaining this level of quality allows the absolute alcohols and xylene rinses to remain color-free.

Replace solution: H&E solution can be reused many times. To determine when to replace the stain solutions, it depends on (1) concentration of dye, (2) volume of staining bath, and (3) number of dips. In addition, it also depends on the thickness and the area of tissue sections.

Common Problems Seen in Hematoxylin and Eosin Stain

- Too much stain
- Too little stain
- Wrong color
- Wrong location

If there is too much stain, use a less concentrated stain for the same staining time or stain for less time with the same concentration, or vice versa. If the color and location are not properly stained, make a new batch of staining solution with the correct pH and concentration. The limitation of hematoxylin staining is that it is not compatible with immunofluorescence. However, it is useful to stain one serial paraffin section from a tissue in which immunofluorescence will be performed. Hematoxylin alone is useful as a counter-stain for many immunohistochemical or hybridization procedures that use colorimetric substance.

30.3.2 Trichrome Stain

Trichrome stain is a general term to describe a histology staining method that uses three colored dyes to differential different tissues. It is widely used to visualize fibrous tissues on tissue sections of tumors, connective tissue diseases, or musculoskeletal disorders.

The most common techniques in trichrome staining are the Gomori trichrome (one-step) and Masson trichrome (multistep). The one-step technique incorporates all of the staining solution except the mordant (Bouin's) and the nuclear stain, whereas the multistep technique utilizes all the mordants and staining solutions individually.

One-Step Technique

The one-step technique (Gomori's or Gieson's method) combines all of the staining dyes and reagents into one single solution that is applied to the specimens for a specific amount of time. The various tissues are stained differentially. As expected, this technique depends on a standardized protocol to obtain consistent results. If changes need to be made, it is recommended that one factor is changed at a time, and that all steps are recorded. Because all the dyes are in one solution, it is difficult to adjust the plasma stain over the fiber stain or vice versa. Protocol must be standardized as changing any of the parameters may result in a different staining pattern. Proper staining is reached by interrupting the progress toward equilibrium at a specified and repeatable point. Remove the specimens from the solution once the desired results are achieved.

> **Key Concepts: The Final Staining Pattern of One-Step Trichrome Stain**
>
> - Erythrocytes: Yellow or red
> - Cytoplasm, fibrin, and muscle: Red
> - Collagen: Light green

Multistep Technique

The Masson trichrome staining (▶ Fig. 30.1) is commonly used in the laboratory setting. It is used to differentiate between muscle fibers and collagen, or to demonstrate a change in the amount of collagen present. In these methods, the dyes are applied sequentially, and staining time is optimized at each step.

> **Key Concepts: The Final Staining Pattern of Multistep Trichrome Stain**
>
> - Cytoplasm, fibrin, and muscle: Red
> - Collagen and bone: Blue (aniline blue with polyacid mixture of phosphotungstic acid/phosphomolybdic acid) or green (polyacid phosphotungstic acid)—depends on the collagen stain utilized

Factors that Affect Trichrome Stain

Fixation and preparation: Treatment with a picric acid solution such as Bouin's after formalin fixation will enhance staining intensity and radiance. Other fixatives such as Bouin's formalin and picro-mercuric alcohol are recommended. Optimal staining can be achieved by using tissue sections of 5 to 10 µm.

pH: Staining solutions prepared in low pH solvent is recommended. In general, staining dye is diluted in aqueous acetic acid. Usually, the concentration of acetic acid matches the concentration of dye (1% dye in 1% acid). The acid pH can help to maximize the amount of dye that will attach to tissue amino groups.

Molecule size of the dyes: Fixative agents react with protein components of a tissue and result in changing tissue permeability. To obtain a better staining, a smaller dye molecule is recommended because it can penetrate and stain a tissue element better.

Utilization of phosphotungstic and phosmolybdic acids: Phosphotungstic and phosmolybdic acids both act as conventional acidifying agents that can optimize collagen staining. These acids can be utilized:

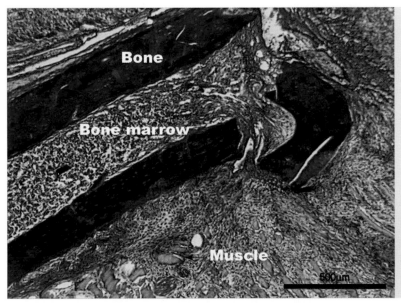

Fig. 30.1 Trichrome staining of fracture callus (a murine tibia fracture).

1. Before treatment with small molecule dye.
2. Combined in solution with the small molecular dye.
3. Before treatment with the large molecule dye.

However, the treatment needs to be stopped at a proper time in order for the collagen to stain when treated with a large molecule dye in the following step.

30.3.3 Safranin-O Stain

Safranin-O staining has been used to demonstrate changes that occur in articular disease. This method is used for the detection of cartilage, mucin, and mast cell granules on tissue sections. Safranin-O is a basic dye that stains acidic proteoglycan present in cartilage tissues. The intensity of safranin-O staining is directly proportional to the proteoglycan content. Fast green is a common contrast stain for safranin-O and strongly stains noncollagen sites. ▶ Fig. 30.2 demonstrates a safranin-O staining with fast green contrast stain.

Key Concepts: The Staining Pattern of Safranin-O Stain

- Cartilage: Red
- Mucin: Orange
- Nuclei: Black
- Background: Bluish green

It is important to choose the correct fixative and decalcifying agent when preparing the specimens. Prolonged exposure to decalcifying agents such as ethylenediaminetetraacetic acid may extract proteoglycans from the tissue and lead to loss of staining. A normal undecalcified articular cartilage should be used as a positive control to show any extraction of proteoglycans by decalcifiers along with the decalcified cartilage.

30.3.4 Fluorochrome Labeling

Fluorochromes are calcium-binding substances that are preferentially taken up at the site of active mineralization of bone, including a site of bone formation or dentin deposition, and also hypertrophic cartilage in the growth plate. They are detected using either epifluorescence or fluorescence microscopy on undecalcified sections. Fluorochrome labeling provides a means to investigate the dynamics of bone formation. By using double or triple sequential labeling, we can detect the rate and extent of bone deposition and resorption during skeletal development and bone regeneration. ▶ Table 30.1 shows the overview of four frequently used groups of fluorochromes.

Sample Preparation

Samples can be fixed in 10% neutral buffer formalin or 4% paraformaldehyde. For larger specimens, a combination of 4% glutaraldehyde and 5% paraformaldehyde is recommended. Samples can be followed with the standard dehydration steps without affecting the staining. However, decalcification should be avoided because it dissolves the fluorochrome label from the bone. To obtain better sections, polymethylmethacrylate embedding is recommended.

Autofluorescence and Photobleaching

Autofluorescence seems to be an issue when immunofluorescene staining is performed. However, it is not a problem when we perform fluorochrome because it is

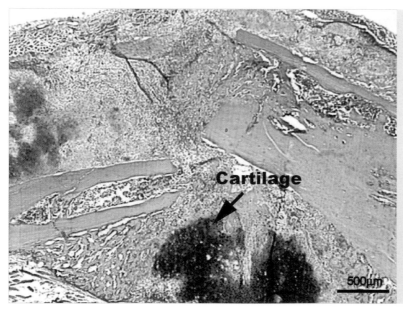

Fig. 30.2 Safranin-O staining of fracture callus (a murine tibia fracture).

Table 30.1 Overview of Four Frequently Used Groups of Fluorochromes

	Solvent	Dosage (mg/kg)	Excitation wavelength (nm)	Emission wavelength (nm)
Tetracyclines	Distilled water, pH 6.0–6.5	25	365–436	570
Calcein green	2% NaHCO3	10	436–495	517–540
Xylenol orange	1% NaHCO3	80	377–570	610–615
Alizarin complexone/red	Distilled water or 2% NaHCO3	25–30	530–580	600–645

not confined to specific regions of bone and can thus clearly be distinguished from the distinct bands that are characteristic for fluorochrome labeling. Photobleaching is the decrease in fluorescence intensity with time under constant exposure to the light used for excitation. Different fluorochromes have different intrinsic photobleaching characteristics, and this process is affected differently depending on the light source used for excitation. In general, photobleaching is not a problem when the samples are properly stored in standard nontransparent boxes.

Further Reading

Bancroft J, Gamble M. Theory and practice of histological techniques. 6 e. London: Churchill-Livingstone; 2008

Blomquist L, Hanngren A. Fluorescence technique applied to whole body sections for distribution studies of tetracyclines. Biochem Pharmacol 1966; 15: 215–219

Carson FL. Histotechnology: a self-instruction text. 2 e. Chicago: ASCP Press; 1997

Lee TC, Mohsin S, Taylor D et al. Detecting microdamage in bone. J Anat 2003; 203: 161–172

Lee TC, Staines A, Taylor D. Bone adaptation to load: microdamage as a stimulus for bone remodelling. J Anat 2002; 201: 437–446

Pautke C, Vogt S, Tischer T et al. Polychrome labeling of bone with seven different fluorochromes: enhancing fluorochrome discrimination by spectral image analysis. Bone 2005; 37: 441–445

Solheim T. Pluricolor fluorescent labeling of mineralizing tissue. Scand J Dent Res 1974; 82: 19–27

31 Immunohistochemistry

Wing-Hoi Cheung and Simon Kwoon Ho Chow

The word "immunohistochemistry" (IHC) is composed of "immuno-," "histo-," and "chemistry," which refer to the application of immunological techniques to the chemical analysis of cells and tissue sections. IHC is a laboratory technique to make use of antibodies with high specificity and subsequently a color-based detection system to identify target antigens of cells of a tissue section.

IHC has wide applications in laboratories and clinical diagnosis, including characterization and localization of particular cells (e.g., platelet endothelial cell adhesion molecule or vascular endothelial growth factor for endothelial cells), diagnosis of abnormal cells (e.g., CD68 for giant cell tumor of bone), and identification of some cell events (e.g., cleaved Caspase 3 for apoptosis).

31.1 Basic Protocol[1]

31.1.1 Materials

1. Reagents: 0.01 M phosphate buffered saline (PBS, pH 7.4), bovine serum albumin, xylene, ethanol, 0.1% trypsin, microwave antigen retrieval solution (for heat method), primary antibody, secondary antibody, 3% hydrogen peroxide (H_2O_2), enzyme substrate (e.g., for peroxidase: avidin-biotin complex [ABC] kit, diaminobenzidine [DAB]), Mayer's hematoxylin
2. Materials: Paraffin-embedded tissue sections, microwave-resistant plastic staining container
3. Equipment: Microwave oven, light microscope

31.1.2 Methods

1. Removal of paraffin and rehydration
   - Dewax sections in xylene with two changes, 10 minutes each.
   - Rehydrate sections in graded ethanol (from 100 to 25%, 5 minutes each).
   - Rinse the slides in running tap water for 30 seconds.
   - Replace in PBS wash bath for further rehydration (30 minutes, room temperature).
2. Antigen retrieval (either enzymatic digestion or heat-based)
   - Enzymatic digestion: Place slides in 0.1% trypsin in 0.1% $CaCl_2$ (pH 7.8) and incubate them at 37°C for 30 minutes. Rinse slides with 1 × PBS three times.
   - Heat-based: Wash the slides with deionized water and place them in a microwave-resistant plastic staining container with the slides fully covered by antigen retrieval solution. Operate the microwave oven at high power for 5 minutes; this process can be repeated two to three times. Cool down the slides at room temperature for at least 20 minutes.
3. Inactivation of endogenous peroxidase
   - Place slides in 3% H_2O_2 in PBS at room temperature for 10 minutes.
   - Wash slides with 1 × PBS three times.
4. Blocking
   - Cover slides with 3% bovine serum albumin and 5 to 10% normal serum (from the same species as the host of the secondary antibody) at room temperature for 1 hour or at 4°C overnight in a humid box, prior to primary antibody application.
5. Primary antibody reaction
   - Drain the slides and carefully wipe each slide using a paper towel.
   - Dilute the primary antibody or negative control reagent in diluent to an optimal dilution, while diluent alone can serve as a negative control. A positive control slide (a tissue known to have the target antigen) should also be run.
   - Apply 100 μL primary antibody solution to cover the tissue sections and make sure the solution is evenly spread on the slides.
   - Incubate at 37°C for 60 minutes, at room temperature for 2 hours, or at 4°C overnight in humidified chamber. Longer incubation may be needed for low-density antigens.
   - Wash slides three times in 1 × PBS for 3 minutes each.
6. Secondary antibody reaction
   - Drain the slides and carefully wipe each slide using a paper towel.
   - Dilute the biotinylated secondary antibody in diluent to an optimal dilution.
   - Apply 100 μL secondary antibody solution to cover the tissue sections and make sure the solution is evenly spread on the slides.
   - Incubate at room temperature for 1 hour in humidified chamber.
   - Wash slides three times in 1 × PBS for 3 minutes each.
7. Color development
   - Prepare ABC reagent according to manufacturer's instructions and apply to cover the sections. (Note: If secondary antibody is conjugated with peroxidase, ABC kit can be skipped; jump to DAB application.)
   - Incubate in a humidified chamber at room temperature for 30 minutes.
   - Wash slides three times in 1 × PBS for 3 minutes each.
   - Place slides in freshly prepared DAB solution and keep in dark for 2 minutes or longer to develop the color.
   - Wash the slides with deionized distilled water to stop the reaction.

8. Counterstain
   - Using hematoxylin: Wash the slides with distilled water, place slides in hematoxylin at room temperature for 0.5 to 5 minutes (depending on strength of hematoxylin), rinse with distilled water, incubate slides in 0.5% NH_4OH (v/v) for 20 seconds, and rinse with tap water.
   - Using methyl green: Wash the slides with distilled water, place slides in methyl green for 1.5 minutes at room temperature, rinse with distilled water, and dip slides 5 to 10 times in acetone with 0.05% acetic acid (v/v).
9. Mounting
   - Dehydrate sections in graded ethanol (from 80 to 100%, 1 minute each).
   - Mount slides with hydrophobic mountant.

31.2 Considerations of Antibodies

31.2.1 Choice of Antibodies: Polyclonal versus Monoclonal

Antibodies play critical roles in the success of IHC and therefore a careful selection of antibodies is essential. Antibodies information can be easily retrieved from online search engines and antibody manufacturers' websites. The first and most common question for the choice of antibodies is the decision between polyclonal antibodies (pAbs) and monoclonal antibodies (mAbs). There is, however, no absolute answer for this question, as this is determined by many factors. The most important one is its intended use and whether the antibody is readily available from commercial suppliers or researchers. In the meantime, the researchers should learn some facts about pAbs and mAbs (▶ Table 31.1).

31.2.2 Polyclonal Antibodies

pAbs are produced by inoculation of animals and derived from different types of immune cells. The animals used are usually rabbits, mice, goats, chicken, horses, and guinea pigs, etc., where rabbits and mice are mostly used (pAbs raised from rabbits usually have higher affinity than from mice). The production cost of pAbs is relatively low and the time scale is short. pAbs have the features of recognizing multiple epitopes on an antigen. Therefore, pAbs show the following advantages and disadvantages.

Advantages: (1) more robust detection due to less sensitive to minor changes in the antigen, (2) a preferred option for denatured proteins, (3) may amplify signals from the antigens with low expression.

Disadvantages: (1) not useful for probing specific domain of antigen, (2) relatively high batch-to-batch variability, (3) may give high background signals due to certain extent of nonspecificity.

31.2.3 Monoclonal Antibodies

mAbs are produced by hybrid cells (hybridoma; i.e., mammalian cells fused with endlessly replicating tumor cells) and derived from a single cell line, whereas mouse and rabbit mAbs are more common. The production cost of mAbs is expensive and the time scale for hybridomas is long. mAbs have the feature of recognizing one epitope on an antigen. Therefore, mAbs show the following advantages and disadvantages.

Advantages: (1) high purity and good consistency when all batches are identical, (2) usually give rise to low background signals due to low cross-reaction with other proteins, (3) can generate reproducible results due to high homogeneity.

Disadvantages: (1) more sensitive to the minor changes in the antigen but this can be improved by using two or more monoclonal antibodies recognizing different epitopes on the same antigen, (2) may be too specific and therefore cannot detect antigens across different species, (3) not preferable for the antigens with low expression.

Apart from these considerations, some precautions should be taken into account when choosing primary and secondary antibodies. Primary antibody host that is the same as the tissue being studied should be avoided because the conjugated secondary antibody against the primary antibody may generate high background signals due to potential cross-reactivity (e.g., primary antibody against a rat protein should not be raised from rat or mouse). Instead, the secondary antibodies host should be the same species as the primary antibody being used. Also, researchers should pay attention to different forms of secondary antibodies, which can be either whole immunoglobulin G, $F(ab')_2$ fragments, and Fab fragments. The whole immunoglobulin G is suitable for most IHC experiments and is most cost-effective, whereas $F(ab')_2$ and Fab fragments can provide better signal-to-noise ratios and

Table 31.1 Polyclonal Antibody versus Monoclonal Antibody

	Polyclonal	Monoclonal
Source	Multiple cell types	Single cell type
Detection	Multiple epitopes	Single epitope
Pros	High robustness	High specificity and reproducibility
Cons	Low specificity High variability and background signal	Low signal strength

sensitivity due to their smaller size and faster diffusion through tissues. Sometimes, pAbs are preadsorbed with serum from various species in order to significantly reduce the cross-reactivity, which is a recommended choice.

31.3 Considerations of Antigen Retrieval

IHC relies on a good immunoreaction between antigens and antibodies. However, the sample fixation process usually affects the protein conformation, leading to partial or complete loss of immunoreactivity. Formalin fixation produces cross-links between the proteins, particularly those formalin-sensitive proteins, and mAbs are more sensitive to the minor changes of antigens. Therefore, an antigen retrieval technique is required to expose the epitopes of target antigens in order to facilitate the binding to antibodies. It was reported that 84% of antibodies needed some type of antigen retrieval for optimal results.[2] Antigen retrieval can reverse some conformational changes and there are two commonly used protocols: enzymatic digestion and heat-based. A combination of these two methods (steam heat with ethylene-diamine-tetraacetic acid buffer and protease digestion) was also reported for antigen retrieval in prostatic epithelium.

31.3.1 Enzymatic Digestion

This is a more conventional approach of antigen retrieval in IHC. The enzymes include trypsin, pepsin, ficin, proteinase K, etc. This method depends on the enzyme concentration, pH, temperature, and exposure time. The disadvantage is the possible risk of damaging some epitopes because the mechanism of action is nonspecific protein digestion.[2] Therefore, fine tuning of the settings may be needed when there is lot-to-lot variation of enzyme purchased. The enzyme digestion time is inversely related to the fixation time.

31.3.2 Heat-based

This is a newer approach of antigen retrieval. This method depends on temperature, pH, and incubation duration. The heat-based procedure requires antigen retrieval solution to cover the slides, and the solution is available with a wide range of pH from many commercial companies. It was recommended to heat the solution at high temperature for a short period rather than low temperature for a longer time.[2] A microwave oven, autoclave, or water bath may be used. The microwave approach can be performed for a short period and repeated for a few times. Heating should be followed

with a cooling process that should take around 20 to 30 minutes. The mechanism is unknown yet Van Hecke reported it to be through hydrolysis of methylene cross-links.[3] Also, researchers need to pay attention to the relationship between fixation and heat-based antigen retrieval, as it was reported that unfixed proteins might be denatured at 70 to 90°C but denaturation could be avoided when the proteins were fixed in formaldehyde solution.[4]

> **Jargon Simplified: Antigen Retrieval**
>
> Antigen retrieval is the heat-induced or enzymatic process that is used to break the cross-links created by formalin fixation in order to expose the antigen for immunoreactivity.

31.4 Considerations of Detection System

The last critical procedure of IHC is the labeling and detection system, which can facilitate the visualization of the signals under microscope. The most common labels in the market are enzymes (e.g., peroxidase, alkaline phosphatase, etc.) that will generate color precipitates in the presence of an appropriate substrate/chromogen. This can be divided into direct and indirect methods (▶ Table 31.2).

31.4.1 Direct Methods

This is a one-step procedure to apply an enzyme-labeled primary antibody to react with the antigen, followed with substrate/chromogen reaction. This method offers the following advantages and disadvantages.

Table 31.2 Direct and Indirect Detection Systems of Immunohistochemistry

	Direct	Indirect
Characteristics	One-step labeled primary antibody	Two steps of unlabeled primary antibody and labeled secondary antibody
Advantage	• Simple and quick • Reduced problems created by the secondary antibodies	• Higher sensitivity
Disadvantage	• Lower sensitivity • Limited availability of labeled primary antibodies	• Higher background signal due to nonspecific bindings of secondary antibodies

Advantages: (1) simple and can be performed quickly, (2) nonspecific binding from secondary antibodies and crossover problems are minimal.

Disadvantages: (1) signal amplification is not allowed, (2) sensitivity may not be sufficient.

With these characteristics, a direct method is applicable when using antibodies with high avidity and for localization of high-density antigens (> 10,000 molecules/cell).[2] This is not a commonly used approach nowadays, and there may not be suitably labeled primary antibodies available commercially.

31.4.2 Indirect Methods

This is a two-step procedure and was developed to increase sensitivity. The method is to apply an unlabeled primary antibody to bind antigen, followed with a secondary antibody labeled with an enzyme, or biotin or fluorophores. This method provides the following advantages and disadvantages.

Advantages: (1) higher sensitivity due to signal amplification, (2) suitable for specimens with low-expression antigens.

Disadvantages: (1) nonspecific reactions may occur if the secondary antibodies cross-react with tissue specimen (can be minimized by using preadsorbed secondary antiserum), (2) may generate high background signals.

With the feature of signal amplification, the indirect method is more commonly used and is recommended for low-density antigens (> 2,000, < 10,000 molecules/cell). Among signal amplification methods, the (Strept) avidin-biotin method is most common. Avidin is a glycoprotein with four binding sites per molecule and high affinity to biotin, thus increasing the sensitivity. ABC is a popular and widely used detection system for IHC. However, avidin may bind to lectins and negatively charged tissues nonspecifically, leading to high background. Avidin is therefore replaced by streptavidin produced by the bacterium *Streptomyces avidinii*. Another commonly used avidin-biotin method is the labeled avidin-biotin or labeled streptavidin-biotin method, which uses a biotinylated secondary antibody and a third reagent of peroxidase (or alkaline phosphatase)-labeled avidin; the sensitivity is higher than the ABC method.[2]

31.4.3 Counterstain

Counterstain is the final step of IHC, and hematoxylin (blue) or methyl green (green) are commonly used ones. The key point to selecting a correct counterstain is to provide a good contrast with the chromogen precipitates. A poor selection of counterstain may cause a difficult analysis of IHC signals by image analysis software that depends on the hue, saturation, and brightness (HSV) system to distinguish the color.

31.5 Considerations of Immunohistochemistry Signal Quantification

31.5.1 Precautions

- To ensure IHC signals are quantified with high precision, reliability, and a fair comparison between groups, images must be captured with consistent and even distribution of light. Too dark or too bright of an image could reduce the clarity and detail of the IHC signal. Blankfield subtraction is recommended to reduce inconsistency across images; this function is usually available within the image-acquire software provided.
- Consistency in magnification is also important for spatial calibration. This is usually precalibrated by the technician during the installation of the microscope and the associated software. Insertion of a scale bar is often available in most software programs.
- Avoid capturing images with different microscopes with different light sources and different optical pieces for the consistency of brightness and intensity of the IHC signals.
- White-balancing should be performed either during image capturing within the microscope software or during later image processing procedures.
- Prior to capturing the first image, researchers are recommended to visually scan through all specimens both by the naked eye and under the microscope to identify any inconsistency and the best microscope settings for image capture.

31.5.2 Choices of Software

After image capturing under the microscope, the images are processed for the subsequent quantification of the IHC signal by image analysis software. There are a number of choices depending on their availability at the researcher's institute. The following is a list of the most popular and powerful image analysis software programs that are either available as paid-license software or freeware. Some of these also have specialized plugins available for automated IHC signal quantification.

- Image-Pro Plus (Media Cybernetics, Bethesda, MD)
- MetaMorph (Molecular Devices, Sunnyvale, CA)
- ImageJ (Wayne Rasband, National Institute of Health, Bethesda, MD)
- Photoshop (Adobe Systems Incorporated, San Jose, CA)

31.5.3 Basic Image Processing and Segmentation

Segmentation is a procedure carried out to select and localize the IHC stained signals based on differences in color between the signal and the counterstain. The most common way to achieve this purpose is by thresholding. Thresholding is typically performed by adjusting or selecting a specific range in the HSB to include as your region of interest (ROI).[5] The hue, saturation, and brightness are three axes in a three-dimensional spectrum that can be visualized as a cylindrical shaped spectrum.

Hue is a description of color with respect to the characteristic colors of red, green, blue, and yellow, commonly presented in a circular polar coordinate or in a 360-degree palette (with rainbow colors in radial distribution). Adjustment in the hue would rotate the degree in the polar coordinate such that the palette of colors are turned, and transform all colors in the image to the same degree to a different color in the visible spectrum. Saturation is a description of the intensity of colorfulness away from white (at the center) along another axis (to the outside) in the three-dimensional spectrum to the specific color in the hue.[6] Finally, the brightness is the vertical axis in the three-dimensional spectrum that determines how far away the color is from total darkness or black. Therefore, segmentation using HSB thresholding is the selection of a subset of colors within this three-dimensional spectrum to include as the ROI.[5] See the sample screenshot showing the adjustment sliders (▶ Fig. 31.1) and the before and after images after HSB thresholding to select the areas stained with DAB (*brown*) signals (▶ Fig. 31.2a,b).

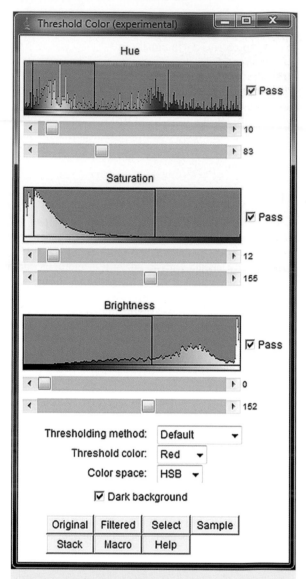

Fig. 31.1 Sample ImageJ dialogue box of the hue, saturation, and brightness sliders. Each thresholding parameter is presented with a gradient of 255 levels.

Jargon Simplified: Segmentation

Segmentation is the thresholding procedure carried out to select the pixels corresponding to the IHC stained signals for later quantification.

31.5.4 Quantification of Immunohistochemistry Signals

After segmentation and selection of the IHC signals, common ways to quantify and analyze these signals depend on the objective of the experiment. For example, some common ways include evaluating the area of stained tissue versus unstained tissue, measuring the signal intensity to investigate the expression quantity of a certain protein in a specific area, and the cell counts of stained nuclei are often the most common objectives.

The area of the IHC signals can be automatically measured by the image analysis software of choice, or the percentage of IHC stained area expressed per ROI area can be computed manually at a later time. An exportable result table presented would typically consist of the following quantitative measurements for the image analyzed:
- Total segmented pixel area or number
- Percentage of segmented area to total image area
- Maximum, minimum, and mean intensities
- Total number of elements
- The mean size of the elements

Different software would implement different rules of counting the segmented area, including the outline options, object-fill options, and size limits of each element. These operator- and application-specific parameters vary from software to software, and the robustness of each is determined greatly by these algorithms. Software distributors provide detailed descriptions in the form of online documentation or tutorials. These settings must also be standardized and performed on all images in the experiment to ensure consistency of the results and fair comparison.

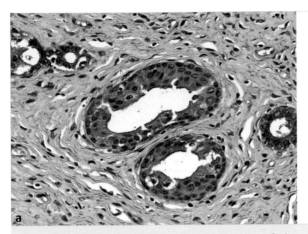 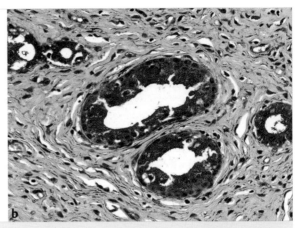

Fig. 31.2 (a) Immunohistochemistry of estrogen receptor-β, diaminobenzidine detection system, on Sprague Dawley rat uterus, captured at 400× magnification by the Leica DFC-495. (b) After hue, saturation, and brightness thresholding, diaminobenzidine signal is selected and highlighted in *red*. The selection can be quantified further for the area, intensity, or number of particles/cells.

31.5.5 Automated Work Flow

There are also many apps, macros, or plugins shared or distributed in the scientific community written for common or popular analytical tasks that consist of highly repetitive and tedious procedures. One example for this type of automated algorithm for the purpose of IHC quantification is the DAB Analysis App for the ImagePro Premier. These types of apps, macros, or plugins are often distributed along with the image analysis software for free, or shared by other scientists working in the same field who have published the related method in detailed descriptions so that the end-user or researcher would be able to understand the procedures and be able to manipulate and fine-tune the method. Once the protocol for processing the images has been preliminarily determined, more programming-experienced researchers may also record their own macros in the image analysis software programs to automate these steps to streamline the work flow from image enhancement to data export.

31.6 Considerations of Immunohistochemistry Result Interpretation

IHC is a staining protocol with multiple steps, where every step may cause problems; therefore, results interpretation should be careful. It is highly recommended to have both positive and negative controls run with every IHC experiment. The results from sample tissues, in comparison with the controls, will provide a more reliable interpretation. Misinterpretation is usually caused by false-positive and false-negative results.

31.6.1 False Positive

False-positive results may be caused by (1) nonspecific binding and cross-reaction of antibodies to other antigens, though preadsorbed antiserum may help to reduce the problem; (2) nonspecific attachment of conjugated antibodies to free aldehyde groups introduced by aldehyde-containing fixatives[2]; (3) inadequate quenching of endogenous peroxidase that may generate false signals; and (4) nonspecific binding of detection system (e.g., ABC), though this can be prevented by using ABC or labeled avidin-biotin solutions at pH 9.4 instead of pH 7.6 where the high pH does not affect the previous binding of primary antibodies or the affinity of avidin to biotin.

31.6.2 False Negative

False-negative results may be caused by (1) underfixation of samples, through which target antigens are lost due to degradation (therefore, all samples that will be used for IHC should be quickly fixed to reduce the ischemic time[2]; (2) overfixation of samples that may generate many cross-links, which can be improved by antigen retrieval procedure or corrected by soaking tissue in concentrated ammonia plus 20% chloral hydrate[2]; (3) insufficient antigen retrieval; and (4) inappropriate and inadequate use of antibodies and detection system, which can be improved by careful antibody concentration optimization and comparison with negative and positive controls.

References

[1] Leung KS, Qin YX, Cheung WH, Qin L, eds. A practical manual for musculoskeletal research. Singapore: World Scientific Publishing Co. Pte Ltd. Singapore; 2008

[2] Ramos-Vara JA. Technical aspects of immunohistochemistry. Vet Pathol 2005; 42: 405–426

[3] Van Hecke D. Routine immunohistochemical staining today: choices to make, challenges to take. J Histotechnol. 2002;25:45-54

[4] Mason JT, O'Leary TJ. Effects of formaldehyde fixation on protein secondary structure: a calorimetric and infrared spectroscopic investigation. J Histochem Cytochem. 1991;39(2):225-9

[5] Ruifrok AC, Katz RL, Johnston DA. Comparison of quantification of histochemical staining by hue-saturation-intensity (HSI) transformation and color-deconvolution. Appl Immunohistochem Mol Morphol 2003; 11: 85–91

[6] Levkowitz Haim. Color theory and modeling for computer graphics, visualization, and multimedia applications. Boston: Kluwer Academic Publishers, 1997

Further Reading

Abcam. Author resources. http://www.abcam.com/index.html?pageconfig=resource&rid=112698&pid=11287 Accessed November 7, 2012

Buchwalow IB, Bocker W, eds. Immunohistochemistry: basics and methods. Berlin: Springer; 2010

Sigma-Aldrich. Author resources. http://www.sigmaaldrich.com/life-science/cell-biology/antibodies/antibodies-application/protocols/immunohistochemistry.html Accessed November 5, 2012

32 Molecular Imaging In Situ Hybridization

Kishan Sokhi Aldridge and Roland Aldridge

Molecular genetics describes the study of gene structure and function at its most basic level; it includes determination of the coding sequence itself, the transmission of this genetic information from deoxyribonucleic acid (DNA) to ribonucleic acid (RNA) to polypeptide, and the regulation of these processes. This introduction to molecular genetics provides a synopsis of these mechanisms. The chapter describes a number of techniques commonly used to study genes, including sequencing, molecular cloning, and hybridization. It aims to provide an introduction to the applications of these techniques in the study of genes and their functions. In doing so, it gives an overview of the paradigm shift in recent years from traditional Sanger sequencing to next-generation sequencing (NGS). Molecular cloning, a method used to amplify a defined DNA fragment to obtain multiple identical copies, commonly used to study gene function, will be discussed. Finally, examples of the many usages of nucleic acid hybridization such as fluorescent in situ hybridization, tissue in situ hybridization, and array comparative genomic hybridization are outlined.

32.1 The Genetic Code

A gene may be defined as a heritable unit occupying a specific locus within the genome; it contains the DNA sequence to direct the formation of a protein or RNA of functional importance. A gene is composed of regulatory sequences, such as the promoter and enhancer regions, that drive gene expression on apposite stimuli. Within the transcribed region of the gene, there are introns interspersed with exons. Introns are those regions that are removed by splicing following transcription in the formation of the mature RNA. An exon, in contrast, refers to any nucleotide sequence remaining in the mature RNA; in the case of messenger RNA (mRNA), it is this product that will act as the template for translation into proteins. However, not all of the exonic sequence will be translated into protein because there is typically a 5' (upstream) untranslated region and a 3' (downstream) untranslated region in the first and last exons.

The DNA polymer forms the foundation of the genetic code and is constructed by the covalent linking of nucleotides. A nucleotide consists of a five-carbon sugar, a phosphate group, and a nitrogenous base. There are four nitrogenous bases: two purines, adenine and guanine, and two pyrimidines, cysteine and thiamine. The sequence of these nucleotides encodes the genetic information.

The double helix DNA molecule exists as two strands held together by the hydrogen bonds that form between a complementary purine and pyrimidine: adenine pairs with thiamine and guanine pairs with cysteine (▶ Fig. 32.1). The sense or coding strand, termed the Crick strand, provides the sequence of the RNA to be transcribed, whereas its complementary antisense or noncoding strand, termed the Watson strand, provides the template on which RNA is constructed.

The structure of RNA is very similar to that of DNA with a linear backbone of repeating phosphate and five-carbon sugar units, with each unit attached to a nitrogenous base. However, most RNA is single stranded. In addition, the ribose sugar residue in RNA possesses a hydroxyl group at the 2' carbon compared to the hydrogen atom in DNA. RNA shares three out of four nucleotides with DNA; the thiamine is replaced with uracil. Mature mRNA exits the nucleus and moves to the ribosome where its genetic code is translated. The code is read as triplicates of nucleotides, termed codons, commencing from the initiation codon AUG, encoding a methionine. Translation will usually start at the first initiation codon in the sequence; however, the surrounding sequence must conform to the Kozak consensus sequence (in eukaryotes) in order to be correctly identified as the translational start site by the ribosome. There are 64 codons, each of which codes either one of the 20 standard amino acids or a sequence terminating stop codon. This process forms the polypeptide, which may then be required to undergo a series of posttranslational modifications in order to correctly perform its function.

32.2 Genetic Variation

Genetic variation within the human genome underlies a significant portion of the phenotypic variation among individuals. A genetic variant can be considered neutral if it does not cause any phenotypic consequence or functional if it imparts an altered phenotype. A functional genetic variant that causes or leads to an increased susceptibility to a disease is considered pathogenic. In single gene disorders, monogenic conditions, it is easier to identify overtly pathogenic variants, whereas in complex polygenic disorders the influence of genetic variation is more subtle.

Genetic variants may be grouped into different subclasses; these include single nucleotide polymorphisms (SNPs), deletions, insertions, translocations, and inversions. The effect of any of these variants depends to a significant extent on their location within the genome and the downstream effects on protein expression, structure, and function.

SNPs are the most common source of genetic variation within the human genome, with an SNP predicted to occur every 1 in 300 nucleotides. An SNP is a nucleotide position within the genome at which one of two or occasionally three bases may be found. These variants may be

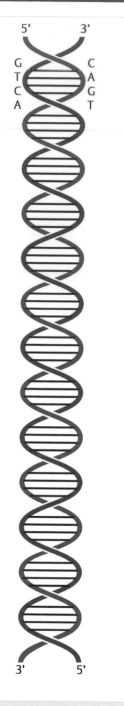

5'   3'

G   C
T   A
C   G
A   T

3'   5'

Fig. 32.1 The double helix deoxyribonucleic acid molecule exists as two strands held together by the hydrogen bonds that form between a complementary purine and pyrimidine: Adenine pairs with thiamine and guanine pairs with cysteine.

sequence but may not affect the amino acid sequence of the protein; these variants are termed synonymous. These synonymous variants may still be pathogenic if they cause anomalous splice sites. SNPs that alter both DNA and amino acid sequence are termed nonsynonymous. Nonsynonymous variants may be missense when the amino acid is changed to another amino acid or nonsense, which occurs when a premature stop site is inserted. There are databases of all known SNPs within the human genome that are easily accessible. Large population studies termed genome-wide association studies commonly use microarrays with up to 3 million known SNPs to examine for association between these variations and human traits (e.g., height) or complex polygenic disease.

Insertions and deletions result in either the gain or loss of nucleotides within the genome. These sequence changes vary in size. Deletions or insertions of single nucleotides within coding regions will cause a frameshift in codon sequence most commonly resulting in a premature stop codon. Large deletions or insertions can result in the loss or duplication of whole genes or groups of genes.

32.3 Sequencing

Gene sequencing has undergone a paradigm shift in recent years. Fredrick Sanger first described his chain termination method for sequencing DNA in 1977 and since then this method has been virtually the sole technique used in genetic sequencing. It was Sanger sequencing that was used to sequence the entire human genome. However, in the last decade, NGS methods have been developed; these methods are also termed massively parallel sequencing, due to the millions of sequencing reactions that occur simultaneously. This advance allows much greater capacity and speed of sequencing while decreasing costs. The developments in sequencing technology have been complemented by advances in bioinformatics in order to analyze the large datasets obtained.

32.3.1 Sanger Sequencing

Sanger sequencing requires a single-strand DNA template upon which DNA polymerase is used to synthesize the complimentary strand in vitro. Using the Sanger sequencing technique, four reactions are set up simultaneously each containing the four deoxynucleotides (dATP, dCTP, dGTP, dTTP) required for DNA synthesis and one of four chain terminating dideoxynucleotides. Dideoxynucleotides are analogous to deoxynucleotides except they lack the hydroxyl group on the 3' carbon required for polymerization and therefore when incorporated will terminate strand elongation. The stochastic incorporation of a dideoxynucleotide, rather than its corresponding deoxynucleotide, will terminate elongation. Identifying the positions of termination by size of the strand will identify the nucleotide present at sequential positions.

common or rare and may be functional or neutral. SNPs may influence gene function through effects on regulatory sequences, intronic sequences with effects on splicing, or exonic sequences. An SNP within the exonic protein-coding region of a gene will result in altered DNA

32.3.2 Next-Generation Sequencing

There are multiple different NGS platforms available, utilizing different technologies, and the field continues to advance rapidly. Despite this, there are commonalities between many of the NGS systems. The majority of the systems require library preparation by the random fragmentation of sample DNA to generate sequences of the appropriate length for the platform. These sequences are then end repaired and short sequences, termed adaptor sequences, are ligated to the ends of the strands. The library is then amplified on a fixed surface; this amplification step spatially separates library fragments to create clusters of amplified template from an individual DNA fragment, each on a separate bead or at a single locus on a glass slide. This spatial separation allows localization of individual fragment reads, whereas the amplification enables the output of nucleotide incorporation to be of sufficient magnitude to be detected.

The majority of NGS systems operate through sequencing by synthesis (i.e., it is recorded each time a nucleotide is incorporated into the newly synthesized chain). This is more efficient than traditional techniques, which separate the synthesis reaction and the sequence determination. Individual nucleotides are sequentially applied to the platform, and, where incorporated into an elongating polymer, this is detected and recorded at each discrete locus. This produces reads (strings of bases) that can be reassembled on a reference sequence to determine origin. In addition, multiplexing allows a number of DNA libraries to be sequenced simultaneously through addition of a distinct "barcode" sequence to each library. This barcode sequence will be appended to each individual sequence read, so they can be accurately ascribed to the different libraries. Several of the NGS technologies currently in use are summarized in the following; this is not exhaustive, and the field remains dynamic.

Sequencing by Synthesis

Pyrosequencing relies on the emission of a pyrophosphate group from the elongating chain during nucleotide incorporation. This pyrophosphate is used for the creation of adenosine triphosphate (ATP) by the enzyme ATP sulphurylase in the presence of adenosine 5-phosphosulphate; the ATP then interacts with the enzyme luciferase to emit light.

Ion semiconductor sequencing is similar to pyrosequencing except it utilizes the release of a hydrogen ion during DNA polymer elongation. The platform uses a semiconductor chip to detect alterations in pH upon hydrogen ion release.

Sequencing by reversible terminator chemistry is utilized by the Illumina HiSeq (San Diego, CA); this is one of the most commonly used platforms due to its speed and efficiency. Unique flowcell technology utilizes a bridge amplification technique to form clusters of the individual library fragments. The sequencing by synthesis chemistry operates through the addition of all four nucleotides simultaneously; each has a different fluorophore attached to the external phosphate group. The fluorophore is cleaved off by the DNA polymerase after detection and therefore will not cause background or stereo chemical inhibition to elongation. There is a block at the 3' hydroxyl group to ensure detection and cleavage of the fluorophore prior to any subsequent base incorporation.

Single molecule real-time sequencing does not use an amplification step but records the real-time incorporation of individual fluorescently labeled nucleotides to a single sequence complexed to DNA polymerase on a smart cell. The smart cell contains multiple zero-mode wavelength guides on which a camera focuses with resolution sufficient to detect single nucleotide incorporation. The fluorophore is again cleaved by the polymerase to prevent stereochemical elongation inhibition.

Sequencing by Ligation

Sequencing by ligation uses fluorescently labeled complementary probes and DNA ligase as opposed to DNA polymerase to determine the fragment sequence.

Other Sequencing Technology

Nanopores are under development through which the DNA fragment is passed; an electric current is simultaneously passed through the nanopore. Each nucleotide blocks the nanopore to a different degree depending on its shape; this results in alterations to the electrical current passing through the nanopore. This in turn can be used to determine the nucleotide sequence.

Applications

The ability to rapidly and comparatively inexpensively sequence vast quantities of DNA has created a wealth of opportunities, and numerous applications of NGS have been described. Whole exome sequencing of patients with rare monogenetic disorders in whom causative mutations have not been identified is now commonly undertaken. The first major success of this approach was the identification of mutations in gene encoding the enzyme dihydroorotate dehydrogenase as a potential cause of a cohort of Miller syndrome.

NGS has been used to examine the modulation of whole transcriptomes by a given treatment or genetic alteration. It has allowed genome-wide study of the binding of regulatory proteins to DNA and interrogation of epigenetic changes such as histone modification or methylation on a global scale across the genome. However, with such large datasets, the work to analyze, validate, and interpret the data is now often more time-consuming than the sequencing itself.

As sequencing technologies and the associated bioinformatics analysis advance, knowledge of genetic influences on disease risk, disease progression, and response to therapy will increase. In the future, this progress in sequencing and the information it brings will enable an individual genetically tailored approach to medical practice.

32.4 Molecular Cloning

Molecular cloning describes the methods used to amplify a defined DNA fragment to obtain multiple identical copies, or clones; it involves construction of recombinant DNA that directs autonomous replication of the fragment in a host organism (most commonly *Escherichia coli*). Molecular cloning has numerous applications, of which some are detailed in the following.

Molecular cloning has been utilized extensively in sequencing of the human genome and the genomes of other organisms. Prior to the development of polymerase chain reaction (PCR), this was the method by which DNA fragments were amplified to enable sequencing, and it remains the method most commonly used to amplify large DNA fragments to allow subsequent sequencing, as was undertaken for the human genome project.

It is commonly used now in the study of gene function and enables the expression of a gene of interest in host cells through insertion of the gene, via a gene cassette, into an appropriate vector. This in turn allows the study of protein function as different protein isoforms and fusion proteins can be expressed.

Molecular cloning is made possible by the production of recombinant DNA, so called because it is the novel unification of the DNA fragment of interest to vector DNA, generally derived from a bacterial plasmid or virus. This process is reliant on two fundamental tools: restriction endonucleases and vectors.

32.4.1 Restriction Endonucleases

Restriction endonucleases, commonly termed restriction enzymes, are naturally occurring bacterial enzymes that cleave DNA at defined sequences. These enzymes are believed to have arisen as a defense mechanism employed by bacteria against invading pathogens such as bacteriophages, or bacteria-infecting viruses. Each restriction enzyme recognizes a specific sequence and cleaves the DNA at a site either within this sequence or in the vicinity. Palindromic recognition sequences (i.e., those that read identically in the 5' to 3' direction on both strands) are commonly cleaved within the sequence itself to leave either a blunt end or a DNA overhang, termed a cohesive or "sticky" end. Blunt ends or complementary cohesive ends may be ligated with DNA ligase, an enzyme that covalently links two DNA molecules. The ability to cleave and religate DNA molecules enables the researcher to insert or remove DNA fragments to or from vectors.

32.4.2 Vectors

Vectors enable DNA to enter host cells without being subject to degradation and allow independent replication of the DNA fragment; fragments of DNA inserted alone will be degraded and will not replicate. Vectors contain an origin of replication that allows this replication; on account of this, vectors are also termed replicons. The majority of vectors are extrachromosomal because they replicate independently of the host chromosome; these vectors have the capacity to replicate several times in a single cell cycle resulting in great increases in copy number compared to the host genome. A vector that integrates into the host chromosome is known as an episome; in this case, replication occurs with host replication. Different types of vector are available and are discussed in the following.

Plasmids

A plasmid is a small DNA molecule that replicates independently; it usually exists in the form of a double-stranded circular DNA molecule. They are naturally occurring in bacterial cells, having evolved as a mechanism to transmit beneficial genes both vertically and horizontally. These naturally occurring plasmids can be modified and used as vectors. A specialized sequence termed a polylinker sequence, or multiple cloning site, which contains multiple sites recognized by restriction enzymes, can be inserted into the plasmid to aid insertion of the DNA fragment of interest. Ideally, these restriction sites are unique to the polylinker sequences and only occur once within the plasmid so that the restriction enzyme produces a single cleavage site. If necessary, other copies of the restriction site elsewhere in the plasmid can be deleted by site directed mutagenesis (see the following). There is a limitation in the size of the DNA fragment that can be inserted into a plasmid due to the increased frequency of recombination events in large plasmids. The insert is usually restricted to less than 5 kilobases (kb).

Artificial Chromosomes (Bacterial Artificial Chromosomes and Yeast Artificial Chromosomes)

Bacterial artificial chromosomes (BACs) and yeast artificial chromosomes enable the cloning of large DNA inserts. BACs are engineered plasmids derived from the *E. coli* F (fertility factor) plasmid. This plasmid contains genes that restrain extrachromosomal replication resulting in low copy number; this limits replication errors associated with rapid replication in high copy number plasmids. This engineered DNA construct can accept DNA fragments ranging from 100 kb to 300 kb. As a result of both their insert capacity and their excellent stability, BACs were commonly used in the human genome project.

Yeast artificial chromosomes are engineered DNA molecules that can be used for cloning DNA in yeast cells; DNA fragments of up to two million bases can be inserted.

Phage Hybrid Vectors

Phage hybrid vectors contain elements derived from bacteriophages, which exist as a simple structure of DNA surrounded by a protein capsid. These phage-plasmid hybrids can act in a similar manner to plasmids but also enable DNA to be packaged in phage capsids. Cosmids are a plasmid hybrid containing the cos sequence derived from the lambda phage. They are able to accept DNA inserts of up to 50 kb; however, they have a high copy number and large inserts are unstable. Fosmids are similar to cosmids but in addition contain the F plasmid genes, used in BACs, which ensures low copy number and result in greatly increased stability.

Viral Vectors

Viral vectors are commonly used to transport genetic sequences of interest into host cells. Viruses have developed techniques to incorporate their genome into the host genome; this is termed transduction. The major advantages of viral vectors include high transduction efficiency and minimal toxicity to the target cell.

A retrovirus is an RNA virus that uses the reverse transcriptase enzyme to convert its RNA sequence into DNA, which can then be stably integrated into the host genome. The viral DNA sequence is then read as part of the host DNA sequence and translated into protein. The viral DNA is replicated along with the host's genome during cell division and maintained within the genome of daughter cells. This system requires actively dividing cells in order to integrate the virus. However, a subclass of retroviridae, known as lentiviruses, have the ability to incorporate their DNA into the host genome of nondividing cells. The viral genome is stable and passed on to further generations.

To increase safety, replication-deficient viral vectors have been developed that do not contain the viral genes required for independent viral replication and packaging. These genes are contained in separate plasmids that are cotransfected with the viral vector into a packaging cell line, commonly HEK293 cells. Virus is produced within these cells utilizing genes expressed from the "helper" plasmids; viral particles can then infect target cells and integrate into the host genome but cannot generate virus within that host.

Cell lines that stably express packaging components have been created for retroviral production; these cell lines are termed "helper-free" as they do not require cotransfection with additional plasmids. The phoenix cell lines, based on the HEK293 line, are widely used; the two principal lines in use are the ecotropic and amphotropic cells. Ecotropic virus has a narrow range of host species that it will infect; ecotropic phoenix cells will generate virus primarily targeted to murine cells. Amphotropic virus has a broader range of host species, and the phoenix amphotropic cell will generate virus capable of infecting human cells. Safety considerations are of importance when undertaking work with viral vectors, particularly amphotropic retrovirus and lentivirus. Lentiviral vectors used in the laboratory are never replication competent, and the components required for replication and packaging are divided between multiple plasmids to minimize the risk that recombination events could lead to replication competent virus.

32.4.3 Molecular Cloning Procedure

As described previously, molecular cloning requires a DNA fragment for insertion and an appropriate vector. The DNA fragment may be obtained by restriction cleavage of the desired genomic region or PCR of short fragments; protein-coding sequences for a gene of interest may be created by PCR of complementary DNA. PCR products should ideally contain restriction sites at either end of the fragment to ease insertion; these can be introduced with the PCR primers, if none are available in the fragment itself. Consideration should be given to the choice of vector and will depend on the planned application of cloned fragment. The host system in which the cloned vector is to be used will influence choice as will the vector's promoter region; certain promoters designed to work optimally for protein expression while others are designed to drive small hairpin RNA (shRNA).

The strategy for insertion of the DNA fragment into the vector should be carefully planned; a fragment cut so as to produce two blunt ends or two identical cohesive ends may insert in either direction, whereas this should not occur if cohesive ends on either side of the fragment are different. If the vector has been cleaved using a single restriction site, it can be treated with alkaline phosphatase to prevent religation of the identical cohesive ends; this removes the phosphate group required for religation.

The DNA fragment and the vector backbone are then ligated utilizing a DNA ligase (▶ Fig. 32.2). This recombinant DNA is then inserted into competent bacterial cells; bacteria are the host used most commonly in molecular cloning. These cells are termed competent as their membranes have been treated either chemically or by electroporation to allow admittance of large molecules. This uptake of foreign DNA is termed transformation. The cells are then plated out on an agar plate and incubated overnight at 37°C. This process will allow distinct colonies to form; each colony will contain multiple bacteria all carrying a single identical recombinant DNA or clone. Colonies can be picked and grown up in liquid culture at 37°C overnight. Plasmid DNA is extracted through alkali cell lysis. This process denatures both bacterial and plasmid DNA; the addition of acetate-containing neutralization

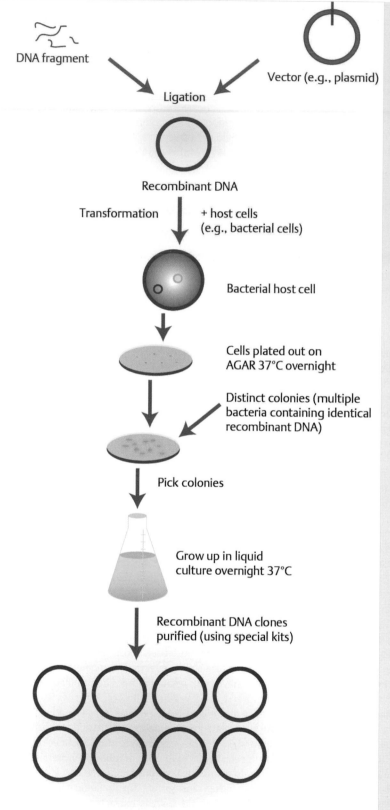

Fig. 32.2 Overview of molecular cloning procedure. The deoxyribonucleic acid (DNA) fragment and vector are prepared using restriction endonucleases and ligated with DNA ligase enzyme. During transformation competent bacteria cells take up the recombinant DNA. The cells are plated out on agar and incubated overnight at 37°C. Distinct colonies form containing multiple bacterial cells carrying a single identical recombinant DNA. The colonies are picked and grown up in liquid culture (37°C) overnight. The recombinant DNA is then extracted using commercial kits.

buffer enables plasmid DNA to renature and supercoil but not the large chromosomal DNA, which precipitates out of solution. The recombinant plasmid DNA in solution can then be purified by anion exchange chromatography. DNA binds tightly to the beads but impurities do not and can be washed away. Purified plasmid DNA is then eluted from the beads.

Screening and Selecting Transformed Host Cells

Molecular cloning methods have the capacity to generate vast numbers of host colonies; however, not all will contain the desired recombinant DNA. There are several strategies available to improve the efficiency of generating and selecting clones carrying the correct recombinant DNA.

The most common approach is to insert a dominant selective marker into the vector backbone such as an antibiotic resistance gene. In order for this to be effective, the host cell must be susceptible to the antibiotic; ampicillin, kanamycin, and chloramphenicol are commonly used. The transformed cells are plated out on agar containing the antibiotic; only those colonies containing the vector should grow due to the antibiotic resistance it confers.

A fluorescent marker gene or the lacz reporter gene system may also be employed to assist clone selection. The lacz gene can be inserted into the vector; the gene product hydrolyses the colorless substrate X-gal to yield a blue compound. The polylinker site is placed so that on insertion of the DNA fragment, the lacz gene is disrupted and therefore cells transformed with vector containing the DNA fragment will be colorless. The blue colonies will contain only the empty vector.

Successful insertion of the DNA fragment of interest can be confirmed by PCR screening, restriction fragment analysis, or definitively by DNA sequencing.

32.4.4 Gateway Molecular Cloning

The gateway system, a recent addition to the molecular cloning toolbox, is a fast and cost-effective cloning technique that has advantages over traditional methods. Restriction and ligation enzymes are redundant in this system, with advantages including increased cloning efficiency, greater ease, and the ability to stably insert larger fragments (>5 kb). The versatile gateway system allows the inserts to be shuttled between vectors while maintaining the reading frame in the correct orientation.

The system operates with the use of complementary recombination sites allowing fragments of DNA to be transferred between vectors with the use of the appropriate enzyme catalyzing the recombination. The desired insert lies between two different recombination sites in an entry vector; these sites each align with their own complementary recombination site in the destination vector. These sites then recombine and there is a transfer of fragments between the vectors, with the insert moving to the destination vector. The destination vector also contains a counter selectable marker "ccdb" that leads to cell death, when transformed into bacteria lacking resistance, if it is not replaced with the fragment of interest. This increases cloning efficiency, with the majority of inserts in the correct reading frame and orientation.

32.4.5 Gene Expression

Molecular cloning can be used to create vectors containing a gene of interest or its protein coding DNA sequence; this therefore enables further interrogation of the functions of that gene or its protein. Utilizing vectors designed to drive expression, proteins can be expressed in target cells and the effect of that expression studied. Protein expression may be transient if the vector remains extrachromosomal, with peak expression at 48 to 72 hours following transfection of the plasmid. Protein levels will then diminish through cell division, cell death, and loss of recombinant DNA. Recombinant DNA can randomly integrate into the host chromosome to derive cells that maintain stable protein expression, with the advantage that this expression is maintained in daughter cells. Retroviral vectors are relatively efficient at causing host integration, plasmids less so. Cells achieving stable integration of the gene of interest can be selected by drug treatment, such as puromycin or blastocidin, with resistance conferred by the recombinant DNA.

32.4.6 Fusion Proteins

Molecular cloning also enables the creation of recombinant or fusion proteins. The protein of interest may be tagged with a fluorescent protein to allow interrogation of its localization in vivo. This is undertaken by inserting the coding sequence of the fluorescent protein in frame, either upstream or downstream of the coding sequence of the protein of interest, tagging either the N-terminal or C-terminal with the fluorescent marker. It is important to note, however, that the addition of any tag may modulate the function, binding, or location of a protein; this is of particular concern when large tags are fused to a protein. Attempts should therefore be made to confirm that a fusion protein acts in a similar manner to endogenous protein.

Small tags such as the myc-tag, HA-tag, and FLAG-tag comprise 10 or fewer amino acids and are commonly fused to proteins as, due to their size, they are considered less likely to modulate function. These tags allow differentiation of the vector-derived protein from endogenous protein. In addition, they are commonly used to enable immunoprecipitation of the protein to examine binding partners or assess protein functions in vitro. Tags may be fused to the N-terminal or the C-terminal of the protein;

again, it should be noted that these could each affect the protein differently. In both cases, the tag should be in frame with the protein with no stop codon between the two proteins. There are numerous vectors available that contain the sequence for fluorescent markers or other tags, with the coding sequence of the protein of interest inserted into these to produce the desired fusion protein.

Molecular cloning techniques also enable the expression of mutant proteins. This allows examination of the function of a protein mutation identified in screening for potential disease causing gene variants; it may assist in determining whether a nonsynonymous mutation is deleterious to protein function. Such mutations may cause the protein to lose function or to gain function, both of which may be pathogenic. In addition, artificial mutations can be created in the protein coding sequence to alter certain domains within the protein to determine the effects of these alterations on protein function; examples include altering residues so that they can no longer undergo modification such as phosphorylation or deleting regions of the protein. These alterations in the protein-coding sequence can be performed by site-directed mutagenesis.

32.4.7 Site-Directed Mutagenesis

Site-directed mutagenesis was traditionally undertaken on single-stranded DNA templates, often obtained from phage vectors, but now is commonly performed on double-stranded plasmids using one of the commercial site-directed mutagenesis kits. In principle, primers are designed over the site of the desired mutation, one designed to the sense strand and one to the antisense. These primers contain the mutation to be inserted. A high fidelity hot start DNA polymerase is used to continue the polymerization of the primers around the whole length of the plasmid in opposite directions. Only the original plasmid DNA acts as template, not the product of the polymerization reaction. Once the appropriate quantity of cycles is complete, the reaction is treated with DpnI, which cleaves the methylated template DNA derived from the bacterial host but not the unmethylated PCR product. The reaction is then transformed into bacteria and the resulting colonies screened for the mutation.

32.4.8 Ribonucleic Acid Interference

An important tool in the study of protein function is the ability to inhibit or knock down protein expression so as to examine the associated phenotype. The discovery of short interfering RNA has made this technique easily accessible.

RNA interference is a mechanism evolved in both animals and plants to protect against viruses and transposable elements. These potential pathogens can produce long double-strand RNA, which is not commonly found in cells. This long double-strand RNA is cleaved by the ribonuclease Dicer within the cell cytoplasm, and the resulting short double-stranded RNA is bound by the argonaute complex, which degrades one strand and uses the remaining strand as a guide to target complementary RNA sequences within the cell for degradation.

This machinery can be commandeered to knock down endogenous mRNA by introducing, into target cells, small (~21 nucleotide) double-stranded interfering RNA (siRNA) that is complementary to the mRNA of the protein, the expression of which is to be inhibited. siRNA can be introduced by poration of the cell membrane, commonly with liposomes. Time taken to precipitate protein knockdown will depend on the stability of the protein, but it may take 48 to 72 hours to obtain maximal reduction in protein, after which levels recover. Knockdown with siRNA rarely leads to complete abrogation of gene expression but can reduce it significantly. An alternate mechanism to induce knockdown using RNA interference is to introduce a plasmid or viral vector expressing shRNA; cells in which this vector stably integrates can then be selected. This can result in a stable reduction in protein levels.

Off-target effects with siRNA are known to occur; therefore, results should be confirmed with more than one siRNA sequence. Further proof that the phenotypic effects are not due to off-target events includes rescuing the phenotype by re-expressing the protein in the target cells. Silent mutations should be inserted into the DNA sequence of this rescue protein, by site-directed mutagenesis, so that the resultant mRNA is not susceptible to the siRNA; the amino acid sequence of the protein should not be altered.

There are several available vectors that contain tetracycline responsive elements. These elements are placed upstream of the vector promoter and drive expression from the promoter on binding of the tetracycline transactivator. Two systems exist: the Tet-On and the Tet-Off. In the Tet-On, the transactivator will only bind the tetracycline responsive elements in the presence of tetracycline or doxycycline, whereas in the Tet-Off system the opposite is true. These systems are commonly used to drive inducible shRNA expression, but can also be utilized to induce expression of proteins.

32.5 Gene Analysis by Hybridization

Nucleic acid hybridization is an important tool in molecular genetics, with common principles underlying all hybridization assays. Oligonucleotides or larger probes are used to hybridize to complementary target sequences; depending on the assay, the avidity of this hybridization can be examined to determine any mismatches between the sequences. The complementary probe and target nucleic acid are denatured to form single-stranded molecules; these can then anneal to form a double-stranded molecule, a hetero-duplex. This hybridization between the probe and the target nucleic acid is often carried out on a solid surface. Either the DNA sample or the probes can be attached to a solid surface, such as a glass slide, whereas the other nucleic acid population remains in solution and are labeled (e.g., by radioisotope, fluorophore, or a chemical group). After hybridization, the surface is washed to remove any nonspecific binding so that only complementary probe-target hetero-duplexes remain. The stability of the hetero-duplex is dependent on the temperature and ionic environment and the stringency of the hybridization assay is determined by the reaction conditions; these include temperature, salt concentration, and pH. Stringency is considered high when hetero-duplexes only occur between fully complementary sequences; lower stringency tolerates a degree of mismatching. Higher annealing temperatures and decreased salt concentration increase the stringency; low salt concentration washes posthybridization result in only highly specific, highly complementary heteroduplexes remaining. Many molecular biology techniques employ hybridization. The following are a few examples of its application.

32.5.1 Fluorescent In Situ Hybridization

Fluorescent in situ hybridization is a cytogenetic technique used to detect the presence or absence of defined DNA sequences on chromosomes and their localization. It employs probes that are complementary to the sequence of interest; these are either directly labeled with a fluorophore or with a reporter molecule such as biotin, which can subsequently be detected by fluorescently labeled antibody. It is commonly used to examine chromosomes in metaphase to detect rearrangements or other aberrations.

32.5.2 Tissue In Situ Hybridization/ Whole Mount In Situ Hybridization

RNA probes known as riboprobes are used to investigate the expression pattern of the gene of interest in either whole tissue samples or tissue sections, through hybridizing to complementary mRNA. The riboprobes are typically labelled with digoxigenin, which can subsequently be detected with antidigoxigenin antibody. The antidigoxigenin antibody is commonly conjugated to a fluorophore or an enzyme (e.g., alkaline phosphatase or peroxidase) so that detection can be performed by fluorescent microscopy or colorimetric assay (▶ Fig. 32.3).

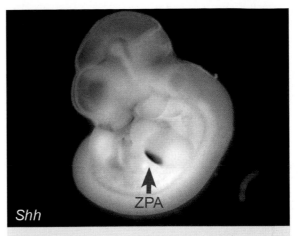

Fig. 32.3 Whole mount in situ hybridization 10.5 days postconception mouse embryo showing Sonic Hedgehog (*Shh*) expression in the zone of polarizing activity (*ZPA*), in the posterior limb bud.

32.5.3 Array Comparative Genome Hybridization

Array comparative genome hybridization is a hybridization protocol employed to compare a genome of interest to a control reference genome, interrogating for areas of loss or gain and thereby copy number variation within the sample. DNA fragments regularly distributed across the genome are annealed to the microarray chip in a precise order. These fragments act as probes and hybridize to the human genome, occurring at a frequency of up to one probe every 500 bases. The control DNA is labeled with one color, and the test sample is labeled with another color. The relative amount that each DNA hybridizes to the microarray is studied using colorimetric analysis; this can identify regions of loss or gain in the test sample.

32.6 Glossary

Amplification: Production of multiple copies.

Anneal: The formation of hydrogen bonds between two complimentary nucleic acids.

Denature: The heat or chemical treatment of double-stranded deoxyribonucleic acid (DNA) to break hydrogen bonds between complimentary bases (i.e., the opposite of anneal).

Competence: The ability of a cell to admit extracellular DNA. This can be natural or induced by treatment with heat, chemicals, or electricity to confer the cells' transient permeability.

Gene cassettes: Distinct elements that normally contain a single gene plus a short sequence that acts as a recombination site. The gene cassettes usually do not have promoters. They typically exist as a linear molecule integrated into a larger DNA molecule such as a plasmid.

Molecular cloning: Molecular cloning involves making an identical copy of a DNA molecule of interest (a clone).

Open reading frame: A sequence of nucleotides that can be translated into a protein polypeptide.

Restriction enzyme: A bacterial enzyme also known as a restriction endonuclease used to cut double-stranded DNA at a specific recognition sequence.

Shh: Sonic Hedgehog gene, involved in limb development.

Transduction: The addition of foreign DNA to a cell using a recombinant virus.

Transfection: Introduction of foreign DNA into a cell without use of a vector.

Transformation: Transferring large naked DNA molecules from the surrounding environment into competent host cells (e.g., bacteria).

Vector: A nucleic acid that contains an origin of replication allowing it to replicate independently in a host cell. It can be used to also replicate a sequence of interest by covalently attaching them.

ZPA: The zone of polarizing activity, posterior region of the limb bud where Sonic Hedgehog is expressed.

Further Reading

Gallagher S, Wiley EA. Current protocols essential laboratory techniques. 2 e. Hoboken, NJ: Wiley-Blackwell; 2012

Green MR, Sambrook J. Molecular cloning: a laboratory manual. 4 e. Cold Spring Harbor, NY: Cold Spring Harbor Laboratory Press; 2012

Strachan T, Read A. Human molecular genetics. 4 e. New York: Garland Science, Taylor and Francis Group, LLC; 2011

33 Laser Scanning Confocal Microscopy and Laser Microdissection

Kwong-Man Lee

Laser scanning confocal microscopy and laser microdissection are the most indispensable cell image acquisition and isolation tools incorporating advanced laser technology into specially designed optical microscopes. In this chapter, we will outline the technical principles and present applications of these two advanced technologies in biomedical sciences. When we look at the Nobel Prizes in the past decade, cellular and molecular biology have been the topics being awarded the Nobel Prize in chemistry, physiology, or medicine almost every year. However, compared to those of nervous and circulatory systems, cellular and molecular studies of bone, cartilage, and tendon cells in the musculoskeletal system are much left behind. Cell-to-matrix interaction seems to be a much more critical issue in bone, cartilage, and tendon as these tissues are always under tensile or compressive forces. With confocal laser scanning microscopy (CLSM), the cellular activities of chondrocyte, osteoblast, or other bone cells can be monitored in situ while these cells are still interacting with their normal surrounding matrix. By applying laser microdissection technique, deoxyribonucleic acid (DNA), ribonucleic acid (RNA), and protein of cells from various site of skeletal tissue, such chondrocytes from resting, proliferative, and hypertrophic zones of the growth plate, can be isolated for advanced molecular analysis.

33.1 Basic Principles and Applications of Laser Scanning Confocal Microscopy

CLSM is a technique to obtain high-resolution and high-contrast optical images by using point illumination and a spatial pinhole to eliminate out-of-focus light in specimens that are thicker than the focal plane. The key feature of confocal microscopy is its ability to acquire in-focus images from selected depths, a process known as optical sectioning. Images are acquired by point-by-point scanning and reconstructed with a computer, allowing three-dimensional reconstructions of topologically complex objects. For opaque specimens, this is useful for surface profiling, whereas for nonopaque specimens, interior structures can be imaged. For interior imaging, the quality of the image is greatly improved when compared to conventional fluorescent microscopy because in-focused image information from multiple depths in the specimen is superimposed.

The principle of confocal microscopy was originally patented by Marvin Minsky in 1957, and it took more than 30 years of development for CLSM to become a standard technique.[1] In 1978, Thomas and Christoph Cremer designed a laser scanning process that scanned the three-dimensional surface of an object point-by-point by means of a focused laser beam and created the overall picture by electronic means similar to those used in scanning electron microscopes. This CLSM design combined the laser scanning method with the three-dimensional detection of biological objects labeled with fluorophore for the first time. During the next decade, confocal fluorescence microscopy was developed into a fully mature cellular and molecular imaging technology.

In CLSM, a laser beam passes through a light source aperture and is then focused by an objective lens into a focal volume within a fluorescent specimen. A mixture of emitted fluorescent light as well as reflected laser light from the illuminated spot is then recollected by the objective lens. The recollected lights then pass through a beam splitter, separating the laser light, which is reflected away from the detector, and the fluorescent light, which is passed through the splitter to the detection apparatus, from the objects. After passing through a pinhole, the fluorescent light is detected by a photo-detector, transformed into an electronic signal that is then transferred to an imaging computer system.

As seen in ▶ Fig. 33.1, the confocal pinhole obstructs the "out-of-focus" fluorescent light. Light rays from below the focal plane come to a focus before reaching the pinhole, and then they expand out so that most of the rays are physically blocked from reaching the detector by the pinhole.[2] In the same way, light from above the focal plane is focused behind the pinhole, so that most of this light also hits the edges of the pinhole and is not detected. However, all the light from the focal plane (*solid red lines*) is focused at the pinhole and passed on to the detector. In turn, a sharper image is obtained when compared with conventional light microscopy because all the information that is not in the focal plane is blocked. The detected light originating from an illuminated volume element within the specimen represents one pixel in the final image. As the laser scans over the plane of interest, a whole image is obtained pixel by pixel and line by line, while the brightness of a final image pixel corresponds to the relative intensity of the detected fluorescent light. The laser beam is scanned across the sample in the horizontal plane using one or more oscillating mirrors. This scanning method usually has low reaction latency, and the scan speed can be varied as slower scans provide a better signal-to-noise ratio and result in better contrast and higher resolution. Information can be collected from

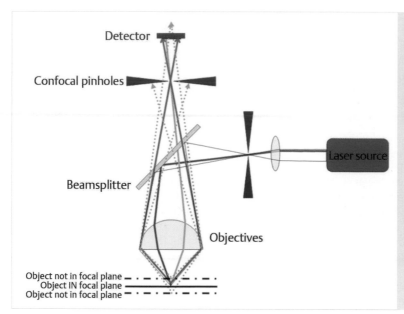

Fig. 33.1 Basic principles of confocal laser scanning microscopy. (From Lee KM, Yeung HY. Application of laser scanning confocal microscopy in musculoskeletal research. In Qin L, Genant HK, Griffith JF, Leung KS, eds. Advanced bioimaging technologies in assessment of the quality of bone and scaffold materials. Berlin: Springer; 2007:173–189.)

different focal planes by raising or lowering the microscope stage. The computer can generate a three-dimensional picture of a specimen by assembling a stack of these two-dimensional images from successive focal planes.

Jargon Simplified: Fluorophore

A fluorophore is a fluorescent chemical compound that can re-emit light upon light excitation.

33.2 Imaging Modes

33.2.1 Two-Dimensional Imaging: Single Optical Section

The simplest single optical sectioning is x-y scanning. The optical section is the basic image unit in confocal microscopy. Data can be collected from fixed and stained specimens in single-, double-, triple-, or multiple-wavelength illumination modes, and the images collected from multiple-labeled specimens will be in register with each other to produce a two-dimensional image. The thickness of the optical section is determined by the magnification, the numerical aperture of the objective used, and the diameter of the pinhole, as shown in ▶ Table 33.1. With most confocal microscopy software packages, optical sections are not restricted to the perpendicular lateral (x-y) plane, but can also be collected and displayed in transverse planes. Vertical sections in the x-z and y-z planes (parallel to the microscope optical axis) can be readily generated by

Table 33.1 Objective Lens Parameters and Optical Section Thickness

Objective		Pinhole diameter	
Magnification	Numerical Aperture	(1 mm)	(7 mm)
60×	1.40	0.4	1.9
40×	1.30	0.6	3.3
40×	0.55	1.4	4.3
25×	0.80	1.4	7.8
4×	0.20	20	100

most confocal software programs. Thus, the specimen appears as if it had been sectioned in a plane that is perpendicular to the lateral axis. In practice, vertical sections are obtained by combining a series of x-y scans taken along the z axis with the software, and then projecting a view of fluorescence intensity as it would appear should the microscope hardware have been capable of physically performing a vertical section.

Jargon Simplified: Optical Sectioning

Optical sectioning is the process by which a suitably designed microscope, such as confocal laser scanning microscope, can produce clear images of a focal plane deep within a thick sample without performing physical sectioning.

33.2.2 Three-Dimensional Imaging: x-y-z Series

A z-series is a sequence of optical sections collected at different levels perpendicular to the optical axis (the z-axis) within a specimen. Z-series are collected by coordinating step-by-step changes in the fine focus of the microscope with sequential image acquisition at each step. Then, a z-series can be further processed into a three-dimensional representation of the specimen using various volume visualization techniques. In terms of three-dimensional reconstructions of topologically complex objects, some models such as surface rendering are useful for surface profiling of opaque specimens, whereas other models can be used for revealing the interior on nonopaque specimens.

33.2.3 Four-Dimensional Imaging: Time Lapse and Live Cell Imaging

Living tissue preparations or other specimens exhibiting dynamic phenomena present the possibility of using CLSM to collect time-lapse sequences of three-dimensional (x, y, and z) data to be combined with time (t) as the fourth dimension. These four-dimensional datasets can be viewed using a four-dimensional viewer program. Such programs allow stereo pairs taken at each time point to be constructed and played back as a three-dimensional movie.

Imaging living tissues with CLSM is substantially more difficult than imaging fixed specimens, and it is not always a practical option because the specimen may not tolerate the conditions involved. ▶ Table 33.2 lists some of the factors to be considered when imaging live cells

Table 33.2 Imaging Fixed and Living Cells with Confocal Laser Scanning Microscopy (Modified from www.microscopyu.com with permission.)

Criteria	Fixed cells	Living cells
Limits of illumination	Fading of fluorophore	Phototoxicity, fading of dye
Antifade reagent	Phenylenediamine, etc.	Not applicable
Mountant	Glycerol ($n = 1.51$)	Water ($n = 1.33$)
Highest numerical aperture lens	1.4	1.2
Time per image	Unlimited	Limited by speed of phenomenon; light sensitivity of specimen
Signal averaging	Yes	No
Resolution	Wave optics	Photon statistics

with CLSM compared with those on fixed cells.[3] Some specimens simply will not physically fit on the stage of the microscope, or they cannot be kept alive on the stage during observation. The phenomenon or structures of interest may not be accessible to the objective lens field of view.

Successful imaging of live cells requires extreme care to be taken throughout the imaging process to maintain tolerable conditions on the microscope stage. Photo damage from the illuminating laser beam can be cumulative over multiple scans, so the exposure to the beam should be kept to the minimum. Antioxidants such as ascorbic acid are commonly added to the culture medium to reduce oxygen, which can be released in the excitation of fluorescent molecules, causing free radicals to form and cell death. It is usually necessary to carry out extensive preliminary control experiments to assess the effects of light exposure on fluorescent-labeled cells. Following the imaging tests, the continued viability of the living specimens should be evaluated. Embryos, for example, should continue their normal development after the imaging process, and any abnormalities caused by the laser scanning should be determined.

In order to minimize the photo toxicity effect, multiphoton confocal fluorescence microscopy has been developed. This special technique allows imaging of living tissue up to a depth of 1 mm.[3] Multiphoton excitation is defined as a process in which the energy for the excitation of a single molecule comes from two or more photons with lower energy and longer wavelength that are absorbed at virtually the same time. Each photon needs to contribute only part of the total energy required for the fluorophore excitation, provided that the combined amount of energy is sufficient. One advantage of this technique is that the excitation light scattering by tissue is reduced as a result of longer wavelengths, allowing excitation to penetrate more deeply into the tissue than visible light.

Specific requirements to sustain the life of cells have to be met for each individual cell type that is to be imaged. Most cell types require a stage heating device and possibly a perfusion chamber in which the proper carbon dioxide level can be maintained through the entire process of imaging.

Many physiological processes and events take place faster than they can be captured by most CLSMs, which have image acquisition rates typically on the order of one frame per second. CLSMs using acousto-optical devices and a slit for scanning are faster than the galvanometer-driven point scanning systems, and are more practical for physiological studies. This is known as a spinning disk confocal microscope. These faster designs combine good spatial resolution with good temporal resolution, which can reach up to 30 frames per second at full screen resolution, near video rate. The conventional slower single point scanning microscope systems can achieve the best temporal resolution only by scanning a much reduced area on the specimen. If full spatial resolution is required, the frames must be collected less frequently, losing some temporal resolution. On the other hand, the confocal systems using disks are capable of imaging fast physiological or other transient events.

33.3 Basic Principles and Applications of Laser Microdissection

As the Human Genome Project offers a lot of basic information about the sequences of the complete genome, researchers now want to examine the functions, expressions, and regulations of gene activity. Some of the most exciting new developments in biomedical research, such as DNA microarrays and proteomics, depend on the isolation of single cells or pure populations of cells with specific phenotypes. Materials for molecular analyses should be collected with great caution to avoid contamination. Slight contamination may be amplified, giving false results or compromising data interpretation. This is even more critical for laser microdissection, because it takes only one unwanted cell to result in a contamination error of 100% if we are testing individual cells.

Jargon Simplified: Proteomics

Proteomics is the large-scale study of proteins, particularly their structures and functions.

Laser microdissection, also called laser capture microdissection or laser-assisted microdissection, is a method for isolating specific cells of interest from microscopic regions of tissue/cells/organisms. A laser is coupled into a microscope and focuses onto the tissue on the slide. By movement of laser beam or the sample holding stage, the focus follows a trajectory that is predefined by the user. This trajectory is then cut out by high energy laser and separated from adjacent tissue.

Microdissection is a well-established advance technology in molecular pathology, cell biology, oncology, and forensic medicine, where minute samples need to be isolated from surrounding materials for contamination-free analysis. For example, histological examination shows that most tumors are composed of mixed cell populations, including tumor cells, inflammatory cells, and endothelial cells, and the tumor cells themselves may be at different differentiation stages. One of the most challenging problems in cancer research is that it is very difficult to isolate DNA or RNA from a pure population of cancerous cells—reducing both the sensitivity and accuracy of any genetic analyses. One solution is to preselect and isolate only cells of interest using laser microdissection.

Automated laser microdissection requires a computer-controlled microscope coupled to a video imaging system with appropriate software and drawing tools.[4] With suitable software, an area, or multiple areas, of interest in a specimen under the microscope may be outlined using a mouse or screen pen, dissected using a laser, and isolated safely for further analysis in a contamination-free environment. There are a variety of laser dissection technologies commercially available, which may differ in the software-user interface, the type of laser used for dissection, and the method of tissue isolation. Key factors in selection of a microdissection system include easy navigation, high precision definition of areas of interest, contamination-free tissue isolation, and preferably, cold laser technology to avoid exposing tissues to heat or radiation that could damage cells.

There are currently four commercially available systems designed specifically for laser capture microdissection: ArcturusXT by Applied Biosystems (Foster City, CA), CellCut Plus by Molecular Machines & Industries (Glattbrugg, Switzerland), PALM MicroBeam by Zeiss (Oberkochen, Germany), and LMD7000 by Leica (Solms, Germany). ▶ Table 33.3 shows the feature comparison of various laser microdissection systems.

Laser microdissection technology has many applications, but its power lies in the selective harvesting of multicellular regions of interest, single cells, or even subcellular structures from histological sections, cytospines, etc. The laser has an extremely high energy density at the small focal point only (focus, 1 µm). To facilitate cutting, microscope slides covered with polyethylene naphthalate membrane are used. This membrane acts as a stabilizing scaffold during cutting and allows larger areas in a single laser shot. Other specialized membranes and consumables are available for fluorescence and live-cell applications.

33.3.1 Procedures for Laser Microdissection

Loading slides and adhesive-cap centrifuge tubes onto the microdissection system:
  Adjust laser focus and intensity
  Automatic laser cutting
  Inspect sample
  Save sample image for future checking
  Perform analyses of DNA, RNA, or protein

33.4 Applications of Laser Microdissection

33.4.1 Ribonucleic Acid Applications

For experimental design involving RNA extraction, there are several important factors one should be aware of before beginning a laser microdissection experiment. RNA is much more susceptible to degradation than DNA. Due to the presence of ribonucleases, both endogenous to

Table 33.3 Comparison of Various Laser Microdissection Systems

	Applied Biosystems	Zeiss	Molecular Machines & Industries	Leica
	Arcturus (Foster City, CA)	**PALM MicroBeam IV** (Oberkochen, Germany)	**CellCut Plus** (Glattbrugg, Switzerland)	**LMD7000** (Solms, Germany)
Laser microdissection technology	Infrared laser enabled laser capture microdissection on CapSure LCM Cap.	Ultraviolet cutting only. Laser pressure catapult cut material into collection cap.	Ultraviolet cutting only. Collect cut material onto adhesive cap.	Ultraviolet cutting only. Gravity collection of cut material into cap.
Collection vessel	CapSure LCM Caps	Microtube cap	Adhesive microtube cap	Microtube cap
Ultraviolet laser cutting	355 nm or 349 nm passive Qswitch diode pumped ultraviolet laser	355 nm solid-state ultraviolet laser	355 nm solid-state ultraviolet laser	249–377 nm solid-state ultraviolet laser
Infrared laser capture	810 nm solid-state near infrared laser			
Microscope	Inverted microscope (Nikon)	Inverted microscope (Zeiss)	Inverted microscope (Olympus or Nikon)	Upright microscope (Leica)
Allowable slide preparation	Any slide type	Any slide type	Membrane slides only	Membrane slides only
Collected sample inspection	Yes	No	Yes	No
Noncontact sample collection	No	Yes	No	Yes

the tissue and from environment surfaces, one must be very careful in protecting the integrity of the sample's RNA. Therefore, membrane slides and any glass surface that will come in contact with the sample should be heat-treated before use, or treated with appropriate solvents.[5]

As a general rule of thumb, the colder and dryer the slides are, the better off the RNA will be. Therefore, when cutting fresh frozen sections in optimal cutting temperature compound (OCT), it is imperative that one keep the slides cold and begin any staining steps quickly. Before microdissection, OCT must be washed away with diethylpyrocarbonate-treated water. Keep staining procedures brief, keep all reagents ice cold, and avoid any prolonged aqueous phase steps because they will allow ribonuclease activity. As long as the samples are fully dehydrated in the final staining steps, the RNA should be stable up to a few hours for the microdissection. Ending a staining protocol with a quick increasing ethanol series with a longer dehydration step in 100% ethanol should keep the ribonuclease activity to a minimum.

Jargon Simplified: Optimal Cutting Temperature Compound

OCT, composed of polyvinyl alcohol and polyethylene glycol, is used to embed tissue samples prior to frozen sectioning on a microtome-cryostat.

33.4.2 Protein Applications

In general, the sample preparation goals for protein applications are quite similar to those of RNA applications. The work flow should be:

Tissue sectioning

Laser microdissection

Protein extraction for analysis

Working quickly and keeping the slides cold and dry will help avoid protein degradation. While sectioning, do not let the slides warm to room temperature and store at −80°C prior to laser microdissection. Fresh frozen tissue will yield the best protein (avoid excess OCT), and minimal fixation is preferred. Ethanol or methanol should be used as fixative rather than formalin. Staining may affect mass spectrophotometry results, so one should try staining an adjacent section for tissue navigation. If staining is critical for target identification, consider stains like hematoxylin alone (avoid eosin), cresyl violet, toluidine blue, methylene blue, or short immunostaining protocols. One can also consider adding protease inhibitors to the staining reagents. Protein quality may degrade rapidly after staining, so minimize the laser microdissection session to less than an hour. Stay consistent in the staining methods and laser microdissection time throughout the sample set. Doing so will ensure consistent levels of protein degradation across the samples.

Table 33.4 Amount of Microdissected Tissue for Various Molecular Assays

Molecule	Methodology/Assay	Cellular yield/Area of microdissection
DNA	Loss of heterozygosity	100–1,000 cells
	Imprinting/DNA methlylation	200 cells
	Genetic mosaic analysis of gDNA	2,000 cells
RNA	cDNA library construction	5,000–25,000 cells (15–90 ng total RNA)
	Gene expression arrays	100 cells from FFPE
	Real-time RT-PCR	1–22,000 cells
	qRT-PCR	100–5,000 cells
Protein	Western blot (optimized blotting procedure)	500 cells
	Western blot	2,500–10,000 cells
	Two-dimensional gel electrophoresis	10,000–100,000 cells
	Two-dimensional DIGE	30,000 cells/40 µl
	Molecular profiling: reverse-phase protein microarray	5,000–30,000 cells
	Mass spectrometry: MALDI or LC/MS-MS	10,000–100,000 cells
	Mass spectrometry: SELDI	1,500–5,000 cells

Abbreviations: cDNA, complementary DNA; DIGE, fluorescence difference gel electrophoresis; DNA, deoxyribonucleic acid; FFPE, formalin-fixed, paraffin-embedded; gDNA, genomic DNA; LC/MS-MS, liquid chromatography-mass spectrometry; MALDI, matrix-assisted laser desorption/ionization; qRT-PCR, quantitative RT-PCR; RNA, ribonucleic acid; RT-PCR, reverse transcription–polymerase chain reaction; SELDI, surface-enhanced laser desorption/ionization.
Modified from Laser Capture for Dummies. http://www.ecu.edu/cs-dhs/internalmed/lasercapture/upload/Laser-Capture-for-Dummies-June-2010.pdf.

33.4.3 Live Cell Applications

Laser microdissection of live cells is possible using specially designed consumables such as Duplex dishes. These dishes have a thin layer of Teflon (DuPont, Wilmington, DE) coated with polyethylene naphthalate membrane.[5]

Theoretically, quantitative reverse transcription–polymerase chain reaction and other sensitive assays can be performed on single cells. However, this can be extremely challenging. One must also be aware that tissue sectioning cuts cells at various planes. The cross section of a cell visible on microscope may only be about half or even less of an entire cell. Therefore, it may be necessary to capture several "cells" to obtain the equivalent of a single cell's biomolecules. Alternatively, multiple laser microdissection samples can be pooled to obtain enough cellular material for assay. ▶ Table 33.4 is a summary table modified from Espina et al's[5] 2006 "Laser-capture microdissection" article, published in *Nature Protocols*, which reported on the amount of microdissected tissue recommended to perform a particular assay.

References

[1] Wouterlood FG, ed. Cellular imaging techniques for neuroscience and beyond. Amsterdam: Elsevier; 2012

[2] Lee KM, Yeung HY. Application of laser scanning confocal microscopy in musculoskeletal research. In Qin L, Genant HK, Griffith JF, Leung KS, eds. Advanced bioimaging technologies in assessment of the quality of bone and scaffold materials. Berlin: Springer; 2007:173–189

[3] Fujimoto JG, Farkas DL, eds. Biomedical optical imaging. Oxford: Oxford University Press; 2009

[4] Conn PM, ed. Laser capture microscopy and microdissection, Vol 356: methods in enzymology. Boston: Academic Press; 2002

[5] Espina V, Wulfkuhle JD, Calvert VS et al. Laser-capture microdissection. Nat Protoc 2006; 1: 586–603

Further Readings

Molecular Expressions. Author resources. http://micro.magnet.fsu.edu/primer/techniques/confocal/index.html

Olympus. Author resources. http://www.olympusconfocal.com/theory/index.html

Centre for Cellular Imaging. Author resources. http://www.cf.gu.se/english/Centre_for_Cellular_Imaging/Techniques/Laser_Microdissection___Pressure_Catapulting

34 Image Analysis Histomorphometry Stereology

Chuanyong Lu, Ralph Marcucio, and Theodore Miclau

> ### Jargon Simplified: Stereology
>
> Stereology is a method to get unbiased quantitative estimation of the first-order stereological parameters in a three-dimensional sample from measurements made on two-dimensional planar sections.

Many systems and techniques have been developed for quantitative analyses in orthopedic research. Bioquant systems (Nashville, TN) are widely used in the field of orthopedic research. Bioquant's Osteo System is ideal for analyzing bone structure, osteoblast activity, and osteoclast activity. Detailed instruction about the Bioquant systems can be found on the company's website at http://www.bioquant.com/. For researchers who are interested in fracture repair and bone regeneration, recently developed stereology technique may have advantages over the Bioquant systems. Stereology is a method to get unbiased quantitative estimation of the first-order stereological parameters in a three-dimensional sample from measurements made on two-dimensional planar sections. These parameters include volume, surface area, length, and number. Stereology allows us to quantify not only the amount of tissue formation, but also many of the regulating mechanisms that underlie bone repair. For example, tissue vascularization and infiltration of inflammatory cells can be accurately measured using stereology technique. In this chapter, we describe our experience of using stereology to quantify fracture healing, tissue vascularization, and inflammation.

34.1 Basic Rules of Stereology

To achieve unbiased estimation in stereology, certain rules have to be followed through the whole process of the assay. The number of samples, the time points of tissue collection, the parameters to be analyzed, and appropriate sampling need to be decided before the experiment even starts. A pilot study will provide information about the variation of the parameters, which can be used to determine the sample size (power analysis) and the adequacy of sampling (coefficient of error). The following are some basic rules of stereology.

34.1.1 Comparable Reference Space

Reference space is the anatomical region in the tissue that contains all the objects of interest. Reference space must be unambiguously defined, and 100% of it should

be available for analysis in each sample. In addition, the reference spaces of the control group and the treated group in one experiment need to be comparable. For later stages of fracture healing (i.e., 7 days or more after injury in a murine tibia fracture model[1,2]), the callus usually has a clear margin and it is reasonable to use the whole callus as the reference space. For early fracture healing (i.e., before 5 days after injury in a murine tibia fracture model[1,2]), it may be difficult to outline the callus because it has no clear margin yet. For samples collected early after fracture, the reference space needs to be carefully defined. One method is to use the whole tibia with all the surrounding soft tissues as the reference space. An alternative approach is to add permanent markers to the tissue before creating bone fracture. The markers will be used to define the reference space.[3] This second approach will be discussed in more detail later.

34.1.2 Isotropic Uniform Random and Vertical Uniform Random Sections

Two types of sections can be used for stereology (▶ Fig. 34.1). Isotropic uniform random sections are sections with complete randomness. On the contrary, vertical uniform random (VUR) sections are prepared by randomly rotating the sample around an axis before embedding. In fracture studies, this axis can be the long bone that is fractured. VUR sections are less random compared to isotropic uniform random sections and are good for tissues with defined orientations. Fracture callus, bone, and cartilage in the callus do not have defined orientation, and the estimation of their volume does not require random sectioning. Blood vessels, however, may have defined orientation, and isotropic uniform random or VUR sections are required for their quantification.

34.1.3 Random Systemic Sampling

This is a central role of stereology. All tissues of interest in the reference space should have the same probability to get analyzed. To achieve this, random systemic sampling is performed, which means a starting point is chosen at random from the sampling frame and selections thereafter are at regular intervals (▶ Fig. 34.1). The intervals between selected sections in one sample have to be consistent; however, a different sample can have different intervals between its selected sections.

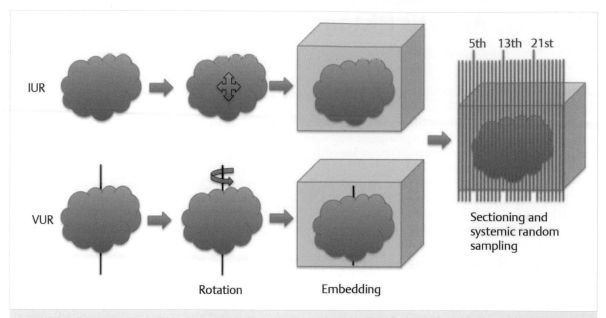

Fig. 34.1 Schematic illustration of the isotopic uniform random (IUR), vertical uniform random (VUR) sectioning, and systemic random sampling. IUR sections are generated by completely randomly rotating the tissue before embedding. VUR sections are generated by randomly rotating the tissue around an axis before embedding. In a long bone fracture, this axis can be the bone. Systemic random sampling is achieved by choosing a starting point of sectioning at random and selections thereafter are at regular intervals. In this example, the random starting point is the surface of the block. The interval is eight sections. A random number of five is chosen between numbers one to eight. The 5th, 13th, and 21st sections are selected for further histomorphometry.

34.1.4 Adequate Sampling

Adequate and efficient sampling is required to capture most of the biological variation in a parameter and to use your time and effort productively. Adequate sampling depends on the heterogeneity of the tissue and the amount of the object of interest in the reference space. It is easy to appreciate that quantification of tissues of high heterogeneity or counting rare events will need a higher fraction of sampling. The adequacy of sampling is measured by the coefficient of error, which is defined as the standard deviation divided by the mean.

As a rule of thumb, analysis of 6 to 10 levels (sections) and counting at least 200 intersections or points of the object of interest are usually enough. To guarantee adequate sampling, researchers may rely on a reasonable degree of oversampling by analyzing at least eight sections or more than 500 counts for each sample.

34.1.5 Choose the Right Probe

Many probes have been developed to analyze different parameters in stereology. One rule of probe selection is that the number of dimensions in the parameter of interest and the probe must have a sum of 3. For example, to estimate the number of cells, which is a zero-dimensional parameter, three-dimensional probes like a physical dissector or optical dissector should be used. To estimate surface area, a two-dimensional parameter, a one-dimensional line probe is used. For length of blood vessels, a two-dimensional planar probe is used as length is a one-dimensional parameter. For total volume, which is a three-dimensional parameter itself, a zero-dimensional point grid will be appropriate.

34.1.6 Follow the Same Protocol of Tissue Processing

Tissue processing has significant effects on the tissues. For example, dehydration steps in paraffin section preparation significantly shrink the tissue. Compared to frozen sectioning, which does not require dehydration, paraffin sectioning gives a lower reading of tissue volume. Tissue processing also affects the quality of histological staining, immunohistochemistry, and molecular analyses. For one analysis in one study, the same protocol of tissue processing, including harvesting, fixation, decalcification, embedding, sectioning, and staining, should be followed. For fracture studying, paraffin sections can be used to quantify the volume of callus, bone, or cartilage. To analyze fluorescent cells or perform immunostaining, frozen sections are usually better.

34.2 Stereology in Research on Bone Regeneration

Stereology is a valuable tool in orthopedic research. It is used to estimate volume. More importantly, stereology allows the unbiased quantification of cells including inflammatory cells and stem cells and tissue vascularization. Based on an Olympus CAST system (Center Valley, PA) and Visiopharm software (Hoersholm, Denmark), we have developed protocols to estimate the volume of tissue, number of cells, and length and surface area of blood vessels during fracture healing. The animal model we used is a murine tibia fracture model.

34.2.1 Creation of Tibia Fractures

Mice are anesthetized and a transverse fracture is created by three-point bending at the midshaft of tibia. Fractures are either left unstabilized or stabilized with a custom-made external fixator.[2] To apply the external fixator, the proximal and distal metaphyses of the tibia are transfixed using two insect pins each, which are oriented perpendicular to the long axis of the tibia. Two rings are secured to the pins and then bridged with three threaded bars (▶ Fig. 34.2). This external fixator provides rigid stability to the fracture. Animals are allowed to ambulate freely after recovery.

34.2.2 Tissue Processing

Animals with tibia fracture are euthanized at day 3 to 28 after injury. The whole tibia from the knee joint to the ankle is collected, skinned, and fixed in 4% paraformaldehyde for 24 hours at 4°C. Muscles are kept intact. Tissues are then decalcified in 19% ethylenediaminetetraacetic acid for 2 weeks at 4°C. Complete decalcification is confirmed by X-ray.

34.2.3 Estimation of Volume
Collect Systemic Random Sections

To estimate the volume of a tissue of interest in fracture callus, systemic random sections are collected. Either frozen or paraffin sections can be used. If immunohistochemistry is not part of the analysis, we routinely choose paraffin sections for their easy handling and better quality of histology. Longitudinal sections are used to estimate the volume of callus, bone, and cartilage within the callus. Section thickness is 10 μm or less. A nonstabilized tibia fracture normally has a large callus and 200 to 400 serial sections can be collected for each callus.[1,3,4,5] Therefore, we choose an interval of 30 sections (equals to 300 μm if each section is 10 μm thick) between two systemic randomly selected sections for histomorphometry. This setting allows us to analyze at least six sections for each sample. ▶ Fig. 34.1 illustrates the strategy of random

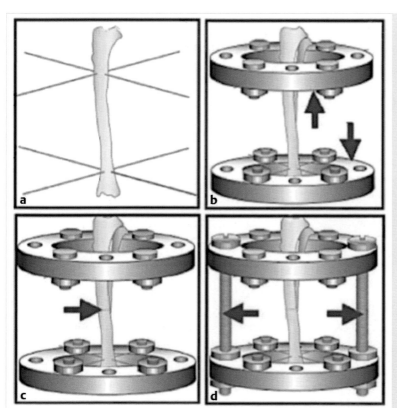

Fig. 34.2 Create a stabilized tibia fracture using an external fixator. (**a**) Two sets of pins are inserted in the proximal and distal tibia. (**b**) Rings are secured to the pins. (**c**) Transverse fracture is created at the midshaft of tibia. (**d**) Threaded rods are used to connect the two rings and stabilize the fracture. Tissues between the two sets of pins will serve as comparable reference space.

systemic sampling. Before the start of sectioning, a random number between 1 and 30 is assigned to each sample. For example, sample X is assigned a random number of 15. The tissue block of sample X is mounted on the microtome. The section thickness is set to 10 μm, and cutting is started. Sections are counted starting at the first cut, even if there is no tissue. The researcher then checks whether there is callus tissue on the 15th section. If there is callus tissue, this section will be collected as the first section for histomorphometry, the 45th section will be second, the 75th the third section, and so on. If there is no callus tissue on the 15th section, the researcher will need to continue cutting to the 45th section. The presence of callus tissue on the 45th section is then checked again, and this will be the first section to be collected if there is callus tissue. If the 45th section still has no callus tissue, the researcher will need to move on to the 75th section. After the first section with callus tissue is collected, every 30th section will be collected throughout the whole callus tissue.

Histological Staining

All collected sections will be subjected to histological staining. Because stereology allows the researcher to determine the tissue type basing on its structure and morphology under microscope, histological staining is not critical. All staining methods available for skeletal tissues can be used. We routinely use hematoxylin and eosin staining or Hall's and Brunt's quadruple staining for this task.[5] Slides stained with safranin-O/fast green staining, which stains cartilage red and bone and soft tissues green, or Mason's trichrome staining, which stains bone blue and soft tissues red, are also good for estimation of tissue volume.[1,4]

Estimate Tissue Volume Using Stereology

Estimation of tissue volume is performed under an Olympus CAST system, which has an automated stage, and Visiopharm stereology software. The volume of tissue of interest is estimated using Cavalieri's principle: "The Cavalieri principle states that the volume of two objects is the same if planes parallel to the base of the two objects intersect the objects to form profiles that have equal areas" (http://www.stereology.info/glossary/). The following is a step-by-step instruction of the analysis (► Fig. 34.3).

1. **Outline the callus.** Open Visiopharm. Outline the fracture callus under low magnification (40×) (► Fig. 34.3a). This will be the region of interest.
2. **Count callus.** Switch to a higher magnification (100×) and apply a proper point probe (i.e., four points/screen) to the region of interest (► Fig. 34.3b). Sample 100% of the outline area and count the points that fall on callus tissues.
3. **Count bone, cartilage, or other tissues.** Under high power (100×), apply a proper point probe with denser points (i.e., 36 points/screen) to the region of interest (► Fig. 34.3c). Sample 100% of the outline area and count the points that overlap with bone, cartilage, or any other type of tissue separately.
4. **Calculate the volume.** The area that each point represents in a setting of point probe can be read from the Visiopharm software. Export the counts of point to an Excel spreadsheet. Calculate the area of the analyzed tissue as: Area (section #) = point counts on that section * area/point. The volume of the tissue analyzed in the sample will be calculated as: Volume = Interval between two adjacent selected sections * Sum of the area of the tissue on all sections.

34.2.4 Quantification of Tissue Vascularization

Blood supply is critical for tissue regeneration. Bone fracture causes injury to blood vessels and disrupts blood supply. During fracture healing, vascularization of fracture callus occurs predominantly through angiogenesis, a

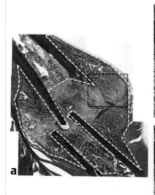
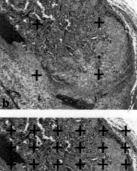
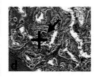

Fig. 34.3 Use point probes to estimate volume. (a) Fracture callus is outlined as the reference volume. (b) A point probe is superimposed to the section. One hundred percent of the outlined area is samples, and all points that fall onto callus tissue are counted. (c) A probe with denser points is used to count bone or cartilage. (d) The right upper quadrant of a cross is used to determine the type of tissue.

process of new blood vessel formation from preexisting ones. In murine tibia fracture, angiogenesis starts early after bone injury. By 3 days, angiogenesis is robust at the fracture site.[6] Stereology is one of the most powerful techniques to quantify blood vessels. Compared to conventional techniques that quantify the number and size distribution of blood vessels on two-dimensional sections, stereology allows us to estimate the length and surface area of blood vessels in a three-dimensional tissue.

Creating Comparable Reference Volume

As described previously, angiogenesis initiates early during fracture healing. At these early time points, fracture callus is obscure with no clear margin. It is a challenge to define comparable reference spaces for studies focusing on early fracture healing. The whole tibia with surrounding muscles could serve as a reference space. However, fracture callus is just a small portion of the whole tibia. Changes in the callus could be difficult to detect due to the large amount of normal tissue included in the reference space. One solution is to add permanent markers to the middle part of the tibia before the creation of fracture.[6] Modified from our procedures for an external fixator, a set of two insect pins is inserted into the proximal and distal tibia separately. The two sets of pins are 11 mm apart. Tissues between the proximal and distal pins are used as the reference space and subjected to analysis by stereology. This procedure allows us to collect comparable tissues from early fractures.

Generation of Vertical Uniform Random Sections

VUR sections are used in our study to analyze tissue vascularization during early fracture healing. Fracture tissues

are fixed with 4% paraformaldehyde and decalcified in 19% ethylenediaminetetraacetic acid at 4°C. Using tibia as the axis, fracture tissue is rotated randomly and embedded in optimal cutting temperature compound (▶ Fig. 34.1). VUR sections (10 μm) are prepared through the whole tissue block. Ten to fifteen VUR sections are then randomly and systemically selected for immunostaining to visualize the blood vessels.

PECAM-1 Immunohistochemistry

In hematoxylin and eosin staining, small blood vessels, especially capillaries, are difficult to identify. We suggest using immunohistochemistry for endothelium to identify blood vessels. Among markers of endothelium like PECAM-1 (CD-31), vWF, and CD34, we found PECAM-1 is superior with consistent results on frozen sections (▶ Fig. 34.4a). Routine protocol of immunohistochemistry is followed for PECAM-1 immunostaining. Briefly, tissues are first incubated with an anti–PECAM-1 antibody (Pharmingen, San Diego, CA; 1:100) overnight at 4°C, then with a second antibody (biotinylated goat anti-rat immunoglobulin G, Pharmingen, San Diego, CA), and finally with streptavidin-horseradish peroxidase (Amersham, Piscataway, NJ). The immune complexes are visualized using diaminobenzidine as the substrate, and the tissues are counterstained with methyl green.

Quantification of the Length Density of Blood Vessels

In stereology, two parameters are commonly used to assess vascularity. Length density refers to the length of blood vessels per unit volume of the reference space. Surface density refers to the area of the surface of blood

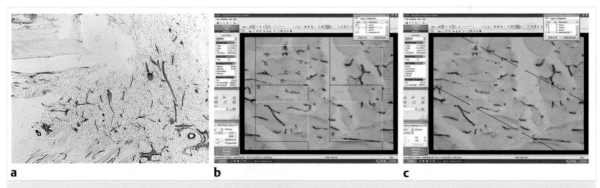

Fig. 34.4 Use counting frames and line segments to estimate the length density and surface density of blood vessels. **(a)** Blood vessels in the callus are visualized by immunohistochemistry for PECAM-1, a marker of endothelium. **(b)** To analyze length density of the blood vessels, the reference volume is outlined and 5 to 10% of it is sampled under 100×. Counting frames are superimposed on each systemic randomly selected field. The number of blood vessels (q, labeled as *C* in the figure) within the fracture callus is counted within each frame. The area of the callus is determined by counting the number of points (p, labeled as *B* in the figure) within the counting frame that fell on callus tissue. **(c)** To analyze the surface density of blood vessels, the reference volume is outlined and 5 to 10% of it is sampled. Randomly oriented line probes with points are then applied to each field. The points that fell onto callus tissue (p, labeled as *D* in the figure) and the number of intersections (I, labeled as *E* in the figure) between the outer surface of blood vessels and the line probes are quantified.

vessels per unit volume of the reference space.[3] Analysis of length density of blood vessels is performed on the Olympus CAST system and software by Visiopharm. All tissues on the VUR sections will be included and outlined as the reference volume at low power (40×) under microscope. The volume of the reference space is estimated using Cavalieri's principle, as described previously. The length density is estimated using high magnification (200×) and a count frame probe (▶ Fig. 34.4b). Depending on the size of the section and the vascularity, 5 to 10% of the outline reference volume is systematically acquired using unbiased uniform random sampling. Four counting frames that covered 50% of the area within a field are overlain on each field (▶ Fig. 34.4b). The number of blood vessels (q) within the fracture callus is counted within each frame. The area of the callus is determined by counting the number of points (p) within the counting frame that fell on callus tissue. The goal of the configuration is to achieve at least 200 counts for blood vessel profiles on all selected sections of one sample, because this is optimal for deriving accurate and precise estimates using stereology. For each configuration, the area per point (a/p) can be read from the Visiopharm software. Length density is calculated as: $Lv = 2^* \Sigma (q) / (\Sigma (p)^* a/p)$.

Determination of the Surface Density of Blood Vessels

The surface density of the blood vessels within fracture callus is determined under high magnification (200×). Approximately 5 to 10% of the outlined reference volume is systematically acquired using uniform random sampling. Randomly oriented line probes with points are then applied to each field (▶ Fig. 34.4c). The points that fell onto callus tissue (p) and the number of intersections (i) between the outer surface of blood vessels and the line probes are quantified. The surface density was calculated as: $Sv = 2^* \Sigma (i) / ((l/p)^* \Sigma (p))$. For each configuration, the length per point (l/p) can be read from the Visiopharm software.

34.2.5 Quantification of Inflammatory Cells

Inflammation plays an important role in fracture healing. Inflammatory cells are recruited to the fracture site and express numerous cytokines and growth factors, regulating angiogenesis, stem cell recruitment and differentiation, and callus remodeling. Inflammation is a promising direction for current orthopedic research. Studying infiltration of inflammatory cells, expression of cytokines, and their role in bone regeneration will improve our understanding of the regulating mechanisms of bone repair. Stereology is a valuable tool in the quantification of inflammatory cells in tissues.

Conventional cell counting techniques can take advantage of the stereology system by using its systemic

random sampling function. To do this, load the thin sections stained with immunohistochemistry for inflammatory cells on the stereology microscope. Open Visiopharm software. Outline the region of interest, and specify the proportion of the region of interest to be analyzed. The system will select systemic random fields for cell counting, which can be done using counting frames (▶ Fig. 34.5). The results will be expressed as number of cells/area of tissue of interest.

For more advanced users, stereology is able to get unbiased estimation of the number of cells in a three-dimensional space. Cells can be counted by either physical dissector or optical dissector. The physical dissector method requires the registration of two serial sections: One is the reference section and the other is the look-up section. Cells that show up in the look-up section but not the reference section are counted. The physical dissector is time consuming and requires high-quality sections. The optical dissector, an extension of the physical dissector, does not require the registration of two physical sections. Instead, the optical dissector is used by creating focal planes with a thin depth-of-field through a thick section. Oil immersion lenses are used to achieve the smallest focal depth under conventional or confocal microscope. To use the optical dissector, thick sections (≥60 μm) need to be prepared. Immunohistochemistry for specific surface markers is performed to visualize the inflammatory cells. The protocol of immunohistochemistry needs to be optimized so the reagents can penetrate the whole thickness of the section. The height of the optical dissector is determined based on the thickness of the section. A thin layer of tissue (about 5 μm) on the surface and at the bottom of the section should be excluded from the optical dissector. Under high magnification, a counting frame is superimposed to the microscopic field. The top surface of the optical dissector will serve as the look-up section and cells that are in focus at this plane will not be counted. Cells that come in focus in the optical dissector will be counted if they are found within the counting frame or hit the inclusion lines but not any of the exclusion lines of the counting frame. The size of the counting frame should be not too large. It is configured to have one to three cells in each counting frame.

34.3 An Alternative Technique of Histomorphometry: Photoshop

Using Photoshop (Adobe Systems Incorporated, San Jose, CA) software is an inexpensive and convenient alternative to Bioquant or stereology systems to estimate volume.[1,4,7,8,9] Tissue sections are generated and selected by systemic random sampling for histological staining. To give bone and cartilage distinct colors, safranin-O/fast green staining is used for cartilage and Manson's

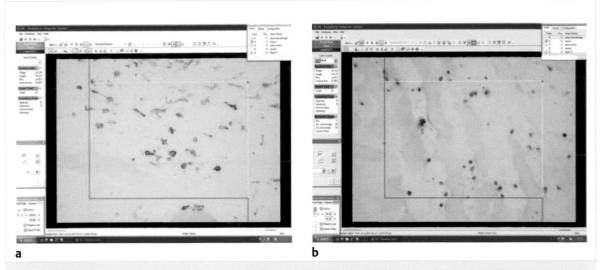

Fig. 34.5 Quantification of inflammatory cells. Immunohistochemistry for F4/80 and Ly6G was performed to visualize macrophages (**a**) and neutrophils (**b**), respectively. The reference volume is outlined, and 1 to 3% of it is sampled under 200 ×. A counting frame is applied to each field. Positive cells are counted if they are within the frame and the reference volume but not hitting the *red exclusion line*. The area of tissue analyzed is estimated by counting the left lower and right upper corners of the counting frame if they are within the reference volume.

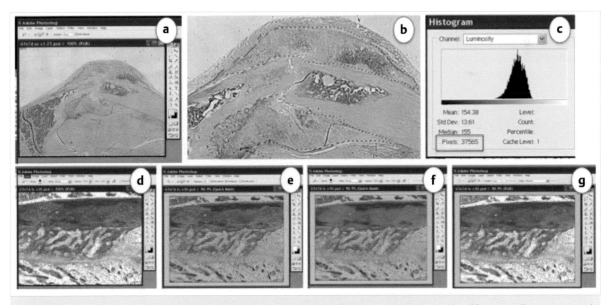

Fig. 34.6 Quantify tissue area using Photoshop (Adobe Systems Incorporated, San Jose, CA). Micrographs of fracture callus are imported into Photoshop. (**a**) Use the Lasso Tool to outline the callus. (**b**) The outlined callus. (**c**) Histogram shows the pixel counts of the outline area. (**d**) On sections of trichrome staining, use the Magic Wand Tool to select a blue color that represents bone. Note preexisting cortical bone is also selected, which needs to be deselected as we are only interested in the newly formed bone. (**e**) To erase the selection of cortical bone, add Quick Mask. (**f**) Use Eraser to remove unwanted selection of cortical bone. (**g**) Undo Quick Mask and now only newly formed bone is selected. Pixel count of the selected bone is read from Histogram as shown in (**c**).

trichrome staining for bone. Micrographs of fracture callus are imported into Photoshop. To achieve the best results, micrographs covering the whole fracture callus should be taken at a relatively high magnification (i.e., 40 to 100×). All micrographs for the same section are imported into Photoshop and photomerged into one large image. Histomorphometry is then performed on this image using the tools of Photoshop (► Fig. 34.6).

To estimate the volume of the fracture callus, the callus tissue is traced with the Lasso Tool and the number of pixels in the outlined area is read from the Histogram Panel. To convert the pixel numbers to area, a 1 mm × 1 mm square will be created in a new image with scales bars at the same magnification as that is used for micrographs. The number of pixels of this 1 mm^2 square is read from the Histogram Panel, which is then used to convert pixel numbers to area. The total volume of the callus is calculated as: $Vcallus = h*(Acallus_1 + Acallus_2 + ... + Acallus_n)$, in which h is the distance between two sections, and A is the area of callus on each section.

Cartilage or bone tissue on the image of fracture callus is selected with the Magic Wand Tool based on color similarity. Safranin-O/fast green stains cartilage red. Use the Magic Wand Tool to pick a red color representing cartilage and then select the similar color. Specify the tolerance to make your selection more accurate. Use the Magic Wand Tool to add more tissue or use the eraser to remove selection that is not cartilage. The pixels of the traced area are read from the Histogram and converted to area and volume using the same calculation as described previously for callus tissue. Bone appears blue on modified Milligan's trichrome staining so blue color is used to select bone tissue in Photoshop.[1] Because Photoshop selects bone or cartilage based on the color of tissue, quality control of staining is important.

In conclusion, many techniques of histomorphometry are available. The choice is dependent on the goal of your research and the data you want to collect to support your theory.

References

[1] Lu C, Miclau T, Hu D et al. Cellular basis for age-related changes in fracture repair. J Orthop Res 2005; 23: 1300–1307

[2] Thompson Z, Miclau T, Hu D, Helms JA. A model for intramembranous ossification during fracture healing. J Orthop Res 2002; 20: 1091–1098

[3] Lu C, Hansen E, Sapozhnikova A, Hu D, Miclau T, Marcucio RS. Effect of age on vascularization during fracture repair. J Orthop Res 2008; 26: 1384–1389

[4] Lu C, Miclau T, Hu D, Marcucio RS. Ischemia leads to delayed union during fracture healing: a mouse model. J Orthop Res 2007; 25: 51–61

[5] Lu C, Xing Z, Yu YY, Colnot C, Miclau T, Marcucio RS. Recombinant human bone morphogenetic protein-7 enhances fracture healing in an ischemic environment. J Orthop Res 2010; 28: 687–696

[6] Lu C, Saless N, Hu D et al. Mechanical stability affects angiogenesis during early fracture healing. J Orthop Trauma 2011; 25: 494–499

[7] Hu D, Lu C, Sapozhnikova A et al. Absence of beta3 integrin accelerates early skeletal repair. J Orthop Res 2010; 28: 32–37

[8] Xing Z, Lu C, Hu D, Miclau T, III, Marcucio RS. Rejuvenation of the inflammatory system stimulates fracture repair in aged mice. J Orthop Res 2010; 28: 1000–1006

[9] Xing Z, Lu C, Hu D et al. Multiple roles for CCR2 during fracture healing. Dis Model Mech 2010; 3: 451–458

Further Reading

Baddeley AJ, Gundersen HJ, Cruz-Orive LM. Estimation of surface area from vertical sections. J Microsc 1986; 142: 259–276

Dorph-Petersen KA. Stereological estimation using vertical sections in a complex tissue. J Microsc 1999; 195: 79–86

Howard CV, Reed M. Unbiased stereology: three-dimensional measurement in microscopy. New York: Springer-Verlag; 1998:107–132

Mouton PR. Principles and practices of unbiased stereology: an introduction for bioscientists. 1 e. Baltimore: The Johns Hopkins University Press; 2002

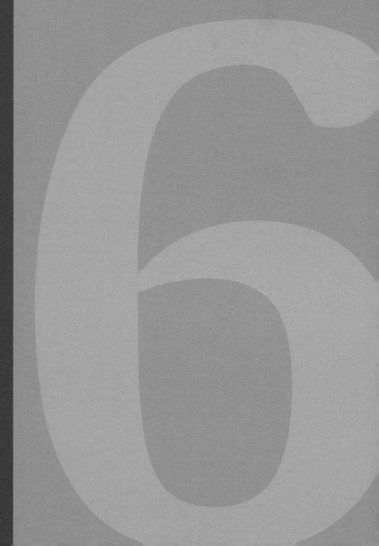

Part 6
Cellular Studies

35 Cell Culture Research

Franz Jakob, Barbara Klotz, Birgit Mentrup, Torsten Blunk, Andre F. Steinert, and Regina Ebert

Musculoskeletal diseases are increasingly important in all age groups with respect to injuries and degenerative diseases. The latter are particularly relevant in developed and aging societies, where mobility is an essential part of independence, especially in higher age. Degenerative diseases of bone, joints, and muscle like osteoporosis, osteoarthritis, and sarcopenia are common in the elderly and are main causes of dependence and disability. The burden of disease is extremely high and is second after mental and behavioral disorders worldwide with respect to years lived with disability. Injuries and degenerative conditions of tendons and ligaments are also increasing both in sport and in age-associated degenerative diseases and here regenerative therapeutic strategies are even less developed.

Jargon Simplified: Cell Line

A cell line is a cell culture that will proliferate indefinitely given appropriate fresh medium and space. It is immortalized and thereby escapes the Hayflick limit of population doublings. Cell lines may be looked upon as resembling neoplastic cells. In contrast, primary cells have a limited lifespan and undergo replicative senescence if they reach the Hayflick limit of population doublings.

Cell culture of mesenchymal cells has become an indispensable research tool. Transformed cell lines are commercially available and can be used as reproducible models for various scenarios. Primary cells can be isolated from various sources such as bone marrow, trabecular bone, cartilage, tendons, ligaments, and muscle. Being closer to physiology compared to cell lines derived from tumorous tissues, their disadvantage is their limited number and lifespan in culture. Their donor-dependent variability may both be an advantage and a disadvantage with respect to the reproducibility of experimental settings and their potential to get insights for individualized medicine, respectively. Immortalized and reprogrammed primary cells are coming into focus based on new technologies that are developed for genetic engineering and reprogramming.

The last three decades have seen an incredible increase in cell culture techniques and research with mesenchymal stem cells (MSC) from various sources to describe their potency, differentiation, and plasticity, and to develop stem cells as a tool for cell-based therapies. The techniques developed have reached a basis of state-of-the-art routine and offer a huge potential for future improvement.

The transition from two-dimensional to three-dimensional culture is key for many questions to be addressed. In order to mimic the physiological environment of the cells in vivo with respect to their microenvironment in terms of, for example, extracellular matrix (ECM), oxygen tension, and mechanical conditions, respective techniques will have to be refined and co-cultures with other cell types will have to be established. Reprogramming techniques will be helpful to avoid senescence and to get closer to individualized medicine. Enhanced bioreactor techniques will allow for reconstitution of a physiological environment in vitro to set up complex new experiments.

35.1 Mesenchymal Stem Cells

MSCs are adult stem cells scattered all over the organism. They reside in protected niche microenvironments and give rise to regenerative populations of precursors, capable of forming repair tissues upon injury or degeneration. By asymmetric cell division, the pool of stem cells ideally is unchanged, while daughter cells are amplified and form new tissue, together with precursors for vascularization where needed. The sequential phases of repair—blood clot–derived growth factors and precursor amplification, inflammation, modeling, and remodeling—are quite uniform throughout various tissues and for both regeneration and healing.[1,2]

MSCs are the most important source for tissue regeneration in mesenchymal tissues and as a support for non-mesenchymal tissues.[3,4] MSCs are multipotent precursor cells that can give rise to osteoblasts, chondrocytes, adipocytes, and other mesenchymal offspring upon specific stimuli for lineage-specific commitment. The nature and homogeneity of cell populations assigned as MSCs has been discussed since their first description.[5,6] The biology of commitment and differentiation for bone, fat, and cartilage formation has been largely unraveled, whereas the way from MSCs to muscle, tendon, and ligament cells is less well characterized but is under intensive research. As demonstrated by Sacchetti and coworkers,[7] CD146 + MSCs could establish a complete bone plus bone marrow microenvironment in vivo, indicating that the multipotency of at least some distinct MSC populations goes beyond a simple trilineage capacity of forming bone, cartilage, and fat.

What we culture and amplify is not the stem cell itself but the offspring (so called transient amplifying pool) generated by asymmetric cell division, which is prone to commitment and ages in culture.

35.2 Primary Cultures of Mesenchymal Stem Cells and Related Precursor Cell Populations

35.2.1 Core Definition of Mesenchymal Stem Cells: How to Establish a Mesenchymal Stem Cell Culture

Primary mesenchymal precursor populations can be established from outgrowth populations of bone marrow aspirates, mashed pieces of trabecular bone (bone chips), adipose tissue, pieces of tendon and ligaments, and almost any other tissue. The "gold standard" of MSC populations are those retrieved from bone marrow, whereas other populations are very similar but also significantly different in their transcriptome signature and multipotency.

After several days of primary culture, mesenchymal precursors start to grow in the dishes; they tightly adhere to plastic, which is a simple and effective selection criterion for MSC. The populations obtained are predominantly spindle cell–like cultures that show self-renewal and can give rise to several mesenchymal lineages derived from mesenchyme (▶ Fig. 35.1). Consensus conferences have been held (e.g., by The International Society for Cellular Therapy) that defined a minimum requirement for the definition of MSCs.[8] Cells must be plastic adherent when cultured under standard conditions and express the surface markers CD73, CD90, and CD105, and they should not express CD45, CD34, CD14, CD11b, CD79, or CD19 and HLA-DR. Finally, they must be capable of in vitro differentiation into osteoblasts, adipocytes, and chondrocytes, as described subsequently in the section of trilineage differentiation tests (▶ Table 35.1).

Having met all these criteria, one can work with these cultures as accepted true MSC cultures (▶ Fig. 35.1). However, these populations are still heterogeneous. The various cell types that grow in such cultures may be MSCs in variable stages of multipotency, lineage commitment, presenescence, or even senescence, or may be "contaminated"

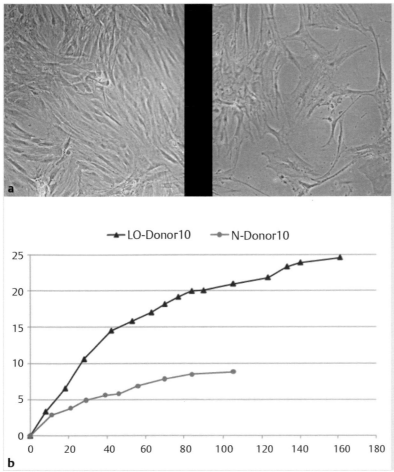

Fig. 35.1 Mesenchymal stem cells in culture. (a) On the *left*, human bone marrow–derived cells in passage 1 are depicted showing a typical spindle cell–like morphology. On the *right*, a presenescent culture is demonstrated showing more rounded cells that are not confluent and stop dividing. (b) Mesenchymal stem cells from human bone marrow of the femoral head show enhanced cumulative population doublings and a prolonged lifespan when cultured in low oxygen (3%) (*black triangles*) compared to "normal" oxygen (21%) (*gray dots*). The graph shows a remarkable difference depending on the oxygen concentration in this individual donor. Similar results are described in the literature.[14]

Table 35.1 Mesenchymal Stem Cell Types and Characteristic Marker Proteins

Cell Type	Source	Differentiation marker/Capacity	Literature
MSC minimum requirement definition and extended markers			
MSC	Bone marrow, trabecular bone chips, adipose tissue, cord blood, ligaments, teeth	Plastic adherence, self-renewal, production of colony-forming units; CD73++, CD90++, CD105++ CD45-, CD34-, CD14-, CD11b-, CD79-, CD19-, HLA-DR-; Trilineage differentiation potential (osteogenic, chondrogenic, adipogenic)	8,25
MSC	See above	Extended markers: CD13++, CD29++, CD44++, CD49e++, CD54++, CD71++, CD73++, CD90++, CD105++, CD106++, CD166++, HLA-ABC++ CD14-, CD31-, CD34-, CD45-, CD62E-, CD62L-, CD62P-, HLA-DR-	26
Mesenchymal precursors, extended definitions/specific subpopulations/other species			
MSC	Perivascular space, adjacent to vascular smooth muscle, "pericytes"	CD146++, CD105++, CD49a++, CD73++, CD90++, CD140b++, capable of reconstituting bone and bone marrow	7,25
MSC	Adipose tissue	CD117 (c-kit)++, HLA-DR++, CD34+/–, CD13+, CD29+, CD54++, CD73++, CD90++, CD105++, MHC I++; CD34+ higher proliferation, CD34- higher plasticity?	27
MSC	Muscle, nonsatellite stem cells	Sca1+, PDGFR-α++, PDGFR-β++, CD45-, CD31-; multipotency, but own myogenic capacity not demonstrated	20
MSC	Wharton's jelly	CD146++, CD59++; Oct-4++, SSEA4++, nucleostemin++, SOX-2++, Nanog++; CD105++/CD31–/KDR– cells have myogenic capacity	28
MSC	Bone marrow, umbilical cord blood	Sca1+, CD133+, Lin-, CD45-; Enriched for Oct4++, Nanog++, SSEA++ Very small embryonic–like stem cells, extended multipotency for hematopoietic stem cells, MSCs, lung epithelial cells, cardiomyocytes, and gametes	29
Pluripotent triploblastic "MSC"	Bone marrow	SSEA-3++, CD105++, triploblastic differentiation, "Muse cells" (multilineage-differentiating stress enduring)	30,31
Murine MSCs highly clonogenic	Bone marrow flushing and bone chips	LNGFR++, THY-1++, and VCAM-1++; rapidly clonogenic subpopulations, isolation produces genetically stabile populations and separates highly senescence prone populations	32
Murine MSCs (PαS cells)	Perivascular space, adjacent to vascular smooth muscle	PDGFR-α++, Sca-1++; Ang-1++, CXCL12++	25
Murine MSCs	Bone marrow, small subset of nonhematopoietic stromal cells in the perivascular space	Nestin++, overlap with PαS cells	33

Comprehensive reviews.[8,26,34,35]

Abbreviations: MSC, mesenchymal stem cell; CD, cluster of differentiation; HLA, human leukocyte antigen; SCA1, spinocerebellar ataxia type 1; PDGFR, platelet-derived growth factor receptor; Oct-4, octamer-binding protein 4; SSEA, stage-specific embryonic antigen; SOX-2, SRY (sex determining region Y)-box 2; KDR, kinase insert domain receptor; LNGFR, low-affinity nerve growth factor receptor; THY-1, thymocyte antigen 1; VCAM, vascular cell adhesion molecule; Ang-1, angiopoietin 1; CXCL12, chemokine (C-X-C motif) ligand 12; PαS, PDGFRα + Sca-1 + .

with, for example, endothelial precursors. Taking passage 1 of cultures is usually the time point where the plastic adherence criterion has worked out and other contaminating cells have been removed. Cell preparations from bone marrow in passage 0, for example, contain mature B cells that adhere to MSC but disappear after the first passage. Expression of immunoglobulin light or heavy chains is usually a reasonable criterion to proof if B cells have been removed from the cultures (our unpublished results).

35.2.2 Enhancing the Homogeneity of Mesenchymal Stem Cell Cultures

There is no single molecule that characterizes a true MSC and that would allow for highly specific sorting. Several groups have described MSC subpopulations with specific attitudes such as preferential osteogenic potential or high colony-forming capacity, but there is no accepted standard of selection that would allow for a standard operating procedure to get robust and homogeneous populations for defined purposes. In the future, the trend will be toward more defined MSC populations, which can be obtained by combined selection procedures (▶ Table 35.1). Selection for CD146, platelet-derived growth factor receptor (CD140), and stem cell antigen 1 (LY6A/E) expression may enhance the quality of cultures and provide more homogenous populations with respect to their multipotency. Selection for low-affinity nerve growth factor receptor (CD271), THY-1++(CD90), and vascular cell adhesion molecule 1 (CD106) expression was reported to separate highly stable and clonogenic populations from senescence prone ones that accumulate deoxyribonucleic acid damage.

The classical way of selecting more homogenous cell populations is preparative fluorescence activated cell sorting. Analytical fluorescence activated cell sorting procedures allow for more extensive nonpreparative characterization of the sorted populations using, for example, multicolor applications.

Jargon Simplified: Fluorescence Activated Cell Sorting

Fluorescence activated cell sorting analysis is a fluorescent antibody–based flow cytometry technique that allows analysis of single cells as to their pattern of membrane-associated proteins (intracellular proteins may less frequently also apply for this measure) even in heterogenous mixtures. It is used both for diagnostic cell phenotyping and preparative sorting of specific cell populations.

Selection of cell subpopulations is based on targeting cell type–specific surface molecules, but may also perform as "negative selection," which specifically removes contaminating populations. In addition, antibody-based immobilization procedures are commercially available such as magnetic bead–based applications, which do not require high tech equipment and are less expensive.[9] Another way to clonally select subpopulations of MSCs is the colony forming assay in several variations. This assay is based on picking single clones that arise from colonies in, for example, three-dimensional agarose environment and may also be used in combination with other methods of selection and characterization.[10]

35.3 Media and Serum

The routine experimental setting is that we use commercially available media in combination with serum, the latter being usually fetal calf serum (FCS). If heading for translational settings for therapeutic strategies, the use of nonhuman materials and well-defined media is a major obstacle, which should be avoided from the beginning, and well-defined media are desired. Before buying larger batches of FCS, screening for the efficacy of respective batches is recommended. Commercially available media can be very variable and especially variably expensive, ranging from basic media to so called stem cell media, which often comprise unknown growth factors that considerably influence the cell biology and cell signatures. The decision for the experimental setup should be carefully discussed ahead of the start of cell cultures (see ▶ Table 35.2).

Serum-free media are being developed for MSC propagation, especially for cultures that are produced for therapeutic purposes. Standard operating procedures that meet the regulations for good medical practice are being developed for future cell-based clinical applications using MSC large-scale amplification methods.[11,12] There is a research need about industrial production methods for MSC production and banking.[13]

35.4 Oxygen Tension in Cell Culture

Oxygen tension in routine cell culture is 21% corresponding to the atmospheric oxygen pressure. In vivo, the respective tissue oxygen tensions are extremely variable depending on the vascularization/availability of erythrocytes as oxygen carriers or the distance of a respective microenvironment to capillaries. Truly hypoxic conditions are usually around or below 1.5% oxygen, and low oxygen conditions may be defined around 3%. Oxygen tension has repeatedly been reported to modulate stemness and differentiation in culture and certainly also in vivo. These well-known facts are neglected worldwide, which may be due to the necessity of respective

Table 35.2 Trilineage Differentiation

	Expansion	Osteogenic	Adipogenic	Chondrogenic
Medium	DMEM F12 10% FCS 50 µg/mL L-ascorbic acid-2-phosphate 1% PenStrep	DMEM high glucose 10% FCS 1% PenStrep 10 mM β-glycerophosphate 100 nM dexamethasone 50 µg/mL L-ascorbic acid-2-phosphate	DMEM high glucose 10% FCS 1% PenStrep 1 µM dexamethasone 500 µM IBMX 1 µg/mL insulin 100 µM indomethacin	DMEM high glucose 1% PenStrep 50 µg/mL L-ascorbic acid-2-phosphate 100 nM dexamethasone 100 µg/mL pyruvate 40 µg/mL L-proline 1% ITS-1 10 ng/mL TGF-β1
Marker genes		Alkaline phosphatase Osteopontin Osteocalcin Bone sialoprotein Collagen 1A1	Fatty acid binding protein Lipoprotein lipase Peroxisome proliferator-activated receptor gamma	Collagen II Collagen IX Collagen X Aggrecan
Staining		Alizarin red Alkaline phosphatase	Oil Red O	Alcian blue

Abbreviations: DMEM, Dulbecco's Modified Eagle Medium; FCS, fetal calf serum; IBMX, 3-isobutyl-1-methylxanthine; ITS + 1, Insulin-transferrin-sodium selenite; TGF, transforming growth factor; PenStrep, penicillin streptomycin.

incubators, which are more expensive and cannot be used universally for any cultures in the laboratory. MSCs can be propagated under low oxygen conditions where their proliferation and their lifespan are enhanced (▶ Fig. 35.1).[14] Hence, a "modern" and adequate recommendation would be to generally amplify MSCs under conditions of low oxygen (e.g., 3%) until they are being used for assays, which require different conditions.

35.5 Mechanobiology of Cells in Culture

Control of transcription is mechanosensitive in multiple tissues and cells both during development and adult tissue regeneration. Some special aspects of mechanobiology are covered by Pathak et al in Chapter 38. Stem cell response to physical strain can be modulated by engineering the physical environment. Parameters determining this response include rigidity and topology of the ECM or adhesion substrate, mechanical loading of cells and tissues, and shear stresses associated with fluid flow. MSCs can both be seeded on stretchable dishes and scaffolds and subjected to mechanical strain using newly developed bioreactors in order to induce or to foster lineage commitment and differentiation. Specific mechanobiological conditions can enhance lineage commitment as it has been demonstrated for myogenic differentiation including cell fusion events by applying, for example, 11% cyclic uniaxial strain, 0.5 Hz, 1 h/day to adipose tissue–derived MSCs in culture and for osteogenic commitment.

35.6 Lineage Commitment and Multipotency Assays

35.6.1 Trilineage Differentiation of Mesenchymal Stem Cells

Basal trilineage tests (osteogenic, adipogenic, chondrogenic differentiation) are very commonly used to demonstrate the multilineage capacity of mesenchymal precursors (▶ Fig. 35.2). Trilineage differentiation of MSCs is induced by switching from stem cell expansion medium to specific differentiation media described by Pittenger et al[6] (▶ Table 35.2). When osteogenic and adipogenic differentiations are induced in two dimensions, it is important to start with a confluent MSC monolayer culture. Chondrogenic differentiation is classically performed in three dimensions in high density pellet culture, where 2×10^5 cells are centrifuged in a conical tube at $250 \times g$ for 5 minutes. The medium composition applied in the different laboratories did not change too much during the last decades, although some authors use single ingredients in different concentrations. In terms of osteogenic differentiation, a recent publication suggests switching from β-glycerophosphate to $Na_xH_{3-x}PO_4$ as a different phosphate source; other authors add growth factors such as basic fibroblast growth factor (FGF2), bone morphogenetic protein (BMP)2, BMP9, hepatocyte growth factor, epidermal growth factor, or platelet-derived growth factor. The use of 1,25-vitamin D3 is discussed controversially as some authors report lipid droplet formation in otherwise osteogenic cultures. Umbilical

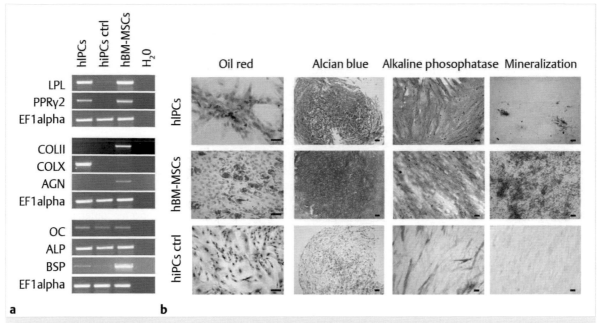

Fig. 35.2 Trilineage tests from human mesenchymal precursors derived from bone marrow of the femoral head (*hBM-MSC*) and from human pancreatic islets (*hiPCs*) in comparison. While both populations show comparable mesenchymal features in terms of surface markers and, for example, vimentin expression (*not shown*), the trilineage test is positive for hBM-MSC but hiPCs show moderate adipogenic differentiation and only marginal capacities for osteogenic and chondrogenic differentiation (**b**). Reverse transcription–polymerase chain reaction of some typical marker genes mirrors the results demonstrated in **a**. These data indicate that mesenchymal stem cell precursors that accompany the endocrine pancreas are different from mesenchymal stem cells derived from bone marrow with respect to their multipotency (reproduced from Limbert et al, 2010 with permission).

cord blood serum or platelet-rich plasma are discussed to support osteogenic or adipogenic differentiation better than the routinely used FCS. In chondrogenic pellet cultures, transforming growth factor (TGF)-β growth factors are mandatory as they are inductors of chondrogenesis. Other supplements belong to the group of promoting factors as BMP2, BMP4, BMP6, BMP7, and insulin-like growth factor 1, and are used by some authors to support chondrogenic differentiation.

35.6.2 Osteogenic Commitment and Differentiation

Osteogenic differentiation leads to the development of cell types that compose bone structure. The largest population of bone cells are osteocytes, cells that keep in touch and communicate with each other by developing multiple filamentous cell membrane extensions and produce high amounts of ECM, which is mineralized. Other cells that constitute bone are those that cover the surface of, for example, bone trabeculae, the so called lining cells. It is probably a subpopulation of these cells that is part of the protected niche for hematopoetic stem cells. The process of osteogenic differentiation is complex, and several partially overlapping phases can be observed. Roughly,

the crude phases from MSCs to terminally differentiated osteocytes comprise osteogenic commitment to "becoming an osteoblast," gradual loss of migration and proliferation capacity, expression of specific genes to create ECM (mainly collagen 1A1) and to regulate mineralization processes, and finally the transition to become an osteocyte, which is accompanied by the acquisition of expression of osteocyte specific markers such as sclerostin (SOST) and dentin matrix protein 1 (DMP-1). Osteogenic commitment is achieved through the combined and interactive activity of osteogenic signaling pathways such as parathyroid hormone receptor 1 signaling, BMPs and their receptors of the TGFβ family, and components of the wnt/frz/LRP5/6 pathway. Several other systems are potent contributors, and the reader is referred to respective review articles about osteoblast/osteocyte biology for detailed information.

From all the complex cellular tasks that could be monitored for the process of in vitro differentiation, the common two-dimensional test procedure monitors the expression of basic osteogenic transcription factors like RUNX2 (runt-related transcription factor 2) and osterix, intermediate or late marker genes for osteogenesis such as osteocalcin and alkaline phosphatase, and finally the mineralization capacity. The two-dimensional test requires 2 to 4 weeks of cell culture using empirically developed "osteogenic" ingredients of media. The main readouts for the test consist of reverse transcription–polymerase chain reaction for the gene expression pattern, staining methods for alkaline phosphatase activity, and staining of mineral using, for example, alizarin red. These readouts are basically qualitatively reported but can be quantified if comparison of modulators for osteogenic differentiation is required in the experimental setting (▶ Fig. 35.2 and ▶ Table 35.2). We have to realize that these test setups are yet insufficient to qualitatively describe the fine tuning of bone formation parameters, and basically the setup can be extended until it reaches conditions of in vitro tissue engineering. At least two important components of osteogenic differentiation and bone formation are lacking in this system, which are endothelial precursors and a three-dimensional environment. Neuronal influences are completely neglected and may be an important third component. Three-dimensional cell culture tests for osteogenic differentiation are not yet routinely established. Using collagen 1A1 gels, it is however possible to rapidly achieve osteogenic differentiation, and the expression of osteocyte specific genes is accelerated. Such three-dimensional gels can be maintained for months and still the cells survive and express osteocyte-specific genes (▶ Fig. 35.3).

35.6.3 Chondrogenic Differentiation and Cartilage Regeneration

Chondrogenic differentiation can be mimicked in culture but is the only process that is traditionally followed in three-dimensional pellet cultures obtained from routinely processed MSC cultures, which are pelleted and not resuspended.[6] The differentiation process is usually induced by TGFβ ligands and empirically established media ingredients in the absence of FCS. The minimum requirement readouts for chondrogenic differentiation are the stainings for collagen II and glycosaminoglycans. Many experimental settings require the demonstration of expression of collagen X, which is a marker for chondrocyte hypertrophy that precedes chondrocyte death. It is, however, increasingly becoming clear that our established in vitro assays are insufficient to describe the complex process of chondrocyte differentiation and cartilage formation and maintenance, as these assays lack important components such as control of hierarchical architecture, oxygen tension, and mechanical strain, which both control tissue quality and maintenance as a balance between synthesis and degradation of ECM components. Therefore, for more differentiated experimental setups, we need the continuously developed cell culture systems toward tissue engineering that finally allow for production of mature hyaline cartilage for therapeutic strategies, for example, in osteoarthritis.[15]

35.6.4 Adipogenic Differentiation

Adipogenic differentiation of MSCs is routinely monitored in vitro using two-dimensional cultures. The media, which also have been empirically found, comprise glucocorticoids and small molecule compounds that induce adipogenic commitment and differentiation. The steroid hormone receptor peroxisome proliferator-activated receptor gamma is a central transcription factor that is assigned to adipogenic differentiation. Several marker genes such as adiponectin, lipoprotein lipase, and fatty acid binding protein are accepted indicators for adipogenic differentiation. Staining of the developing lipid droplets using Oil Red O is commonly used to demonstrate a functional readout for the adipogenic differentiation. This assay is very powerful in terms of demonstrating the adipogenic potency of precursors, but is of course insufficient if it comes to questions like what type of adipose tissue is generated. Three-dimensional methods to grow adipose tissue have been developed for tissue engineering purposes, either directed toward therapeutic application or the generation of three-dimensional tissue models.

Employing the mouse preadipocyte cell line 3T3-L1 and three-dimensional polyglycolic acid fiber meshes, a coherent adipose tissue exhibiting mature adipocytes could be developed in long-term culture over 5 weeks in vitro[16] (▶ Fig. 35.4). In numerous studies, adipogenic induction in cell culture prior to implantation has been shown to be beneficial for the in vivo outcome. However, to date, no adipose tissue constructs have been developed in a clinically meaningful size. It has been widely acknowledged by now that there is a close physiological interplay between adipogenesis and angiogenesis in adipose tissue development.[17] Thus, current developments in adipose tissue regeneration aim to integrate various approaches to enhance tissue vascularization (e.g., by delivering angiogenic growth factors or integrating a vascular pedicle into the implanted construct). Three-dimensional co-cultures (e.g., of adipogenically induced MSCs and endothelial cells) may provide further valuable insights into the underlying mechanisms. Other current approaches in adipose engineering include the application of decellularized ECM structures derived from adipose tissue, demonstrating the instructive function of the biomaterial in the process of cell differentiation in three-dimensional cell culture, an observation that is by no means restricted to adipose tissue.

35.6.5 Tenogenic Differentiation

Mesenchymal precursor cells can be recovered from tendon tissue and may have potential for tendon repair.[18] Their signature is also specifically affected by degenerative diseases. There is not yet an established routine differentiation assay for tenogenic differentiation that is commonly used. Recent publications describe the effect

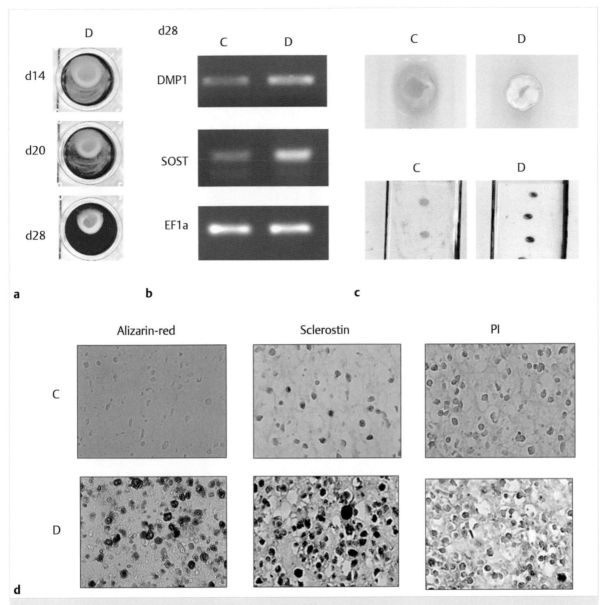

Fig. 35.3 Three-dimensional culture of mesenchymal stem cells (MSCs) in collagen 1 gels.(a) Increasing contraction of collagen gels during osteogenic differentiation (D) of MSCs after 14, 20, and 28 days. (b) Reverse transcription–polymerase chain reaction analysis of MSCs after 28 days of osteogenic differentiation in collagen gels. Even in the controls (C), the osteocytic marker genes dentin matrix protein 1 and sclerostin can be amplified after 28 days in three-dimensional culture. The housekeeping gene *EF1α* was used for reference. (c) Collagen gels with MSCs incubated in differentiation medium (D) appear more compact and more white after 4 weeks in three-dimensional culture in comparison to the controls (*upper lane*); alizarin red staining of gel sections covered on slides is more intensive in the differentiated gels due to increased mineral deposition than in the controls (*lower lane*). (d) Microscopic analysis of differentiated collagen gels (D) and controls (C) after 6 weeks in three-dimensional culture. Alizarin red staining and sclerostin expression is considerably increased in differentiated gels. Control staining with preimmune serum was performed to exclude unspecific signals.

of growth factors such as BMP12; growth differentiation factors (GDF) 5, 6, and 7; endothelial growth factor; basic fibroblast growth factor (FGF2); platelet derived growth factor; and TGFβ1, and ECM alignment combined with mechanical strain on tenogenic differentiation. Specific genes that are associated with tenogenic differentiation are, for example, decorin, tenascin C, and scleraxis. Tenogenic differentiation can be enhanced using mechanical stretching protocols combined with growth and differentiation factors (3% versus 21% oxygen tension, use of GDF5, GDF6, and GDF7).[19]

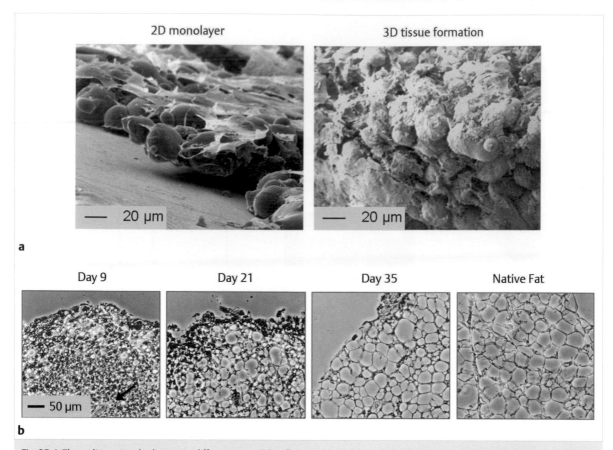

2D monolayer

3D tissue formation

— 20 μm

— 20 μm

a

Day 9

Day 21

Day 35

Native Fat

— 50 μm

b

Fig. 35.4 Three-dimensional adipogenic differentiation. (**a**) Cellular composition of two-dimensional and three-dimensional long-term cell culture (after 5 weeks) as investigated by scanning electron microscopy. Adipogenically induced 3T3-L1 preadipocytes in two-dimensional monolayers (well plates, tissue culture–treated plastic) were loosely connected to each other and extracellular matrix sheets were preferentially deposited on the cell surface. In contrast, three-dimensional differentiated adipocytes (seeded on polyglycolic acid fiber meshes) were situated within a coherent environment featuring three-dimensional cell-cell and cell–extracellular matrix interactions. (**b**) Development of three-dimensional tissue constructs in long-term culture in vitro as analyzed by histological staining (hematoxylin and eosin). Blank spaces within the cells were caused by dissolving lipid inclusions with organic solvents during deparaffinization. Native fat from rat femur is depicted for comparison. (Reprinted from Fischbach C, Spruss T, Weiser B, et al. Generation of mature fat pads in vitro and in vivo utilizing 3-D long-term culture of 3T3-L1 preadipocytes. Exp Cell Res 2004;300[1]:54–64, with permission from Elsevier.)

35.7 Muscle Stem Cells

Satellite stem cells and nonsatellite cells have both been assigned regenerative capacities for muscle regeneration, where a small nonsatellite cell population fulfils the criteria for multipotent MSCs (▶ Table 35.1).[20] The small nonsatellite MSC population is multipotent, seeming to contribute to muscle regeneration after injury, but their effect might be indirect through satellite cells. Their own myogenic differentiation capacity has not been demonstrated and a more deleterious role in pathology settings is discussed. Myogenic differentiation can be enhanced by applying tensile strain.

35.8 Three-Dimensional Cultures

Culturing cells in a two-dimensional monolayer does not really reflect the situation in vivo, where cells are in contact with each other or with cells from lineages characteristic for the particular microenvironment in a totally different spatial architecture. In comparison to conventional monolayer culture, three-dimensional cultures offer a more in vivo–like context including three-dimensional cell-cell and cell-ECM interactions, which can decisively influence shape and structure of the cells as well as the repertoire of genes expressed. Additionally, three-dimensional cultures in bioreactors will provide enhanced chances and tools to grow stem cells and differentiate them in vitro.

For three-dimensional cultures, different kinds of cell carriers can be utilized, the choice of which depends on the experimental goals of the cell culture or the requirements of the therapeutic application. Prefabricated porous three-dimensional scaffolds are widely used for cell seeding, cell culture in vitro, and subsequent implantation. The use of scaffolds offers the advantage that it allows for shape definition and maintenance but it requires surgery. As an alternative minimally invasive cell carrier, cell-encapsulating hydrogels are employed. They can be used as injectables (i.e., cells are suspended in the still liquid materials and gelation occurs after injection in the body). Another large advantage of injectables is their possible use in the filling of irregularly shaped defects. For experimental cell culture purposes, or precultivation in vitro prior to implantation, such cell-encapsulating hydrogels can be gelled also in vitro and subsequently cultured and/or implanted. A third cell carrier option for cell delivery and culture is the use of microparticulate carrier systems. Cells can attach on or within solid or porous microspheres and, similar to hydrogels, these microspheres may then be used as injectables. With regard to cell culture, these carriers even offer the option to preculture the cells in vitro prior to implantation (e.g., utilizing stirred bioreactors) and to still have the carrier in an injectable form (which is in contrast to the hydrogels, where gelation in vitro is a prerequisite for cell culture, but inhibits the use as injectables). Combinations of different kinds of scaffolds are possible (e.g., composite constructs made from solid porous scaffolds in which cells suspended in hydrogel materials are injected, or cell-seeded microspheres encapsulated in hydrogels).

Three-dimensional spheroid cultures may be used as building blocks in tissue engineering applications or as small tissue models for basic research. Advantages include the necessity for only low quantities of cells and a high reproducibility in size and cell number of the culture. Further advantages include an immediate cell-cell interaction and a favorable tissue homogeneity due to the small size. The latter is especially important when it comes to gene expression analysis in basic research, which is easily impaired by gradients in cell differentiation and tissue development when larger three-dimensional cultures are used. Furthermore, the spheroids enable a biomaterial-free three-dimensional cell culture, which may also be beneficial in basic research deliberately excluding the influence of any cell carrier.

As examples from bone research, three-dimensional cultures among others comprise cells embedded in matrices like collagen 1 or hydroxyapatite/tricalcium phosphate biphasic calcium phosphate ceramic particles (e.g., to mimic the mineral composition of bone matrix). MSCs, embedded in three-dimensional collagen 1 hydrogels, can be cultivated up to several months. After evaluation of the optimal cell density and gel concentration, cells are seeded in multiwell plates and incubated with the appropriate medium. This enables monitoring of the differentiation from a multipotent precursor cell to a specialized osteocyte-like cell, expressing marker proteins like DMP-1 or SOST, and coming along with a deposition of mineralized and calcified ECM. Histochemical analyses of sections from collagen gels embedded in paraffin with specific antibodies as well as von Kossa or alizarin red staining can easily be performed at any particular point in time. Furthermore, collagenase digestion enables the release of the cells from the matrix to isolate ribonucleic acid and characterization of the gene expression profile even after several weeks in three-dimensional culture.

Comparing the expression of osteoblast and osteocyte markers during human primary osteocyte differentiation reveals considerable differences for two-dimensional and three-dimensional cell culture. Whereas genes like RUNX2, OPN, PHEX, or DMP-1 are upregulated during the first 2 weeks in three-dimensional culture, the expression in adherent two-dimensional cells is very low.

A three-dimensional environment alone seems to be a stimulus for the MSCs to differentiate toward an osteocyte, as we could detect DMP-1 and SOST expression in three-dimensional–cultivated MSCs without any supplements that typically induce osteogenic differentiation.

Differentiation toward an osteocyte-like cell is often accompanied by contraction of collagen hydrogels, but the extent of reduction can vary considerably. It is remarkable that the murine postosteoblast cell line MLO-A5 displays only marginal contraction of collagen gels and the murine osteocyte cell line MLO-Y4 even no contraction, indicating that the state of differentiation influences this capability (own unpublished data) (▶ Fig. 35.3).

35.9 Embryonic Stem and Induced Pluripotent Stem Cells

Cellular reprogramming is technically rapidly developed and the methods used range from genetic engineering to small molecule approaches.[21,22] Reprogramming enables us to generate pluripotent patient-specific cell lines, that may be useful to establish individualized therapeutic protocols for many diseases.[21] Protocols to develop MSCs and committed offspring from pluripotent cells are also being developed. Human embryonic stem cell culture requires specific supplements and conditions that are described in the literature. Culture conditions to differentiate embryonic stem cells toward chondrocytes for cartilage repair are being reported. Feeder cells and specific ingredients are often required to culture, for example, pluripotent stem cells or embryonic stem cells. Feeder-free substrates are presently being characterized that allow for the development of cell-based clinical applications that are free from animal-derived serum proteins.[23] Overall, such new cell culture methods are important for researchers who work in this field. At present, specialized experts refine such methods to work out robust protocols, which provide sufficiently safe procedures to make sure that any single cell in the induced pluripotent stem cell culture is committed and differentiated toward MSC. Recent publications report that MSC-like cell lines derived from different induced pluripotent stem cell lines exhibit considerable variability in their differentiation capacity.[24]

35.10 Conclusion

Musculoskeletal research during the last two decades has seen a rapid development of methods in cell culture, knowledge in cell biology, and rapid translation into clinical cell based applications. Methods in regenerative medicine are also rapidly developed, including tissue engineering procedures and bioreactor technology. Many new laboratories have been installed and are now run by professional scientists, and this has pushed forward our fascinating field of research. This short introduction into cell culture techniques should raise the interest for more, because there is not enough space to describe sophisticated methods in detail, but it should provide a basic knowledge about what is established in the field.

References

[1] Gerstenfeld LC, Cullinane DM, Barnes GL, Graves DT, Einhorn TA. Fracture healing as a post-natal developmental process: molecular, spatial, and temporal aspects of its regulation. J Cell Biochem 2003; 88: 873–884

[2] Kolar P, Schmidt-Bleek K, Schell H et al. The early fracture hematoma and its potential role in fracture healing. Tissue Eng Part B Rev 2010; 16: 427–434

[3] Ma J, Both SK, Yang F et al. Concise review: cell-based strategies in bone tissue engineering and regenerative medicine. Stem Cells Transl Med 2014; 3: 98–107

[4] Steinert AF, Rackwitz L, Gilbert F, Nöth U, Tuan RS. Concise review: the clinical application of mesenchymal stem cells for musculoskeletal regeneration: current status and perspectives. Stem Cells Transl Med 2012; 1: 237–247

[5] Friedenstein AJ, Chailakhyan RK, Gerasimov UV. Bone marrow osteogenic stem cells: in vitro cultivation and transplantation in diffusion chambers. Cell Tissue Kinet 1987; 20: 263–272

[6] Pittenger MF, Mackay AM, Beck SC et al. Multilineage potential of adult human mesenchymal stem cells. Science 1999; 284: 143–147

[7] Sacchetti B, Funari A, Michienzi S et al. Self-renewing osteoprogenitors in bone marrow sinusoids can organize a hematopoietic microenvironment. Cell 2007; 131: 324–336

[8] Dominici M, Le Blanc K, Mueller I et al. Minimal criteria for defining multipotent mesenchymal stromal cells. The International Society for Cellular Therapy position statement. Cytotherapy 2006; 8: 315–317

[9] Tirino V, Paino F, De Rosa A, Papaccio G. Identification, isolation, characterization, and banking of human dental pulp stem cells. Methods Mol Biol 2012; 879: 443–463

[10] Gronthos S, Zannettino AC, Hay SJ et al. Molecular and cellular characterisation of highly purified stromal stem cells derived from human bone marrow. J Cell Sci 2003; 116: 1827–1835

[11] Jung S, Panchalingam KM, Wuerth RD, Rosenberg L, Behie LA. Large-scale production of human mesenchymal stem cells for clinical applications. Biotechnol Appl Biochem 2012; 59: 106–120

[12] Sensebe L, Gadelorge M, Fleury Cappellesso S. Production of mesenchymal stromal/stem cells according to good manufacturing practices: a review. Stem Cell Res Ther 2013;4(3):66

[13] Thirumala S, Goebel WS, Woods EJ. Manufacturing and banking of mesenchymal stem cells. Expert Opin Biol Ther 2013; 13: 673–691

[14] Fehrer C, Brunauer R, Laschober G et al. Reduced oxygen tension attenuates differentiation capacity of human mesenchymal stem cells and prolongs their lifespan. Aging Cell 2007; 6: 745–757

[15] Tuan RS, Chen AF, Klatt BA. Cartilage regeneration. J Am Acad Orthop Surg 2013; 21: 303–311

[16] Fischbach C, Spruss T, Weiser B et al. Generation of mature fat pads in vitro and in vivo utilizing 3-D long-term culture of 3T3-L1 preadipocytes. Exp Cell Res 2004; 300: 54–64

[17] Christiaens V, Lijnen HR. Angiogenesis and development of adipose tissue. Mol Cell Endocrinol 2010; 318: 2–9

[18] Rothrauff BB, Tuan R. Cellular therapy in bone-tendon interface regeneration. Organogenesis 2014

[19] Raabe O, Shell K, Fietz D et al. Tenogenic differentiation of equine adipose-tissue-derived stem cells under the influence of tensile strain, growth differentiation factors and various oxygen tensions. Cell Tissue Res 2013; 352: 509–521

[20] Boppart MD, De Lisio M, Zou K, Huntsman HD. Defining a role for non-satellite stem cells in the regulation of muscle repair following exercise. Frontiers Physiol 2013;4:310

[21] Malik N, Rao MS. A review of the methods for human iPSC derivation. Methods Mol Biol 2013; 997: 23–33

[22] Wörsdörfer P, Thier M, Kadari A, Edenhofer F. Roadmap to cellular reprogramming—manipulating transcriptional networks with DNA, RNA, proteins and small molecules. Curr Mol Med 2013; 13: 868–878

[23] Sams A, Powers MJ. Feeder-free substrates for pluripotent stem cell culture. Methods Mol Biol 2013; 997: 73–89

[24] Hynes K, Menicanin D, Mrozik KM, Gronthos S, Bartold PM. Generation of functional mesenchymal stem cells from different induced pluripotent stem cell lines. Stem Cells Dev 2014; 23: 1084–1096

[25] Mabuchi Y, Houlihan DD, Akazawa C, Okano H, Matsuzaki Y. Prospective isolation of murine and human bone marrow mesenchymal stem cells based on surface markers. Stem Cells Int 2013a; 2013: 507301

[26] Calloni R, Cordero EA, Henriques JA, Bonatto D. Reviewing and updating the major molecular markers for stem cells. Stem Cells Dev 2013; 22: 1455–1476

[27] Barba M, Cicione C, Bernardini C, Michetti F, Lattanzi W. Adipose-derived mesenchymal cells for bone regeneration: state of the art. Biomed Res Int 2013;2013:416391

[28] Kim DW, Staples M, Shinozuka K, Pantcheva P, Kang SD, Borlongan CV. Wharton's jelly-derived mesenchymal stem cells: phenotypic characterization and optimizing their therapeutic potential for clinical applications. Int J Mol Sci 2013; 14: 11692–11712

[29] Shin DM, Suszynska M, Mierzejewska K, Ratajczak J, Ratajczak MZ. Very small embryonic-like stem-cell optimization of isolation protocols: an update of molecular signatures and a review of current in vivo applications. Exp Mol Med 2013; 45: e56

[30] Kuroda Y, Dezawa M. Mesenchymal stem cells and their subpopulation, pluripotent muse cells, in basic research and regenerative medicine. Anat Rec (Hoboken) 2014; 297: 98–110

[31] Kuroda Y, Wakao S, Kitada M, Murakami T, Nojima M, Dezawa M. Isolation, culture and evaluation of multilineage-differentiating stress-enduring (Muse) cells. Nat Protoc 2013; 8: 1391–1415

[32] Mabuchi Y, Morikawa S, Harada S, et al. LNGFR(+)THY-1(+)VCAM-1 (hi+) cells reveal functionally distinct subpopulations in mesenchymal stem cells. Stem Cell Reports 2013;1(2):152–165

[33] Méndez-Ferrer S, Michurina TV, Ferraro F et al. Mesenchymal and haematopoietic stem cells form a unique bone marrow niche. Nature 2010; 466: 829–834

[34] Boxall SA, Jones E. Markers for characterization of bone marrow multipotential stromal cells. Stem Cells Int 2012; 2012: 975871

[35] Mafi P, Hindocha S, Mafi R, Griffin M, Khan WS. Adult mesenchymal stem cells and cell surface characterization - a systematic review of the literature. Open Orthop J 2011;5(Suppl 2):253–260

Further Reading

Boskey AL, Roy R. Cell culture systems for studies of bone and tooth mineralization. Chem Rev 2008; 108: 4716–4733

Holzapfel BM, Reichert JC, Schantz JT et al. How smart do biomaterials need to be? A translational science and clinical point of view. Adv Drug Deliv Rev 2013; 65: 581–603

Jakob F, Ebert R, Ignatius A et al. Bone tissue engineering in osteoporosis. Maturitas 2013; 75: 118–124

Marie PJ. Signaling pathways affecting skeletal health. Curr Osteoporos Rep 2012; 10: 190–198

Dawson JI, Kanczler J, Tare R, Kassem M, Oreffo RC. Bridging the gap: Bone regeneration using skeletal stem cell-based strategies - Where are we now? Stem Cells 2014;32(1):35–44

36 Cartilage Explants and Organ Culture Models

Innes D.M. Smith

Cartilage is a unique tissue that allows the frictionless motion of a joint while withstanding considerable forces. Unfortunately, for individuals affected by a variety of joint pathology (e.g., osteoarthritis and rheumatoid arthritis), the loss of cartilage is a common end pathway that results in pain, loss of joint function, and subsequent disability. Exciting and challenging aspects of cartilage research may focus on identifying factors that result in cartilage damage and subsequent loss or mechanisms of cartilage regeneration and repair. All basic research in these areas is directed, ultimately, to future clinical benefit. Two particular research methods are considered suitable[1]: cartilage explants[2] and organ culture models. A prerequisite for any individual intending to embark on cartilage research is an understanding of cartilage physiology. This will direct the researcher to identify particular experimental targets. In this chapter, the reader will be introduced to basic cartilage physiology before proceeding to experimental cartilage explant and organ culture methodology.

36.1 Articular Cartilage: Composition

It is considered by many that the most important structure within a synovial joint is articular cartilage, otherwise known as hyaline cartilage. This tissue is the smooth, glistening white material covering the articulating bone ends and serves to provide frictionless joint movement. For the vast majority of individuals, it will act in a trouble-free manner over their lifetime. Cartilage is remarkably resilient to compressive forces, which can exceed 100 atmospheres during standing,[1] yet allows controlled deformation in order to distribute loads. It is all the more remarkable, therefore, that articular cartilage is alymphatic, aneural, and avascular. Furthermore, it is 65 to 80% water by wet weight.[2] Given the avascular nature of cartilage, its nutrition is entirely reliant on the diffusion of metabolites from the synovial fluid.

The chondrocyte is the only cellular component of articular cartilage. Chondrocytes comprise less than 10% of the structure of cartilage and contribute approximately 1% of its volume.[3] They exhibit a very simple rounded shape when viewed under a microscope (▶ Fig. 36.1). Despite their simplistic appearance, however, chondrocytes are actually highly differentiated and specialized mesenchymal cells that are central to the survival of cartilage.[1]

The primary role of the chondrocyte is to synthesize the macromolecular components that constitute the extracellular matrix. These components include collagen, proteoglycans, and noncollagenous proteins.[3] The final addition to these macromolecular components, in the extracellular matrix, is tissue fluid, which is predominantly water. The extracellular matrix is thereby essentially a fiber-reinforced gel. It is the interaction between the macromolecular framework and tissue fluid that provides cartilage with its unique mechanical properties of "stiffness" and "resilience."

Throughout their lifespan, chondrocytes have an intimate relationship with the extracellular matrix. Alterations in the macromolecular composition of the matrix are closely monitored by the chondrocytes and, when necessary, controlled matrix synthesis or breakdown is initiated. Chondrocytes are therefore both the architects and cellular building blocks of articular cartilage.

Chondrocytes are regarded as postmitotic cells, insomuch that once skeletal maturity is reached there is no further cell division detectable in healthy adult articular cartilage.[1] Mature chondrocytes therefore have a long lifespan and are generally expected to remain viable as long as their host.

Once chondrocytes are lost they are not replaced, and when they are lost in large numbers their importance in

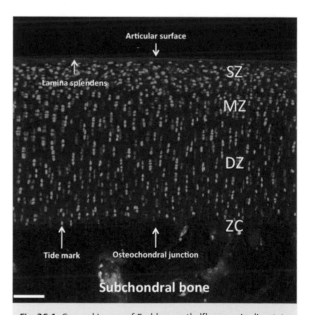

Fig. 36.1 Coronal image of 5-chloromethylfluorescein diacetate and propidium iodide labeled bovine cartilage, acquired using an upright confocal laser scanning microscope coupled with a ×10 dry objective, displaying the superficial (*SZ*), middle (*MZ*), and deep zones (*DZ*) of cartilage along with the zone of calcification (*ZC*). Important histological/microscopic landmarks are also illustrated. 5-chloromethylfluorescein diacetate and propidium iodide label living and dead chondrocytes *green* and *red*, respectively. *White bar* = 100 μm.

the maintenance of cartilage integrity is truly illustrated. Simon et al,[4] investigating the long-term effect of chondrocyte death induced by localized cryotherapy on rabbit articular cartilage in vivo, demonstrated, through histological staining coupled with both normal and polarized light microscopy, that the cartilage was structurally intact at 6 months despite the absence of living chondrocytes. However, by 12 months extensive cartilage fibrillation and softening was evident, changes which are considered to be among the first macroscopic appearances associated with degenerative joint disease.

There is currently no accurate information as to the length of time taken for human cartilage devoid of chondrocytes to degrade. Nevertheless, the progressive degeneration and loss of cartilage will be inevitable. It is therefore extremely important to preserve chondrocyte viability during both acute and chronic pathology, and also during surgical instrumentation.

36.2 Articular Cartilage: Structure

Despite the apparently simplistic composition of articular cartilage, its structure is both complex and heterogeneous. The thickness, cell density, matrix composition, and mechanical properties of articular cartilage vary within the same joint, between joints in the same individual, and between species.[5] Nevertheless, a consistent feature of articular cartilage within synovial joints, regardless of species, is that it has the same overall structure and serves the same function.

The full thickness of cartilage extends from the articular surface to the osteochondral junction (bone-cartilage interface) (▶ Fig. 36.1). Between these two points, articular cartilage is loosely divided into four distinct zones on the basis of depth-associated variation in cell morphology and extracellular matrix properties[1]: the superficial zone,[2] the middle zone,[3] the deep zone,[4] and the zone of calcification (▶ Fig. 36.1).[3] The demarcation between each zone, however, can often be difficult to define.

The superficial (tangential) zone is the smallest zone, accounting for approximately 0 to 10% depth from the articular surface and typically consists of two layers (▶ Fig. 36.1).[5] The first of these layers is an acellular sheet of fine fibrils that is known as the lamina splendens.[3] Deep to this layer, flattened ellipsoid-shaped chondrocytes lie within a matrix that has a low proteoglycan and high collagen content.[6] The dense network of collagen fibers, which, along with the chondrocytes, are orientated parallel to the articular surface, provide the tissue with tensile strength and stiffness. This arrangement is also considered to act as a sieve by allowing the passage of nutrients from the synovial fluid into the cartilage while, at the same time, preventing the ingress of potentially damaging larger molecules of the immune system.[3]

The middle zone provides a functional and anatomical bridge between the superficial and deep zones. It accounts for approximately 10 to 40% depth from the articular surface (▶ Fig. 36.1). The chondrocytes within this zone are at lower density and are more spherical in shape in comparison to the superficial zone. The collagen fibers have a greater diameter and, in contrast to the superficial zone, arch obliquely in relation to the articular surface. Furthermore, there is a greater concentration of proteoglycans within the matrix of this zone but, conversely, there is a lower water and collagen content.[5] Functionally, the middle zone offers the first line of resistance to compressive forces and thereby acts as a "shock absorber."

Immediately below the middle zone lies the deep zone, which accounts for approximately 40 to 100% depth from the articular surface (▶ Fig. 36.1). It is characterized by spherical chondrocytes that organize themselves into columns, sometimes referred to as "Benninghoff's arcades," that are perpendicular to the articular surface. The adjacent collagen fibers, which have the widest diameter of all collagen fibers embedded within articular cartilage, extend into the tidemark, the boundary between uncalcified and calcified cartilage.[3] The main function of this zone, which contains the highest concentration of proteoglycans and the lowest water content, is to provide the maximum resistance to compressive forces.[2]

The deepest layer of cartilage is the zone of calcification, otherwise known as the zone of calcified cartilage, and this layer separates articular cartilage from subchondral bone (▶ Fig. 36.1). This zone is characterized by a sparse population of spherical chondrocytes that are of a lower volume than those from the deep zone. The chondrocytes are surrounded by uncalcified lacunae and radial collagen fibers that are anchored within a calcified matrix in which there is an absence of proteoglycans.[6] The zone of calcification plays a crucial role in tethering cartilage to bone.

36.3 Cartilage Repair

It is well recognized that articular cartilage has a very poor regenerative capacity following injury. There are two likely explanations for this phenomenon. Firstly, as mentioned previously, the literature to date suggests that cellular division does not take place in healthy articular cartilage chondrocytes once skeletal maturity has been reached. Chondrocyte loss, as a consequence of injury or disease, in adulthood is therefore not replaced. Secondly, cartilage is an avascular tissue. In well-vascularized tissues such as skin and liver, the healing process follows an established pattern of necrosis, inflammation, and repair. An adequate blood supply is essential for the inflammation and repair phases of the response. Necrosis has been shown to be present in partial thickness articular cartilage injuries but no healing process has subsequently been identified.[7] However, if the injury extends beyond the zone of calcification (see the previous discussion), blood seeps into the wound from the vascularized subchondral bone, thereby delivering the necessary inflammatory mediators, growth factors, and reparative cells, such as fibroblasts and mesenchymal stem cells, for healing to occur. Nevertheless, the healing process that ensues is rudimentary and the defect is filled with mechanically inferior fibrocartilage. This suboptimal tissue has been shown to degenerate quickly once mechanical load is applied with the eventual formation of an isolated osteoarthritic lesion that may subsequently result in pain and disability.[7]

36.4 In Vivo Cartilage and In Vitro Isolated Chondrocyte Studies

The ever-rising prevalence of osteoarthritis in the population commands research attention. Osteoarthritis is fundamentally a disease of articular cartilage loss, a loss in a tissue that has minimal capacity for healing and regeneration. Research in this area is crucial and exciting not least because of its unique challenges.

The experimental study of cartilage has largely been conducted on animal models, isolated chondrocytes, or cartilage explants. Animal models have the advantage of allowing the analysis of cartilage within a living joint. The obvious advantage of such studies is that the results obtained reflect a closer correlation and relevance to the clinical setting.

Nevertheless, there are disadvantages to the use of live animal models. The strong and often complex host immune response, inherent in an animal model, can make the assessment of experimental variables difficult. For example, when assessing the impact of a particular bacterial strain on cartilage in an animal model of septic arthritis, it is difficult to distinguish what proportion of the resulting cartilage damage is due to the bacterial toxins and what proportion is due to the host immune response. Albeit, some of these difficulties can be overcome with the use of animals, such as mice, bred with selective absence of various components of the immune response. Animals are expensive to purchase and maintain, which is a not inconsiderable factor. Animal studies also necessitate the acquisition of animal handling licenses and ethical approval, both of which are time-consuming and associated with considerable paperwork.

In some research circumstances, it is important to remove the host immune response from the experimental environment in order to more accurately evaluate the primary effect of particular "challenges" on articular cartilage. Accordingly, it is necessary to distance the research model from the living animal. One such model is the use of isolated chondrocytes.

In the absence of a host immune response, isolated chondrocytes have the advantage of allowing easier control of experimental variables. However, in relative comparison to other isolated cell types, chondrocytes are challenging. Despite their apparently stable appearance within healthy living cartilage for many decades, once chondrocytes are isolated within an experimental vessel such as a petri dish (i.e., taken out of their native environment), they rapidly attempt to change their phenotype. They develop a "fibroblast-like" flattened and elongated shape, enter a proliferative cycle, and alter the characteristics of the synthesized collagen. In order to avert this undesirable change in phenotype, isolated chondrocytes must be rapidly embedded within agarose gels, thereby making their isolation less simplistic.

36.5 Cartilage Explants

Articular cartilage explants are simply pieces of cartilage of variable size that are extracted from a synovial joint. In comparison to isolated chondrocytes, they allow the assessment of cartilage as a tissue, intact with its cellular and matrix components, while also permitting tight control of experimental variables in the absence of a host immune response. Cartilage explants, sourced from various animals, have frequently been used for research purposes.

> **Jargon Simplified: Cartilage Explants**
>
> Cartilage explants are defined as harvested pieces of articular cartilage, of variable size, for the purpose of in vitro culture. In comparison to isolated chondrocytes, they permit the study of cartilage as a tissue (i.e., with intact cellular and extracellular components and thus more accurately mimic the in vivo environment).

Some studies have utilized human cartilage explants. However, there are several potential problems associated with their use. Similar to live animal studies, ethical permission is again required and, additionally, patient consent is required. Human cartilage is traditionally obtained from the femoral condyles or tibial plateaus of patients undergoing total knee joint replacement or the femoral heads of patients either undergoing total hip replacement or hemiarthroplasty for osteoarthritis and femoral neck fracture. Because these patients are invariably elderly, the common pathology is osteoarthritis and it is therefore extremely difficult to source healthy nondegenerate cartilage from such surgical discard. In a study by Amin et al,[8] which investigated the chondroprotective effect of raised irrigation solution osmolarity in a human cartilage explant model of sharp mechanical trauma, the femoral condyles of only four patients out of a total of 30 (87% rejection rate) recruited for the study were deemed nondegenerate and suitable for experimental purposes. A further consideration against the use of human cartilage is that studies have demonstrated similar responses by bovine and human cartilage to a variety of experimental challenges.[9]

36.6 Cartilage Explant Harvesting

A recommended and reliable source of healthy, nondegenerate, articular cartilage for experimentation is the metacarpophalangeal joint of bovine feet (▶ Fig. 36.2). Although bovine cartilage is thinner than human cartilage, it does share many of the characteristics of human cartilage in terms of composition, chondrocyte function, and matrix interactions.[3] Following the abattoir slaughter of cows, bovine feet are routinely removed from the animals as part of the meat production process. Most large abattoirs will invariably generate a potentially large quantity of cartilage for research. Beneficially, no animals are specifically sacrificed for experimentation purposes and no ethical permission is required because the material is classed as "abattoir discard."

The procedure for harvesting cartilage explants from the bovine metacarpophalangeal joint is outlined in ▶ Fig. 36.2. When the joint is opened, it is important to closely inspect the cartilage for any signs of degeneration, which include fissures and regions of ulceration, and if judged to be present the specimen should be discarded. Cartilage explants are harvested from the convex articular surface of the proximal aspect of the joint with the "rocking motion" of a number-24 scalpel blade (▶ Fig. 36.2). Explants may also be harvested with an osteotome or punch biopsy instrument. It is recommended that a full osteochondral explant (▶ Fig. 36.3; i.e., full thickness of cartilage including 1 to 2 mm of subchondral bone) is obtained whenever possible because the shearing of the collagen fibers anchoring the cartilage to the bone results in marked "curling" of the cartilage explant, thereby rendering the subsequent preparation of histological sections and microscopy more difficult. Ideally, cartilage explants should be harvested from the metacarpophalangeal joint within 12 hours of slaughter. If, for logistical reasons, this is not possible, healthy cartilage can still be harvested from feet stored at 4°C for up to 48 hours.

36.7 Cartilage Explant Culture

The stages at which cartilage explants are harvested from the joint will vary depending on the experiment. In some cases, the cartilage may be deliberately injured while still on the joint. For example, experimentation to assess the effect of drilling on cartilage will necessitate the drilling of the cartilage on the joint prior to extraction of an explant containing the drill hole. In other cases, cartilage explants are harvested from the joint prior to experimentation (e.g., the assessment of chondrocyte viability and matrix integrity in acidic conditions, whereby culture medium pH is altered and an experimental time course established).

All cartilage explants will ultimately end up in culture medium, whether it is for fluorescent staining purposes or long-term culture. A recommended and well-established cartilage culture medium is Dulbecco's Modified Eagle's Medium (DMEM). Penicillin (50 U/mL DMEM) and streptomycin (50 μg/mL DMEM) should be added to the DMEM in order to reduce the chance of infection, unless a specific bacterial infection is desired as part of the experiment. As long as the medium is changed regularly, cartilage explants can be kept alive for several weeks. A good indicator for culture medium replacement is when the DMEM, which contains phenol red, becomes orange in color. Phenol red is pH-sensitive and progresses from red (pH 7.4) through to yellow as the pH becomes more acidic. Thus, as the concentration of the acidic by-products of cartilage metabolism builds, the DMEM changes color.

36.8 Experimental Assessment: Chondrocytes

There are two potential experimental targets when assessing cartilage explants[1]: chondrocytes[2] and the extracellular matrix. Chondrocytes have traditionally been assessed by standard histological staining techniques.[4] However, a technique for the assessment of in situ chondrocytes that is becoming increasingly popular is confocal laser scanning microscopy (CLSM) (see Chapter 33). A major benefit of CLSM is that fluorescently labeled living or fixed in situ chondrocytes can be directly visualized in three dimensions. An array of designated responses can be quantified, using both low- and high-power objectives (▶ Fig. 36.4), within a defined region of cartilage (i.e., superficial zone), using a variety of specialized software packages. There are a vast number of highly specific fluorescent stains available and those chosen will depend on the particular study. For example, the fluorescent stains 5-chloromethylfluorescein diacetate and propidium iodide, which stain living and dead cells green and red, respectively, can be used to perform chondrocyte viability assays on explants following either mechanical, chemical, or biological trauma (▶ Fig. 36.4).

36.9 Experimental Assessment: Extracellular Matrix

As mentioned earlier in the chapter, the major constituents of the extracellular matrix are (1) tissue fluid, (2)

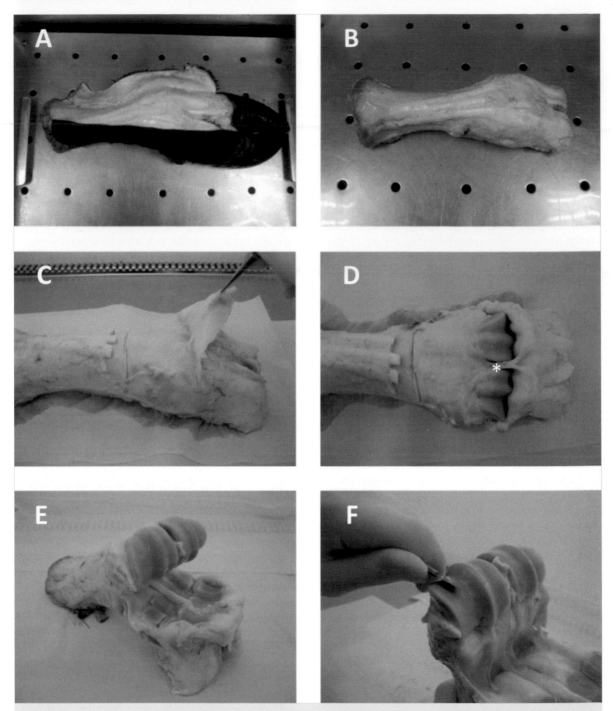

Fig. 36.2 The harvesting of osteochondral explants from the bovine metacarpophalangeal joint (anterior approach). (a) The bovine foot is washed in running water to remove excess dirt and skinned using a number-24 scalpel. (b) The hoof is removed and the skinned specimen is sprayed with 70% ethanol to reduce the risk of cartilage contamination upon opening the joint. (c) The extensor tendons are divided, exposing the underlying joint capsule. (d) The joint capsule is dissected at its proximal margin and reflected distally to expose the joint. Care should be taken not to injure/contaminate the articular surface with the dissection instruments. The collateral and intra-articular (*asterisk*) ligaments are divided in order to permit adequate joint exposure. (e) The articular surface is carefully inspected for evidence of degenerative disease/cartilage injury and, if necessary, the joint is discarded. (f) If the articular surface appears healthy, osteochondral explants are harvested with a fresh number-24 scalpel. (Photographs kindly provided by Mr. Joseph Winstanley.)

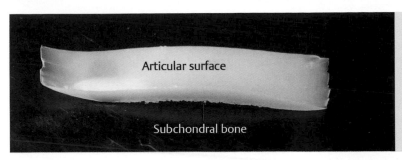

Fig. 36.3 A bovine osteochondral explant. The acquisition of 2 to 3 mm of subchondral bone maintains explant integrity and prevents cartilage "curling."

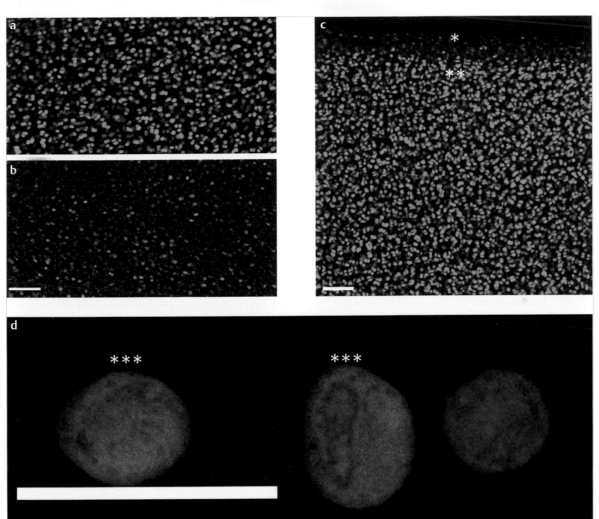

Fig. 36.4 Examples of the use of confocal laser scanning microscopy for the analysis of in situ chondrocytes following experimental challenge. (**a, b**) Axial sections (× 10 dry objective) of 5-chloromethylfluorescein diacetate and propidium iodide labeled bovine cartilage (5-chloromethylfluorescein diacetate and propidium iodide stain living and dead chondrocytes green and red, respectively), imaging chondrocytes within the superficial zone only, following a 40-hour culture in Dulbecco's Modified Eagle's Medium (DMEM) alone (**a**) or DMEM inoculated with *Staphylococcus aureus* (**b**). In comparison to the explant cultured in noninfected DMEM, there is marked chondrocyte death in the explant cultured in the presence of bacteria (**b**). (**c**) An axial section (× 10 dry objective) of bovine cartilage incorporating a scalpel cut (*asterisk*), which induces a band of cell death extending from the cut margin. (**d**) A high power image (× 64 oil immersion objective) of chondrocytes at the interface between healthy and dead cells (**) illustrates cells in the process of dying (***), which may not be evident on low power images. *White bar* in **b** and **c** = 100 μm. *White bar* in **d** = 10 μm.

collagen, and (3) proteoglycans. Damage to the extracellular matrix can be assessed in several different ways. The most simplistic approach is to measure cartilage explant water content, which is usually on the order of 65 to 80%, as it has been demonstrated that an increased cartilage water content is a sensitive indicator of matrix disruption.[10] This can be achieved by obtaining the (a) wet and (b) dry weights of the explants and using the following equation to calculate percentage water content: $((a - b)/a) \times 100$.

Collagen and proteoglycan content can be investigated in a number of ways. Firstly, the content of either component can be indirectly performed by specific histological stains. Alternatively, another method is based on the premise that when the matrix degrades in response to experimental challenge, these components are released directly into the surrounding culture medium and can be directly measured by specific assays. Finally, the chondrocyte release of degradative enzymes from such collagenases, metalloproteases, and aggrecanases, which will contribute to matrix breakdown in response to injury, can also be measured.

> **Jargon Simplified: Glycosaminoglycan and Aggrecan Assays**
>
> In some studies, glycosaminoglycan and aggrecan assays are performed as a measure of extracellular matrix damage. Proteoglycans are formed by a core protein to which are attached sulfated sidechains of glycosaminoglycan. In cartilage, the key core protein is aggrecan. Thus, glycosaminoglycan and aggrecan assays are essentially measures of proteoglycan breakdown.

36.10 Organ Culture Models

Undoubtedly, one of the major benefits of cartilage explants is their simplicity. They are easy to harvest, maintain, and conduct experiments upon. They do have several limitations, however. Explants inherently allow only a relatively small area of cartilage for experimentation. For example, cartilage explants would not be suitable for assessing the integration of autologous stem cell grafts into large cartilage defects. Furthermore, and perhaps most importantly, they do not allow a more accurate representation of the in vivo joint environment in respect of constant variations in both load and movement.

Organ (joint) culture models are, by definition, the culture (37°C) of an intact joint in vitro. They are undoubtedly more complex than cartilage explants to work with as research tools, a difficulty that may explain their relatively infrequent use in the field of articular cartilage research. However, despite these difficulties, once the experimental technique is established the researcher can

be rewarded with an experimental tool that has the potential to mimic a joint environment similar to that in vivo, albeit without an immune response and an active blood supply to the subchondral bone. The same experimental assessment techniques for the assessment of cartilage explants (i.e., CLSM and proteolytic enzyme assays) can be used to analyze joint culture model experiments.

Joint culture models can be established from the joints of a variety of animal species. The bovine metacarpophalangeal joint (▶ Fig. 36.2), which has been mentioned previously, is an excellent choice for establishing such a model as it has a size not dissimilar to the human knee joint. The joint should be skinned, de-hoofed, and skeletalized, sparing the intra-articular ligament (▶ Fig. 36.5), and the bones proximal and distal to the joint cut at the junction of the metaphysis and diaphysis in order to allow complete immersion in culture medium (DMEM including 10% fetal calf serum) within the experimental vessel. Thereafter, a magnetic stirrer can be used to circulate culture medium around the joint. If the culture medium is changed regularly, and bacterial or fungal infection is prevented, then the organ culture model can be kept "alive" for several weeks.

Organ culture models are highly adaptable. ▶ Fig. 36.5 provides an illustration of both a static and dynamic organ culture model of the bovine metacarpophalangeal joint. The static model simply sits within the culture vessel while the rotating wheel and attached lever arm allows continuous joint motion in the dynamic model. Both models are ideal for the study of cartilage response and repair in the absence of the complexities of the host immune response. If desired, a defined load can also be applied to both models with the use of a mechanical loading rig.

> **Jargon Simplified: Organ (Joint) Culture**
>
> Organ (joint) culture is defined as the culture of an entire organ (joint) in vitro. While complex, such a model enables the establishment of a joint environment similar to that in vivo, but without the complexities of a host immune response. Organ (joint) culture models are ideally suited for the study of cartilage injury and the assessment of novel cartilage healing strategies (i.e., autologous stem cell grafts).

36.11 Conclusion

Despite its complex structure, the simplistic composition of articular cartilage allows clearly defined experimental assessment targets: chondrocytes and the constituents of the extracellular matrix. Many basic science research questions may potentially be answered using either cartilage explants or organ culture models. The answers to whatever these questions may be are important and

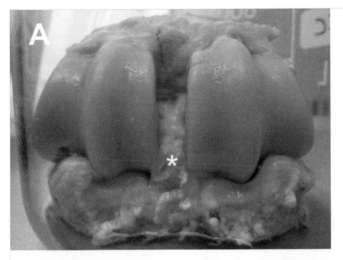
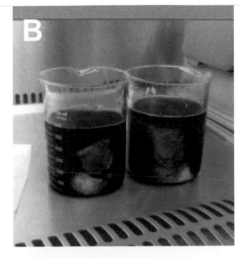
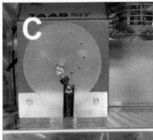
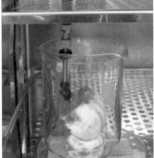
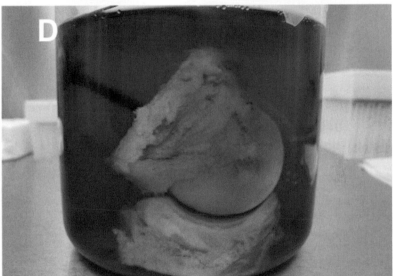

Fig. 36.5 Static (**a, b**) and dynamic (**c, d**) joint culture models established from the bovine metacarpophalangeal joint. The bone is cut proximal and distal to the joint (**a**) to allow submersion in culture medium within a suitable experimental vessel (**b**). The joint is skeletalized (**a**) with sparing of the intra-articular ligament (*asterisk*), which provides joint stability. (**c, d**) The attachment of a lever arm to an electronic rotating wheel allows controlled motion of the joint. (Photographs kindly provided by Mr. Yicheng Lin.)

contributory in their own right. Ultimately, however, the knowledge and information acquired has to be taken from the laboratory bench to the living animal with all its inherent challenges and difficulties.

References

[1] Muir H. The chondrocyte, architect of cartilage. Biomechanics, structure, function and molecular biology of cartilage matrix macromolecules. BioEssays 1995; 17: 1039–1048

[2] Pearle AD, Warren RF, Rodeo SA. Basic science of articular cartilage and osteoarthritis. Clin Sports Med 2005; 24: 1–12

[3] Buckwalter JA, Mankin HJ. Articular cartilage. Part I: tissue design and chondrocyte-matrix interactions. J Bone Joint Surg Am 1997; 79: 600–611

[4] Simon WH, Richardson S, Herman W, Parsons JR, Lane J. Long-term effects of chondrocyte death on rabbit articular cartilage in vivo. J Bone Joint Surg Am 1976; 58: 517–526

[5] Buckwalter JA, Mankin HJ, Grodzinsky AJ. Articular cartilage and osteoarthritis. Instr Course Lect 2005; 54: 465–480

[6] Poole CA. Articular cartilage chondrons: form, function and failure. J Anat 1997; 191: 1–13

[7] Mankin HJ. The response of articular cartilage to mechanical injury. J Bone Joint Surg Am 1982; 64: 460–466

[8] Amin AK, Huntley JS, Patton JT, Brenkel IJ, Simpson AHRW, Hall AC. Hyperosmolarity protects chondrocytes from mechanical injury in human articular cartilage: an experimental report. J Bone Joint Surg Br 2011; 93: 277–284

[9] D'Lima DD, Hashimoto S, Chen PC, Lotz MK, Colwell CW, Jr. In vitro and in vivo models of cartilage injury. J Bone Joint Surg Am 2001; 83-A Suppl 2: 22–24

[10] Buckwalter JA, Mankin HJ. Articular cartilage. Part II: degeneration and osteoarthritis, repair, regeneration, and transplantation. J Bone Joint Surg Am 1997; 47: 487–504

Further Reading

Amin AK, Huntley JS, Bush PG, Simpson AHRW, Hall AC. Osmolarity influences chondrocyte death in wounded articular cartilage. J Bone Joint Surg Am 2008; 90: 1531–1542

Buckwalter JA, Mankin HJ, Grodzinsky AJ. Articular cartilage and osteoarthritis. Instr Course Lect 2005; 54: 465–480

de Vries-van Melle ML, Mandl EW, Kops N, Koevoet WJLM, Verhaar JAN, van Osch GJVM, An osteochondral culture model to study mechanisms involved in articular cartilage repair. Tissue Eng Part C Methods 2012; 18: 45–53

37 Fluid Flow and Strain in Bone

Petra Juffer, Astrid D. Bakker, Richard T. Jaspers, and Jenneke Klein-Nulend

It has been well established that lack of physical exercise leads to bone loss, though this can be prevented by mechanical stimulation. Bone mass in athletes performing high-impact activities such as running, basketball, or tennis is much higher when compared to bone mass in sedentary people.[1] The process of bone remodeling allows bones to adapt their mass and structure to mechanical loading.[2] During bone remodeling, bone resorption by osteoclasts is followed by bone deposition by osteoblasts.[3] Current scientific insights strongly suggest that mechanical adaptation by osteoclasts and osteoblasts is orchestrated by osteocytes.[2] The osteocyte is a stellate-shaped cell with numerous processes, embedded within the mineralized bone matrix. Osteocytes are connected to each other via their processes, forming a network through very thin canals, the canaliculi. Of all cells in mature bone, over 90% are osteocytes.[2] In response to a mechanical stimulus, osteocytes transduce the mechanical signal into a biochemical signal (i.e., production of growth factors, cytokines, and reactive nitrogen and oxygen species). These signaling molecules activate osteoblasts to form new bone.[2] In the absence of a mechanical stimulus, osteocytes produce molecules that stimulate osteoclast development and activity.[2] Osteoblasts themselves are able to respond to mechanical loading as well.[4]

Mechanical loading on bone causes tiny deformations in the stiff mineralized bone matrix. The cells that are attached to the deforming bone matrix will deform as well (▶ Fig. 37.1). Quantitative studies on animal and

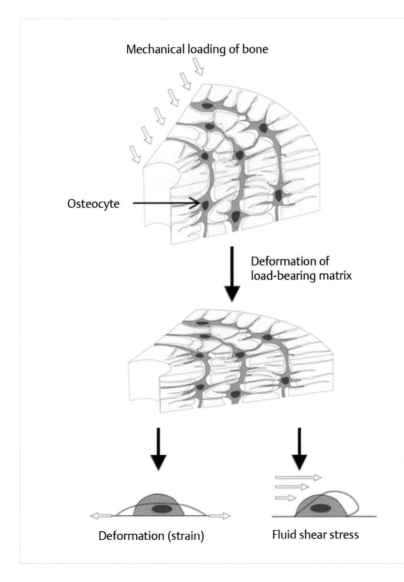

Fig. 37.1 Mechanical loading of bone causes deformation of the load-bearing matrix. This load can be transmitted to the cells directly, causing cell deformation (strain), or indirectly through fluid flow resulting in fluid shear stress that can be sensed by the osteocytes.

Mechanical loading of bone

Osteocyte

Deformation of load-bearing matrix

Deformation (strain)

Fluid shear stress

human bones found maximal loading-induced strains (matrix deformation) of 0.2 to 0.3%.[5] These deformations are very small, and one can wonder whether they are sensed at all by the cells. However, because bone is not a homogenous material, the magnitude of global (end-to-end) strain that is applied on bone will be different from the local strains within the bone matrix.[6] Strain distributions in bone are highly heterogeneous, and therefore the strains that osteocytes experience in vivo might be much higher than the applied strain to bone.

When bones are loaded, the resulting deformation will drive a thin layer of fluid through the canaliculi around the network of osteocytes.[2] This can be compared with squeezing a stiff, water-soaked sponge. The fluid flows from regions under high pressure to regions under low pressure, and results in a fluid shear stress, ranging from 0.8 to 5 Pa.[7]

In vitro studies have demonstrated that bone cells are sensitive to both fluid shear stress and tensile stress, and that these two types of mechanical stimuli have different effects on bone cells with respect to their biological response.[8] In the next paragraphs, two in vitro methods are described that can be used to study the effect of fluid flow and tensile strain on bone cells in a two-dimensional environment. Increasing our knowledge of how bone cells respond to mechanical loading in vitro will help to better understand the processes involved in the in vivo–induced adaptation of bone mass and structure in response to mechanical loading.

37.1 Mechanical Loading of Bone Cells in Vitro

37.1.1 Parallel-Plate Flow Chamber

The effect of physiological flow regimes on the biochemical response of bone cells can be studied using a parallel-plate fluid flow chamber (▶ Fig. 37.2). A cell monolayer attached to a glass slide is subjected to fluid flow by forcing the medium to flow between two parallel plates, creating a pressure gradient along the chamber. The shear stress (τ) induced by a specific flow is mainly determined by the flow rate (Q) of the culture medium, the fluid viscosity (μ), the width (b) of the channel, and the height (h) difference between the two parallel plates: $\tau_{wall} = \frac{6\mu Q}{bh^2}$. For details about the required dimensions of the chamber, and characterization of the chamber for dynamic fluid flow experiments, see Bacabac et al.[9]

37.1.2 Membrane Stretch

The biochemical response of bone cells to strain can be investigated in vitro using a Flexcell Tension Plus System (Flexcell Corporation, McKeesport, PA). This system uses vacuum to deform a flexible-bottom culture plate

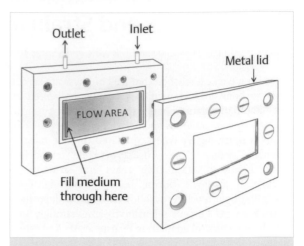

Fig. 37.2 A parallel plate flow chamber consisting of an inlet (where fluid enters the flow chamber), a flow area, an outlet (where fluid leaves the flow chamber), and a metal lid to cover the glass slide with the cells facing the flow area. Fill the flow chamber with flow medium through one side of the flow area.

(▶ Fig. 37.3). The precision, accuracy, and repeatability of the strains controlled by the system, resulting in deformations to growing cells, are essential to analyze and interpret the results accurately. It is therefore recommended to validate the system before starting experiments (Note 37.1 (p.297)).

37.2 Mechanical Loading of Bone Cells by Pulsatile Fluid Flow

Jargon Simplified: Pulsatile Fluid Flow

Mechanical loading of bone cells by pulsatile fluid flow results in a dynamic fluid shear stress onto the cells. This fluid shear stress mimics in vivo loading on bone cells that are located in the canalicular network of bone.

37.2.1 Materials

Cell Culture Media and Solutions

1. Culture medium: alpha-Modified Eagle's Medium (22571, GIBCO, Paisley, UK), supplemented with 10 µg/mL penicillin (Sigma-Aldrich, St. Louis, MO), 10 µg/mL streptomycin (Sigma-Aldrich), 50 µg/mL fungizone (GIBCO), and 10% serum (10% heat-inactivated fetal bovine serum [FBS] when using the MC3T3-E1 cell line; 5% FBS plus 5% heat-inactivated calf serum [CS] when using the MLO-Y4 cell line). When using other cell types, change the contents of the medium according to the requirements of that specific cell type.

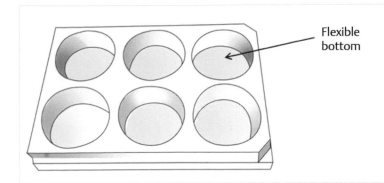

Fig. 37.3 Bioflex plate: A six-well cell culture plate with a flexible silicone elastomer membrane (Flexcell International Corporation, Hillsborough, NC).

Flexible bottom

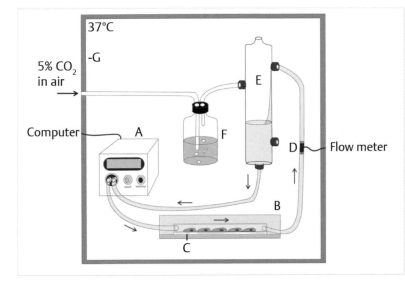

Fig. 37.4 Fluid flow apparatus: *A*: Pump. *B*: Flow chamber. *C*: Glass slide with cells (only part of the slide containing the cells is exposed to fluid flow). *D*: Flow probe. *E*: Medium reservoir. *F*: Water bottle. *G*: Incubator.

37°C

5% CO_2 in air

-G

Computer

A

F

E

D — Flow meter

B

C

2. Flow medium: alpha-Modified Eagle's Medium supplemented with 10 µg/mL penicillin, 10 µg/mL streptomycin, 50 µg/mL fungizone, and 2% serum (2% FBS when using the MC3T3-E1 cell line; 1% FBS plus 1% CS when using MLO-Y4 cell line).
3. Sterile phosphate-buffered saline (PBS), pH 7.4.
4. Trypsin-tetra sodium ethylenediamine tetraacetic acid (EDTA) solution consisting of 0.25% trypsin and 1 mM EDTA 4Na.
5. 70% ethanol.
6. Griess reagent for determination of nitric oxide (NO) production. Solution A: 2% sulfanylamide and 5% phosphate in water. Solution B: 0.2% naphtylethelene diamine HCl in water. Store the solutions separately in a refrigerator and protect from light.
7. 0.1 M $NaNO_2$ in water (stock solution) for quantification of NO production.

37.2.1.2. Instruments

1. 75 cm^2 tissue culture flasks
2. 94/16 mm cellstar petri dishes
3. Fluid flow apparatus (▶ Fig. 37.4):
   a) 37°C incubator

b) Water reservoir
c) Gas phase of 5% CO_2 in air (or use CO_2 independent medium)
d) Parallel-plate flow chamber (▶ Fig. 37.2). The chamber provides a controlled laminar flow over the cells (Note 37.2 (p. 298)).
e) Poly-l-lysine-coated (50 µg/mL) or collagen-I–coated glass slides
f) Medium reservoir
g) Microannular gear pump (Mikrosysteme GmbH, Germany) (Note 37.3 (p. 298))
h) Flow probe

37.2.2 Methods

Make sure that all materials are sterilized before use. Work in a laminar flow cabinet as much as possible.

Cell Culture

Culture cells in T75 flasks in a humidified atmosphere of 5% CO_2 in air at 37°C in culture medium, and refresh culture medium every 3 to 4 days. Trypsinize the cells upon 90% confluency:

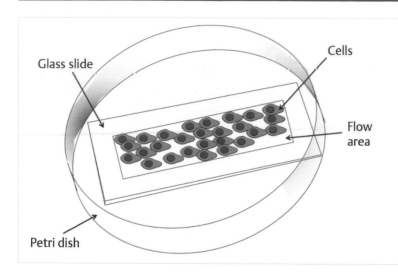

Fig. 37.5 Seeding bone cells on glass slide: Seed cells only on the area that will be exposed to fluid flow (flow area).

Glass slide

Cells

Flow area

Petri dish

1. Remove the culture medium and wash the cells in T75 flasks thoroughly with 5 mL PBS.
2. Remove PBS and add 1 mL of trypsin-EDTA at 37°C.
3. Incubate the cells in trypsin-EDTA up to 10 minutes at 37°C. Make sure that all cells are loose by tapping the flask gently on the side.
4. Add 8 mL of culture medium to the trypsin/cell suspension in the flask and transfer the cell suspension to a 15 mL plastic sterile tube.
5. Centrifuge the cell suspension at 1,000 g for 10 minutes.
6. Discard supernatant, resuspend cells in 1 mL culture medium, and count the cells with an automatic cell counter or a cell counting chamber.
7. Seed 2×10^5 cells in a new T75 flask to keep cells in culture, and culture until the cell layer reaches 90% confluence again, or seed the cells on a glass slide for treatment with fluid flow.

Seeding Cells on Glass Slide

1. Place a poly-l-lysin–coated glass slide in a sterile petri dish. We use slides of 25×65 mm. Other sizes are possible, depending on the parallel-plate flow chamber used.
2. Seed cells on the exact area of the glass slide that will be exposed to the laminar fluid flow when placed inside the flow chamber (▶ Fig. 37.5). Use 0.5 mL cell suspension containing 2 to 3×10^5 cells to fill the area that will be exposed to the fluid flow. End up with a rectangular layer of medium containing the cells on the glass slide that matches the area that will be exposed to a laminar fluid flow.
3. Allow the cells to adhere for 1 hour at 37°C with 5% CO_2.
4. Check cell adherence under the microscope and fill the petri dish with 12.5 mL of culture medium.
5. Incubate overnight at 37°C with 5% CO_2.

Application of Pulsatile Fluid Flow

1. Make fresh flow medium (as described in section 37.2.1. step 2) before assembling the fluid flow system and keep at 37°C.
2. In the computer that is connected to the pump: Set the loading regime at the needed frequency, mean shear stress, pulse amplitude, and duration.
3. Connect one silicone tube (10 cm) onto the inlet as well as the outlet of the flow chamber (▶ Fig. 37.2), and fill the flow chamber with 2 mL flow medium using a 2 mL syringe.
4. Fill the medium reservoir with 11 mL of flow medium. Turn on the pump to fill the flow system with flow medium, and turn it off when the flow system is filled with flow medium. The silicone tube attached to the outlet of the pump must be filled with flow medium.
5. Pick up a glass slide containing the cells using a sterile pincet, and lower the glass slide on top of the medium in the rectangular flow area of the flow chamber. Make sure the cells are facing down and no air bubbles are trapped underneath the glass slide. Hold the glass slide at a 45-degree angle. Let the bottom side touch the flow chamber. Slowly lower the other side of the glass slide until the whole flow area underneath the glass slide is filled with flow medium.
6. Position the metal lid over the glass slide and place screws to tightly close the glass slide.
7. Remove the silicone tube from the inlet of the chamber, and connect the medium-filled tube (step 4) attached to the pump to the inlet of the chamber. Make sure no air bubbles are trapped within the system.
8. Connect the silicone tube that is still attached to the outlet of the chamber to the flow probe to monitor the flow rate. If no probe is available, remove the silicone tube from the outlet and connect the silicone tube that is attached to the medium reservoir to the outlet of the flow chamber. Place the chamber in the incubator with the cells facing up.

9. Turn on the pump to start the fluid flow treatment.
10. Take medium samples from the medium reservoir with a 2 mL syringe at 5, 10, 15, and 30 minutes to assess signaling molecules produced by the cells. For NO measurement, see section 37.2.1. Samples can be stored for 3 months at −20°C.
11. As a static control for the mechanically stimulated cells, place a glass slide containing the same number of cells in a petri dish containing 12 mL of fresh flow medium at 37°C in a humidified atmosphere. Take medium samples as described in step 10.
12. After the fluid flow treatment, remove the parallel-plate flow chamber from the fluid flow system. Remove the glass slide from the chamber, lyse the cells, and isolate ribonucleic acid (RNA) and/or proteins for analyzing genes and/or proteins whose expression/production in osteocytes is modified by mechanical loading (e.g., COX-2, RANKL, and osteoprotegerin).

37.2.3 Analysis of the Cellular Response to Fluid Flow

Nitric Oxide

Mechanical forces trigger a series of biochemical responses in bone cells. An important early response to mechanical loading is production of NO.[10] Quantification of NO production using Griess reagent is described in the following. NO is a gas that quickly reacts with culture medium to form NO_2^-. This method is based on determining NO_2^- concentrations in the medium.

1. Dilute the 0.1 M $NaNO_2$ stock solution in culture Alpha-Modified Eagle's medium (GIBCO) to make a standard curve of the following concentrations: 100, 50, 25, 10, 5, 2.5, and 1.25 μM.
2. Pipet 75 μL standard, blank, or unknown sample in each well of a 96-well plate.
3. Mix 4 mL Griess reagent part A with 4 mL Griess reagent part B immediately prior to use. Add 75 μL Griess reagent per well.
4. Incubate at room temperature for 15 minutes on a microplate shaker.
5. Measure the absorbance at 540 (up to 570) nm using an enzyme-linked immunosorbent assay plate reader. In cell lines such as MLO-Y4 and MC3T3-E1, fluid flow increases NO production by five-fold.[11] In primary bone cells, you may expect a two-fold upregulation.

Ribonucleic Acid Isolation/Polymerase Chain Reaction

Total RNA can be isolated using RiboPure Kit (Applied Biosystems, Foster City, CA) or standard RNA isolation methods. Taqman gene expression assays (Applied Biosystems) can be used to measure messenger RNA levels of genes in which expression in osteocytes is modified by mechanical loading (e.g., COX-2, RANKL, osteoprotegerin). Note that RNA samples can be stored without loss at −80°C for 1 year.

37.3 Application of Cyclic Strain

> **Jargon Simplified: Cyclic Strain**
>
> Mechanical loading by cyclic strain results in a dynamic deformation of the substratum to which the cells are attached. This deformation mimics the in vivo deformation of the load-bearing bone matrix.

37.3.1 Materials

Cell Culture Media and Solutions

1. Culture medium: Alpha-Modified Eagle's Medium (22571, GIBCO), supplemented with 10 μg/mL penicillin (Sigma-Aldrich), 10 μg/mL streptomycin (Sigma-Aldrich), 50 μg/mL fungizone (GIBCO), and 10% serum (10% heat-inactivated FBS when using the MC3T3-E1 cell line; 5% FBS plus 5% heat inactivated CS when using the MLO-Y4 cell line). If using other cell types, change the contents of the medium according to the requirements of that specific cell type.
2. Strain medium: α-MEM supplemented with 10 μg/mL penicillin, 10 μg/mL streptomycin, 50 μg/mL fungizone, and 2% serum (2% heat-inactivated FBS when using the MC3T3-E1 cell line; 1% FBS plus 1% heat-inactivated CS when using the MLO-Y4 cell line) to be used for the fluid flow experiments.
3. Sterile PBS, pH 7.4.
4. Trypsin-tetra sodium EDTA solution consisting of 0.25% trypsin and 1 mM EDTA 4Na.
5. 70% ethanol.

Instruments

1. 75 cm^2 tissue culture flasks
2. Bioflex collagen-I–coated six-well culture plates (Flexcell International Corporation, Hillsborough, NC)
3. Flexcell Tension System (Flexcell International Corporation, Hillsborough, NC; ► Fig. 37.6)
   a) Computer
   b) Tension FlexLink
   c) Vacuum base plate
   d) Vacuum pump
   e) Gaskets
   f) 25 mm loading stations
   g) Loctite silicone lubricant (Loctite, Dusseldorf, Germany)

(For specifications, see FX-4000 T components and specifications.)

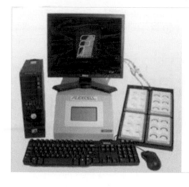
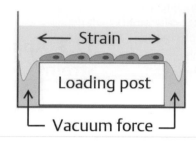

Fig. 37.6 Flexcell Tension System (Flexcell International Corporation, Hillsborough, NC): A computer-regulated bioreactor that uses vacuum pressure to apply cyclic or static strain to cells cultured on flexible-bottomed culture plates.

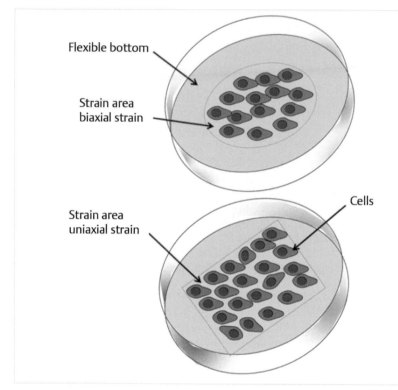

Fig. 37.7 Seeding bone cells on Bioflex plate (Flexcell International Corporation): Seed cells only on the area that will be uniformly exposed to the applied strain. This area is a somewhat smaller than the surface of the loading post.

37.3.2 Methods

Make sure that all materials are sterilized before use. Work in a laminar flow cabinet as much as possible.

Cell Culture

Culture cells in a humidified atmosphere of 5% CO_2 in air at 37°C in culture medium, and refresh culture medium every 3 to 4 days.

1. Trypsinize the cells upon 90% confluency as described in section 37.2.1. steps 1 to 7.
2. Seed 2×10^5 cells in a new T75 flask and culture until the cell layer reaches 90% confluence again, or seed the cells on a Bioflex six-well plate for treatment by cyclic strain.

Seeding Cells on a Collagen-I–Coated Bioflex Six-Well Plate

1. Seed cells on the exact area of the flexible membrane that will be exposed to the cyclic strain when placed on the loading posts (▶ Fig. 37.7). Use 0.5 mL cell suspension containing 1.5 to 2×10^5 cells to fill the area that will be exposed to the cyclic strain. End up with a rectangular (for uniaxial strain) or circular (for biaxial strain) layer of medium containing the cells on the flexible membrane that matches the area that will be exposed to the cyclic strain.
2. Allow the cells to adhere for 1 hour at 37°C with 5% CO_2.
3. Check cell adherence under the microscope and fill the wells with 2.5 mL culture medium/well.
4. Incubate overnight at 37°C with 5% CO_2.

Cyclic Strain

1. Make fresh strain medium (as described in section 37.3.1 step 2) before assembling the Flexcell apparatus and keep at 37°C.
2. In the computer that is connected to the Flexcell apparatus: Set the loading regime at the appropriate frequency, deformation, and duration, according to the manufacturer's manual.
3. Lubricate the gaskets and loading posts with silicone lubricant. Note that for optimal sliding between loading post and the flexible bottom of the Bioflex culture plate, it is very important to use Loctite silicone lubricant (Note 37.4 (p. 298)).
4. Remove the culture medium from the cells and wash the cells once with PBS.
5. Pipette 3 mL strain medium into each well.
6. Place the culture plate in the gasket, and place the gasket on the loading stations in the vacuum base plate.
7. Make sure the flexible membranes of the culture plate touch the loading posts.
8. Check the connections between the gaskets and the vacuum base plate to ensure that no air can leak from the system.
9. Turn on the vacuum pump.
10. Start the Flexcell treatment.
11. As a static control for the mechanically stimulated cells, seed the same amount of cells on a Bioflex culture plate, and incubate cells for the same duration at 37°C with 5% CO_2 in air.
12. After the treatment, remove the strain medium from the cells. For protein measurements, strain medium can be stored at −20°C for at least 3 months. Lyse the cells and isolate RNA for analyzing expression levels of genes that are well known to be involved in mechanical loading-induced bone adaptation (e.g., COX-2, collagen I, c-jun, and c-fos; see section Ribonucleic Acid Isolation/Polymerase Chain Reaction).

37.4 Conclusion

This chapter describes in vitro methods for investigation of mechanosensing by bone cells at the cellular level. Many insights in bone mechanobiology have been gained using in vitro applications of fluid flow and tensile strain to bone cells. It is important to note that culturing cells in a monolayer on a two-dimensional surface does not represent an in vivo three-dimensional environment. Nonetheless, the responses of bone cells to these in vitro applications of mechanical loading correspond to those events that occur in vivo.[10,12] Increasing our knowledge of how bone cells respond to fluid flow and tensile strain at the cellular level will help us to improve our understanding of the processes involved in the adaptation of bone mass and structure to mechanical loading in vivo.

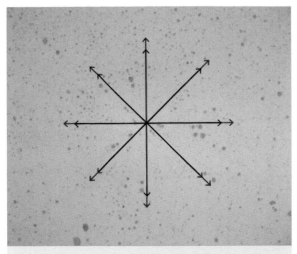

Fig. 37.8 Deformation of the flexible membrane. Landmarks in the form of a speckled pattern were created on the membrane of Bioflex plates (Flexcell International Corporation) using an airbrush. The actual membrane deformation was calculated by the following formula, where *l* is the distance between two speckles:

$$\text{Actual Membrane Strain} = \frac{l(\text{strain}) - l(\text{static})}{l(\text{static})} * 100\%$$

37.5 Notes

37.1. Validation of the Flexcell system: To determine whether the strain programmed in the Flexcell system matches the actual membrane strain applied to the cells, landmarks in the form of a speckled pattern were created on the membrane of Bioflex plates using an airbrush (▶ Fig. 37.8). Plates were subjected to strains ranging from 0 to 20% while photos were taken. The actual membrane deformation was calculated by the following formula, where *l* is the distance between two speckles (▶ Fig. 37.8b):

$$\text{Actual Membrane Strain} = \frac{l(\text{strain}) - l(\text{static})}{l(\text{static})} * 100\%$$

The programmed strain correlates with the actual membrane strain (▶ Fig. 37.9). Before starting experiments, adjust the programmed strain to the actual membrane strain using a calibration method.

To determine whether cells actually respond to the mechanical stimulus, MLO-Y4 osteocytes were seeded on a Bioflex plate and subjected to strains ranging from no strain to 20% strain for 1 hour. Subsequently, the cells were lysed, ribonucleic acid was isolated, and messenger ribonucleic acid levels of the early mechanotransduction marker c-fos were measured (▶ Fig. 37.10). Cyclic strain increased c-fos messenger ribonucleic acid levels in MLO-Y4 osteocytes. This effect was positively correlated with the magnitude of the applied cyclic strain.

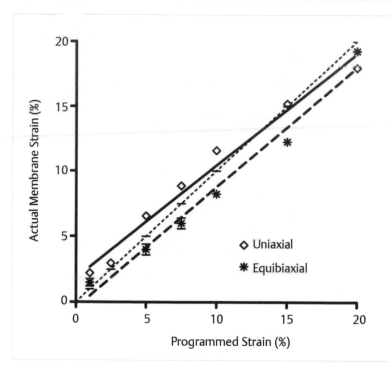

Fig. 37.9 Validation of programmed strain. Bioflex plates (Flexcell International Corporation) containing a speckled pattern were subjected to uniaxial strains and biaxial strains ranging from no strain to 20% strain while photographs were taken. Actual membrane strains were calculated and plotted against programmed strains. The programmed strain correlates with the actual membrane strain (*dotted line*: y = x).

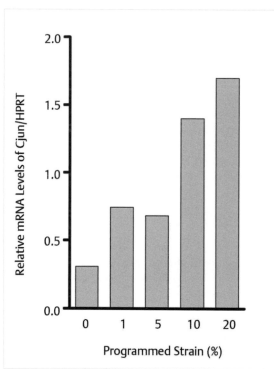

Fig. 37.10 Biological response of bone cells to cyclic strain. MLO-Y4 osteocytes were seeded on a Bioflex plate (Flexcell International Corporation) and subjected to strains ranging from no strain to 20% strain for 1 hour with a frequency of 1 Hz. Messenger ribonucleic acid (mRNA) levels of c-fos were measured. Cyclic strain increased c-fos mRNA levels in MLO-Y4 osteocytes. This effect is positively correlated with the magnitude of the applied cyclic strain. HPRT, hypoxantine phosphoribosyltransferase.

37.2. The parallel plate flow chamber used in this chapter is custom-made, but several parallel-plate flow chambers are commercially available. See for instance the µSlide chamber (Ibidi GmbH, Munich, Germany) or Flex-Flow Shear Stress Device (Flexcell, Hillsborough, NC).

37.3. Instead of the microannular gear pump (Mikrosysteme GmbH, Germany), a simple peristaltic pump can be used to create a pulsatile fluid flow.

37.4. It is very important to use the right silicon lubricant (Loctite Silicone Lubricant) for the application of strain. This lubricant provides equal strain distributions of the flexible bottom of the Bioflex culture plate (Note 37.1 (p.297)).

37.5. With the setups described in this chapter, we generally do not encounter cell death or detachment removal of cells from the glass slides of Bioflex plates. Cell loss by application of mechanical loading can be easily assessed by visual inspection of the cultures before and after application of fluid flow or cyclic strain. The total amount of protein or deoxyribonucleic acid of the cells can be measured (as described in Chapter 38), and this number should be similar to cells kept under static unloaded culture conditions.

37.6. Not much is known about the magnitude of load applied to the cells in vivo. Frequency spectra of hip joint forces during normal walking and jogging have been calculated,[13,14] and theoretical models have been developed.[7,8] This may help the researcher decide what type of loading regime to use (i.e., amplitude, frequency). It is important to realize the limitations of each system and to be careful in interpreting any results.

References

[1] Ginty F, Rennie KL, Mills L, Stear S, Jones S, Prentice A. Positive, site-specific associations between bone mineral status, fitness, and time spent at high-impact activities in 16- to 18-year-old boys. Bone 2005; 36: 101–110

[2] Burger EH, Klein-Nulend J. Mechanotransduction in bone—role of the lacuno-canalicular network. FASEB J 1999; 13 Suppl: S101–S112

[3] Andersen TL, Sondergaard TE, Skorzynska KE et al. A physical mechanism for coupling bone resorption and formation in adult human bone. Am J Pathol 2009; 174: 239–247

[4] Mullender MG, Huiskes R. Osteocytes and bone lining cells: which are the best candidates for mechano-sensors in cancellous bone? Bone 1997; 20: 527–532

[5] Burr DB, Milgrom C, Fyhrie D et al. In vivo measurement of human tibial strains during vigorous activity. Bone 1996; 18: 405–410

[6] You L, Cowin SC, Schaffler MB, Weinbaum S. A model for strain amplification in the actin cytoskeleton of osteocytes due to fluid drag on pericellular matrix. J Biomech 2001; 34: 1375–1386

[7] Price C, Zhou X, Li W, Wang L. Real-time measurement of solute transport within the lacunar-canalicular system of mechanically loaded bone: direct evidence for load-induced fluid flow. J Bone Miner Res 2011; 26: 277–285

[8] McGarry JG, Klein-Nulend J, Mullender MG, Prendergast PJ. A comparison of strain and fluid shear stress in stimulating bone cell responses—a computational and experimental study. FASEB J 2005; 19: 482–484

[9] Bacabac RG, Smit TH, Cowin SC et al. Dynamic shear stress in parallel-plate flow chambers. J Biomech 2005; 38: 159–167

[10] Mullender M, El Haj AJ, Yang Y, van Duin MA, Burger EH, Klein-Nulend J. Mechanotransduction of bone cells in vitro: mechanobiology of bone tissue. Med Biol Eng Comput 2004; 42: 14–21

[11] Juffer P, Jaspers RT, Lips P, Bakker AD, Klein-Nulend J. Expression of muscle anabolic and metabolic factors in mechanically loaded MLO-Y4 osteocytes. Am J Physiol Endocrinol Metab 2012; 302: E389–E395

[12] Klein-Nulend J, Semeins CM, Ajubi NE, Nijweide PJ, Burger EH. Pulsating fluid flow increases nitric oxide (NO) synthesis by osteocytes but not periosteal fibroblasts—correlation with prostaglandin upregulation. Biochem Biophys Res Commun 1995; 217: 640–648

[13] Bergmann G, Deuretzbacher G, Heller M et al. Hip contact forces and gait patterns from routine activities. J Biomech 2001; 34: 859–871

[14] Bacabac RG, Smit TH, Mullender MG, Dijcks SJ, Van Loon JJ, Klein-Nulend J. Nitric oxide production by bone cells is fluid shear stress rate dependent. Biochem Biophys Res Commun 19 2004;315 (4):823–829

38 Biomechanics of Bone Cells

Janak L. Pathak, Ineke D.C. Jansen, Nathalie Bravenboer, Jenneke Klein-Nulend, and Astrid D. Bakker

Mechanosensitive bone cells translate mechanical stimuli into a biological response. The bone cell response to mechanical stimuli varies from one individual to another depending on age, sex, as well as physiological and pathological conditions.[1] In the absence of mechanical stimuli, such as during disuse, stasis of interstitial fluid in bone occurs leading to a lack of fluid shear stress on the osteocytes.[2] Osteocytes produce pro-osteoclastogenic signals in the absence of mechanical loading, leading to a stimulation of bone resorption.[3] In the presence of mechanical stimuli, osteocytes produce factors that inhibit osteoclastogenesis and/or decrease the production of osteoclast-stimulating signals.[4] The most well-known soluble factors affecting osteoclastogenesis are receptor activator of nuclear factor kappa-B ligand (RANKL) and macrophage colony-stimulating factor (M-CSF), which stimulate osteoclast formation, and osteoprotegerin (OPG), which inhibits osteoclast formation. Under disuse conditions, osteocytes produce RANKL, M-CSF, and OPG. In response to mechanical stimulation, osteocytes produce factors (e.g., matrix extracellular phosphoglycoprotein) that decrease RANK, and increase OPG production[5] (▶ Fig. 38.1).

To study the communication between mechanically stimulated osteocytes and osteoclast precursors in vitro, one requires a source of osteocyte-like cells, a method for mechanical stimulation, and a source of osteoclast precursors. Mechanical stimuli can be applied to osteocytes in vitro through various methods, such as pulsating fluid flow (PFF). The protocol for performing PFF is described

in Chapter 37. Osteocyte-like cells of human origin can be obtained by culturing human primary bone cells as outgrowth from long bones. Because osteocytes are terminally differentiated cells of the osteoblast lineage, mechanosensitive human osteoblast cell lines can be used as a model for osteocytes. In studies where it is appropriate to use cells of animal origin, the mouse osteocyte cell line MLO-Y4 can be used or osteocytes can be isolated from the calvariae of chickens. Basic principles of culturing bone cells are described in Chapter 35. Bone marrow and peripheral blood mononuclear cells (PBMC) are an excellent source of osteoclast precursors. PBMCs can be easily isolated from human peripheral blood, and when cultured with RANKL and M-CSF, these cells fuse and form multinucleated osteoclasts.[6,7] The formation of osteoclasts in vitro can be quantified relatively easily as osteoclasts are multinucleated and produce high levels of the enzyme tartrate-resistant acid phosphatase (TRAcP), which can be visualized by a TRAcP staining.[7,8] In addition, PBMCs cultured on a bone or dentin slice become active, bone-resorbing osteoclasts and form a resorption pit on the slice. These resorption pits can be visualized by a Coomassie Brilliant Blue (CBB) staining after removal of the cells[9] (▶ Fig. 38.2).

Culture medium taken from PFF-stimulated or statically cultured osteocytes (conditioned medium) contains growth factors produced by the osteocytes. Control medium (medium that has not been in contact with osteocytes) lacks osteocyte-growth factors. Compared to control medium, culturing osteoclast precursors with

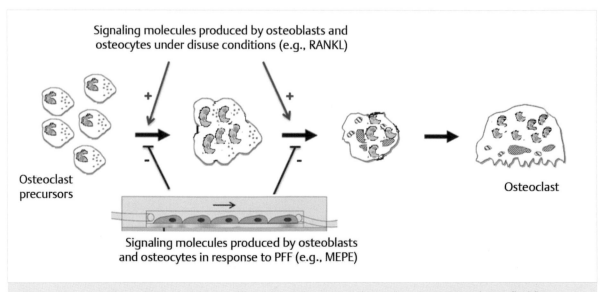

Fig. 38.1 Biomechanical stimulation of osteocytes affects osteoclastogenesis and osteoclast activity. PFF, pulsating fluid flow.

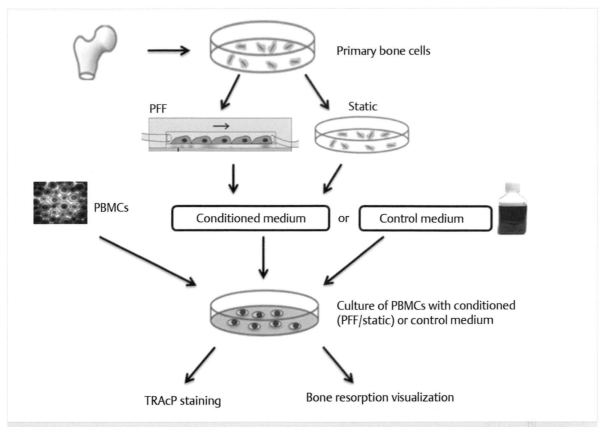

Fig. 38.2 Experimental setup for studying the effect of biomechanical stimulation of osteocytes on osteoclastogenesis and osteoclast activity in vitro: Conditioned medium is collected from pulsating fluid flow (*PFF*) or statically cultured primary bone cells. Peripheral blood mononuclear cells (*PBMCs*) are cultured with conditioned medium or control medium. The effect of conditioned medium on osteoclast formation and osteoclast activity is analyzed by tartrate-resistant acid phosphatase (*TRAcP*) staining and the resorption pit assay, respectively.

static conditioned medium enhances osteoclast formation, whereas culturing osteoclast precursors with conditioned medium of PFF-stimulated osteocytes reduces osteoclast formation.[5]

In the first half of this chapter, we focus on in vitro methods that can be used to analyze the effect of conditioned medium of osteocytes on osteoclast formation and osteoclast activity. In the second half of this the chapter, we focus on in vitro methods for analyzing the effect of conditioned medium on proliferation and osteogenic differentiation of mesenchymal stem cells (MSCs). Under physiological conditions, osteocytes produce signaling factors that enhance osteogenic differentiation of stem cells (e.g., bone morphogenic proteins and Wnts) in response to mechanical loading[10] (▶ Fig. 38.3). MSCs are the progenitors of bone-forming cells. They are often derived from bone marrow or adipose tissue for in vitro experiments.

In this chapter, we describe a protocol for the culture of human bone marrow–derived MSCs with conditioned medium of osteocytes or control medium, and the subsequent analysis of proliferation and osteogenic differentiation of the MSCs. Cell proliferation is estimated by measuring the cell number via quantification of deoxyribonucleic acid (DNA) content. Osteogenic differentiation of MSCs can be determined by quantifying gene expression of osteogenic markers via polymerase chain reaction (see Chapter 39). Mature, active osteoblasts deposit mineralizing matrix in culture, which can be visualized by alizarin red or von Kossa-staining. Osteocalcin and serum procollagen type 1 amino-terminal propeptide are released in the culture medium and can be analyzed by enzyme-linked immunosorbent assay (▶ Fig. 38.4).

38.1 Materials and Reagents

All reagents, materials, and culture medium used for cell purification and cell culture should be sterile.

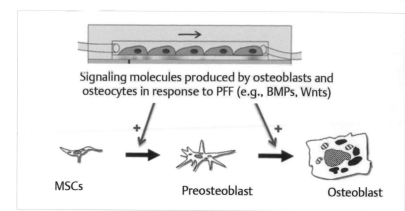

Fig. 38.3 Biomechanical stimulation of osteocytes affects the differentiation of mesenchymal stem cells (*MSCs*) toward osteogenic cells. BMP, bone morphogenetic protein; PFF, pulsating fluid flow.

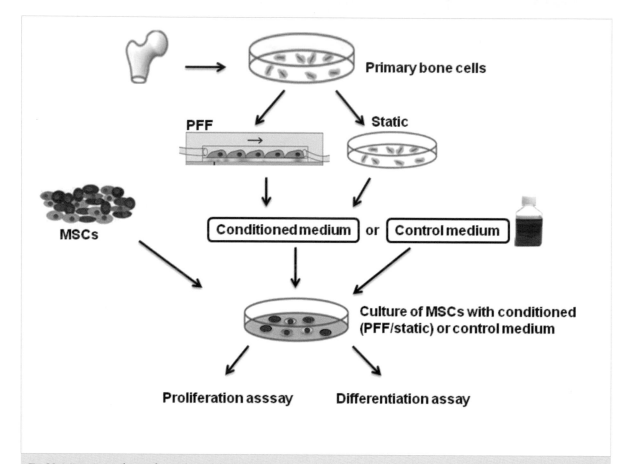

Fig. 38.4 Experimental setup for studying the effect of the biomechanical stimulation of osteocytes on mesenchymal stem cells (*MSCs*) differentiation toward osteogenic cells in vitro: Conditioned medium is collected from pulsating fluid flow (*PFF*) or statically cultured primary human bone cells. MSCs are cultured with conditioned medium or control medium. The effect of conditioned medium on MSC proliferation is analyzed by deoxyribonucleic acid quantification. The effect of conditioned medium on osteogenic differentiation of MSCs is analyzed by measuring alkaline phosphatase activity, osteogenic gene expression (e.g., OCN, OPN, RUNX2, DMP1), and mineral deposition and matrix formation (alizarin red staining and quantification).

38.1.1 Osteoclastogenesis and Osteoclast Activity Assays

Osteoclast Precursor (Peripheral Blood Mononuclear Cell) Isolation

1. Buffy coat or venipuncture blood with anticoagulant (e.g., ethylenediaminetetraacetic acid or heparin).
2. 1% phosphate buffered saline (PBS)-citrate: Mix 10 mL citrate stock in 1,000 mL PBS at room temperature (RT), and put the bottle on ice until use.
3. Citrate stock: Dissolve 456 g of sodiumcitrate-dihydrate (molecular weight = 294) and 21.4 g of citrate-monohydrate (molecular weight = 192.12) in up to 1 L of Milli-Q water (Millipore Corporation, Billerica, MA) and autoclave.
4. Lymphoprep (Ficoll).
5. 50 mL tubes.
6. Pasteur pipettes.
7. Cell culture flasks (T75) and 96-well plates.

Peripheral Blood Mononuclear Cell Culture

1. Dulbecco's Modified Eagle's Medium (DMEM)
2. Fetal clone serum (FCS) (see Note 38.1 (p. 307))
3. Penicillin-streptomycin-fungizone (PSF; Sigma #A-5955, St. Louis, MO)
4. M-CSF (R&D Systems #216-MC, Minneapolis, MN)
5. RANK-L (Peprotech #310–01, Rocky Hill, NJ)
6. Conditioned medium: Collect the conditioned medium after 60 minutes of PFF/static culture of primary human bone cells and store the medium at −20°C (see Note 38.2 (p. 307))
7. Control medium: DMEM + 10% FCS + 1% PSF + M-CSF (50 ng/mL) + RANK-L (80 ng/mL); make fresh control medium each time
8. 96-well culture plates (Greiner # 655180, Monroe, NC) (see Note 38.3 (p. 307))

Tartrate-resistant Acid Phosphatase Staining

1. Leukocyte acid phosphatase TRAcP kit (Sigma #387A-1 kt)
2. PBS-buffered 4% formaldehyde
3. Milli-Q water
4. Potassium sodium tartrate solution (1 mol/L); dissolve 2.8 g in 10 mL Milli-Q water
5. 4′, 6-diamidino-2-phenylindole (DAPI), stock = 100 mg/mL in PBS, dilute 100 × to make a working solution (see Note 38.4 (p. 307))

Bone Resorption Visualization

1. Bovine cortical bone slices (thickness 0.5 mm).
2. PBS.

3. 70% ethanol.
4. Medium: DMEM + 10% FCS + 1% PSF.
5. Forceps.
6. 10% ammonium hydroxide (NH_4OH) solution.
7. Approximately 10% water saturated alum [$KAl(SO_4)_2{}^*12H_2O$]; filter before use.
8. CBB (PhastGel Blue R, Pharmacia, Uppsala, Sweden). Dissolve 1 tablet in 80 mL water for 5 minutes and add 120 mL methanol. The solution is stable for a couple of months in the refrigerator. Dilute 1:1 in 20% acetic acid directly before use. Filter this solution (Wattman) before use.

38.1.2 Proliferation and Osteogenic Differentiation of Mesenchymal Stem Cells

Mesenchymal Stem Cell Culture

1. Human MSCs, bone marrow (Lonza Cologne GmbH, Long Branch, NJ).
2. DMEM.
3. FCS.
4. PSF (Sigma #A-5955).
5. 20 mM β-glycerophosphate (Sigma); dissolve 14.79 g/50 mL PBS (1 M), heat at 50°C for 10 minutes to dissolve. Filter and divide in 1 mL aliquots, and store at −20 °C. Dissolve in 50 mL medium to make a final concentration of 20 mM.
6. 100 μM ascorbic acid (Sigma); dissolve at 5 mg/mL PBS, filter, and add 1 mL to 50 mL medium to make a final concentration of 100 μM (make fresh solution before each use).
7. 48-well culture plates.

Deoxyribonucleic Acid Quantification

1. PBS
2. Milli-Q water
3. CyQUANT NF Cell Proliferation Assay Kit (Invitrogen, Carlsbad, CA)

Alkaline Phosphatase Activity

1. ALP IFCC liquid assay (Roche, Basel, Switzerland)
2. Protein assay (BCA; Bio-Rad, Hercules, CA)

Analysis of Osteogenic Gene Expression

1. Ribonucleic acid isolation spin columns (e.g., RNeasy, QIAGEN, Venlo, Limburg)
2. Random primers
3. Reverse transcriptase kit (e.g., SuperScript VILO cDNA Synthesis Kit, Life Technologies, Carlsbad, CA)
4. Primers and master mix for SYBR green (e.g., SYBR Green Supermix, Bio-Rad)

5. Light cycler system to quantify amplified complementary DNA (e.g., LightCycler 480, Roche)

Alizarin Red Staining

1. 4% formaldehyde
2. 40 mM alizarin red S; dissolve 500 mg of alizarin red in 40 mL dH$_2$O; adjust pH to 4.1 with 0.5% ammonium hydroxide

Alizarin Red Staining Quantification

1. 10% acetic acid
2. Cell scraper
3. Parafilm or mineral oil
4. 0.5% ammonium hydroxide
5. Opaque-walled, transparent-bottom 96-well plates

38.2 Methods

38.2.1 Osteoclastogenesis and osteoclast activity

In short, preparations for this experiment are as follows: Obtain human trabecular bone (e.g., surgical waste material) and mince into small pieces. Incubate bone pieces at 37°C collagenase type II (Worthington, NJ) for 2 hours. After washing several times with PBS, transfer the bone pieces to a culture flask with DMEM + 10% FCS + 1% PSF. Primary bone cells will grow out of the bone pieces and reach confluence within 3 to 4 weeks. Subject the primary human bone cells to PFF or static control culture and analyze the production of known signaling molecules (e.g., nitric oxide and prostaglandin E$_2$), as described in Chapter 37. Collect the conditioned medium and store as described in step 38.1.1 of this chapter.

Isolation of Peripheral Blood Mononuclear Cells from Buffy Coat or Venipuncture

1. Prepare 1% PBS-citrate from the citrate stock at RT.
2. Transfer the buffy coat to a T 75 cm^2 flask (see Note 38.5 (p. 307)) and dilute 1:1 with the 1% PBS-citrate (e.g., add 50 mL PBS-citrate solution to 50 mL buffy coat). Mix very gently (do not shake).
3. Fill four 50-mL tubes with 15 mL of Lymphoprep (Axis-Shield, Oslo, Norway) (Ficoll, GE Healthcare, Cleveland, OH) per tube at RT.
4. Layer the buffy coat on the Lymphoprep (Ficoll) in the tubes. Do this carefully, drop by drop, with a 25 mL pipette. Do not mix the cells with the Lymphoprep (most tricky step). Layer two tubes with 25 mL buffy coat and two tubes with 20 mL buffy coat. Discard the remaining buffy coat.

5. Centrifuge four tubes for 30 minutes at 800 xg at RT. Do not use brakes to stop the centrifuge.
6. Carefully take off the interphase containing monocytes and lymphocytes with a Pasteur pipette and transfer to two 50-mL tubes.
7. Fill the tubes with 1% PBS-citrate up to 50 mL.
8. Centrifuge for 10 minutes at 400 xg at RT.
9. Discard the supernatant carefully so you will not discard the cells.
10. Very gently resuspend the cell pellet of bottom of each tube in 5 mL 1% PBS-citrate at RT, and fill with 1% PBS-citrate (4°C) up to 50 mL (mix gently). Never shake your tubes as this will activate the monocytes and lower the yield.
11. Centrifuge the tubes for 5 minutes at 400 xg at 4°C.
12. Repeat steps 9 to 11 three times, until the supernatant is completely clear (colorless).

Culture of Osteoclast Precursors with Conditioned Medium and Control Medium

1. Dilute the PBMCs obtained from section 38.2.1 to 1.3×10^7 cells/mL with control culture medium.
2. Pipette 75 μL cell suspension per well in a 96-well plate. Add 75 μL PFF-conditioned medium or 75 μL static-conditioned medium or 75 μL DMEM culture medium without serum. Final cell density: 1×10^6 cells/well; final M-CSF concentration: 25 ng/mL; final RANK-L concentration: 40 ng/mL; final volume per well in 96-well plate: 150 μL.
3. Gently refresh the medium with 1:1 diluted medium every 3 days in consecutive wells: 150 μL conditioned medium (diluted with control medium) and 150 μL control medium (diluted with DMEM).
4. Continue to culture for 3 weeks.

Visualization of Osteoclasts by Tartrate-resistant Acid Phosphatase Staining

1. Wash the cells with PBS and fix the cells with PBS-buffered 4% formaldehyde.
2. Wash the cells with 37°C Milli-Q water.
3. Mix 25 μL of fast garnet GBC base and 25 μL of sodium nitrate solution from the kit.
4. Prepare mix solution:
   - Milli-Q water at 37°C 4.5 mL
   - Solution from point 3 50 μL
   - Napthol AS-BI solution 50 μL
   - Acetate solution 200 μL
   - Tartrate solution 1 M 250 μL
5. Cover the cells with mix solution (50 μL in a 96-well plate). Incubate for 30 minutes at RT in the dark.
6. Wash the cells gently with tap water and stain the nuclei with DAPI for 2 minutes.

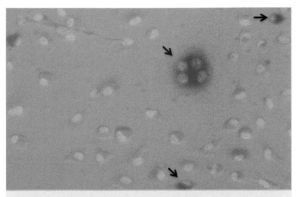

Fig. 38.5 Tartrate-resistant acid phosphatase–positive multi-nucleated cell (i.e., osteoclast, *red arrow*) and tartrate-resistant acid phosphatase–positive mononuclear cells (*black arrows*).

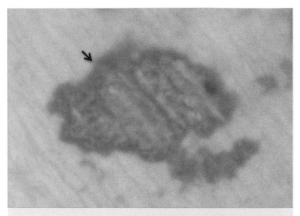

Fig. 38.6 Resorption pit (*blue*) made by an active osteoclast on the bone surface visualized by light microscopy.

7. Wash the cells gently with tap water at RT. TRAcP-positive cells stain dark red with light blue nuclei (DAPI), as shown in ▶ Fig. 38.5.
8. Categorize TRAcP-positive cells: mononuclear cells and multinuclear cells. Subcategorize the multinucleated TRAcP-positive cells: three nuclei, three to six nuclei, more than six nuclei.
9. Count the number of TRAcP-positive cells per well according to categories using a microscope with 20 × objective.

Analysis of Osteoclast Activity by Resorption Pit Assay

1. Wash the bone slices (stored in 70% ethanol) several (at least three) times with PBS before use. Put the bone slices in a 96-well plate with sterile forceps, add the medium, and put for at least 30 minutes in the incubator.
2. Seed the osteoclast precursor cells (as described in step 38.2.1 of this chapter, and replace the media as described in step 38.2.1 of this chapter).
3. After 3 weeks, wash the bone slices with water. If necessary, the slices can be stored after this step for up to 1 month in the refrigerator.
4. Pipette the water from the bone slices and sonicate for 30 minutes in 10% NH_3OH on ice.
5. Wash the bone slices twice with water in the wells in a fume cabinet (ammonium hydroxide is toxic), and bring back to the laboratory bench. Dry bone slices on a filter paper, but do not allow them to dry completely. Store the slices in tap water if you have a large series of experiments.
6. Transfer the bone slices to a new well of a 96-well plate, wash them with a small volume of water-saturated alum, and subsequently incubate for 10 minutes in fresh water. Make sure that both sides of the bone

chip have been covered by the alum by placing the bone chips vertically in the well.
7. Wash the slices thoroughly again, twice with tap water. Leave the bone slices in tap water. Pick up a bone slice, one by one, and splash once with a strong spurt (water siphon).
8. Completely dry both sides of the bone slices between filter paper. Pick up the bone slices, one by one, and splash once with a strong water spurt rinse of CBB solution to both sides of the bone slice using a Pasteur pipette. Decant excess of CBB on the side of the tube and dry immediately between filter paper; press on it. Transfer to a clean well in a well plate. Bone resorption is visible as blue resorption pits (▶ Fig. 38.6); visualize the pits using a light microscope.

38.2.2 Proliferation and Osteogenic Differentiation of Mesenchymal Stem Cells

Mesenchymal Stem Cell Culture

1. Prepare osteogenic medium: DMEM + 10% FCS + 1% PSF + 20 mM β-glycerophosphate + 100 µM ascorbic acid (see Note 38.6 (p. 308)).
2. Dilute the MSCs (see Note 38.7 (p. 308)) to 4×10^4 cells/mL with osteogenic medium.
3. Pipette 125 µL cell suspension per well in 48-well plates. Add 125 µL PFF-conditioned medium, static-conditioned medium, and osteogenic-conditioned medium in consecutive wells. So, final cell density: 5×10^3 cells/well; final β-glycerophosphate concentration: 10 mM; final ascorbic acid concentration: 50 µM; final volume in 48-well plate: 250 µL.
4. Refresh the media with 1:1 diluted media every 3 days in consecutive wells; 250 µL conditioned medium (diluted with osteogenic medium) and 250 µL osteogenic medium (diluted with DMEM).

5. Measure DNA content on days 5, 7, 10, and 14.
6. Measure alkaline phosphatase activity on days 5, 7, 14, 21, and 28.
7. Isolate total ribonucleic acid on days 5, 7, 14, 21, and 28.
8. Perform alizarin red staining on days 14, 21, and 28 because osteogenic cells produce mineralizing matrix at these late time points.

Deoxyribonucleic Acid Quantification

1. Wash the cells with PBS.
2. Lyse the cells with 0.5 mL ice cold Milli-Q water and collect the lysate.
3. Sonicate the lysate twice for 30 seconds.
4. Centrifuge for 5 minutes at 5,000 rpm, collect the supernatant, and analyze directly or store at −20°C.
5. Analyze the total DNA content from the supernatant according to the manufacturer's protocol; CyQUANT NF Cell Proliferation Assay Kit (Invitrogen) (see Note 38.8 (p. 308)).

Alkaline Phosphatase Activity

1. Take the supernatant of the lysate from step 38.2.2 of this chapter. Avoid freeze-thaw cycles.
2. Analyze alkaline phosphatase activity from the cell lysate using the ALP IFCC liquid assay (Roche) kit according to the manufacturer's instruction.
3. Analyze total protein from the cell lysate using the Bio-Rad protein assay according to the manufacturer's instruction.

4. Calculate alkaline phosphatase activity per amount of protein.

Analysis of Osteogenic Gene Expression

1. Isolate total ribonucleic acid using commercially available ribonucleic acid isolation spin columns kit.
2. Synthesize complementary DNA from total ribonucleic acid using random primers, as described in Chapter 39.
3. Analyze osteogenic gene expression by using specific primers listed in ▶ Table 38.1, SYBR Green Supermix in the LightCycler 480. Commonly used housekeeping genes (see Note 38.9 (p. 308)) are glyceraldehyde-3-phosphate dehydrogenase, TATA-box binding protein, and tyrosin-monooxygenase activation protein.

Alizarin Red Staining

1. Carefully aspirate the medium from each well. Be careful to not aspirate the cells.
2. Wash cells once with 2 mL PBS.
3. Fixate cells by covering with 4% formaldehyde and incubating at RT for 15 minutes.
4. Carefully remove the fixative and rinse cells three times (5 to 10 minutes each) with Milli-Q water. Wash gently to avoid disturbance of the monolayer.
5. Remove water and add 0.5 mL/well alizarin red staining solution. (Von Kossa staining can also be used instead of alizarin red staining.)
6. Incubate at RT for at least 20 minutes.
7. Wash four times with Milli-Q water by gently shaking for 5 minutes to remove excess dye.

Table 38.1 Primer Sequences for Determination of Osteogenic Differentiation Through Polymerase Chain Reaction

Target gene		Oligonucleotide sequence	Annealing temperature (°C)	Product size (bp)
ALP	Forward Reverse	5′ GCTTCAAACCGAGATACAAGCA 3′ 5′ GCTCGAAGAGACCCAATAGGTAGT 3′	58	101
OPN	Forward Reverse	5′ TTGCTTTTGCCTCCTAGGCA 3′ 5′ GTGAAAACTTCGGTTGCTGG 3′	60	430
OCN	Forward Reverse	5′ GCTACCTGTATCAATGGCTG 3′ 5′ GGAAGAGGAAAGAAGGGTG 3′	56	222
RUNX2	Forward Reverse	5′ ATGCTTCATCGCCTCAC 3′ 5′ ACTGCTTGCAGCCTTAAAT 3′	60	165
DMP-1	Forward Reverse	5′ AGCATCCTGCTCATGTTCCTTT 3′ 5′ CCAAATGACCCTTCCATTCTTC 3′	60	102
MEPE	Forward Reverse	5′ GAGTTTTCTGTGTGGGACTACTCT 3′ 5′ TCTGCTCTTCCACACAGCTTTG 3′	60	101
GAPDH	Forward Reverse	5′ ATGGGGAAGGTGAAGGTCG 3′ 5′ TAAAAGCAGCCCTGGTGACC 3′	60	68

Abbreviations: ALP, alkaline phosphatase; DMP1, dentin matrix acidic phosphoprotein 1; GAPDH, glyceraldehyde-3-phosphate dehydrogenase; MEPE, matrix extracellular phosphoglyco-protein; OCN, osteocalcin; OPN, osteopontin; RUNX2, core-binding factor α 1, also known as CBFA1.

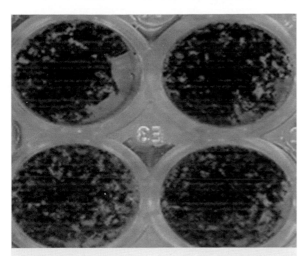

Fig. 38.7 Alizarin red staining of mineralized matrix formed by osteoblasts.

8. Add 0.5 to 1 mL water to each well to prevent the cells from drying. The plate is now ready for visual inspection and/or image acquisition under light microscope. Cells that have differentiated into osteoblasts (showing mineral formation and matrix deposition) produce bright red nodules, as shown in ▶ Fig. 38.7.

Quantification of Alizarin Red Stained Mineral and Matrix

1. Add 200 μL of 10% acetic acid to each alizarin red stained well of a 48-well plate and incubate for 30 minutes under gentle shaking.
2. The cell monolayer will now be loosely attached. Gently scrape the cells from the plate and transfer cells and acetic acid to a 1.5 mL microcentrifuge tube.
3. Vortex vigorously for 30 seconds.
4. Heat to 85°C for 10 minutes. To avoid evaporation, seal the microcentrifuge tube with parafilm or overlay the sample with 200 μL mineral oil.
5. Transfer the tube to ice for 5 minutes. Do not open the tube until fully cooled.
6. Centrifuge the slurry at 20,000 xg for 15 minutes.
7. Prepare alizarin red standard serial dilutions from alizarin red solution with Milli-Q water (2 mM, 1 mM, 500 μM, 250 μM, 125 μM, 62.5 μM, 31.3 μM, and blank). You can change standard dilutions according to cells staining intensity.
8. After centrifugation transfer 200 μL of the supernatant to a new 1.5 mL microcentrifuge tube.
9. Neutralize the pH with ~75 μL of 0.5% ammonium hydroxide (sample/standard). Take a small aliquot and test the pH to ensure that it is in the range of 4.1 to 4.5.
10. Pipette 100 μL of the standard/sample (25 μL sample + 75 μL Milli-Q water) to an opaque-walled, transparent bottom 96-well plate.

11. Measure the optical density at 405 nm.
12. Plot the standard curve according to concentration versus optical density of the standards.
13. Quantify the alizarin red stained mineral and matrix according to standard curve and optical density of your samples.

38.3 Conclusion

Studies on the response of osteocytes to mechanical stimuli are highly important in order to gain insight as to how bone homeostasis is disturbed in diseases such as rheumatoid arthritis, osteoarthritis, or osteoporosis. In Chapter 37, the protocol for subjecting mechanosensitive bone cells to mechanical stimuli in vitro has been described in detail. In the current chapter, a protocol is provided that allows investigation of the effect of mechanical stimulation on the production of factors by osteocyte-like cells that affect bone resorption and bone formation. These in vitro experiments may help clinicians and researchers to unravel how biomechanics of bone cells varies from one individual to another depending on age, sex, and physiological and/or pathological conditions, and how biomechanics of bone cells affects bone homeostasis.

38.4 Notes

38.1. The exact constitution of serum batches can vary strongly, thereby influencing the outcome of cell culture experiments. It is therefore of utmost importance to test several serum batches (e.g., culture peripheral blood mononuclear cells with different batches and measure the effect on osteoclast formation), choose the batch that performs best, and use the same batch of serum during experiments.

38.2. The signaling molecules produced by bone cells on the response to pulsating fluid flow (PFF) will generally be released within 60 minutes after the start of PFF. In order to study the effect of signaling molecules produced de novo by osteocytes in response to PFF, or to concentrate the amount of proteins in the conditioned medium, continue the cell cultures for 2 to 48 hours after PFF before collecting the conditioned medium.

38.3. The 96-well plates have a high clarity for optimal microscopic examination and have undergone a physical surface treatment that improves cell adhesion.

38.4. Potassium sodium tartrate and 4', 6-diamidino-2-phenylindole are toxic. Use gloves and take general safety measures during the use of these chemicals.

38.5. Osteoclast precursors can be obtained from peripheral blood, but also from bone marrow. Due to the invasive medical procedure needed to get human bone marrow and the low amount of bone marrow that can be obtained, peripheral blood mononuclear cells are a preferable source of human osteoclast precursors for in vitro experiments.

38.6. Platelet lysate enhances osteogenic differentiation of mesenchymal stem cells better and faster than fetal calf serum, theerefore 5% platelet lysate can be used instead of 10% fetal calf serum.

38.7. Bone marrow is not the only source of mesenchymal stem cells. Adipose tissue obtained by liposuction is also a good source of mesenchymal stem cells and is often available in relatively large quantities.

38.8. The deoxyribonucleic acid content in the cell lysate is directly proportional to cell number. Deoxyribonucleic acid quantification can thus serve as an estimate of cell proliferation. An alternative method for determining cell number is the XTT assay (XTT proliferation kit II; Roche, Basel, Switzerland). In addition, one can measure markers for proliferation during polymerase chain reaction, such as Ki67 and PCNA.

38.9. Housekeeping genes are essential for basic cellular function. These genes are expressed at relatively constant level in all cells of an organism under normal and pathophysiological conditions. To measure the effect of a stimulus (e.g., bone morphogenetic proteins, Wnts) on target gene expression (e.g., ALP, OCN), the target gene is divided by housekeeping gene expression as an indirect correction for cell number.

References

[1] Squire M, Brazin A, Keng Y, Judex S. Baseline bone morphometry and cellular activity modulate the degree of bone loss in the appendicular skeleton during disuse. Bone 2008; 42: 341–349

[2] Price C, Zhou X, Li W, Wang L. Real-time measurement of solute transport within the lacunar-canalicular system of mechanically loaded bone: direct evidence for load-induced fluid flow. J Bone Miner Res 2011; 26: 277–285

[3] Tatsumi S, Ishii K, Amizuka N et al. Targeted ablation of osteocytes induces osteoporosis with defective mechanotransduction. Cell Metab 2007; 5: 464–475

[4] Tan SD, de Vries TJ, Kuijpers-Jagtman AM, Semeins CM, Everts V, Klein-Nulend J. Osteocytes subjected to fluid flow inhibit osteoclast formation and bone resorption. Bone 2007; 41: 745–751

[5] Kulkarni RN, Bakker AD, Everts V, Klein-Nulend J. Inhibition of osteoclastogenesis by mechanically loaded osteocytes: involvement of MEPE. Calcif Tissue Int 2010; 87: 461–468

[6] Teitelbaum SL. Osteoclasts: what do they do and how do they do it? Am J Pathol 2007; 170: 427–435

[7] Bloemen V, Schoenmaker T, de Vries TJ, Everts V. Direct cell-cell contact between periodontal ligament fibroblasts and osteoclast precursors synergistically increases the expression of genes related to osteoclastogenesis. J Cell Physiol 2010; 222: 565–573

[8] Perez-Amodio S, Jansen DC, Tigchelaar-Gutter W, Beertsen W, Everts V. Endocytosis of tartrate-resistant acid phosphatase by osteoblast-like cells is followed by inactivation of the enzyme. Calcif Tissue Int 2006; 78: 248–254

[9] de Vries TJ, Mullender MG, van Duin MA et al. The Src inhibitor AZD0530 reversibly inhibits the formation and activity of human osteoclasts. Mol Cancer Res 2009; 7: 476–488

[10] Vezeridis PS, Semeins CM, Chen Q, Klein-Nulend J. Osteocytes subjected to pulsating fluid flow regulate osteoblast proliferation and differentiation. Biochem Biophys Res Commun 2006; 348: 1082–1088

Further Reading

Bacabac RG, Smit TH, Cowin SC et al. Dynamic shear stress in parallel-plate flow chambers. J Biomech 2005; 38: 159–167

Bonewald LF. The amazing osteocyte. J Bone Miner Res 2011; 26: 229–238

Helfrich MP, Ralston SH. Methods in molecular biology: bone research protocols. 2 e. New York: Springer; 2012

Klein-Nulend J, van der Plas A, Semeins CM et al. Sensitivity of osteocytes to biomechanical stress in vitro. FASEB J 1995; 9: 441–445

Robling AG, Turner CH. Mechanical signaling for bone modeling and remodeling. Crit Rev Eukaryot Gene Expr 2009; 19: 319–338

Part 7

Molecular Techniques in Bone Repair

39 Molecular Testing

Esther M.M. Van Lieshout

Measuring expression of specific proteins can be valuable when assessing local reactions at fracture sites or when assessing progression of healing. Proteins can be measured directly, either at a tissue level (using immunohistochemistry) or in homogenized tissues (using Western blotting or enzyme-linked immunosorbent assays), but expression can also be measured at the deoxyribonucleic acid (DNA) or ribonucleic acid (RNA) level. Depending on the research question, one may be interested in studying a single gene, but more complex research questions may also require studying the entire genome. Single gene studies are most applicable for measuring changes in expression of a single gene over time, or for studying differences in gene expression between treatments. They are generally regarded as hypothesis-testing studies. Genome-wide assessments are preferable in hypothesis-generating studies, for instance for identifying which gene expression pathways are switched on or off in particular patients or treatment groups. This may help, for instance, in visualizing what the difference in gene expression is in patients that progress to higher disease stages versus those that remain stable, or in patients who show impaired fracture healing versus those who heal uncomplicated. This chapter provides an overview of frequently used molecular techniques in trauma and orthopedic surgery.

39.1 Isolation of Nucleic Acids

Isolation and purification of DNA or RNA is a critical step, because it delivers the input material for all molecular analyses. DNA and RNA can be isolated from any living or dead organism. Common sources used in orthopedic trauma research include whole blood, bone, or tissue samples like biopsies or surgical specimens. The preferred isolation method depends on the source, age, and size of the sample. Despite differences between the methods, their basic principle is to separate DNA or RNA present in the cell from other cellular components.

39.1.1 Deoxyribonucleic Acid Isolation

DNA isolation is a routine procedure. First, cell lysis breaks cells open and allows for release of nucleic acids from the nucleus. This can be achieved by chemical and physical blending, grinding, or sonicating the sample. Hard tissues like bone require mechanical homogenization. Lysis is carried out in a salt solution that contains detergents (e.g., sodium dodecyl sulphate, for dissolving membrane lipids) and proteases (e.g., proteinase K, for denaturing proteins). Adding RNase is optional but advisable if the molecular assay detects RNA.

Next, DNA needs to be purified, because the presence of proteins, lipids, polysaccharides, and (in)organic compounds in the DNA preparation can interfere with molecular assays. The oldest methods to separate DNA from protein use organic solvents. Lysed samples are mixed with phenol, chloroform, and isoamylalcohol to denature proteins. After centrifugation, DNA is retained in the aqueous (upper) layer, whereas phenol is at the bottom of the tube and denatured proteins form a cloudy interface. DNA is precipitated with alcohol (ice-cold ethanol or isopropanol), resulting in a DNA pellet after centrifugation. After washing the pellet with ultrapure alcohol four to five times, DNA is resolubilized in Tris–ethylenediaminetetraacetic acid (EDTA) or ultra-pure water.

Alternatively, commercial DNA isolation kits can be used. The common lysis solution contains sodium chloride, Tris (to retain constant pH), ethylenediaminetetraacetic acid (binds metal ions), sodium dodecyl sulphate (detergent), and proteinase K. DNA purification involves spin columns, which are packed with ion exchange or silica-based matrices that bind negatively charged DNA. Unbound material is removed with washing buffer, and DNA is eluted using water or a neutral pH salt solution to break down the resin-DNA bonding. Commercial isolation kits tend to take a shorter time and result in higher yield of the purified DNA.

Isolated DNA can be stored at 4°C for short-term storage or at −20°C to −80°C for intermediate-term storage. Long-term storage (more than 1 year) is best done in liquid nitrogen.

39.1.2 Ribonucleic Acid Isolation

RNA isolation follows essentially the same protocol as DNA isolation; however, protecting RNA from degradation by adding an RNase inhibitory agent is critical. The method of cell or tissue disruption affects the yield and quality of the isolated RNA. RNA is best protected if the lysis buffer is in contact with cellular contents immediately when the cells are disrupted. This could be problematic if the tissue sample is hard (e.g., bone) or if sample processing is delayed (e.g., it takes time to go to the laboratory). Therefore, samples should be frozen in liquid nitrogen or on dry ice immediately after harvesting. Larger samples may require homogenization in a dounce homogenizer. Storing samples in an RNA stabilizing solution like RNAlater reagent (storage at 4°C; Sigma-Aldrich, St. Louis, MO), RNAlater-ICE (Sigma-Aldrich), or TRIzol (storage at −20°C or −80°C; Life Technologies, Carlsbad,

CA) allows postponement of RNA isolation up to months without compromising the RNA integrity.

Three techniques can be used for the subsequent RNA extraction: (1) In organic extraction methods, samples are homogenized in a phenol-containing solution. Centrifugation separates the sample into a lower organic phase, a middle phase that contains denatured proteins and genomic DNA, and an upper aqueous phase that contains RNA. RNA is collected from the aqueous phase by alcohol precipitation and rehydration. (2) Filter-based, spin basket formats are the second option: Following lysis in an RNase inhibitor–containing buffer, the lysate is loaded onto a membrane (glass fiber, silica, or ion exchange membrane) that binds RNA. Centrifugation passes unbound lysate through the membrane. After washing, RNA is eluted from the membrane and collected in a tube by centrifugation. (3) In magnetic particle methods, samples are lysed in a solution containing RNase inhibitors and allowed to bind to 0.5 to 1 µm magnetic particles. Magnetic particles with bound RNA are collected by applying a magnetic field. After washing, RNA is released into an elution solution and the particles are removed.

Because isolated RNA is sensitive to RNase degradation, samples should be stored in an RNase-free environment, preferably in single-use aliquots (to prevent degradation due to repeated freezing and thawing). For short-term storage, RNase-free water (with 0.1 mM EDTA; treated with diethylpyrocarbonate) or Tris-EDTA buffer (10 mM Tris-HCl, 1mM EDTA, pH 7.0) are mostly used as storage solution. RNA is generally stable at −80° C for up to a year without degradation. For long-term storage, RNA samples may also be stored at −20°C as ethanol precipitates (in 50%, 70%, or 80% ethanol). Complementary DNA (cDNA) (see next section) is more stable and can be kept at −20°C.

39.1.3 Complementary Deoxyribonucleic Acid Synthesis

Although most molecular assays are designed for studying DNA, they can also be used for RNA. In such cases, RNA first has to undergo reverse transcription (RT). In the RT reaction, single-stranded RNA is reverse transcribed into cDNA. For the RT reaction, 1 to 2 µg of RNA (total cellular RNA or poly[A] RNA) is first incubated with a primer (either oligo[dT], random [hexamer] or gene-specific primer) at 70°C to denature the RNA secondary structure, and then quickly cooled on ice to allow the primer to anneal to the RNA. Next, deoxynucleotide triphosphates, RNase inhibitor, reverse transcriptase, and RT buffer are added to the reaction. The RT reaction is extended at 42°C for 1 hour, followed by a final heating to 70°C to inactivate the enzyme. If necessary, the template RNA can be removed by treating the RT reaction with RNase H. The cDNA resulting from the RT reaction is ready for use in molecular assays.

39.1.4 Quality Control of Isolated Deoxyribonucleic Acid and Ribonucleic Acid

It is advisable to perform three quality controls on isolated DNA and RNA. The first is to determine the quantity, the second is to check the purity, and the third is to confirm integrity.

DNA and RNA concentrations and purity are traditionally assessed using ultraviolet spectroscopy. Absorbance is measured in quartz cuvettes at 260 and 280 nm (A_{260} and A_{280}). DNA and RNA have their absorption maximum at 260 nm, and their concentration is linearly related to the A_{260}. An A_{260} reading of 1 is equivalent to a concentration of 50 µg/mL double-stranded DNA, 40 µg/mL single-stranded RNA, and 37 µg/mL single-stranded DNA. Because the A_{260} is most accurate between 0.1 and 1, it may be necessary to dilute the sample. DNA and RNA may also be quantified using fluorescence tagging methods with dyes that are specific to DNA or RNA. This improves the sensitivity, but is also more expensive and time-consuming.

The A_{260}/A_{280} ratio reflects the sample purity. Pure DNA and RNA have A_{260}/A_{280} ratios of 1.8 and 2, respectively. A ratio of 1.8 to 2.1 indicates sufficient purity of the sample. It is good to note that at higher pH, the A_{280} decreases while the A_{260} is unaffected, resulting in an increased ratio. Because spectroscopy does not discriminate between RNA and DNA, it may be necessary to treat RNA samples with RNase-free DNase to remove contaminating DNA.

For small samples, the NanoDrop ND-1000 UV-Vis Spectrophotometer (Thermo Fisher Scientific Inc., Waltham, MA) may be preferred. It provides a scan of the absorbance from 200 nm up to 350 nm, and therefore provides data on both the nucleotide concentration and purity. A sample as small as 1 to 2 µL is pipetted directly onto the measurement pedestal. Within 10 seconds, the absorbance scan, A_{260}, A_{280}, A_{260}/A_{280} ratio, and nucleotide concentration is shown on screen and archived on the computer.

Because most RNA-based analyses are quantitative assays, excellent RNA integrity is critical. RNA integrity is commonly checked with the Agilent 2100 Bioanalyzer instrument (Santa Clara, CA), which uses a combination of microfluidics, capillary electrophoresis, and a fluorescent dye that binds to nucleic acids. The Agilent RNA 6000 Nano System can quantify 25 to 500 ng/µL of RNA, whereas the Agilent RNA 6000 Pico Chip System can quantify 50 to 5,000 pg/µL of RNA. Samples and a six-band RNA ladders are loaded on the Bioanalyzer Lab Chip. Size and mass information are provided by the fluorescence of RNA molecules as they move through the channels of the chip. The instrument software generates both a gel-like image and an electropherogram (▶ Fig. 39.1), and compares the peak areas from unknown RNA samples to the peaks of the RNA ladder to determine the concentration of the unknown samples. When assessing total

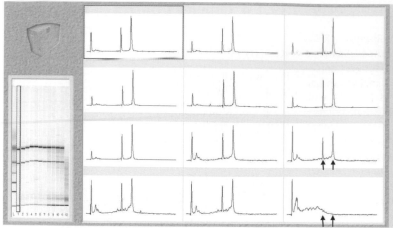

Fig. 39.1 Ribonucleic acid (RNA) integrity testing using the Agilent 2100 Bioanalyzer instrument (Santa Clara, CA). The *left panel* shows a gel-like image that contains the RNA ladder (L, most left lane) and the 12 unknown RNA samples. The *right panel* shows electropherograms for the 12 individual samples. Sample 12 (most right lane on the gel and lower right electropherogram) is degraded, as seen by the absence of the RNA peaks (indicated with *arrows*).

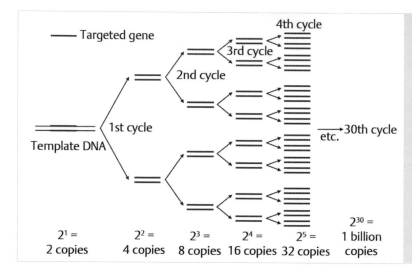

Fig. 39.2 Schematic overview of polymerase chain reaction principle, with each cycle (exponentially) duplicating the number of copies of the target sequence.

RNA, integrity is expressed by the RNA integrity number, with a maximum value of 10. Significant decreases in the RNA integrity number indicate degradation of total RNA.

39.2 Polymerase Chain Reaction

39.2.1 What is Polymerase Chain Reaction?

Polymerase chain reaction (PCR) was developed only in 1983. PCR is sometimes called "molecular photocopying" because it amplifies (copies) a single or a few copies of a specific short piece of DNA sequence across several orders of magnitude, generating thousands to millions of copies of that particular DNA sequence. PCR is the most common technique used in medical and biological research laboratories including trauma and orthopedic surgery. Because most molecular and genetic analyses require significant amounts of DNA, most assays are nearly impossible without PCR amplification.

39.2.2 How Does Polymerase Chain Reaction Work?

PCR is the most simple and straightforward method for measuring gene expression. It relies on repeated heating (for DNA melting) and cooling (for enzymatic replication of the DNA) (▶ Fig. 39.2). PCR generally amplifies DNA targets that are 100 to 1,000 base pairs long. The amplified product is called an amplicon. PCR is carried out in 200 to 500 μL volume reaction tubes in a thermal cycler. For optimal temperature conduction, thin-walled reaction tubes are preferred. Most thermal cyclers have heated lids to prevent condensation at the top of the reaction tube. Alternatively, a layer of oil on top of the reaction mixture will also suffice.

The PCR amplification mixture (usually 20 to 200 μL volume) typically contains:

a) DNA template that contains the DNA target region to be amplified.

b) Two oligonucleotide primers: These are stretches of single-stranded DNA of 20 to 30 nucleotides with sequences complementary to the flanking regions of the target sequence. Primers anneal to flanking regions by hydrogen bonding (G binds C, A binds T).

c) Thermostable DNA polymerase (*Taq* polymerase; temperature optimum at around 70°C).

d) Deoxynucleotide triphosphates (dNTPs; nucleotides containing triphosphate groups), the building blocks from which the DNA polymerase synthesizes a new DNA strand.

e) Reaction buffer containing magnesium ions and other components, providing a suitable chemical environment for optimum activity and stability of the DNA polymerase.

The amplification typically consists of the following steps:

1. **Initialization (90 to 95°C, 1 to 10 minutes):** The two DNA strands carrying the target sequence separate due to breakage of the hydrogen bonds holding them together.

2. **Denaturation (94 to 98°C, 30 to 60 seconds):** This is the first regular cycling event. Heating causes melting of the double-stranded DNA template by disrupting the hydrogen bonds between complementary bases, yielding single-stranded DNA molecules.

3. **Primer annealing (50 to 65°C, 30 to 60 seconds):** Temperature lowering allows annealing of the primers to the single-stranded DNA template. These primers are complementary to either end of the target sequence but lie on opposite strands. The annealing temperature is about 3 to 5°C lower than the melting temperature of the primers used. The polymerase binds to the primer-template hybrid and begins DNA formation.

4. **Primer extension/elongation (72°C, 30 to 60 seconds):** At 72°C and in the presence of an excess of dNTPs (DNA "building blocks" A, C, G, and T), *Taq* DNA polymerase synthesizes two new strands of DNA, using the original strands as templates. The extension time depends on the DNA polymerase used and on the length of the DNA fragment to be amplified. At its optimum temperature, DNA polymerase will polymerize 1,000 bases per minute. Under optimum conditions, the amount of DNA target should be doubled at the end of this step.

5. **Repetition:** Steps II to IV are repeated 30 to 40 times, depending on the number of copies of the target sequence in the original DNA sample.

6. **Final elongation (70 to 74°C, 5 to 15 minutes):** This (optional) step is performed at elongation temperature to ensure that any remaining single-stranded DNA is fully extended.

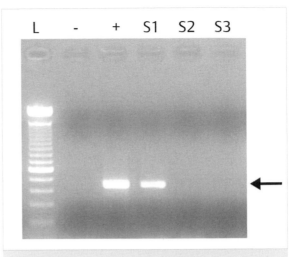

Fig. 39.3 Ethidium bromide-stained polymerase chain reaction products after agarose gel electrophoresis. Sample S1 shows an amplicon with the expected size (same as positive control; see *arrow*), implying presence of the targeted sequence in the sample. Samples S2 and S3 lacked the targeted sequence. L, 100-base pair ladder; -, negative control sample; +, positive control sample.

Following PCR, the amplification product can be detected using agarose gel electrophoresis. The percentage of agarose in the gel is inversely related to the amplicon size. The size of PCR product is determined by comparison with a DNA ladder (i.e., a molecular weight marker with DNA fragments of known size) that is run on the same gel (▶ Fig. 39.3). Presence of a band with the expected amplicon size indicates the presence of the target sequence in the original DNA sample. Similarly, absence of such a band may indicate that the original sample lacked the target sequence. PCR may be prone to (preventable) contamination, which may lead to false-positive or -negative results. Therefore, it is crucial to always include a positive and negative reference DNA standard when performing PCR.

39.2.3 Alternative Polymerase Chain Reaction Techniques

There are numerous variations to the basic PCR protocol given previously. It is beyond the scope of this book to give also details on these techniques. The most commonly used include:

1. Allele-specific PCR: Used for detecting single nucleotide polymorphisms (SNPs), which are single-base differences in DNA.

2. Assembly PCR or polymerase cycling assembly: Can be used for amplifying very long stretches of DNA.

3. Hot start PCR: This uses a specific type of polymerase and can be used to reduce nonspecific amplification during the initial cycles of the PCR.

4. Methylation-specific PCR: This is used to detect methylation of CpG islands in genomic DNA as a measure of the gene activation status.

5. Multiplex ligation-dependent probe amplification: This permits multiple targets to be amplified with only a single primer pair.

6. Multiplex-PCR: This uses multiple primer sets within a single PCR mixture to produce amplicons of varying sizes that are specific to different DNA sequences.

7. Nested PCR: A second PCR is carried out using a PCR product as template to enhance signal-to-noise balance and to increase the amount of amplicon.

8. Quantitative PCR: This is used to quantify the amplicon, commonly in real time.

9. Reverse transcription PCR (RT-PCR): This combines cDNA synthesis (reverse transcription) with PCR amplification and is widely used to quantify gene expression.

10. Touchdown PCR or step-down PCR: This variant of PCR aims to reduce nonspecific background by gradually lowering the annealing temperature as PCR cycling progresses.

39.3 Gene Expression Analysis

Many research questions require monitoring changes in gene expression. One may be interested in the effect of treatment A versus B on the expression of a particular gene.[1,2] In other situations, one may be interested in investigating which genetic pathways are activated or inactivated. The first question can be solved using a single target assay (using quantitative PCR), whereas the second question requires expression profiling of the entire genome (by DNA microarray). These two modern methodologies for measuring gene expression are described in the following paragraph. Northern blot can also be used, but will not be described in this book.

39.3.1 Single Target Assays (Quantitative Polymerase Chain Reaction)

Comparing gene expression between treatments or over time requires a sensitive and quantitative assay. The expression level of a specific gene in a cell is reflected by the number of copies of the messenger RNA transcripts of that gene in the sample. Due to low copy numbers and small sample sizes, amplification is often needed. Therefore, expression of single genes is studied using quantitative real-time PCR (qPCR). In the past, this technique was often abbreviated as RT-PCR (RT for real-time), which was confusing as RT-PCR is also used for reverse transcription PCR. Nowadays, qPCR is consistently used for quantitative PCR. The input material for the PCR is cDNA, generated by reverse transcribing isolated messenger RNA. Following is an overview of the commercially available qPCR instruments:

- Bio-Rad iCycler (Hercules, CA)
- Roche LightCycler (Roche, Basel, Switzerland)
- Perkin Elmer ABI Prism 7700 Sequence Detection System (Waltham, MA)
- Perkin Elmer ABI Prism 7900HT Sequence Detection System
- Perkin Elmer GeneAmp 5700 Sequence Detection System

qPCR combines traditional PCR amplification with quantification of the amount of amplicon formed. As in traditional PCR, the reaction mixture contains a DNA template, a pair of primers, dNTPs, and Taq polymerase (or other thermostable DNA polymerase) in a buffer solution. The key feature of qPCR is that the amount of amplified DNA is detected as the reaction progresses in real time, as opposed to the standard PCR where the amplification product is detected only at the end. In order to quantify in real time, a substance labeled with a fluorophore is added to the reaction mixture. The qPCR is run in a thermocycler that is equipped with sensors for measuring the fluorescence of the fluorophore following excitation at a fluorophore-specific wavelength.

Two strategies can be used. The first is adding nonspecific fluorescent dyes to the PCR reaction mixture. The most commonly used dyes are SYBR-Green-I dye (Molecular Probes, Life Technologies, Carlsbad, CA), SYTO dyes (Invitrogen, Carlsbad, CA), and ResoLight dye (Roche, Basel, Switzerland). These dyes emit fluorescence upon intercalation with any double-stranded DNA (▶ Fig. 39.4a). Fluorescence can be detected once intercalated; unbound dyes do not emit fluorescence. The second real-time recording strategy uses sequence-specific DNA probes (i.e., oligonucleotides labeled with a fluorescent reporter and a quencher; ▶ Fig. 39.4b). The probe, with a sequence complementary to a stretch on the target gene located in between the PCR primers, is added to the PCR reaction mixture. The fluorescent reporter permits detection only after hybridization of the probe with its complementary sequence. After hybridization, the probe is incorporated in the amplicon. During elongation, the quencher is trimmed and no longer blocks the reporter fluorescence. In the unbound probe, a quencher molecule quenches the fluorescent reporter molecule.

In both methods, the amount of fluorescence is related to expression of the target gene in the unknown sample. The amount of fluorescence is measured at the end of each PCR cycle. Computer software is used in order to calculate the messenger RNA expression in the sample. Quantity can either be an absolute number of copies or a relative amount. For the relative expression, the expression of the gene of interest is expressed relative to a normalizing gene. Such normalizing genes (also known as housekeeping genes) are characterized by their almost constant expression rate. Commonly used normalizing genes are glyceraldehyde-3-phosphate dehydrogenase, tubulin, and ribosomal RNA.

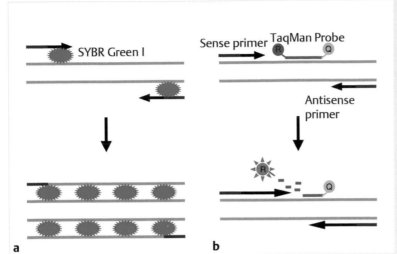

Fig. 39.4 Quantitative polymerase chain reaction using an intercalating fluorescent dye (**a**) or a probe labeled with a fluorophore and a quencher (**b**). The fluorescent dye used in panel (**a**) emits a bright fluorescence only when intercalated (bound) between the double-stranded deoxyribonucleic acid. Unbound dye hardly fluoresces. The probe used in panel (**b**) does not fluoresce while the probe is intact. Upon binding to its complementary deoxyribonucleic acid sequence, the fluorophore is trimmed off, and starts to fluoresce. As the polymerase chain reaction progresses, fluorescence increases in both assays.

39.3.2 Gene Expression Profiling (Gene Chips)

Gene expression profiling or genome-wide microarray analysis is a powerful tool for simultaneous measurement of expression of tens of thousands of genes in a single RNA sample. If one is interested to find out the molecular mechanism underlying the response of bone to osteoinductive stimuli (e.g., to growth factors like bone morphogenetic proteins), gene expression profiling is the preferred method.

The basic principle of cDNA microarray is that every nucleic acid strand recognizes its complementary sequence through base pairing. This type of research requires advanced technical skills and should only be done by (or in close collaboration with) experts. Providing an elaborate protocol for gene expression profiling would be a book on its own. Detailed protocols describing the process from scratch until statistical analysis are available online.[3,4,5] An overview of commonly used protocols and instruments follows:

- General Microarray Protocols
  - Pat Brown's Laboratory—Stanford
  - DeRisi Laboratory—University of California, San Francisco
  - John Quackenbush protocols (TIGR)
  - Microarray Protocols (Oak Ridge National Laboratories)
  - Microarray Core Facility (Baylor College of Medicine)
- Deoxyribonucleic Acid Amplification and Purification
  - Preparation of deoxyribonucleic acid samples (Brown Laboratory—Stanford)
  - National Human Genome Research Institute
  - QIAquick 96 PCR Purification Kit (Qiagen, Venlo, Limburg)
  - MinElute 96 UF PCR Purification Kit (Qiagen)
  - Montage PCR Cleanup Filter Plates (Millipore)
- Slide Array Preparation and Printing

- National Human Genome Research Institute
  - Poly-l-lysine coating of slides (Brown Laboratory—Stanford)
  - Preparation of poly-lysine slides (DeRisi Laboratory—University of California, San Francisco)
  - Printing Microarrays (DeRisi Laboratory—University of California, San Francisco)
  - Slide array preparation and printing (QUANTIFOIL, Jena, Germany)
- Ribonucleic Acid Isolation
  - Fast Track mRNA Isolation (Brown Laboratory—Stanford)
  - FastTrack 2.0 mRNA Isolation Kit (Invitrogen, Carlsbad, CA)
  - Micro-FastTrack 2.0 mRNA Isolation Kit (Invitrogen)
  - mRNA isolation kits and reagents (Ambion, Inc.)
  - RNA Catcher (Invitrogen)
  - RNA Extraction (National Human Genome Research Institute)
  - QIAquick PCR Purification Kit (Qiagen)
  - TRIzol Reagents (Invitrogen)
- Ribonucleic Acid Amplification
  - RNA Amplification (Brown Laboratory—Stanford)
  - Amino Allyl MessageAmp aRNA Kit (Ambion, Inc., Austin, TX)
  - MessageAmp II aRNA Amplification Kit (Ambion, Inc.)
  - BDSmart mRNA Amplfication Kit (BD Biosciences Clontech, Franklin Lakes, NJ)
- Probe Labeling
  - Amino-Allyl Reverse Transcription (Brown Laboratory—Stanford)
  - Amino Allyl cDNA Labeling Kit (Ambion, Inc.)
  - FairPlay II Microarray Labeling Kit (Stratagene, La Jolla, CA)
  - Labeling Human RNA (Brown Laboratory—Stanford)
  - LabelStar Array Kit (Qiagen)
  - Label IT μArrayCy/Cy Labeling Kit (Mirus Bio Corporation, Madison, WI)

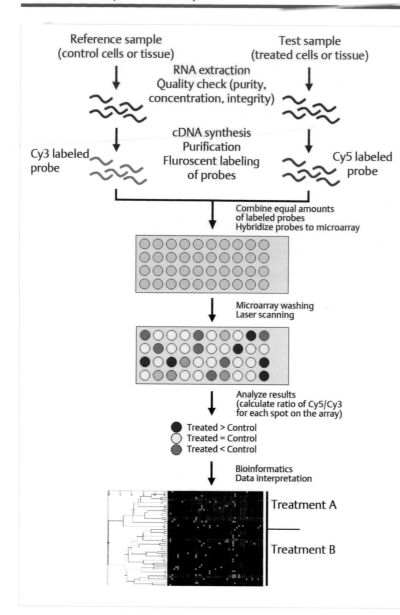

Reference sample
(control cells or tissue)

Test sample
(treated cells or tissue)

RNA extraction
Quality check (purity,
concentration, integrity)

cDNA synthesis
Purification
Fluroscent labeling
of probes

Cy3 labeled
probe

Cy5 labeled
probe

Combine equal amounts
of labeled probes
Hybridize probes to microarray

Microarray washing
Laser scanning

Analyze results
(calculate ratio of Cy5/Cy3
for each spot on the array)

Treated > Control
Treated = Control
Treated < Control

Bioinformatics
Data interpretation

Treatment A

Treatment B

Fig. 39.5 Schematic overview of gene expression profiling. Overview of all steps in microarray analysis. Combined Cy3 and Cy5 labels result in a range of fluorescence ranging from green only (Cy3) to red only (Cy5). Analysis software generates a heatmap in which samples of which expression pattern are most alike cluster together. In this example, samples from treatment A and B separate nicely based on their expression pattern. Each row in the heatmap represents a single sample, the consecutive *small blue* (Cy3) or *red* (Cy5) *squares* show the relative expression of individual gene targets on the array. cDNA, complementary deoxyribonucleic acid; RNA, ribonucleic acid.

- Hybridization and Washings
  - Array Washing Protocol (QUANTIFOIL)
  - Array Hybridization (DeRisi Laboratory—University of California, San Francisco)
  - Array Hybridization—Human (Brown Laboratory—Stanford)
  - Hybridization (National Human Genome Research Institute)
  - Hybridization/Washing Glass Slide Arrays (QUANTIFOIL)
- Scanning
  - Array Scanning (DeRisi Laboratory—University of California, San Francisco)

This overview contains commercial and academic protocols. It is of course far from complete.

Despite the technical complexity, the basic idea is rather simple and can be summarized into the following steps (see also ▶ Fig. 39.5):

1. **Generation of the array:** DNA fragments or oligonucleotides representing specific gene coding regions are spotted (also called "arrayed") onto a glass slide or membrane; Initially, cDNA clones were applied manually, but nowadays robotic spotting of up to 5,000/cm² of DNA clones or synthetic oligonucleotides is mostly used.

2. **Probe labeling and hybridization:** Purified RNA (the test sample) is labeled with a fluorescent dye and hybridized to the slide or membrane. Optionally, a second RNA pool (known as reference RNA or reference sample) can be hybridized simultaneously with the test sample. In addition to providing information on

the expression pattern in each sample, this double hybridization also allows comparison of data across multiple experiments.

3. **Quantification of fluorescence:** Following thorough washing steps, the fluorescence is measured using laser scanning imaging. The amount of fluorescence for a particular DNA fragment represents the amount of gene expression of the encoded gene in the rest sample.

4. **Data analysis:** The resulting data are entered into a database and can be analyzed with a number of advanced statistical methods. The analysis will result in a list of gene targets that are either overexpressed or underexpressed in the target sample. The critical part of data interpretation begins here. Commonly used software packages include:

- Microarray Design/Management Software
  - Array Genetics (μArrayDB; Newtown, CT)
  - BioConductor (Whitehead Institute, Massachusetts Institute of Technology, Cambridge, MA)
  - BioDiscovery (CloneTracker; Miranda del Ray, CA)
  - Silicon Genetics (GeNet; Redwood City, CA)
- Annotation/Data Standards
  - GenMapp (University of California, San Francisco)
- Data Analysis Software
  - Applied Maths (GeneMaths XT; Sint-Martens-Latem, Belgium)
  - Array Genetics (AffyMate)
  - Axon Instruments (Acuity 4.0; Sunnyvale, CA)
  - Axon Instruments (GenePix Pro 6.0)
  - BioDiscovery (ImaGene)
  - DNA-Chip Analyzer (dChip) (Wong Laboratory—Harvard University)
  - GeneCluster 2.0 (Broad Institute, Massachusetts Institute of Technology)
  - MediaCybernetics (ArrayPro Analyzer; Rockville, MD)
  - Predictive Patterns Software (GeneLinker; Vancouver, BC, Canada)
  - SAS Microarray (Cary, NC)
  - SNOMAD (Johns Hopkins Schools of Medicine and Public Health, Baltimore, MD)
  - Spotfinder (TIGR)
  - Spotfire (Spotfire, Somerville, MA)
  - TreeView (Eisen Laboratory—Stanford/University of California, Berkeley)
  - Venn Mapper (University Medical Center Rotterdan, The Netherlands)

▶ Table 39.1 gives an overview of suppliers of microarray scanners and analysis packages.

As mentioned previously, gene expression profiling is in theory straightforward, but in practice it is one of the most advanced molecular techniques. The use of robotic spotting and hybridization techniques and the use of commercialized kits for almost every step in the process (for RNA isolation, cDNA synthesis and labeling, hybridization, and washing)

Table 39.1 Overview of Suppliers of Microarray Scanners and Data Analysis Packages

Supplier	Website
Affymetrix	www.affymetrix.com
Agilent Technologies	www.agilent.com
Applied Precision	www.appliedprecision.com
Axon Instruments	www.axon.com
BioDiscovery	www.biodiscovery.com
BioGenex	www.biogenex.com
Bio-Rad	www.bio-rad.com
Genomics Solutions	www.genomicsolutions.com
Hitachi Genetic Systems	www.miraibio.com
Incyte Genomics	www.incyte.com
Molecular Dynamics	www.mdyn.com
OmniViz	www.omniviz.com
Perkin Elmer Life Sciences	www.perkinelmer.com/life-sciences
Research Genetics	www.resgen.com
Rosetta Biosoftware	www.rosettabio.com
Silicon Genetics	www.sigenetics.com
Spectral Genomics	www.spectralgenomics.com
Spotfire	www.spotfire.com
Vysis	www.vysis.com

has advantages such as greater consistency and reproducibility.

Data analysis is aimed at converting hybridization signals (i.e., fluorescence) into differences in gene expression between groups of samples. The most widely used method of microarray data interpretation is by hierarchical clustering (i.e., by grouping samples according to similarity in expression profiles). Clustering analysis yields trees that look like phylogenetic trees that are used for describing the evolution of species. Differences in expression between clusters indicate which genes or molecular pathways have been altered by the treatment under study. Interpreting these data is a critical step that often requires extensive literature study.

39.4 Single Nucleotide Polymorphism Analysis

Abnormal expression of genes may have different causes; it may be due to exposure to specific treatment, but genetic variations in DNA sequence may also play a role.

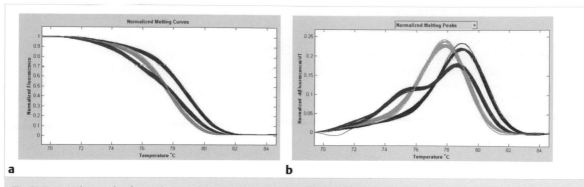

Fig. 39.6 Typical example of a single nucleotide polymorphism assay, with fluorescence (**a**) or its first derivative (**b**) plotted against temperature. Sequence variations in the sample deoxyribonucleic acid cause the melting temperature to change; the drop in fluorescence shows a different pattern. This way, three genotypes can be discriminated; a person may have two common alleles (*blue line*), a common and a rare allele (*gray line*), or two rare alleles (*red line*).

Variations in the DNA sequences of humans can affect how humans develop diseases and respond to pathogens or treatment. As an example, genetic variation in genes of the innate immune system may play a role in susceptibility of severely injured patients for the onset and course of infections, as a subset of patients may be unable to produce relevant proteins.[6,7]

Thousands of small genetic variations between persons exist. The most commonly occurring variation is called a single nucleotide polymorphism (SNP). An SNP is a DNA sequence variation that occurs when a single nucleotide (i.e., A, T, C, or G) in a gene differs between persons or between the paired chromosomes within one person. The most frequently found genetic variant is called the common allele, as opposed to the rare allele that is found in a certain (low) percentage of persons. The vast majority of SNPs is located in noncoding regions of the DNA, and most of these have no consequence at all. SNPs in coding regions, on the other hand, may result in an amino acid substitution in the protein that the gene encodes. If that is the case, the protein may have a different tertiary structure that may alter the expression level of the encoded protein or its tertiary structure.

SNPs can be analyzed using molecular techniques. If one is interested in evaluating the role of a single SNP, a single-target assay is preferred. If there is no a priori notice as to which SNPs are relevant, genome-wide SNP array should be used.

39.4.1 Single-Target Single Nucleotide Polymorphism Assays (Polymerase Chain Reaction)

SNP assays for single targets are easy and straightforward. The assay is merely a qualitative, standard PCR with a small amplicon as final PCR product. The protocol is essentially as described previously and uses a fluorescent DNA-intercalating fluorophore. The 20 nucleotides on either side of the polymorphic nucleotide are used as the forward and reverse primer, respectively. The amplicon size in this case is 41 base pairs (2×20 nucleotides used as primer + 1 polymorphic nucleotide). This is the case both for the common and the rare allele; these products differ only in the polymorphic nucleotide in the middle. Discriminating the common from the rare allele is done by high-resolution melting analysis (HRMA). HRMA is a precise warming of the PCR product from 50°C up to around 98°C. At some point during this heating, the melting temperature of the amplicion is reached; at that temperature, the two strands of DNA separate (they "melt" apart). The fluorophore used binds specifically to double-stranded DNA; it fluoresces brightly as long as the PCR product is double-stranded, but ceases to do so once the two strands melt apart. In HRMA, the amount of fluorescence rapidly drops when the melting temperature of the amplicon has been reached. The HRMA machine is equipped with a camera that quantifies fluorescence, and the software plots the fluorescence versus the temperature. The melting point of any amplicon is determined by the DNA sequence and is therefore highly predictable. Sequences of the common and rare allele differ in one nucleotide, and this causes a shift in the melting temperature of the amplicon (▶ Fig. 39.6). This fixed relation between differences in DNA sequence and differences in melting temperature allows scientists to evaluate presence/absence of common and rare alleles. For newly designed SNP assays, the different amplicons should be confirmed using direct sequencing.[6,7]

39.4.2 Whole Genome Assays (Single Nucleotide Polymorphism Chip)

The HRMA analysis as described in the previous section can only be used if the SNP of interest is known and if one is interested in only a limited number of SNPs. If the researcher does not know up front which SNPs are relevant, a hypothesis-generating experiment is more sensible. In that case, a genome-wide approach is needed. As for expression analysis, genome-wide SNP arrays are currently available. Such SNP arrays can be used for genome-wide association studies, which may help to identify genetic risk profiles or susceptibility genes.[8,9]

39.5 Conclusion

Several molecular methods exist for measuring gene expression or for assessing the relevance of genetic variation between persons. For both types of studies, protocols for single target as well as genome-wide assessment exist. As the numbers of molecular targets evaluated in a single assay increases, the complexity of the method increases. Single-target assays can be done with limited supervision of a molecular biologist, but genome-wide studies are technically demanding. They require a true team effort, including molecular biologists and statistical experts.

References

[1] Li R, Nauth A, Li C, Qamirani E, Atesok K, Schemitsch EH. Expression of VEGF gene isoforms in a rat segmental bone defect model treated with EPCs. J Orthop Trauma 2012; 26: 689–692

[2] Wagegg M, Gaber T, Lohanatha FL et al. Hypoxia promotes osteogenesis but suppresses adipogenesis of human mesenchymal stromal cells in a hypoxia-inducible factor-1 dependent manner. PLoS ONE 2012; 7: e46483

[3] Hegde P, Qi R, Abernathy K et al. A concise guide to cDNA microarray analysis. Biotechniques 2000; 29: 548–554

[4] Schena M, Shalon D, Davis RW, Brown PO. Quantitative monitoring of gene expression patterns with a complementary DNA microarray. Science 1995; 270: 467–470

[5] Kwosk-Sui L, Qin L, Cheung W-H, eds. A practical manual for musculoskeletal research. 1 e. Singapore: World Scientific Publishing Company; 2008

[6] Bronkhorst MWGA, Lomax MAZ, Vossen RHAM, Bakker J, Patka P, van Lieshout EMM. Risk of infection and sepsis in severely injured patients related to single nucleotide polymorphisms in the lectin pathway. Br J Surg 2013; 100: 1818–1826

[7] Bronkhorst MWGA, Boyé NDA, Lomax MAZ et al. Single-nucleotide polymorphisms in the Toll-like receptor pathway increase susceptibility to infections in severely injured trauma patients. J Trauma Acute Care Surg 2013; 74: 862–870

[8] Liu SL, Lei SF, Yang F et al. Copy number variation in CNP267 region may be associated with hip bone size. PLoS ONE 2011; 6: e22035

[9] Guo Y, Tan LJ, Lei SF et al. Genome-wide association study identifies ALDH7A1 as a novel susceptibility gene for osteoporosis. PLoS Genet 2010; 6: e1000806

Further Reading

The Basics. RNA isolation. http://www.lifetechnologies.com/nl/en/home/references/ambion-tech-support/rna-isolation/general-articles/the-basics-rna-isolation.html

qPCR Education. http://www.lifetechnologies.com/nl/en/home/life-science/pcr/real-time-pcr/qpcr-education.html

40 Genetically Modified Models for Bone Repair

Rana Abou-Khalil and Céline Colnot

Delayed fracture repair and nonunions represent a major clinical challenge due to the lack of understanding of the causes for skeletal repair defects and limited approaches to correct these defects. Basic research in bone biology has had major impacts on the field of orthopedic surgery. The discovery of Bone Morphogenetic Proteins (BMPs) and the purification of BMP7 and BMP2 revolutionized the field of orthopedic research and led to new treatments of long bone fractures and spinal fusion.[1] Bone autografts or allografts are largely used worldwide, yet stem cell–based approaches are not yet generalized, although several clinical trials are under way to test the efficacy of bone marrow–derived mesenchymal stromal cells. There are many efforts under way in numerous biology and bioengineering research laboratories to better understand the cellular and molecular bases of skeletal regeneration. These efforts are based on in vitro approaches to improve the conditions for stem cell transplantation, or to define the molecular regulation of cell differentiation in the osteogenic and/or chondrogenic lineages, the two cell lineages that produce the bone and cartilage matrices indispensable for fracture consolidation. In parallel, in vivo approaches are required to place these in vitro data back in the context of endogenous bone repair, which cannot be entirely modeled in vitro due to the numerous cell types involved, and the complex interplay among these cell types and the supporting vasculature. Therefore, animal models, and more specifically genetically modified mouse models, are essential to define the roles of specific cell types and molecular pathways, and to test new therapies prior to their application in humans.

> ### Jargon Simplified: Genetically Modified Mouse Model
>
> A mouse whose genetic material (deoxyribonucleic acid [DNA]) has been modified using genetic engineering tools. Genetic modifications may include mutation, insertion, or deletion of genes.

40.1 Advantages of Mouse Models to Study Bone Repair

Although large animal models are essential to test new orthopedic devices and for clinical trials due to their size and anatomy closer to human, smaller animal models and in particular mice have become very popular in basic orthopedic research. Mice are more cost-effective and have a shorter gestation time than large animal models.

Many physiological processes, including bone repair, are accelerated but share common features between mice and human, justifying the use of mouse models to study diseases and to test the efficacy of new drugs for disease conditions like cardiovascular diseases, neurological disorders, diabetes, and cancer. In the skeletal system, mouse models are employed to elucidate the genetic bases of rare bone diseases, and the mechanisms responsible for osteoarthritis, osteoporosis, or skeletal repair.

The stages of bone repair can be described in both human and mouse in four phases beginning with the inflammatory phase, followed by soft callus formation, hard callus formation, and the remodeling phase. Careful analyses of the cellular and molecular processes regulating these stages of repair have revealed that these processes can be extrapolated from mouse to human.

> ### Jargon Simplified: Genetic Modification Terms
>
> - Genetic Screen: Large-scale mutagenesis (via exposure to irradiation, mutagens, or random DNA insertion into the genome) of an animal population followed by phenotypic analyses and genotyping in order to identify new genes involved in a given biological function (for example genes involved in bone formation).
> - Transgenesis: Alteration of the genome of an organism via insertion of an exogenous gene, called a transgene, into the genomic DNA. This transgene is then transmitted to the organism offspring.
> - Targeted Gene Deletion (KO Mouse Model): Deletion of a specific gene in the whole organism, which can be achieved by deleting either the entire gene sequence on the chromosome or a small portion of the gene (leading to misexpression or interruption of the gene sequence).
> - Conditional KO Mouse Models: Mouse carrying a targeted gene deletion in a cell-, tissue-, or organ-specific manner, so that only one cell type, tissue, or organ is affected by the mutation (the Cre-Lox system is the most common tool used to generate conditional mouse KO models).
> - Inducible Gene Inactivation (Inducible KO): Targeted gene deletion at a given time point (for example at the time of bone injury) in order to bypass the effects of the mutation during embryonic development. The Cre-Lox system allows both conditional and inducible gene inactivation, thanks to tamoxifen-inducible CreER. Following tamoxifen injection into the mouse, CRE recombinase is expressed and causes gene inactivation in the tissue/cell of interest.

Over the past decade, mouse genetics has allowed scientists to identify key genes involved in embryonic bone development based on genetic screens and has provided the ability to mutate specific genes in the genome to study the phenotypic consequences of these mutations. This genetic research is directly relevant to human skeletal development and diseases as mouse and human genomes share 95% homology. These advances have been possible thanks to various technologies such as transgenesis and the ability to culture embryonic stem cells for targeted gene deletion via homologous DNA recombination (knockout [KO] mouse models). More elaborated genetic technologies have been subsequently developed to induce specific mutations in particular cell types or tissues (conditional KO mouse models), and have even offered the possibility to induce mutations at a particular time during the life of the genetically modified animal (inducible gene inactivation). Combined with reporter mouse models, these tools also allow gene expression analyses and cell lineage tracing in vivo. Following are detailed descriptions of these various mouse models illustrated by specific examples of orthopedic applications.

40.2 Transgenic and Reporter Mouse Models

Using transgenesis, DNA encoding a specific gene sequence under its own regulatory gene sequence or another promoter can be introduced directly into the fertilized egg via microinjection and is inserted randomly into the mouse genome. The injected eggs are then implanted into a pseudo-pregnant female, which will generate mice carrying the inserted DNA sequence in every cell of the organism and capable of transmitting this DNA sequence to the next generation. Using this technique, a given gene can be overexpressed in a specific cell type if placed under the control of a specific promoter of this cell type such as collagen type 2 promoter for chondrocyte, collagen type 1 promoter for osteoblasts, and tartrate-resistant acid phosphatase promoter for osteoclasts.[2] The gene of interest can be a reporter gene such as *LacZ* (encoding beta-galactosidase) or green fluorescent protein expressed under a cell- or tissue-specific promoter to visualize gene expression on tissue sections. Chen et al[3] reported the expression of the *LacZ* transgene controlled by a c-*fos* minimal promoter and TCF-binding motifs to show the spatial and temporal activation of the WNT pathway, which is essential for bone formation and fracture repair. Using a combination of various reporter genes, several specific cell types can be visualized simultaneously on a given tissue section of the fracture callus to better describe the interrelations of osteoblasts, chondrocytes, endothelial cells, and osteoclasts during bone repair.[4]

40.3 Knockout Mouse Models

KO mouse models are genetically engineered mice carrying a targeted deletion of a specific gene. Targeting DNA vectors are produced in vitro and electroporated into mouse embryonic stem cells. Following homologous recombination between the targeting vector and the endogenous gene sequence, the endogenous gene allele is replaced by a mutated allele causing gene disruption (KO allele).[2] This rare event can be selected in vitro followed by the amplification of the embryonic stem cell clones carrying the targeted mutation. Selected embryonic stem cells clones can be microinjected into the blastocyst (eight cell stage) of wild-type mouse embryos and are then incorporated into the developing embryo formed of both wild-type and mutated cells (i.e., chimeric). These blastocysts are re-implanted into pseudo-pregnant females, and give rise to chimeric mice. Because embryonic stem cells can participate in the formation of the germline in these chimeric mice, the mutation can be transmitted to the next generation of mice, which will carry the mutation in every cell. These mice are heterozygote for the targeted mutation in the first generation and can be crossed to produce homozygote mutant mice (KO mice).

The use of classical KO mouse models for fracture studies has been extensively illustrated in the literature but relies on the ability of the mutant mice to survive embryonic development, skeletal formation, and bone growth in order to analyze the consequence of gene mutations during fracture healing. One of the first examples of such an approach was described in 2003 with the inactivation of matrix metalloproteinase 9, a key matrix metalloproteinase involved in the endochondral ossification process during fracture repair.[5] *Mmp9* KO mice exhibit a growth plate phenotype at birth characterized by an enlarged hypertrophic zone due to a delay in vascular invasion, and accompanied by impaired osteoclast recruitment and bone formation. As many other members of the matrix metalloproteinase family and other extracellular proteases are expressed during the postnatal stage in the developing long bones, compensatory mechanisms cause this phenotype to resolve leading to almost normal bone length in adult mice. This allowed for the analysis of fracture healing in these *Mmp9* KO mice, which exhibit delayed callus angiogenesis, delayed removal of hypertrophic cartilage, and decreased ossification mimicking hypertrophic nonunion in human. As the fracture healing phenotype resembles many aspects of the skeletal development phenotype in *Mmp9* KO mice, these results also provided the first functional evidence that adult skeletal repair and skeletal development share similar mechanisms.

Another example of classical KO approach is the *Cox2* KO mice.[6] The COX2 enzyme is essential for prostaglandin production, a key inflammatory factor released in the early stages of bone repair. In the absence of *Cox2* gene, fracture healing is severely impaired; detailed analysis of the phenotype revealed that *Cox2* inactivation directly affects osteoblast differentiation. These results had a significant clinical impact because they suggested that nonsteroidal anti-inflammatory drugs might have detrimental effects on bone repair. Numerous other KO mouse models have now been described in the literature and lack specific genes involved in one of the steps of bone repair from the initial inflammatory response to chondrocyte and osteoblast differentiation, extracellular matrix remodeling, and matrix mineralization.

40.4 Conditional Knockout Mouse Models

The use of germline deletion or KO mice has been widely useful in the past few years to investigate bone repair. However, this approach deletes the gene of interest in every cell of the body during embryonic stages and throughout the life of the mouse. Due to the lethality of many KO mice and because the majority of genes involved in skeletal development are also essential for skeletal repair, conditional gene inactivation is now indispensable to address important gene functions during bone repair by preventing any adverse consequences of the mutation during development and growth of the animal. This conditional gene inactivation approach requires the production of two distinct mouse lines: (1) one mouse line obtained usually via transgenesis, carrying the *Cre* gene encoding the CRE recombinase enzyme under the control of a cell- or tissue-specific promoter; and (2) one mouse line obtained via homologous recombination (see previous discussion) carrying two loxP sites (34–base pair recognition site for the CRE enzyme) flanking a critical portion of the target gene (floxed allele). When the two mouse lines are crossed, the CRE enzyme

allows recombination and excision of the DNA sequence between the loxP sites and therefore inactivation of the target gene (▶ Fig. 40.1). This system not only allows gene deletion, but also gene replacement/insertion (knockin models), point mutations, or chromosomal translocation.

This approach was employed to study the role of BMP2 during fracture repair, as *Bmp2* inactivation using classical KO approach leads to embryonic lethality due to the essential role of BMP2 in organogenesis. Tsuji et al[7] crossed *Bmp2* fl/fl mice carrying the floxed alleles for the *Bmp2* gene with the Prx1-Cre mice that allows limb-specific Cre recombination. *Bmp2* KO mice (cKO mice) exhibit normal skeletogenesis in the limb, indicating redundancy among BMP family members during long bone development. However, *Bmp2* cKO mice exhibit spontaneous fractures with absence of callus formation, demonstrating that BMP2 is indispensable for bone repair. Wang et al[8] further exploited this *Bmp2* cKO model using bone transplantation to demonstrate the important role of BMP2 in the activation of progenitor cells in the periosteum. The genetic mouse models thus allow extensive manipulation of fracture tissues along with genetic manipulations in order to determine the cellular targets and timing of BMP action, which will be essential to improve their clinical application.

Another key signaling pathway for bone repair is the WNT/beta-catenin signaling pathway, which is already tested clinically. Using the beta-catenin conditional KO approach, Chen et al[3] crossed beta-catenin fl/fl mice with col1a1-Cre mice to show that fracture repair was inhibited when beta-catenin is inactivated in osteoblasts. In the same study, Chen et al[3] generated mice expressing a stabilized form of beta-catenin to show that activation of the WNT/beta-catenin pathway in osteoblasts is beneficial for fracture repair but detrimental at the early stages of repair, indicating that the timing of WNT pathway activation is crucial to improve bone repair therapeutically.

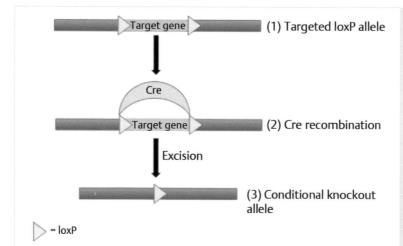

Fig. 40.1 Cre-loxP–mediated conditional gene knockout. Cre recombinase induces recombination of the loxP sites, allowing excision and deletion of the targeted gene.

40.5 Inducible Gene Inactivation and Lineage Tracing

The conditional gene targeting approach may still lead to detrimental effects of the gene mutation during skeletal development. Therefore, inducible gene targeting approaches have proven to be very useful to study gene function during bone formation and may also be used to study bone regeneration.[9] This sophisticated tool allows precise spatial and temporal control of gene modification and/or gene expression. The inducible gene inactivation approach is based on modifications of the Cre/loxP system, where the Cre-ERt protein results from the fusion of the Cre enzyme and the estrogen receptor ligand-binding domain (ERt). When expressed, the Cre-ERt protein is localized into the cytoplasm and is therefore inactive. When exposed to the synthetic estrogen receptor ligand tamoxifen or 4-hydroxytamoxifen, the Cre-ERt protein is translocated into the nucleus and becomes active, allowing recombination of the loxP sites of the targeted gene (▶ Fig. 40.2).

When combined with reporter genes, the inducible Cre/loxP system allows cell lineage tracing to follow the fate of various cell types during fracture repair. The reporter mouse strain contains loxP sites and a transcriptional stop neo cassette preventing the expression of the lacZ (encoding beta-galactosidase) or any other fluorescent transgene (green fluorescent protein, yellow fluorescent protein, red fluorescent protein, etc.). Following synthetic ligand exposure (tamoxifen), Cre recombination induces irreversible expression of the reporter gene in a specific cell type or cell population as well as every cell derived from this cell type or cell population, therefore allowing tracing of cells during the process of bone repair (▶ Fig. 40.3). This approach was used to show that pericytes expressing smooth muscle actin could contribute as a source of progenitor cells during fracture healing.[10] Although these approaches are potentially very powerful tools to define the origins of skeletal progenitors during bone repair, future advances will rely on the identification of new specific markers for genetic labeling of these progenitors.

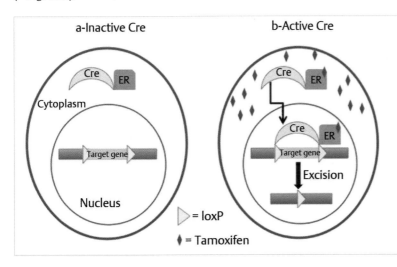

Fig. 40.2 Tamoxifen-inducible CreERt-loxP–mediated conditional gene knockout. Cre recombinase is fused with the ligand-binding domain of estrogen receptor (ER). (a) In the absence of tamoxifen (the synthetic ligand of ER), Cre recombinase is sequestrated into the cytoplasm, keeping Cre inactive with no gene recombination occurring. (b) In the presence of tamoxifen, binding to the ER induces CreER translocation into the nucleus allowing Cre recombination and excision of the targeted gene.

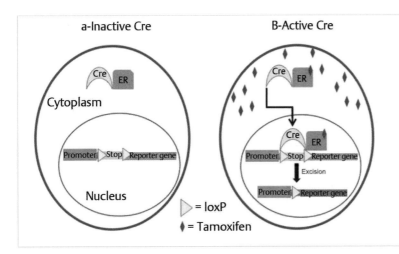

Fig. 40.3 CreERt-loxP–mediated reporter gene expression for lineage tracing. A floxed stop sequence is placed between the promoter (ubiquitous) and the reporter gene. Cre recombinase (expressed under a gene-specific promoter) induces recombination of the loxP sites, allowing excision of the stop sequence and expression of the reporter gene under the promoter.

40.6 Conclusion

Over the past decade, genetically modified mouse models have been instrumental in establishing our current understanding of bone repair. Approaches rely on specific gene deletion or the use of cell- or tissue-specific gene recombination using the Cre/loxP system. These sophisticated genetic tools required many years of research to be developed, but have proven to be very effective to elucidate specific gene functions during bone repair and to provide new insights for the orthopedic field. Future developments of these genetically modified models will further enhance our understanding of the biology of bone repair and will be essential to propose new drug-based or cell-based therapies for enhancing bone repair in human.

40.7 Acknowledgments

This work was supported by INSERM ATIP-AVENIR, Sanofi, FP7 Marie Curie, Osteosynthesis and Trauma Care Foundation, and NIH-NIAMS R01 AR053645 to C.C.

References

[1] Axelrad TW, Einhorn TA. Bone morphogenetic proteins in orthopaedic surgery. Cytokine Growth Factor Rev 2009; 20: 481–488

[2] Elefteriou F, Yang X. Genetic mouse models for bone studies—strengths and limitations. Bone 2011; 49: 1242–1254

[3] Chen Y, Whetstone HC, Lin AC et al. Beta-catenin signaling plays a disparate role in different phases of fracture repair: implications for therapy to improve bone healing. PLoS Med 2007; 4: e249

[4] Ushiku C, Adams DJ, Jiang X, Wang L, Rowe DW. Long bone fracture repair in mice harboring GFP reporters for cells within the osteoblastic lineage. J Orthop Res 2010; 28: 1338–1347

[5] Colnot C, Thompson Z, Miclau T, Werb Z, Helms JA. Altered fracture repair in the absence of MMP9. Development 2003; 130: 4123–4133

[6] Zhang X, Schwarz EM, Young DA, Puzas JE, Rosier RN, O'Keefe RJ. Cyclooxygenase-2 regulates mesenchymal cell differentiation into the osteoblast lineage and is critically involved in bone repair. J Clin Invest 2002; 109: 1405–1415

[7] Tsuji K, Bandyopadhyay A, Harfe BD et al. BMP2 activity, although dispensable for bone formation, is required for the initiation of fracture healing. Nat Genet 2006; 38: 1424–1429

[8] Wang Q, Huang C, Xue M, Zhang X. Expression of endogenous BMP-2 in periosteal progenitor cells is essential for bone healing. Bone 2011; 48: 524–532

[9] Kamiya N, Ye L, Kobayashi T et al. BMP signaling negatively regulates bone mass through sclerostin by inhibiting the canonical Wnt pathway. Development 2008; 135: 3801–3811

[10] Grcevic D, Pejda S, Matthews BG et al. In vivo fate mapping identifies mesenchymal progenitor cells. Stem Cells 2012; 30: 187–196

Further Reading

Capecchi MR. Generating mice with targeted mutations. Nat Med 2001; 7: 1086–1090

Colnot C, Zhang X, Knothe Tate ML. Current insights on the regenerative potential of the periosteum: molecular, cellular, and endogenous engineering approaches. J Orthop Res 2012; 30: 1869–1878

Granero-Moltó F, Weis JA, Miga MI et al. Regenerative effects of transplanted mesenchymal stem cells in fracture healing. Stem Cells 2009; 27: 1887–1898

Nagy A. Cre recombinase: the universal reagent for genome tailoring. Genesis 2000; 26: 99–109

Rosen V. Harnessing the parathyroid hormone, Wnt, and bone morphogenetic protein signaling cascades for successful bone tissue engineering. Tissue Eng Part B Rev 2011; 17: 475–479

Part 8

In Vivo Models

41 General Considerations for an In Vivo Model

Leanora Anne Mills and Hamish Simpson

The American National Research Council Committee on Animal Models for Research and Aging drafted the following definition: "An animal model for biomedical research is one in which normative biology or behaviour can be studied, or in which a spontaneous or induced pathological process can be investigated, and in which the phenomenon in one or more respects resembles the same phenomenon in humans or other species of animals."

The three Rs is a principle aimed at trying to reduce the unnecessary use of animals in research while still recognizing the need for animal models: reduction of animals, replacement of animals, and refinement of procedures (▶ Table 41.1). It is also essential that the design of any animal experiment is optimized, as discussed in Chapter 2.

According to Einhorn,[1] there are three fundamental aspects that a bone repair or restoration model must comply with:

- It must closely reflect the mechanics and physiology of the parallel human clinical scenario.
- It must fail to heal of its own accord.
- It must not heal by the application of simpler strategies.

There are several hundreds of animal models described in the scientific literature. Broadly, they can be divided into three types: exploratory, explanatory, and predictive. Other ways that animal models have been classified are as induced, spontaneous, transgenic, negative, and orphan (▶ Table 41.2). These terms are more for academic discussion than practical implication but are worth considering when choosing the most appropriate model for a specific piece of research. In orthopedic research, the animal models most likely to be required will be induced or spontaneous. Another term used in the literature is fidelity, which refers to how closely the model reflects the human scenario.

41.1 Mode of Interrupting Normal Healing/Physiology

Numerous factors contribute to delayed repair. They include host, local, mechanical, biological, and infective factors, which need to be taken into account when selecting a model of impaired healing.

Table 41.1 The Three Rs Principle

The Three Rs	Definition	Example
Reduction	Using the fewest number of animals possible to obtain meaningful results	Using a validated appropriate model with minimal potential for variation Using genetically identical strains
Replacement	Live animals should be replaced by inanimate or lower sentience where possible	Monoclonal antibody production no longer requires tumor inducement in mice
Refinement	Animal welfare is optimized with pain, distress, and harm minimized	Adequate analgesia and anesthesia, appropriate housing and care Use of purpose bred species Unstabilized fractures are no longer considered acceptable

Table 41.2 Overview of Disease Models

Disease model	Definition	Example
Induced (experimental)	A healthy model in which a diseased state is being created	Inoculation with infection; induced diabetic model
Spontaneous (genetic)	Naturally existing genetic mutations or disease in animals that correspond to human pathology	Muscular dystrophy gene in specific dog breeds Athymic mouse
Transgenic	Embryonic manipulation of deoxyribonucleic acid to produce a specific disease	Knockout mice
Negative	A species or breed in which a particular disease does not develop	
Orphan	A disease that exists in other species but has yet to be found in humans	Historically scrapie in sheep but now used as a human spongiform encephalitis model

41.1.1 Control Positive/Negative

All animal models require a positive and/or negative control. The requirements will depend on various factors including the hypothesis of the study, the model type (e.g., induced or transgenic), the type of bone healing scenario (nonunion, delayed union, etc.), and whether the model is well validated in the literature.

41.1.2 Time Scale of Model

The model (simple fracture, delayed union, nonunion), type of fixation, choice of animal (for its natural time to healing and life expectancy), and aims of study will all directly influence how long the model should be run. Clearly, if the model is not allowed to run for a sufficient period of time, the data will not be valid, especially in the case of a nonunion. However, it is a humane and fundamental principle in the use of animals in research that they should not be exposed to any unnecessary or prolonged periods of stress or suffering. The time scale of the model must be discussed with the departmental head veterinarian and is often a clause in the project license that has been granted.

41.1.3 Numbers Required

For an animal study to show a significant result, a certain number of animals will need to be used. The correct number should be decided upon using power calculations and allowing for potential complications prior to undertaking the study. The number will depend upon the species, model type, and controls. It is vital that such calculations are done, otherwise the study may be invalid or conclude with a false result (type II/ beta error). This topic is considered further in Chapter 52.

41.1.4 Regulatory Aspects

Each institution will have to adhere to strict rules for performing in vivo studies. The project and experimental procedures will have to meet ethical standards and be fully justified. It may be necessary to obtain a project license from the local regulatory authority. The individual performing the procedures also has to meet certain requirements. It may be essential for this person to have attended animal welfare and handling courses and to have a personal license. Obtaining the necessary project and personal licenses can take a number of months, and it is essential to have early discussions with the local animal unit.

41.1.5 Animal Housing and Care

Each housing unit will have its own rules and guidelines, and there should be at least one veterinarian overseeing the unit. It is important to have several meetings with the staff of the housing facility so that aspects such as bedding, water, chow, and analgesia can be discussed. The study animals need to acclimatize to their environment and typically should be in their new housing for at least a week prior to undergoing surgery.

Some species can be housed in groups (e.g., mice), whereas others require separate housing due to their territorial behavior (male rats); this has both financial and space implications. The housing should be in a suitable environment that is overseen by a senior veterinarian. The team looking after the animals needs to be aware of what the model will entail, the presence of surgical wounds, and possible side effects to be aware of afterwards.

In considering animal welfare in the postoperative recovery period, consider the need for subcutaneous fluid to compensate for blood loss and anesthesia, warming lamp and mat to prevent hypothermia, subcutaneous or intravenous analgesia, and separation from the rest of the group.

In the subsequent postoperative period, animals should be weighed daily initially then twice weekly thereafter. Weight loss is an important sign of animal distress; up to 10% weight loss can be expected postoperatively, but more than this or ongoing weight loss is concerning. Analgesia may be required for a few days or weeks postoperatively depending on the model, again this can be decided in collaboration with the veterinarian, an opiate dissolved into dessert jelly and cut into cubes works well in smaller animals. The data available regarding the effect that postoperative use of anti-inflammatory agents for pain relief is mixed but the overall recommendation is that it should be avoided if possible.

Any animals showing signs of distress or wound infection should be urgently discussed with the on-call veterinarian for the unit.

41.1.6 Handling

Depending on the age, species, and exposure that the animals have had to humans, they will respond very differently to being handled. Rats in particular will become more tame with increased handling and attention.

Anyone who is involved in the handling of animals should attend an animal handling course to learn how to handle the relevant species correctly. This is usually a compulsory part of the personal license.

41.1.7 Anesthesia

The license will outline when an animal can be given a general anesthetic. If an anesthetic is required for purposes other than the initial surgery (e.g., delayed introduction of a chemotherapeutic agent into the fracture site, debridement of the fracture, removal of sutures or taking of radiographs), ensure that it is included in the project license.

The anesthetic required should be discussed with the senior veterinarian. In some institutions, there will be a veterinarian to perform the anesthetic, in others the surgeon will be expected to perform it, in which case it is vital that the surgeon has a good understanding of the anesthetic agent and equipment. During the procedure, warmth (warming mat and lights), analgesia, and fluids (volume will be dependent upon species type and weight) will be required.

41.1.8 Perioperative Antibiotics

Antibiotics are not routinely used in small animal models, even in the case of metalware implantation; the emphasis to reduce the risk of infection is on aseptic techniques and appropriate tissue handling. If the operation is prolonged, there maybe justification for a single intravenous shot of clindamycin. In large animals, the AO Institute recommends antibiotics only if the procedure time exceeds 90 minutes, metal implants are used, or extensive soft tissue injury is present, in which case it should be administered prior to the initial surgical incision or inflation of a tourniquet if being used.

41.1.9 Investigations

The ability to assess how a model is progressing may require sequential radiographs at specific time periods (e. g., weekly). Other investigations during the study may also be necessary such as computed tomography scans or blood tests. The feasibility of such investigations and accessibility to equipment should be considered part of deciding which animal model to choose. It is likely that the animal will require a further anesthetic or sedation depending on the species and test. The best situation would be to have an X-ray machine or image intensifier

beside the anesthetic equipment in the animal house; the investigator may be required to undergo training in the safe use of the equipment and assessment of the room where the radiographs will be taken. The requirements of a general anesthetic for nonsurgical reasons (e.g., radiographs) must be included in the project license.

41.2 Animal Model Considerations

41.2.1 Age

To minimize the number of animals necessary and maximize the significance of the results, consistency of age of the animal is important, and previous studies show that the age of an animal affects both bone quality and fracture repair. Most models describe the use of adult animals; however, the age of physeal closure is variable and can remain open in certain species after sexual maturity.[2] It is important to know that the animals are of the same age; equally, if the study is for a lengthy period of time, it is necessary to know the natural life expectancy of the animal. In some species, particularly sheep, the microscopic infrastructure of the bone is known to change with age (▶ Table 41.3).

Meyer et al[3] showed that fracture healing in a 6-week-old rat closed femoral fracture took significantly less time than a 1-year-old rat. Similar findings have been shown in mice with increased time to healing and lower osteogenic potential (Bergman et al[4] and Lu et al[5]). There is limited evidence regarding the effect of age on bone density and fracture healing in species other than rats and mice (it is suggested that the rhesus monkey is the only nonhuman animal found to develop osteoporosis naturally); however, there are many osteoporosis models available in the literature, and they are not age related but induced by other means (e.g., ovariectomy and steroids).[6]

Table 41.3 Animal Models

Animal	Physeal closure (tibia) (months)	Age at sexual maturity (months)	Life expectancy (months)	Expected time to union of simple fractures (weeks)
Mouse (imprinting control region)	5	1	18 to 36	3
Rat (Sprague-Dawley)	11	2	30 to 48	4 to 6
Rabbit (New Zealand white)	6.8 tibia	4 to 9	84 to 96	6 to 7
	5.3 femur			
Dog (greyhound)	7.5 tibia	7 to 10	108 to 168	10 to 13
	7.3 femur			
Sheep (Suffolk × Dorset)	17	5.5	180	10 to 14

Age is also important from a practical perspective; a 2-month-old male rat weighs around 200 g, whereas a 6-month-old weighs 500 to 600 g and is significantly larger. If internal plates or external fixators are being applied, the size of the device will have to reflect the size of the animal.

41.2.2 Sex

Consistently using the same sex is vital, and the choice between male and female should be given some consideration. There is little available in the literature regarding the effect of sex on bone; however, the hormonal and reproductive cycles in the female can significantly influence bone repair and turnover, and this has been most extensively studied in rats.[7] In the rat, bone mineral density and endochondral growth is greatly suppressed in the reproductive cycle, particularly with the first litter and lactation. Rats have an accelerated catch up period between each cycle but fail to equalize that of the nulliparous females.[8] Ovariectomized rats have delayed healing of femoral fractures and reduced bone mineral density (especially in the older test group) due to alteration of their hormonal cycle.

It is because of these issues that males are more commonly used; however, the advantage female rats and other female species have over males is that they are less territorial and can often be housed in the same cage, making them a more economic option.

41.2.3 Size

Size is relevant to animal handling, housing, surgical technique, choice of form of fixation device, and cost. It is discussed in the relevant sections.

41.2.4 Choice of Animal[9]

A paper in 2001 by Martini et al[10] showed that (in 21,500 mammal studies) the most popular choice was the rat: rats (36%), mice (26%), rabbits (13%), dogs (9%), primates (3%), and sheep and cats (both 2%). A similar study in 1996[11] found that 35% of musculoskeletal animal studies had used rabbits, 27% rats, and 13.5% sheep, with only 7% using a murine model, suggesting that preferences had changed toward > the rat (▶ Table 41.4).

The first decision is of that between a large and small animal model; in some situations only one may be necessary and in others both may be required. The advantages

Table 41.4 Choice of Animal

Species	Advantages	Disadvantages	Bone structure compared to human bone
Small animal			
Mouse	Low cost Validated studies Short breeding cycle Specific genetic variants Antibody assays	Size Operative handling Validity of biomaterial testing Cost of microimplants/-scanner	Lack haversian canal system
Rat	Low cost Validated studies Short breeding cycle Adequate size for operative techniques	Housing males separately Variable female bone mass Prolonged open epiphyses High bone turnover	Different biochemical bone composition Minimal haversian system
Large animal			
Rabbit	Early skeletal maturity Ease of handling Genetic homogeneity	Limited size for biomaterial implants High bone turnover	Primary osteonal
Dog	Tame/biddable Specific exercise program Bone composition	Ethical issues	Plexiform bone Increased mineral density Very similar bone composition
Sheep	Size Housed as a flock	Digastric Seasonal fluctuation in bone mass Age-related bone structure changes	Young: plexiform and primary osteonal; greater bone mass Old: similar bone structure
Minipig	Size Similar estrogen cycle Similar bone to human	Cost Aggressive	Lamellar bone structure Similar bone composition

that the small animal model has are the practical and logistical aspects of obtaining an animal license, having access to the correct housing facilities, costs, social acceptance, and official approval. Rats and mice are genetically well defined; there are genetically manipulated breeds and specific monoclonal antibodies available enabling specific parts of the bone healing process to be scrutinized. The advantages larger animals have are size (enabling easier design of bone fixation devices) and similarity of bone micro- and macrostructure to humans. In general, the larger the animals, the more exactly the mechanical environment can be controlled.

Mice

The mouse model is attractive due to low cost, ease of handling, availability of knockout varieties, and increasing knowledge of their genetic blueprint, although the low cost of the animal and upkeep may be offset by the high cost of the minifixation devices and the highly sensitive biomechanical testing equipment or micro-computed tomography scan required for analysis. All methods of fixation have been described and validated.[12] Concerns that exist are because of their size and issue of validity to the human situation particularly when testing any fixation devices or bone substitute scaffolds on such a small scale. In such situations, it would be important to follow-up the small animal model with a large animal model.

Rats

Rats are a popular choice for both long bone and calvarial models and as a consequence there are many validated rat models available in the literature. They are hygienic, easy and economical to house (several females can be kept in one cage), large enough for the majority of fixation devices, and tolerate external fixation well, although a habit of chewing certain materials including plaster of Paris and polyethylene has been encountered. The criticism of rats as a small animal model is their delayed physeal closure and differing bone physiology from humans (e.g., differences in secondary remodeling). If using female rats, it is important to ensure that their age and reproduction history is known and consistent between animals.

Rabbits

Rabbits have also been used in many studies. They are easy to handle, and both their front and hind legs have been used in bone repair models. They have the advantage of having a larger skeleton than rodents but are still easily housed and require low maintenance compared to larger mammals. However, despite being classed as a large animal if being used to test implants or biomaterials, there is clear size limitation when compared to the dog, sheep, or pig. They reach skeletal maturity at a relatively young age and have a significantly fast bone turnover rate, which may not be suitable for certain studies.

Cats

Cats are an uncommon choice, with greater preference being for dogs. They have been used historically for non-union models, but their domesticity makes feline research models relatively socially unacceptable.

Dogs

Dogs have the advantage of being less expensive and more manageable than other large animal species. There are many canine models described in the literature for implants, nonunion models, osteoporosis, and osteomyelitis, and they are well validated for osteoarthritis. Dogs are considered to be the species with the closest commonality with humans for orthopedic research. They have a long life expectancy, reach skeletal maturity at a relatively young age, are monogastric, and have many similarities in their bone microstructure to humans. Their postoperative weight-bearing status can be dictated by the use of splints, slings, and fixators, and they can be made to weight bear in a controlled manner through the use of treadmills or similar. The disadvantages include public perception of canine models and cost.

Sheep

As a large animal, sheep have many advantages: Their long bones and mass are on a scale similar to that of humans, enabling human devices to be tested on them, they are relatively easy to handle and can be housed in large herds, and public acceptance as a model seems to be greater. Sheep have a similar immune system, which aids biocompatibility of biomaterials, but have a different digestive system, which prevents their use for testing orally absorbed agents. Their bone microstructure differs with age, which the researcher must be aware of. It has been reported that they are associated with a high risk of stress fractures predominantly due to poor surgical technique. which if appreciated can be avoided.

Pigs

Pigs are less easy to handle than sheep and have a higher body mass than humans (often in excess of 150 kg), but they do have a similar bone structure to humans on both a macro- and microscopic scale. Minipigs which have an upper weight limit of around 60 kg are easier to house and handle. They have the advantage over other large animals of being monogastric and omnivores but are still relatively specialized, which is reflected in their cost.

41.2.5 Bone Physiology

It is well recognized that there is wide variation (biochemical, biomechanical, and anatomical) of normal bone and healing processes between and within species, and it is important that the investigator is aware of the limitations of their model.[9,13]

Human bone is comprised of a combination of cortical and trabecular bone with secondary osteonal formation in adults (the primary osteons are replaced by remodeling with cutting cones and secondary osteons, which have larger blood vessels and surrounding cement lines are formed). Primary osteonal systems lack haversian canal systems. Other animals have varying amounts of cortical and trabecular bone volume and varying degrees of primary and secondary osteonal architecture.

Other species have plexiform bone. This is a bone type almost never found in humans (except in the mandible), it is similar to woven bone as it forms rapidly but is much stronger, and it has a brick-like structure consisting of layers of lamellar and nonlamellar (woven) bone around vascular plexuses.

The mouse lacks a haversian canal system altogether[12] and has a primitive bone architecture. However, in the fracture model they do form callus and woven bone.

Rat bone differs from that of humans in composition and density; it is predominantly primary osteonal in structure with longitudinal bone tissue and minimal numbers of poorly developed haversian systems.

Rabbits have similar bone density and mineral composition. They have haversian canals and osteons; however, the microstructure does differ because they are predominantly primary osteonal[14] histologically and they have a far more rapid turnover and remodeling of bone.

Dogs have a combination of plexiform, lamellar, and trabecular bone, with osteons closer to the center of the bone and lamellar bone toward the periphery. This and their fast, highly variable[13] remodeling reflects the speed at which they grow when young. Canine biochemical properties are very similar[9] to that of humans but their biomechanical properties differ.[15,16]

Minipig long bone is both morphologically similar and has a similar bone regeneration rate to that of humans; they have lamellar bone and some similarity in composition and density but a far denser trabecular network.

Sheep bone structure and remodeling changes with age. In the first few years, they have predominantly plexiform bone but with increasing age secondary remodeling and haversian canals can be found. Sheep have a similar bone mineral composition but a far greater bone density than humans.

References

[1] Einhorn TA. Clinically applied models of bone regeneration in tissue engineering research. Clin Orthop Relat Res 1999 Suppl: S59–S67

[2] Kilborn SH, Trudel G, Uhthoff H. Review of growth plate closure compared with age at sexual maturity and lifespan in laboratory animals. Contemp Top Lab Anim Sci 2002; 41: 21–26

[3] Meyer RA, Jr, Meyer MH, Tenholder M, Wondracek S, Wasserman R, Garges P. Gene expression in older rats with delayed union of femoral fractures. J Bone Joint Surg Am 2003; 85-A: 1243–1254

[4] Bergman RJ, Gazit D, Kahn AJ, Gruber H, McDougall S, Hahn TJ. Age-related changes in osteogenic stem cells in mice. J Bone Miner Res 1996; 11: 568–577

[5] Lu C, Miclau T, Hu D et al. Cellular basis for age-related changes in fracture repair. J Orthop Res 2005; 23: 1300–1307

[6] Newman E, Turner AS, Wark JD. The potential of sheep for the study of osteopenia: current status and comparison with other animal models. Bone 1995; 16 Suppl: 277S–284S

[7] Bowman BM, Miller SC. Skeletal mass, chemistry, and growth during and after multiple reproductive cycles in the rat. Bone 1999; 25: 553–559

[8] Naylor KE, Iqbal P, Fledelius C, Fraser RB, Eastell R. The effect of pregnancy on bone density and bone turnover. J Bone Miner Res 2000; 15: 129–137

[9] Aerssens J, Boonen S, Lowet G, Dequeker J. Interspecies differences in bone composition, density, and quality: potential implications for in vivo bone research. Endocrinology 1998; 139: 663–670

[10] Martini L, Fini M, Giavaresi G, Giardino R. Sheep model in orthopedic research: a literature review. Comp Med 2001; 51: 292–299

[11] Neyt JG, Buckwalter JA, Carroll NC. Use of animal models in musculoskeletal research. Iowa Orthop Trauma 2009; 23–5 Suppl: 31–38

[12] Holstein JH, Garcia P, Histing T et al. Advances in the establishment of defined mouse models for the study of fracture healing and bone regeneration. J Orthop Trauma 2009; 23 Suppl: S31–S38

[13] Turner CH, Roeder RK, Wieczorek A, Foroud T, Liu G, Peacock M. Variability in skeletal mass, structure, and biomechanical properties among inbred strains of rats. J Bone Miner Res 2001; 16: 1532–1539

[14] Wang X, Mabrey JD, Agrawal CM. An interspecies comparison of bone fracture properties. Biomed Mater Eng 1998; 8: 1–9

[15] Pearce AI, Richards RG, Milz S, Schneider E, Pearce SG. Animal models for implant biomaterial research in bone: a review. Eur Cell Mater 2007; 13: 1–10

[16] Kuhn JL, Goldstein SA, Ciarelli MJ, Matthews LS. The limitations of canine trabecular bone as a model for human: a biomechanical study. J Biomech 1989; 22: 95–107

Further Reading

Russell WMS, Burch RL. The principles of humane experimental technique. London: Methuen; 1959

Auer JA, Goodship A, Arnoczky S et al. Refining animal models in fracture research: seeking consensus in optimising both animal welfare and scientific validity for appropriate biomedical use. BMC Musculoskelet Disord 2007; 8: 72

Reinwald S, Burr D. Review of nonprimate, large animal models for osteoporosis research. J Bone Miner Res 2008; 23: 1353–1368

Tsukamoto T, Pape HC. Animal models for trauma research: what are the options? Shock 2009; 31: 3–10

42 Animal Models for Bone Healing

Hamish Simpson and Leanora Anne Mills

An experimental model for studying bone repair needs to reflect the biomechanics and the physiology of the particular clinical scenario in man. However, frequently models are used that do not meet this criterion. Fresh critical-size-defect (CSD) models are employed to represent a nonunion, despite the fact that most human nonunions do not have a large defect and, by definition, are not fresh.

The clinical scenarios can be considered under the following headings:
1. normal fracture repair: direct/indirect healing
2. delayed union
3. established hypertrophic non-union (HNU)
4. established atrophic nonunion (ANU): stiff or mobile (pseudarthrosis)
5. fracture with a segmental defect
6. fracture at risk of delayed/nonunion: (a) high-energy and open fractures, (b) infected fractures, and (c) fracture healing in the compromised host

In addition, fractures may have to heal in the presence of infection in the compromised host, these are dealt with in later chapters.

Models for these scenarios will be addressed in turn, but first general aspects of bone repair models (i.e., the method of stabilization and the method of bone division) will be considered.

42.1 Methods of Fixation/ Stabilization

When choosing a method of fixation, it is important to consider various aspects of the model and how these variables will influence the final results: for example, whether the "fracture site" should remain a closed, sealed environment; the need for clear serial radiological assessment of the site of interest throughout the study period (may be blocked by fixators or plates); whether direct or indirect bone healing is desired; and if products (e.g., growth factors or scaffolds) are to be injected/introduced to the fracture site.

42.1.1 Intramedullary Nail Technique

Intramedullary (IM) nailing is used in animals of all sizes, mice included. It is a popular method and in a simple fracture model results in indirect repair with callus formation. By intentional undersizing of the nail diameter or omitting of the locking mechanism, the nail can also be used to induce fracture instability and a HNU. IM nailing

has been described for use in open, closed, simple, and comminuted fracture models, in delayed union, nonunion, and CSD. The IM nail enables minimal soft tissue disruption, the fracture site can be either performed as an open or closed procedure, and it is good for being able to assess callus formation radiographically. The main disadvantages of IM nails are (1) that removing the nail postmortem will interrupt the site of interest and may affect the histological, radiological, and biomechanical conclusions taken from the study; and (2) that the contribution of the IM contents to the fracture healing process cannot be studied.

42.1.2 Plate Fixation

Internal fixation by way of plating has also been described in most animal species used for experimental models. In the mouse, it can be technically challenging and requires very small and specialized instrumentation. Plating is an open technique that results in local stripping of the soft tissues but does allow direct visualization of the fracture site; unlike the IM nail method, it allows grafts and other materials or substances to be placed between the bone ends. It can be used in simple and comminuted fractures, in inducing delayed and nonunion, and for CSD models. A wide plate may make radiographic visualization of the bone during the test period difficult, and the residual screw holes can be points of failure for mechanical testing once the plate has been removed.

42.1.3 External Fixation

External fixation, both unilateral fixators and circular frames, are popular choices in animal models. They have the advantage of being distant from the fracture site, they are easy to remove, and they will not interfere with histological, radiological, or mechanical assessment postmortem. The fracture can be achieved using a closed technique so that the site remains entirely free from surgical interference. Plastic ring fixators have been used in the literature to reduce the weight of the frame, but in our experience the plastic may be chewed through; however, this can be overcome by using a lightweight metal such as aluminum instead. The unilateral fixator can result in unwanted excessive micromotion and instability in small animal models, which may lead to an unpredictable number of HNUs.

42.1.4 Ipsilateral Bone Stabilization

The method of relying on the ipsilateral bone (usually the ulna, radius, or tibia) for stability is well described in the

Table 42.1 Modes of Fixation

Mode of fixation	Open or closed fracture technique	Advantages	Disadvantages
Intramedullary nail	Both	Minimal soft tissue stripping Easy radiographic assessment	Difficulty in removing nail postmortem for histology/mechanical testing Placing test substances in the osteotomy site
Plate	Open	Anatomical reduction of osteotomy Direct access into osteotomy site Good stability	Obscured radiographic views Soft tissue handling
External fixation	Both	Away from fracture site Minimal soft tissue stripping	Animal awareness of fixator Potential for instability
Ipsilateral bone	Both	No foreign materials Good radiographic views Low cost Not technically demanding	Unpredictable Unstable Potential for fracture
Plaster cast	Both	Low cost Not technically demanding	Instability Risk of fracture Poorly tolerated by animal Pressure sores

literature. It has the advantages of not introducing foreign materials, enabling good X-ray views, and in the case of a closed fracture model not requiring any "surgical" intervention at all; it has the added benefit of low cost due to the lack of kit required. However, there are concerns that there is the potential of unpredictable results (angular deformity, HNU, and nonweight bearing) is common. It often requires the need for plaster cast immobilization to prevent fracturing of the ipsilateral intact bone. It is therefore not as straightforward as it may seem.

42.1.5 Plaster Cast Stabilization

Plaster (or fiberglass) cast stabilization can be applied rapidly and is noninvasive but has the disadvantage of not always being well tolerated. The casts can be chewed off by the animal (a particular problem in rats), become soiled, and create pressure sores. Although seemingly simple, they may result in numerous unnecessary anesthetics for the animal (▶ Table 42.1).

42.2 Mode of Fracture

42.2.1 Open versus Closed Technique

A popular technique described by Bonnarens and Einhorn[1] using a guillotine and IM nail is regularly used to achieve a closed fracture. This technique can also be utilized with other forms of fixation including the external fixator or ipsilateral bone stabilization. The guillotine method is a closed technique; it prevents the need for surgical disruption at the fracture site and allows

containment of the fracture hematoma. However, with their technique, the fracture is not directly visualized.

The open technique allows direct visualization of the fracture site and aids good bone alignment. Further, any compounds to be introduced locally can be correctly placed. However, the open technique theoretically creates an open fracture and introduces the risks and variables associated with a surgical procedure.

42.2.2 Osteotomy versus Fracture Technique

By employing a manual/guillotine/impact device, the fracture is given more inherent stability from the soft tissue envelope and from the interdigitating bony fragments. Forceps can be used or an osteotomy performed using a burr, saw, osteotome, or Gigli (depending on the size of the animal); these techniques give a cleaner, more controlled break, but the burr or saw in particular may create unwanted thermal damage at the osteotomy site.

An osteotomy model should be used with caution in a trauma model; significant differences have been found between an open osteotomy and a closed fracture model in bone healing, both histologically and biomechanically.

42.2.3 Soft Tissue and Periosteal Involvement

One of the most important factors in orthopedic trauma is the extent of soft tissue and periosteal injury associated with the bony injury; it should therefore be a major consideration when choosing a clinically relevant model. High-energy injuries can be mimicked by stripping or excising periosteum from around the fracture site, crushing or removing muscle, ligating arteries, and dividing nerves.

42.3 In Vivo Models for Different Clinical Scenarios of Bone Healing

42.3.1 Simple Fracture

The majority of fractures occur in healthy patients and heal without problems. The key feature of this model type is that it heals without delay or need of an adjunct. It is often used as a control to evaluate new agents or intervention. Aspects of this model, which have already been discussed, are deciding between an open or closed technique and between a fracture or osteotomy technique. Most of the models heal by indirect repair with callus. However, Savaridas et al[2] have described a model of primary bone repair in the rat. A transgenic model should be considered for studies that are evaluating the effect of the host genotype on fracture repair. Knockout mice with diseases such as diabetes or with deficiencies in the immune system (nude mice/rats, SCID mice) are available.

42.3.2 High-Energy, Comminuted, and Open Injury Models

High-energy and comminuted injuries result in greater soft tissue trauma and an increased risk of delayed or nonunion. For testing certain therapeutic agents such as bone morphogenic proteins, it is important to have a model that reflects the severity of the soft tissue and periosteal injury. High-energy injuries can be mimicked in models by stripping or excising periosteum from the fracture site, crushing or removing muscle, ligating arteries, and dividing nerves. Some models aiming at creating delayed or nonunion may also employ these techniques.

42.3.3 Delayed Union

Delayed union encompasses situations of bone repair (fractures, osteotomies) where the bone does not unite within the expected time frame but does eventually heal with return of structural integrity and function to the bone, often as a result of poor stability and malreduction. Delayed union is a clinical diagnosis and relies on establishing the expected time of healing. This results in wide interobserver variation. A survey of orthopedic surgeons found a huge variation in the time surgeons defined as delayed union and nonunion of the tibia. The expected time to union of a simple fracture in an animal model will depend on many factors, similar to that of human

fractures; rats generally heal by 4 to 6 weeks with full torsional stiffness achieved by 8 weeks, mice take 3 weeks, rabbits 6 to 7 weeks, and dogs 10 to 13 weeks. However, these figures will depend upon the individual characteristics of the fracture and treatment; therefore, it is important that the delayed union model has a positive control group of normal time to fracture union employing a similar method of fixation/osteotomy but without the additional insult leading to the delayed union (▶ Table 42.2).

42.3.4 Nonunion

There are many models of nonunion; however, some reflect the clinical situation more closely than others. The nonunion of a bone can be further categorized into (1) hypertrophic, (2) stiff atrophic, or (3) mobile atrophic. Nonunions are also referred to as pseudarthroses, but only in the latter category of mobile ANU is there a genuine false joint cavity.

Established Hypertrophic Nonunion

HNU is defined by abundant callus formation visible radiographically that does not bridge the fracture. The repair is not freely mobile, but union and strength have not been achieved. Histologically, fibrocartilaginous tissue bridges the fracture site. In the clinical situation, this is as a consequence of excess motion at the fracture site.

HNU can be induced by using an IM nail omitting the proximal cross screw or by relying on the parallel bone alone for stabilization.

The problems with these models are that they are not highly accurate in achieving HNU, there is a high rate of ANU also created either from the outset or after a period of time[3] and hypertrophic fibrous nonunion.[4] The models also require the use of foreign materials such as wax that can interfere with histological studies.[3] Bone wax has been found to prevent osteogenesis; a thin fibrotic membrane formed and there was a minimal inflammatory response mounted. Hietaniemi's model[3] reported the greatest success in creating an HNU model; however, by 1 year the abundant callus formation had become atrophic and the model has been utilized as a pseudarthrosis model in other studies.

Atrophic Nonunion Models

ANU is a well-accepted concept but is not so easy to define. It is broadly defined as when a fracture shows no attempt at healing or callus formation after an acceptable time lag. This is usually judged on radiographs where there is a lack of callus and rounding off of the fracture ends seen. However, there is a wide spectrum of what is considered an acceptable time frame between orthopedic surgeons. In animal models of nonunion, it has been

Table 42.2 In Vivo Models.

	Normal fracture	Delayed	Hypertrophic	Stiff atrophic	Mobile atrophic	High energy/comminuted	Critical size defect	Infected
Intramedullary nail	Holstein (mouse) Mannigrasso (mouse) Bonnarens (rat) Pelker (rat) Schemitsch (sheep)	Aro[a] (rat) Patterson[a] (dog)	Hietaniemi (rat)	Oetgen (mouse) Fujita[a] (rat) Kokubu (rat) Latterman (rabbit) Oni (rabbit)	Hietaniemi (rat)	Schindeler (mouse) Utvag (rat) Claes (rat) Claes (sheep)	Lindsey (dog) Pluhar (sheep)	Worlock (rabbit)
Open reduction and external fixation	Grongroft (mouse) Histing (mouse) Savaridas (rat) Keller (rabbit) Lewallen[a] (dog) Perren (sheep)			Garcia (mouse)		Richards (dog) Claes (sheep)	Drosse (mouse) Yasko (rat) Oakes (rat) Rozes (sheep)	Chen (rat) Southwood (rabbit)
External fixation	Cheung (mouse) Reed (rat) Hart (dog) Goodship (sheep)	Rontgen[a] (mouse) Park (rabbit) Schell[a] (sheep)		Choi[a] (mouse) Dickson (rat) Reed (rat) Brownlow (rabbit) Markel (dog)	Cullinane[a] (rat) Harrison (rat)	Park (rabbit) Claes (sheep)	Drosse (mouse) Einhorn (rat) Johnson (dog)	Chen (rat)
Ipsilateral bone	Waters[a] (Rabbit)	Rijal[a] (rabbit)	Aro[a] (rat) Altner[a] (dog) Dos Santos Neto[a] (dog)				Ibiwoye (rat) Cook (rabbit) Bolander (rabbit)	
Plaster cast			Heckman (dog)	Boyan (dog)				

[a]Variable results

335

defined as being a fracture that will not heal in the lifetime of that animal.

In many small animal studies, 16 weeks has been accepted as a reasonable period of observation as it well exceeds the expected time to union.

There are two types of ANU: stiff and mobile. These terms are often used interchangeably in animal models without differentiation. The stiff ANU shows no radiographic signs of healing but histologically there is tissue across the fracture site and some mechanical stiffness is apparent. Mobile ANU offers no mechanical stability or radiographic suggestion of bridging, and histologically there is a mobile cystic cavity, a genuine pseudarthrosis; this is less frequently found than stiff ANU. The importance of differentiating between these model types is that clinically they require different approaches to treatment in order to obtain union.

Establishing ANU without creating a CSD requires significant insult to the bone and soft tissues; this has been achieved in many ways, some reflecting the human clinical scenario more closely than others.

Stiff Atrophic Nonunion

There are several models of stiff ANU in the literature; although some are modifications of other authors' models, in most cases 100% nonunion was achieved but by a diverse variety of techniques. Those that apply a CSD method are addressed separately.

The use of foreign materials to isolate the fracture from surrounding soft tissues is a popular and straightforward technique that gets good rates of ANU but does not parallel the clinical setting. Lattermans et al's model[5] utilizing silastic tubing ran to 64 weeks with only 1 in 24 rabbits developing complications of infection and almost no callus formation.

Markel et al[6] created a 5 mm gap with double application of liquid nitrogen to the end of the distal fragment. They achieved a 100% ANU rate. Several other authors have used cautery as an alternative thermal insult. Kokubu et al[7] used three-point bending followed by 4 mm circumferential cautery and IM nail fixation. A 100% nonunion rate was achieved with no hypertrophic callus or attempt at bridging. Tiedeman et al[8] employed an unilateral external fixator, 6 mm defect, and cautery to the bone ends. They reliably achieved ANU and their control group only had a 0.5 mm defect (which all healed), so it is not possible to be certain how much healing would have occurred with the 6 mm defect alone. Dickson et al[9] have reported a delayed/nonunion model; this incorporated an osteotomy with endosteal stripping and periosteal diathermy that was stabilized with an unilateral external fixator in compression. The model ran for 14 weeks and 96% developed stiff nonunions.

Muscle interposition is used in some models and is a recognized cause of nonunion in the human clinical situation. Fujita et al[10] used muscle interposition with a closed fracture technique and obtained nonunion that persisted for the 2-year study period. No agents or tissue stripping were employed at the fracture site; unfortunately, they did not provide any quantitative results or indications of problems encountered over the 2 years.

Some models rely on motion and reoperation at the fracture site; Boyan et al[11] elevated periosteum and removed 3 mm of bone from a dog radius, and the animal was splinted and allowed to mobilize (these models are adaptations of Mullers' original nonunion model in 1968). One week later, the animal was anaesthetized, and the repair tissue from the fracture gap was excised. The animal was splinted and mobilized. At 12 weeks, they reported 100% ANU and reported no complications. This method has the disadvantage of requiring a second operation.

Brownlow and Simpson[12] and Reed et al[13] validated similar models in the rabbit and rat. They stripped the endosteum and periosteum from around the osteotomy site after application of an external fixator and achieved 100% ANU. No problems were reported with the nonunion. Choi et al[14] and Garcia et al[15] both describe murine ANU models; Choi et al[14] utilized a distraction technique, creating nonunion in 60% by eliminating the latency phase and tripling the distraction rate, and they found that eliminating the latency period alone led to delayed union. Garcia et al[15] studied two sizes of defect (0.8 and 1.8 mm) with or without periosteal stripping and concluded that even with a 1.8 mm defect stripping was required to achieve a consistent nonunion.

Mobile Atrophic Nonunion (Pseudarthrosis)

Cullinane et al[16] devised a "neoarthrosis" model by application of an external fixation and controlled daily motion. Histologically, four of the six animals developed rounded cartilage-capped bone ends with histological similarity to that of articular cartilage. Harrison et al's model[17] resulted in a gap bridged with hypocellular fibrous tissue and no mechanical strength. Hietaniemi, Peltonen, and Paavolainen[3] described a model that they termed a HNU a few years later. They used a similar model without cautery, which led to a cartilage-filled gap, nonbridging callus, and 100% nonunion.

42.4 Critical Size Defect

The definition of CSD is the minimum amount of bone loss that will not heal by bone formation in the lifetime of that animal. Hollinger et al[18] defined it as a defect that had less than 10% bony regeneration in the lifetime of the animal (or practically within 1 year). The differentiation between a CSD and a nonunion model is that in a CSD the gap created is too wide to be bridged; in a nonunion bone bridging is not achieved because of an inability to mount an adequate fracture repair response or the local environmental factors are preventing the usual process of repair (e.g., poor vascularity, stability). The advantages of CSD is that it is reproducible, there is one single cause for the lack of repair, and there is no need for insults such as foreign body insertion or thermal damage.

The CSD model was first proposed by Key (Key's hypothesis) in 1934, who stated that segmental bone loss 1.5 times the diaphyseal diameter would lead to nonunion. Since then, Toombs et al[19] have suggested that Key may have overestimated the bone loss required.

As would be expected, there is species related variation in the gap size created. In sheep, a long bone CSD of at least 30 mm is required, dogs 21 to 30 mm, rabbit studies suggest that 15 mm defect in the radius/ulna/tibia gives a good result, and 6 mm from a rat or mouse femur is an adequate defect size.

The CSD model is commonly used in investigating bone regeneration because it is a simple way of developing bony nonunion. The model's primary application is to test the osteoinductive and conductive capabilities of growth factors and proteins in association with bone scaffolds and grafts. A CSD mimics situations where there has been substantial bone loss either due to trauma or through surgery for tumor or infection; it does not reflect the clinical circumstances where the pathway to osseous regeneration has been arrested in some way (e.g., due to instability or metabolic disturbance).

42.5 Models of Osteoporosis

Due to the variation in bone composition and structure between different species, the 1994 US Food and Drug Administration guidelines require an ovariectomized rat model and a large animal model with intracortical bone remodeling for testing of all agents for osteoporosis before they can be evaluated in a clinical trial.

42.6 Models of Infection

These are considered in Chapter 44.

42.7 Compromised Host Models

Multiple host and clinical factors are known to impair fracture healing (see Gaston and Simpson),[20] including diabetes, hypothyroidism, malnutrition, alcohol, smoking, and drugs such as nonsteroidal anti-inflammatory drugs.

For each of these situations, animal models of bone repair have been described.

For studies evaluating the effect of the host genotype on fracture repair, strains of mice in which specific genes are suppressed are valuable. Mice with specific genes knocked out are available for diseases such as diabetes, for example, as are ones with deficiencies in the immune system (nude mice/rats, SCID mice) or animals that enable certain cells to be tracked (green fluorescent protein mice).

Fracture healing in the impaired host is discussed further in Chapter 43.

References

[1] Bonnarens F, Einhorn TA. Production of a standard closed fracture in laboratory animal bone. J Orthop Res 1984; 2: 97–101

[2] Savaridas T, Wallace RJ, Muir AY, Salter DM, Simpson AH. The development of a novel model of direct fracture healing in the rat. Bone Joint Res 2012; 1: 289–296

[3] Hietaniemi K, Peltonen J, Paavolainen P. An experimental model for non-union in rats. Injury 1995; 26: 681–686

[4] Altner PC, Grana L, Gordon M. An experimental study on the significance of muscle tissue interposition on fracture healing. Clin Orthop Relat Res 1975: 269–273

[5] Lattermann C, Baltzer AW, Zelle BA et al. Feasibility of percutaneous gene transfer to an atrophic nonunion in a rabbit. Clin Orthop Relat Res 2004: 237–243

[6] Markel MD, Bogdanske JJ, Xiang Z, Klohnen A. Atrophic nonunion can be predicted with dual energy x-ray absorptiometry in a canine osteotomy model. J Orthop Res 1995; 13: 869–875

[7] Kokubu T, Hak DJ, Hazelwood SJ, Reddi AH. Development of an atrophic nonunion model and comparison to a closed healing fracture in rat femur. J Orthop Res 2003; 21: 503–510

[8] Tiedeman JJ, Connolly JF, Strates BS, Lippiello L. Treatment of nonunion by percutaneous injection of bone marrow and demineralized bone matrix. An experimental study in dogs. Clin Orthop Relat Res 1991: 294–302

[9] Dickson GR, Geddis C, Fazzalari N, Marsh D, Parkinson I. Microcomputed tomography imaging in a rat model of delayed union/nonunion fracture. J Orthop Res 2008; 26: 729–736

[10] Fujita M, Matsui N, Tsunoda M, Saura R. Establishment of a non-union model using muscle interposition without osteotomy in rats. Kobe J Med Sci 1998; 44: 217–233

[11] Boyan BD, Caplan AI, Heckman JD, Lennon DP, Ehler W, Schwartz Z. Osteochondral progenitor cells in acute and chronic canine nonunions. J Orthop Res 1999; 17: 246–255

[12] Brownlow HC, Simpson AH. Metabolic activity of a new atrophic nonunion model in rabbits. J Orthop Res 2000; 18: 438–442

[13] Reed AA, Joyner CJ, Isefuku S, Brownlow HC, Simpson AH. Vascularity in a new model of atrophic nonunion. J Bone Joint Surg Br 2003; 85-B: 604–610

[14] Choi P, Ogilvie C, Thompson Z, Miclau T, Helms JA. Cellular and molecular characterization of a murine non-union model. J Orthop Res 2004; 22: 1100–1107

[15] Garcia P, Holstein JH, Maier S et al. Development of a reliable non-union model in mice. J Surg Res 2008; 147: 84–91

[16] Cullinane DM, Fredrick A, Eisenberg SR et al. Induction of a neoarthrosis by precisely controlled motion in an experimental mid-femoral defect. J Orthop Res 2002; 20: 579–586

[17] Harrison LJ, Cunningham JL, Strömberg L, Goodship AE. Controlled induction of a pseudarthrosis: a study using a rodent model. J Orthop Trauma 2003; 17: 11–21

[18] Hollinger JO, Kleinschmidt JC. The critical size defect as an experimental model to test bone repair materials. J Craniofac Surg 1990; 1: 60 68

[19] Toombs JP, Wallace LJ, Bjorling DE, Rowland GN. Evaluation of Key's hypothesis in the feline tibia: an experimental model for augmented bone healing studies. Am J Vet Res 1985; 46: 513–518

[20] Gaston MS, Simpson AH. Inhibition of fracture healing. J Bone Joint Surg Br 2007; 89: 1553–1560

Further Reading

Müller J, Schenk R, Willenegger H. [Experimental studies on the development of reactive pseudarthroses on the canine radius] Helv Chir Acta 1968; 35: 301–308

Park SH, O'Connor K, Sung R, McKellop H, Sarmiento A. Comparison of healing process in open osteotomy model and closed fracture model. J Orthop Trauma 1999; 13: 114–120

43 Models for Impaired Healing

Joseph Borrelli, Jr.

Fracture healing occurs by one of two well-described ways. Direct fracture healing, which is believed to be uncommon in nature, involves the direct remodeling of lamellar bone, haversian canals, and blood vessels. Indirect bone healing occurs much more commonly in nature and combines endochondral and intramembranous bone healing in the overall process.

43.1 Indirect Bone Healing

This occurs when some instability remains between the fracture ends when healing begins. This process is seen when long bone fractures are treated nonoperatively, with intramedullary nailing or with external fixation, and also with plate fixation in the setting of a comminuted fracture. The initial phase of this process is the formation of a hematoma as blood seeps into the area from the surrounding soft tissues as a result of the concomitant injury and from the intramedullary canal. The clot that results from bleeding of the bone at the time of fracture ultimately acts as the template for subsequent callus formation. A highly regulated inflammatory phase generally follows within the next 24 hours. This inflammatory phase involves many known inflammatory cytokines and many still yet undiscovered compounds that will subsequently lead to tissue (in this case bone) regeneration. Proinflammatory factors include TNK-alpha, interleukin (IL)-1, -6, -11, and -18, with IL-1 and IL-6 of extreme importance in this process. These inflammatory factors serve to recruit additional cells into the area and promote angiogenesis. For further bone regeneration to occur mesenchymal stem cells must be recruited into the area. Mesenchymal stem cells are recruited from the surrounding soft tissues, bone marrow, and possibly from the systemic circulation in response to bone morphogenic proteins, stromal cell–derived factor 1, and other cytokines. Once in the area, they proliferate and differentiate into osteogenic cells. Cartilaginous callus begins to form between the fracture ends and external to the periosteum. In rats, rabbits, and mice, peak cartilage formation can be found 7 to 9 days following the fracture, providing increased stability to the fracture site. Simultaneously, intramembraneous ossification is occurring subperiosteally directly adjacent to the distal and proximal ends of the fracture. A molecular cascade that stimulates the production of collagen I and II and several signaling peptides follows. The transforming growth factor superfamily including transforming growth factor-B1, -B2, -B3, and GDF-5 are involved with chondrogenesis and endochondral ossification, while several bone morphogenetic proteins (BMPs; BMP-5 and -6) induce cell proliferation in intramembraneous ossification at periosteal sites. Revascularization of the callus occurs by the in growth of blood vessels from surrounding tissues and the new growth of blood vessels. These processes are regulated by angiopoietin and vascular endothelial growth factor, respectively. To permit revascularization of the callus, chondrocyte apoptosis and degradation of the cartilage also has to occur. Mineralization of the callus follows neovascularization and is regulated by a host of peptides including Wnt-family, macrophage–colony-stimulating factor including kappa-B ligand (RANKL), osteoprotegerin, and tumor necrosis factor-alpha. Mineralization of the soft callus and development of woven bone is then followed by a second resorptive phase with sequential removal of the hard callus and formation of lamellar bone structure with a central medullary cavity. This phase is orchestrated by cytokines including IL-1, TNK-alpha, and BMP2 as the resorption is performed by the osteoclasts and bone deposition is performed by the osteoblasts. This process may take quite some time to complete and requires the presence of a good blood supply.

43.2 Direct Fracture Healing

The process of direct fracture healing varies significantly from indirect fracture healing and occurs considerably less commonly in nature. Direct fracture healing occurs by direct remodeling of the lamellar bone, haversian canals, and local blood vessels. For direct fracture healing to occur, the fracture fragments must be brought into very close proximity and be held there rigidly during the healing process. That being said, two types of direct fracture healing are known to occur. One type of direct fracture healing is referred to as "contact healing," which occurs when the fracture ends are no more than 0.02 mm apart and there is no more than 7% intrafragmentary strain. In this scenario, cutting cones formed by leading osteoclasts and trailing osteoblasts pass across the fracture area at a rate of 50 to 100 um/d. The osteoclasts are responsible for removing bone debris and necrotic bone, whereas the osteoblasts are responsible for laying down new bone across the fracture site. "Gap healing" occurs when a residual gap between the fracture fragments is no more than 0.8 to 1.0 mm; the gap is preliminary filled by woven bone that is oriented perpendicular to the long axis of the bone. Secondary osteonal reconstruction then takes place within this bone, which undergoes secondary remodeling resembling the contact bone healing that is occurring in other areas of the fracture as described previously.

43.3 Animal Models for Studying Fracture Healing

"Animal studies still represent an essential tool to analyze the biology of fracture healing."[1] However, the differences in the anatomy and metabolism of animals compared to humans must be considered in the experimental setup and in the interpretation of the experimental results.[1] Additionally, although there are considerable advantages (size, costs, availability, genetic modifications) to using small rodents (mice, rats) to study fracture healing, their primitive bone structure is not representative of our own. This being said, the majority of the of fracture healing studies use either a mouse tibia fracture model as originally described by Hiltunen et al or the rat femur fracture model, or a similar model modified for mice femurs.[2,3] Because the mechanical environment of the healing fracture affects the cellular and molecular mechanisms of fracture healing, considerable thought must be given to the type of fracture model employed. Stabilization of the fractures can be performed with thin pins,[3] intramedullary locking nails,[4] compression screws, external fixators, pin clip devices, and locking plates[3,4,5] (▶ Table 43.1).

Table 43.1 Commonly Used Animal Models for Studying Fracture Healing

Animal models	
Mouse tibial model	Hiltun A, 1993[a]
Rat femur model	Bonnarens F, Einhorn TA, 1984[2]
Mouse femur model	Manigrasso MB, 2004[3]
Fixation models	
Thin pins	Manigrasso MB, 2004[3]
Intramedullary locking nails	Holstein JH, 2008[a]
Compression screws	Mehta M, 2010[a]
External fixators	Cheung KM, 2003[a]
Pin clip devices	Garcia P, 2008[a]
Locking plates	Matthys, 2008[a]
Physiological compromise models	
Diabetes	Kayal RA, 2007,[7] 2009,[a] 2010[a] Albow J, 2009[a]
Aging	Lu C, 2005,[9] 2008[12] Xing Z, 2010
Hypovitaminosis	Delgado-Martinez AD, 1998[14] Melhus G, 2007[15] Tanaka K, 2010[16] Holstein JH, 2010[17] Aleantara-Martos T, 2007[a]

[a]Not referenced.

43.4 Assessment of Healing Response

Many different means for assessing healing in rodent long bone fractures have been developed and well described. Biomechanical analysis of the mouse long bone is a considerable challenge; to assure accurate results, these tests must be performed with attention to detail and consistency. Generally, three- and four-point bending and torsion tests have proven to be applicable for assessing fracture stability in the murine fracture model. To account for differences in bone properties between animals and side-to-side differences in the same animals, the results of these biomechanical tests are usually expressed as a percentage of the contralateral intact bone.

Imaging techniques to assess healing, gene expression, protein degradation, cell migration, and cell death have been widely published. These techniques include micro–positron emission tomography, micro–magnetic resonance imaging, bioluminescence, near infrared fluorescence, and nuclear and magnetic resonance imaging. High-resolution radiography including two-dimensional and three-dimensional microcomputed tomography (MCT) permits measurement of callus mineral density, bone volume, and bone volume/fracture callus.

Histological analysis allows the assessment of the presence of cytokines and cell markers within the fracture callus. As with biomechanical testing of these small bones, much care must be taken to orient the specimens correctly during sectioning and processing to allow a reproducible calculation of the size and tissue composition of the callus. Cytological and molecular analysis with immunohistochemical methods allows further analysis of the presence of cytokines, markers of cellular metabolism, and cellular surface markers. A host of semiquantitative methods exist such as Western blot, enzyme-linked immunosorbent assay techniques, in situ hybridization, Northern blot, reverse transcription–polymerase chain reaction, cell counting methods, and the assessment of apoptosis with in situ labeling of nuclear DNA fragments using the TdT-mediated duTP-biotin nick end labeling technique.

To assess fracture healing and rehabilitation of the mouse further, gait analysis methods have also been developed. These techniques, in addition to giving the investigator insight into the healing process, indicate whether the means of treatment are interfering with the normal gait of the animal.[6]

43.5 Specific Models to Assess Conditions Known to Impair Fracture Healing

With normal fracture healing occurring as a result of an intricate sequence of events, an alteration in any of these steps can cause a delay or prevent fracture healing.

Table 43.2 Items to Consider When Developing a Small Animal Fracture Investigation

Animal	• Size • Ease of handling • Heartiness • Antibody production • Availability of genetically altered animals
Type of bone healing to be assessed	• Endochondromal • Intramembraneous
Fixation	• Absolute stability • Relative stability
Parameters to assess healing	• Imaging: X-ray, microcomputed tomography, magnetic resonance imaging • Histological • Specific proteins • Biomechanical properties

Conditions known to alter the normal fracture healing response include diabetes, aging, and hypovitaminosis. With the use of animal fracture models, investigators are exploring how these and other conditions alter normal fracture healing (▶ Table 43.2).

43.5.1 Diabetes

Clinical and basic science investigations have confirmed that diabetes delays fracture healing in humans and animal models. In the study of how diabetes affects fracture healing, wild-type mice are routinely rendered diabetic by administration of intraperitoneal injections of streptozotocin (40 mg/kg). In most such studies, animals underwent creation of a closed femur or tibia fracture using one of the previously validated methods. Generally, animals were euthanized at intervals between 7 and 28 days after fracture. Assessment of the quality of fracture healing typically includes radiology, histomorphology, and immunohistochemistry, and quantitative real-time polymerase chain reaction to assess messenger ribonucleic acid levels of each gene of interest related to inflammation, osteoclastogenesis, matrix degradation, and cartilage formation. Although the exact mechanism by which diabetes alters the body's ability to heal a fracture has not been completely delineated, it appears that increased chondrocyte apoptosis and osteoclastogenesis that accelerates the loss of the cartilage callus plays an important role in the fracture healing delay.[7,8]

43.5.2 Aging

Many clinicians agree that aging delays fracture healing. This perception has been confirmed in basic science investigations utilizing small animal fracture models.[9,10,11]

To study the effects of aging on fracture healing, it is important to use animals of the appropriate age. In humans, the ratio of age at growth plate closure to life expectancy is about 20%. This ratio is comparable to that of mice, but is considerably different than that of other species such as rats (30%), rabbits, dogs, and sheep (5 to 10%).[11] When investigating the effects of aging on fracture healing in mice, generally juvenile mice are considered those that are 4 weeks old, middle-aged mice are considered 6 months old, and elderly mice are approximately 18 months of age. Lu et al[12] compared the molecular, cellular, and histological progression of skeletal repair in juvenile (4 weeks old), middle-aged (6 months old), and elderly (18 months old) mice at 3, 5, 7, 10, 14, 21, 28, and 35 days postfracture using a nonstabilizing tibia fracture model. They found a sharp decline in fracture healing potential between juvenile and middle-aged animals, and a more subtle decrease in fracture healing potential between middle-aged mice and elderly mice.[12]

In an effort to delineate how aging negatively influences fracture healing additional studies were performed. Mehta et al[13] studied the effects of age on vascularization during fracture healing. Again, they used a nonstabilized tibial fracture model in juvenile (4 weeks old), middle-aged (6 months old), and elderly mice (18 months old). Stereology, immunohistochemistry, and in situ hybridization were used to assess fracture callus. As a result of this investigation, they found that age affected vascularization during fracture healing, and the changes observed were directly correlated with altered expression of biochemical factors that regulate the process of angiogenesis. In an effort to better understand the role of the aging inflammatory system on fracture repair in aged mice, Xing et al[10] created chimeric mice by bone marrow transplant after lethal irradiation. In this animal model, the chondrocytes and osteoblasts in the fracture regenerate were found to be derived exclusively from host cells, whereas the inflammatory cells were derived from the donor. They found that middle-aged mice receiving juvenile bone marrow had larger calluses and more bone formation during the early stages and faster callus remodeling at late stages of fracture healing, indicating that inflammatory cells derived from the juveniles bone marrow accelerated bone repair in the middle-aged animals. In contrast, they found that transplanting bone marrow from middle-aged mice to juvenile mice did not alter the process of fracture healing in juvenile mice. They concluded that the roles of inflammatory cells in fracture healing may be age-related, suggesting the possibility of enhancing fracture healing in aged animals by manipulating the inflammatory system.[10]

43.5.3 Hypovitaminosis

To study the effects of hypovitaminosis, investigators have utilized a variety of small animal fracture models. Delgado-Martinez et al[14] studied the effects of 25-OH-vitamin D on fracture healing in elderly rats (18 months old). Using a femoral shaft fracture model, they found a positive correlation ($p < 0.01$; $r = 0.55$) between blood levels of the 25-OH-vitamin D at the time of euthanasia and mechanical strength of the fracture callus at 5 weeks postfracture in those animals that received vitamin D during the healing process compared to controls.[14] Surprisingly, Melhus et al[15] were unable to demonstrate a significant effect of vitamin D deficiency in ovarectomized rats. Using a tibial shaft fracture model involving Wistar rats, the animals were either ovarectomized and exposed to a vitamin D–deficient diet or a sham operation and normal diet were studied. Mechanical strength of the callus was assessed at 6 weeks after fracture and bone loss and callus formation was monitored with dual-energy X-ray absorptiometry, whereas serum levels of estradiol and vitamin D3 were measured and histomorphometric analyses were performed.[15] The investigators were unable to demonstrate a difference either in bone mineral density or in the mechanical properties of the callus between the groups.

The effects of vitamin A, folate, and B12 and have also been studied in different animal models. Tanaka et al[16] studied the effects of vitamin A deficiency on BMP2 expression and bone repair in a "drill hole injury." In this unusual model, a 1 mm drill hole was drilled into the femoral diaphysis of vitamin A–deficient mice (10 weeks old). The investigators understood that this model represented an intramembranous ossification model as opposed to the more commonly utilized endochondral ossification model. Retardation of bone repair was realized in the vitamin A–deficient mice when MCT and histomorphometry were used to assess healing. The investigators also found suppression of BMP2 messenger ribonucleic acid production in the defect and the reduction of additional cytokines within the defect as well. This deficiency was reversed when BMP2 was added directly into the defect at the time of its creation.[16] Holstein et al[17] used a stabilized closed femur fracture model in mice to study the effects of folate and vitamin B12 deficiency on fracture healing. Three-point bending tests showed no significant difference in callus stiffness between bones of folate and B12-deficient animals and controls, and histomorphometry showed comparable size and tissue composition of the fracture callus.[17] Alcantara-Martos et al[18] investigated the effects of vitamin C on fracture healing in elderly (18 months old) rats. They created unstable bilateral middle third femur fractures in these animals and then exposed them to different rates of vitamin C intake. The groups with a lower vitamin C intake demonstrated a lower mechanical resistance of the healing callus and a lower histological grade while supplementary vitamin C improved the mechanical resistance of the fracture callus in elderly rats.[18]

References

[1] Holstein JH, Garcia P, Histing T et al. Advances in the establishment of defined mouse models for the study of fracture healing and bone regeneration. J Orthop Trauma 2009; 23 Suppl: S31–S38

[2] Bonnarens F, Einhorn TA. Production of a standard closed fracture in laboratory animal bone. J Orthop Res 1984; 2: 97–101

[3] Manigrasso MB, O'Connor JP. Characterization of a closed femur fracture model in mice. J Orthop Trauma 2004; 18: 687–695

[4] Holstein JH, Menger MD, Culemann U, Meier C, Pohlemann T. Development of a locking femur nail for mice. J Biomech 2007; 40: 215–219

[5] Cheung KM, Kaluarachi K, Andrew G, Lu W, Chan D, Cheah KS. An externally fixed femoral fracture model for mice. J Orthop Res 2003; 21: 685–690

[6] Seebeck P, Thompson MS, Parwani A, Taylor WR, Schell H, Duda GN. Gait evaluation: a tool to monitor bone healing? Clin Biomech (Bristol, Avon) 2005; 20: 883–891

[7] Kayal RA, Tsatsas D, Bauer MA et al. Diminished bone formation during diabetic fracture healing is related to the premature resorption of cartilage associated with increased osteoclast activity. J Bone Miner Res 2007; 22: 560–568

[8] Kayal RA, Alblowi J, McKenzie E et al. Diabetes causes the accelerated loss of cartilage during fracture repair which is reversed by insulin treatment. Bone 2009; 44: 357–363

[9] Lu C, Miclau T, Hu D et al. Cellular basis for age-related changes in fracture repair. J Orthop Res 2005; 23: 1300–1307

[10] Xing Z, Lu C, Hu D, Miclau T, III, Marcucio RS. Rejuvenation of the inflammatory system stimulates fracture repair in aged mice. J Orthop Res 2010; 28: 1000–1006

[11] Kilborn SH, Trudel G, Uhthoff H. Review of growth plate closure compared with age at sexual maturity and lifespan in laboratory animals. Contemp Top Lab Anim Sci 2002; 41: 21–26

[12] Lu C, Hansen E, Sapozhnikova A, Hu D, Miclau T, Marcucio RS. Effect of age on vascularization during fracture repair. J Orthop Res 2008; 26: 1384–1389

[13] Mehta M, Strube P, Peters A et al. Influences of age and mechanical stability on volume, microstructure, and mineralization of the fracture callus during bone healing: is osteoclast activity the key to age-related impaired healing? Bone 2010; 47: 219–228

[14] Delgado-Martínez AD, Martínez ME, Carrascal MT, Rodríguez-Avial M, Munuera L. Effect of 25-OH-vitamin D on fracture healing in elderly rats. J Orthop Res 1998; 16: 650–653

[15] Melhus G, Solberg LB, Dimmen S, Madsen JE, Nordsletten L, Reinholt FP. Experimental osteoporosis induced by ovariectomy and vitamin D deficiency does not markedly affect fracture healing in rats. Acta Orthop 2007; 78: 393–403

[16] Tanaka K, Tanaka S, Sakai A, Ninomiya T, Arai Y, Nakamura T. Deficiency of vitamin A delays bone healing process in association with reduced BMP2 expression after drill-hole injury in mice. Bone 2010; 47: 1006–1012

[17] Holstein JH, Herrmann M, Schmalenbach J et al. Deficiencies of folate and vitamin B12 do not affect fracture healing in mice. Bone 2010; 47: 151–155

[18] Alcantara-Martos T, Delgado-Martinez AD, Vega MV, Carrascal MT, Munuera-Martinez L. Effect of vitamin C on fracture healing in elderly Osteogenic Disorder Shionogi rats. J Bone Joint Surg Br 2007; 89: 402–407

44 In Vivo Models for Bone and Joint Infections

Volker Alt, Christoph Henkenberens, and Reinhard Schnettler

Bone and joint infections do not represent a uniform disease, but a heterogeneous group of diseases that require complex treatment algorithms. The integral part is certain highly standardized surgical procedures.

Even in modern times, bone and joint infections are still associated with a high morbidity and mortality rate resulting in high direct and indirect medical costs, which are increasingly important in the course of the rationalization of health care systems in the Western industrialized nations. To meet these issues, joint and bone infections must be prevented and treated more effectively through improved prophylaxis and therapy algorithms. This results in a constantly increasing importance of in vivo animal studies.

The premise for a good animal model is that it reflects as closely as possible a complex clinical situation. Thus, the first crucial step for in vivo animal studies of bone and joint infection is the selection of the best available model or development of a new animal model that closely reflects the clinical scenario. The more precisely an animal model mimics the clinical situation, the more transferable the results will be from the animal model to clinical practice. To achieve this step, it is necessary firstly to avoid systemic complications that lead to the loss of animals and secondly to induce bone and joint infection reliably. The aim of this chapter is to give the reader a guide with simple basic criteria for orientation in the field of in vivo animal models and studies of bone and joint infections.

44.1 General Requirements

Infection experiments have to be approved by the local authorities, particularly regarding ethical aspects. Approval is subject to numerous conditions. This includes the restriction to the minimum number of animals. Infection experiments can be a heavy burden on laboratory animals. As mentioned previously, the inoculation dose is a compromise between reliable induction of the infection and avoiding systemic complications, with the exception that systemic side effects are investigated. For this reason, no animal should be exposed to avoidable pain and suffering. Adequate anesthesia and analgesia must be provided.

Relevant changes in the study design must be reported immediately to the local authorities. Under certain circumstances, you will be asked to submit a new request. A copy of the approval of the local authorities may need to be submitted with the manuscript. Inconsistencies will lead to the rejection of the manuscript. In addition, the authorities will evaluate future projects more critically and possibly refuse permission.

The animals must be housed in a suitable and approved animal laboratory. Animals should be housed individually after the inoculation to prevent mutual chewing and infecting. The cage floor should be covered with absorbent sheets. Classic litter can get into wounds and promote secondary contamination and thus lead to false results.

The laboratory must meet the minimum safety standard S2 due to the work with biological materials that pose a potential danger for the employees. This standard applies throughout the world. Sometimes more strict state-specific certificates are required, and appropriately qualified and certified personnel must be provided. Before an application is sent to the local animal protection authorities, it is advisable to inquire about the structural and personnel standards of the animal laboratory. Failure to meet these standards results in rejection of the application by the local authorities.

Surgical procedures both for operative interventions on the animals and for euthanasia must be carried out under aseptic conditions in order to prevent contamination with other bacteria (▶ Fig. 44.1).

44.2 Guidelines for Study Planning

Before a systematic action guideline is presented, two terms need to be defined: osteitis and osteomyelitis. In osteomyelitis, the bone marrow is infected first; in contrast, in osteitis there is a centripetal infection with spread of germs from outside the bone to inside. This means that with osteitis, the cortex and/or cancellous bone are infected first and a bone marrow infection occurs secondarily, so that some authors use the term secondary osteomyelitis in the case of an osteitis. In German-speaking countries, the term osteitis is commonly used, whereas in the Anglo-American literature no distinction is made between osteitis and osteomyelitis, and it is generally spoken of as osteomyelitis, which is used in this chapter.

44.2.1 Clinical Situation and Research Target

First, the clinical situation of a joint or bone infection has to be characterized in detail to deduce the clinical problem. AlphaThe exact research question can be formulated only when the clinical problem is exactly identified and described in sufficient detail. The research question should then indicate the research target. Therefore, at least one main parameter and maybe one or several secondary outcome parameters have to be quantified to

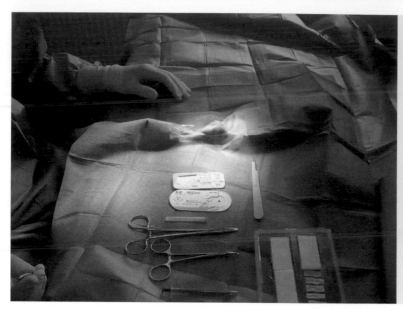

Fig. 44.1 Sterile surgical setup with sterile drapage of the operated limb that will be contaminated with bacteria for infection induction.

compare the findings of the performed animal study with other animal studies to draw a conclusion and transfer the results back to the clinical situation. In vivo models can either be used to investigate the prevention or treatment of joint and bone infections. This has to be stated in the research question, because this may be associated with a different burden on the animals and thus is relevant for the approval of the animal study.

These infections are first divided into a primary bone infection or primary joint infection; they are then differentiated with respect to their exact etiology, pathology, clinical manifestation, and timeline. A pure joint infection should be considered as an infectious synovitis of the joint membrane that does not involve the adjacent bone (e.g., hematogenous or early postarthroscopic infection). The same is true for bone infections. A pure bone infection should not be complicated with a joint infection. An example is the group of blood-borne bone infections (e.g., acute staphylococcal hematogenous osteomyelitis). Currently, in the industrialized nations, the study of implant-associated bone and joint infections is in the foreground, such as joint prosthesis infections. Foreign materials as an important pathogenetic factor in bone and joint infection significantly affect the progression of infections and clinical outcome. However, there are pathophysiological overlaps between the clinical scenarios.

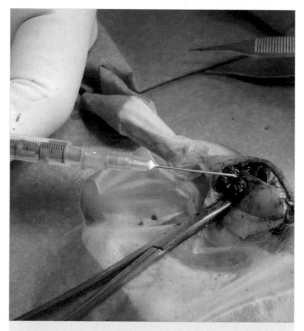

Fig. 44.2 Inoculation of *Staphylococcus aureus* into the osteotomy gap of the tibial diapyhsis for induction of an infected nonunion.

44.2.2 Bacteria

Both bone infections and joint infections—with the exception of some special forms—are caused by bacteria, viruses, fungi, and parasites of endogenous or exogenous origin, and can progress acutely or chronically according to their pathogenicity and the immune status of the host organism. Most commonly, bone and joint infections are due to bacteria. Staphylococci in general are the most common pathogens in acute bone, chronic bone, and all joint infections. Strains of *Staphylococcus aureus* are frequently the focus of in vivo animal research due to their increasing antibiotic resistance (▶ Fig. 44.2).

The selection of a suitable strain plays a key role. Besides the use of "own" isolates, a plurality of commercially available strains exists. The most important criterion is the clinical scenario from which the strain originates. Accordingly, in bone and joint infections the used bacterial strain should derive from an equivalent clinical setting.

Before the main study, a pilot study is highly recommended to evaluate an appropriate bacterial strain in a proper inoculation dose. A proper inoculation dose reliably leads to a high infection rate in the control group. This should be titrated to reduce the number of required animals of the entire study: Statistically significant differences are more likely to be found between the control and the treatment group if there is a high infection rate in the control group, and this helps to ensure that the sample size calculation produces the smallest number. However, excessive inoculation doses have to be avoided due to systemic infection complications, including death of animals in the worst case. Thus, because the inoculation dose can vary widely from species to species, a pilot study should not be skipped. In addition, positive effects in the treatment group can be negated by an overcontamination.

Bioluminescent strains of bacteria are available, and they have almost completely replaced radioactive labeling techniques. Bioluminescent strains have a higher generation time than nonbioluminescent strains. Therefore, the induction of an infection is more difficult, requires higher inoculation doses, and increases the probability of the infection failing to persist due to the elimination of the bacteria by the host's immune system.

44.2.3 Animals

An optimal experimental animal for in vivo study of bone and joint infections does not exist. Most commonly, rats and rabbits are used. Both are large enough to carry out more complex models and thus allow for the use of implants and other materials relevant for clinical use. This leads to a certain degree of standardization of the model and increases the transferability of the results to the clinical situation in humans. Moreover, they can be kept in groups, which is cost-effective. Mice and hamsters are usually too small for implant-related studies, whereas large animals (e.g., sheep or dog) are in most cases too costly and are less ethically accepted than small animals.

44.3 Classification

The classification of osteomyelitis or joint infection is a prerequisite for selection of a suitable animal model, which should represent as accurately as possible a clinical scenario. There exists a variety of criteria by which an animal model can be selected. Special forms, such as sclerosing and cellular plasma osteomyelitis, which are difficult to classify due to their specific and partially unknown pathology, are not discussed in this chapter. For simplicity, this chapter narrows down to two criteria:

1. Etiology
2. Chronological sequence

The first criterion—the etiology—fundamentally determines further planning.

44.3.1 Endogenous Infection

An osteomyelitis or a joint infection can arise endogenously or exogenously. Endogenous infections are usually caused by hematogenous metastatic bacterial colonies in the bone or joints, or by encroachment from a neighboring infection (by continuity). Common sources are purulent infections in the head and neck area, lungs, and soft tissues. Endogenous bone and joint infections are less frequent than exogenous bone infections in the Western world. In endogenous infections, bacteria can pass through the protective growth plate via transepiphyseal blood vessels and settle down in the epiphyseal bone resulting in a simultaneous bone and joint infection. Thus, the strict distinction between bone and joint infections cannot be maintained in every clinical setting.

44.3.2 Exogenous Infection

An exogenous bone or joint infection results from bacterial contamination from the environment such as in open fractures or intraoperative contamination of the surgical site commonly when implants are inserted such as total joint replacement or osteosynthesis devices.

As mentioned previously, the detailed description of the clinical situation is the basic prerequisite in in vivo orthopedic and trauma infection research. This forms the basis for deriving the research questions. From this the animal model is chosen, which should simulate the genesis of the clinical situation as closely as possible.

The second criterion—the chronological sequence—also helps to determine the model and the duration of the experiment. Acute infections are differentiated from chronic infections: By definition, when the infection occurs for the first time, it is initially classified as acute. If the infection persists for a certain time, the infection is defined as chronic. This means that each model of chronic infection is also a model of acute infection. But not every animal model of an acute infection leads inevitably to a chronic infection, because acute infections can be self-limiting. There is no clear definition for the definitive time span for a chronic infection. However, a period of 4 weeks postinfection is favored.

Confirmation of Infection

Clinical and microbiological methods

First, the macroscopic changes should be described (▶ Fig. 44.3). These are mainly clinical signs of infection (lameness, swelling, redness, warmth, exudation, pus

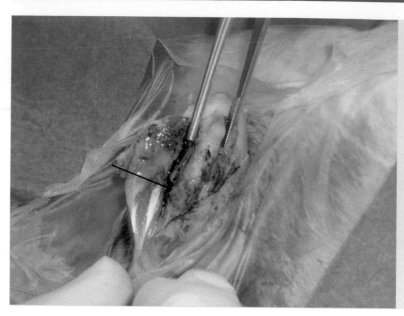

Fig. 44.3 Macroscopic appearance of an infected nonunion of the tibial shaft (*arrow*) with pus formation and nonbridging of the former osteotomy gap.

drainage, deformation). In addition, blood inflammatory markers (c-reactive protein, white blood cells, interleukin-6) can be measured and blood cultures can be set up. Because the infection is mostly restricted to the extremities, blood cultures are often negative.

Tissue samples of the infected region are suitable to culture bacteria on nutrient media. In case of positive bacterial growth, the bone or joint infection is confirmed. To provide semiquantitative microbiological evidence, weighed tissue can be converted into a liquid and processed in a dilution series on agar plates. The number of colony-forming units is determined to quantify the severity of the infection microbiologically.

It is necessary to confirm that the selected bacterial strain caused the infection and that secondary contamination is precluded—this may only be possible at the time of euthanasia. This can be done on a descriptive level by cultivation of bacteria on nutrient media or on a quantitative level to determine the bacterial load via cytogenetic methods such as polymerase chain reaction, pulsed field gel electrophoresis, and fluorescence in situ hybridization.

Imaging and nuclear medicine techniques

Imaging techniques are extremely important for assessing the infection. Conventional radiographs show lack of bone healing and bone destruction. These changes can be quantified using sectional imaging methods (computed tomography, micro-computed tomography). Magnetic resonance imaging is superior in identifying the inflammation of the bone marrow and adjacent soft tissues.

The cellular changes are examined by histological methods. Standard staining using hematoxylin and eosin and toluidine blue may be supplemented by immunohistochemical staining, which enables almost all of the components of pro- and eukaryotic cells to be selectively visualized. Quantification of the bony changes can be provided by using histomorphometry of bone sections, which is still regarded as the reference method.

Scanning electron microscopy is the standard method to visualize bacterial colonies and biofilm formation on implants (▶ Fig. 44.4). In addition, the morphology of bacteria (e.g., cocci) can be analyzed.

With bioluminescent bacterial strains, the infection can be longitudinally quantified in vivo without the use of radioactive markers. Nuclear medicine scintigraphy alternatives are often relatively costly.

Finally, there are some elaborate special procedures for the investigation of specific issues. Metabolic processes can be assessed by positron emission tomography/computed tomography and small vessels can be demonstrated, as a sign of incipient bone formation, by using perfusion computed tomography.

44.4 Specific Animal Models

In the Western industrialized nations, pure bone infections decreased in frequency during the last four decades due to improved hygiene standards and effective antibiotic therapy schemes. However, implant-associated infections have become of greater interest in preclinical bone and joint infection research, because implanted foreign materials provide a potential adhesive surface for bacteria where typical bacteria, like *S. aureus*, form a biofilm on the implant's surface that consistently leads to a failure of well-accepted antimicrobial therapy algorithms.

44.4.1 Bone Infection Models

Essentially three types of animal models for the induction of an exogenous osteomyelitis can be distinguished.

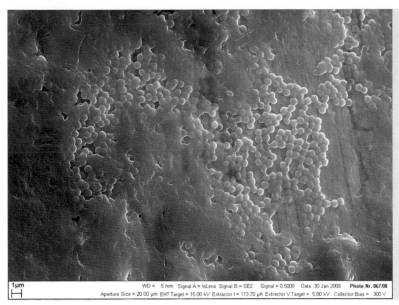

Fig. 44.4 Formation of biofilm by *Staphylococcus aureus* on a K-wire in a rat tibia infection model.

These are models of (1) pure bone infection, (2) posttraumatic implant-associated infection, and (3) prosthesis infection. A strict separation of these models is not possible, as a major intersection of the models lies in the use of foreign materials, which contribute decisively to the emergence and persistence of bone infection

In 1885, the first successful induction of an endogenous/hematogenous osteomyelitis in rabbits after intravenous injection of a bacterial suspension was described.[1] However, a high sepsis rate required refinement of this model leading to the use of sclerosing agents such as sodium morrhuate,[2] which can be injected percutaneously into the bone or into a drilled hole in the bone. All these models lack clinical relevance because sclerosing agents are rarely used in patients; therefore, these models should only be used in instances of specific questions on sclerotic agents.

The highest importance in animal infection research should be given to models that represent the most important entity, which is implant-related infections.

For the study of implant-associated infections, numerous very similar animal models are available. These animal models are based on the principle that a foreign material is introduced into the medullary canal of a bone and the medullary canal is directly contaminated with different bacteria.[3,4,5,6] The advantage of these models is that they are simple and easy to perform, but they do not represent the complex pathophysiology of implant-associated infections sufficiently, because the clinical indication for the implant is not simulated.

Andriole et al[7] introduced the first implant-related bone infection model based on a tibial shaft fracture induced by a three-point clamp onto which bacteria were inoculated via a metaphyseal drill hole. A steel wire was introduced into the medullary canal. This model represented the first attempt to simulate an implant-associated bone infection after a long bone fracture.

Currently, Alt et al[8] have achieved the best possible approximation for a posttraumatic infection after an open fracture stabilized with an imtramedullary rod. In their model, the osteotomized tibia of a rat was directly contaminated and stabilized with an intramedullary stainless steel needle. This model allows the modulation of all established as well as novel treatment modalities in the clinic ranging from the implant material to the antibiotic treatment and the effects of growth factors. Depending at which time interventions are performed, acute and chronic infection can be investigated, because these models are characterized by a persisting infection.

There are only few animal models for true prosthetic joint infections. As mentioned previously, animal models for a prosthetic joint infection do not allow the separation between an infection of the joint or the bone, because the prosthesis connects the bone with the joint. In contrast to all the other models, a two-compartment model with consecutive interaction of the joint with the bone results. In addition, an implant-associated infection is generated by the foreign material. A simple model includes an implant introduced into the medullary canal of a long bone with one implant end reaching into the joint cavitiy.[9] Blomgren and Lindgren[10] describe a complete and Schurman et al[11] a partial knee replacement with resection of the articular surfaces and filling of the defect with gentamicin-containing poly(methyl methacrylate) in rabbits. The cement was investigated in situ to prevent hematogenous infections after intravenous injection of *S. aureus* and *Escherchia coli*. The model does not provide for direct contamination of the knee, and therefore does not simulate the most common cause of artificial joint infections, the intraoperative contamination. A direct contamination of the knee joint is described for a knee hemiarthroplasty with replacement of the tibial component with a commercial available silicone-customer implant for the arthroplasty of the first metatarsophalangeal joint[12] to investigate different antibiotics as a treatment of infection in this context.[13,14]

44.4.2 Joint Infection Models

Models for the induction of endogenous/hematogenous joint infection are strongly analogous to the models of endogenous/hematogenous bone infection.[15,16,17] The bacterial inoculation is also achieved by selective puncture of a vessel. These models have three disadvantages. First, some of the animals die due to septic complications; second, the infection can manifest at each joint; and third, the rate of successful induced joint infections is low. Another research focus for these models is less in the orthopedic and trauma surgery field, but more in the immunological field and focuses on the changes in the synovial fluid in aseptic and reactive arthritis after transient bacteremia.

The induction of an exogenous infection can be achieved by joint puncture and intracavitary injection of bacteria. Depending on the bacterial virulence, a septic arthritis evolves. Most common inserted pathogen is *S. aureus*.

44.5 Limitations

Sometimes the selected bacterial strain—independent of the inoculation dose—induces no infection, although this bacterium was isolated from a clinical comparable setting. Generally, animals require higher inoculation doses than humans, with the result that regardless of the chosen inoculation dose the virulence of a bacterium is not sufficient to produce a bone or joint infection in the host. In addition, excessive doses can also negate positive effects in the treatment groups, although these would be otherwise clinically relevant. A change of the strain and a new pilot study is recommended. In the opposite case, that too many animals suffer septic complications, the inoculation dose should be lowered.

As a general rule, the findings of an animal study—no matter how good the quality of the study—cannot be transferred one to one to the clinical situations in humans. The probability that the findings do indeed exist can be increased by a further animal study in another species. This also holds well for the opposite case: The results are not statistically significant. The change of the species might come to the confirmation of the hypothesis. Positive results must always be confirmed by testing in human experiments.

Overall, there is an 8% chance of a new therapy being approved and the product finally getting to the market. In the vast majority of cases, lack of efficacy or unfavorable

Table 44.1 Summary of practical guidelines

Clinical situation	State clearly the situation and its problems
Research question	Derive clear research question from the clinical problem you want to address Define research target and parameters
Animal model	Select an appropriate model for your research question
Bacteria	Use an appropriate strain from similar clinical settings
Pilot study	Conduct pilot study to determine an adequate inoculation dose Confirm the infection
Study design	Define control and treatment groups Conduct proper statistical sample size calculation
Evaluation	Assess the infection Confirm or reject your hypothesis

pharmacokinetics of the new substance in humans are the reason for this.[18] In contrast, only about 10% of all drugs fail in clinical trials due to unexpected side effects in humans, as the data obtained from animal experiments have a high consistency regarding the observed toxic effects in animals and allow for a sufficient medical-ethical risk assessment in humans. However, the unavoidable residual uncertainty remains.[19]

References

[1] Rodet A. Etude experimentale sur l'osteomyelite infectieuse. Compt Rend Acad Sci 1884; 99: 569–571

[2] Norden CW, Kennedy E. Experimental osteomyelitis. I. A description of the model. J Infect Dis 1970; 122: 410–418

[3] Petty W, Spanier S, Shuster JJ, Silverthorne C. The influence of skeletal implants on incidence of infection. Experiments in a canine model. J Bone Joint Surg Am 1985; 67: 1236–1244

[4] Melcher GA, Claudi B, Schlegel U, Perren SM, Printzen G, Munzinger J. Influence of type of medullary nail on the development of local infection. An experimental study of solid and slotted nails in rabbits. J Bone Joint Surg Br 1994; 76: 955–959

[5] Sanzén L, Linder L. Infection adjacent to titanium and bone cement implants: an experimental study in rabbits. Biomaterials 1995; 16: 1273–1277

[6] Eerenberg JP, Patka P, Haarman HJTHM, Dwars BJ. A new model for posttraumatic osteomyelitis in rabbits. J Invest Surg 1994; 7: 453–465

[7] Andriole VT, Nagel DA, Southwick WO. A paradigm for human chronic osteomyelitis. J Bone Joint Surg Am 1973; 55: 1511–1515

[8] Alt V, Lips KS, Henkenbehrens C et al. A new animal model for implant-related infected non-unions after intramedullary fixation of the tibia in rats with fluorescent in situ hybridization of bacteria in bone infection. Bone 2011; 48: 1146–1153

[9] Bernthal NM, Stavrakis AI, Billi F et al. A mouse model of post-arthroplasty Staphylococcus aureus joint infection to evaluate in vivo the efficacy of antimicrobial implant coatings. PLoS ONE 2010; 5: e12580

[10] Blomgren G, Lindgren U. Late hematogenous infection in total joint replacement: studies of gentamicin and bone cement in the rabbit. Clin Orthop Relat Res 1981: 244–248

[11] Schurman DJ, Trindade C, Hirshman HP, Moser K, Kajiyama G, Stevens P. Antibiotic-acrylic bone cement composites. Studies of gentamicin and Palacos. J Bone Joint Surg Am 1978; 60: 978–984

[12] Belmatoug N, Crémieux AC, Bleton R et al. A new model of experimental prosthetic joint infection due to methicillin-resistant Staphylococcus aureus: a microbiologic, histopathologic, and magnetic resonance imaging characterization. J Infect Dis 1996; 174: 414–417

[13] Crémieux AC, Mghir AS, Bleton R et al. Efficacy of sparfloxacin and autoradiographic diffusion pattern of [14C]Sparfloxacin in experimental Staphylococcus aureus joint prosthesis infection. Antimicrob Agents Chemother 1996; 40: 2111–2116

[14] Saleh Mghir A, Cre'mieux AC, Bleton R, et al. Autoradiographic pattern of 14C-teicoplanin and efficacy of teicoplanin in an experimental staphylococcus infection [abstract no A38]. In: Program and abstracts of the 36th Interscience Conference on Antimicrobial Agents and Chemotherapy (New Orleans). Washington, DC: American Society for Microbiology, 1996: 8

[15] Cai XY, Yang C, Zhang ZY, Qiu WL, Ha Q, Zhu M. A murine model for septic arthritis of the temporomandibular joint. J Oral Maxillofac Surg 2008; 66: 864–869

[16] Hultgren OH, Stenson M, Tarkowski A. Role of IL-12 in Staphylococcus aureus-triggered arthritis and sepsis. Arthritis Res 2001; 3: 41–47

[17] Verdrengh M, Tarkowski A. Inhibition of septic arthritis by local administration of taurine chloramine, a product of activated neutrophils. J Rheumatol 2005; 32: 1513–1517

[18] Kubinyi H. Drug research: myths, hype and reality. Nature Rev Drug Disc 2003;2:665–669

[19] Greaves P, Williams A, Eve M. First dose of potential new medicines to humans: how animals help. Nat Rev Drug Discov 2004; 3: 226–236

45 In Vivo Models for Articular Cartilage Repair

Paul Hindle

The translation of basic science research requires rigorous investigation prior to human clinical trials. An important step in this process is the use of in vivo animal models.[1,2,3,4] They allow the efficacy and safety to be tested in a biological and mechanical environment that aims to protect patients from unsafe drugs or procedures.

The main areas that can be investigated include:

- Foreign-body reactions to new materials (biocompatibility)
- Effects of materials on healing
- Immunological response to cells, autologous and allogeneic
- Effect of growth factors, drugs and other compounds
- Safety and efficacy of new treatments
- Mechanical response to nonbiological implants
- Biological pathways assessment by up- and downregulation of genetic expression
- Mechanical loading of healing tissues

Despite the use of in vitro methods and the promise of technologies, such as induced pluripotent stem cells, there is not a sufficient alternative to in vivo studies at this time. The use of animals unable to consent raises ethical and social concerns that vary from country to country. In the United Kingdom, animal research is legislated by the Animals (Scientific Procedures) Act 1986 and regulated by the Home Office.

Before any research is undertaken, the question and hypothesis need to be clearly defined. This allows three vital questions to be answered. The first is "Has this work been undertaken before?" A thorough review of the literature is mandatory to ensure that animals are not used superfluously; this includes the foreign literature where practicable. The second question is "Can this question be answered using an in vitro laboratory technique without the use of live animals?" For short-term experiments (up to 3 to 4 weeks), sometimes cadaveric tissue will suffice as cells will function postmortem and can provide valid results in appropriate experiments. The third is "Is my experimental model robust enough to provide sufficient data to justify the use of live animals?" There is no excuse for poorly planned experiments wasting animals' lives to no scientific or clinical benefit.

Researchers planning on undertaking animal research need to be fully aware of and trained and supported by appropriate veterinary staff to ensure that disruption to the welfare of the animals is reduced as much as possible. The relative cost and time frame compared to in vitro work needs to be considered.

45.1 Animal Models

To determine the most appropriate animal to use, a number of key factors need to be determined. The first is the model of cartilage repair to be used. The options include heterotopic, cartilage defect, and arthritic or articular fracture, and are described in greater detail below.

After promising in vitro results, a heterotopic model of chondrogenesis should be considered. This would typically be subcutaneous, intramuscular, or intraperitoneal. The rat xiphoid has also been proposed as a potential nonjoint model for cartilage regeneration strategies. Animals used for these studies include nude mice, syngenic mice, rats, and rabbits. Cells can be implanted directly, injected, or introduced within a diffusion chamber. These studies allow researchers to look at the biological effect of the cells being in vivo without the need to use an articular cartilage defect model.

There are two types of cartilage defect models to be considered, partial or full thickness, which relate to whether or not the subchondral plate is breached.[5,6] The choice depends on the hypothesis to be tested. Breaching the subchondral bone when not intended will release bone marrow (including clotting factors and stem cells), which can invalidate the technique being investigated.

Generalized arthritis can be induced by a number of methods. The most common of these include mechanical resection of ligaments, including the anterior cruciate or the cranial cruciate ligament (the Pond-Nuki model), or menisci, which is resection of the medial meniscus inducing medial compartment arthritis. Other possible methods include treatment of spontaneous disease, obesity models, hormone deficiency (ovariectomy), chemical damage (direct cartilage degradation and indirect metabolism inhibition), limb immobilization, hypermotility, and scoring grooves in the cartilage.

Rodent models have also been used in a model of articular fracture healing.

45.2 Animal Selection

Animals are usually categorized into small or large models. Small animals include mice, rats, rabbits, and guinea pigs, and large animals include dogs, pigs, minipigs, sheep, goats, and horses. The International Society for Cartilage Repair recommends that while small animal models are useful for initial studies and proof-of-concept work, a large animal study is required for pivotal studies.[4]

Species selection will be affected by the type of model to be used; heterotopic models typically use small animal models. Cartilage defect and arthritis models can use small and large animal models. Small animals are more appropriate for proof-of-concept work or looking at the effect of drugs, compounds, or alterations in genetic expression. Surgical techniques are better assessed with a large animal model.

The advantage of using small animals such as rodents and rabbits includes ease of use, reduced cost, easier husbandry, and the ability to view the entire joint on one histological slide. Their disadvantages include their relatively smaller joints, thinner cartilage, and problems with postoperative care.

Large animals also have their associated benefits and problems. The use of dogs is socially unacceptable in the United Kingdom due to their status as companion animals. Despite having thicker cartilage, pigs are hard to work with and seldom used as the minipig is easier to work with. Goats have been widely used due to their anatomical shape and cartilage thickness; they are, however, hard to work with and may have been affected with prion disease causing early arthritis leading to early termination of experiments. The sheep is easy to handle and relatively amenable. They have thinner cartilage than some of the other animals but have been successfully used for autologous chondrocyte implantation despite this. Horses have the thickest cartilage and the largest joints, making them the best comparison to human joints,[7] and they themselves have problems with osteochondral disease. Horses are, however, very expensive if large numbers are required and they need to be kept for a long time. There are also similar issues as for the dog due to their status as companion animals. Injured horses that are destined for euthanasia may be considered more appropriate for studies of treatment.

As well as the type of model to be used, species selection will be determined by a number of other factors. The literature will suggest if one particular species has been used for a particular area; if this is the case, using the same species will allow results to be comparable. Local expertise, animal availability, and housing facilities also have to be considered. Other factors to be considered include cartilage thickness, skeletal maturity, and the differing in vitro biology of chondrocytes if they are to be used in the repair.

Cartilage thickness varies from study to study. Simon[8] looked at the variation between species and joint (▸ Table 45.1) and observed the stress across the joint; he also related the thickness to the elasticity of the cartilage.[9] Much more recently, Frisbie et al[10] compared the thickness between humans and varying species but also compared various sites within the stifle joint (▸ Table 45.2).

The skeletal maturity of the animals to be used also has to be considered. Immature cartilage in skeletally immature animals has a greater potential to heal and therefore does not represent the condition found in human adults. The age of sheep has been found to affect the behavior of cultured chondrocytes.

Each species has its relative benefits and problems, and no one species is ideal for all stages of research. Our opinion is that mice may be most appropriate for heterotopic models, rabbits for proof-of-concept work, and sheep for large animal studies.

Table 45.1 Interspecies and Joint Variation in Articular Cartilage Thickness[8]

Average maximum cartilage thickness (mm)						
Species	Hip	Knee	Patella	Ankle	Shoulder	Elbow
Cow	2.49	3.17	3.13	1.43	3.03	1.44
Sheep	1.36	1.68	1.65	0.27	1.39	0.62
Dog	1.19	1.30	1.10	0.06	0.98	0.76
Rat	0.091	0.165	0.060	0.038	0.188	0.095
Mouse	0.053	0.030	0.024	0.023	0.038	0.034

Table 45.2 Interspecies and Intrajoint Variation of the Articular Cartilage Thickness of the Stifle/Knee Joint[10]

Species/Location	PMT	LT	DMT	PMC	DMC
Dog	524 ± 30	530 ± 30	530 ± 30	771 ± 30	731 ± 30
Equine	1832 ± 30	2162 ± 30	1761 ± 30	2215 ± 30	2203 ± 30
Goat	799 ± 30	699 ± 30	786 ± 30	1279 ± 30	1510 ± 30
Human	2596 ± 43	2877 ± 33	2461 ± 43	2411 ± 30	2523 ± 30
Rabbit	221 ± 30	314 ± 30	306 ± 30	341 ± 30	271 ± 30
Sheep	559 ± 30	707 ± 30	559 ± 30	542 ± 30	609 ± 30

[Mean ± SEM in micrometers for the sum of calcified cartilage and the noncalcified cartilage in each location for each species.]
Abbreviations: SEM, standard error of the mean; PMT, proximal medial trochlear; LT, lateral trochlear; DMT, distal medial trochlear; PMC, proximal medial condyle; DMC, distal medial condyle.

45.3 Models of Articular Cartilage Defect

45.3.1 Joint and Defect Location

If an articular cartilage defect model is to be used, there are a number of options available. The first is the joint to be used and the location of the defect within the joint. The stifle joint is most analogous to the knee and therefore the most commonly used; the intra-articular anatomy[11] and the relative cartilage thickness[10] of various animals compared to the human knee have been described. Within the stifle joint, the options are the femoral condyles, the intercondylar groove, or the patella.

The location of the defect needs to take into account the orientation of the animal's limb. There will be differences between the loading characteristics of the human knee (upright biped) and the hind limb of a quadruped that may well be held in a much more flexed position. There is an argument that the patella-femoral joint should be used for three reasons: (1) ease of access in animals such as the sheep; (2) they are harder to repair, making significant results more rigorous; and (3) their orientation and loading profile is more analogous to the tibiofemoral joint in humans due to the orientation of the limb.

Using the sheep as an example, there is little variation in the cartilage thickness within the joint, and the tibiofemoral contact forces during walking are about 2.1 times body weight compared to 2.8 to 3.8 in humans. This helps to validate the use of the femoral condyles for defect location. The osseous anatomy and the kinematics of the ovine stifle joint are also well described.

45.3.2 Defect Creation

Because focal cartilage defects only progress when they reach a critical size, it is most appropriate to use defects that are of a critical size. The size varies between species; it is 7 mm in sheep and 9 mm in horses. Consistent defects can be created using single-use punch biopsies that come in a range of diameters. This allows a circular defect that will create a partial- or full-thickness defect. The cartilage can then be removed using a sharp curette. The use of a drill creates an added thermal injury, which may introduce a confounding factor.

Acute versus Chronic Defects

If investigators are not waiting for arthritis to develop before their intervention, they need to decide whether to do a delayed repair. The advantages of creating a defect and immediately repairing are that only one operation is required. The problem with this is that the homoeostasis around a fresh cartilage defect may be very different from the situation of established defect in an animal or human patient; therefore, results may not be considered comparable. If defects are left for approximately 6 weeks, they are considered to represent chronic defects.

45.3.3 Unilateral versus Bilateral

There are both ethical and practical considerations when deciding upon multiple repairs in a single joint or the use of a single lesion in bilateral joints. While the advantage of being able to use fewer animals is obvious, the other attraction of an internal control in either the same joint or in the contralateral limb is scientifically attractive. The problems with this include the possibility that having multiple lesions or a bilateral model will cause increased morbidity and will affect the purity of the model. Anterior cruciate ligament deficiency in the contralateral limb was shown to increase medial compartment arthritis, and having bilateral lesions may introduce a confounding factor that cannot be controlled for. There are also ethical and regulatory issues that increased lameness to the animal may be considered unacceptable.

45.4 Methods of Repair

Animal models have been used to investigate a wide variety of strategies to repair articular cartilage. These can be split into the following categories.

45.4.1 Grafting of Biological Material

These models allow researchers to investigate the potential to use a patient's own tissue as is done in mosaicplasty (autograft) or the potential for cadaveric tissue (allograft). As articular cartilage is immunoprivileged, it does not elicit a significant immunological reaction when transplanted. This allows the potential of using a xenograft model to test other species' tissues in vivo in an animal model.

45.4.2 Autologous Chondrocyte Implantation

First-generation autologous chondrocyte implantation uses periosteal flaps sutured to the cartilage, which are associated with a flap delamination rate of about 67% in the goat; this was reduced to 10% when fascial flaps were used. Matrix-assisted autologous chondrocyte implantation seeds the cells onto a collagen matrix prior to implantation and has been used to good effect in the sheep. The ability of a patient to (generally) follow postoperative controlled weight bearing cannot be matched in animal studies. Surgical techniques need to allow unrestricted weight bearing, and minimally invasive techniques are most likely to be successful.

45.4.3 Factors to Induce Cartilage Healing

Much research has been done to look at the potential to alter the environment to assist the cartilage to heal itself. Examples of this include the use of microfracture to allow bone marrow blood to enter the environment and platelet-rich plasma to introduce a concentrated amount of growth factors to the area. Other examples include the use of hyaluronic acid, bone morphogenic proteins, interleukins, hormones, and tissue growth factors. The advantage of these techniques is that they can be introduced using intra-articular injection.

45.4.4 Stem Cells

Cartilage arises from the mesoderm and therefore mesenchymal stem cells have the ability to differentiate into chondrocytes. Different sources have been suggested for obtaining these cells including bone marrow, adipose tissue, synovium, periosteum, muscle, and peripheral blood. In addition to mesenchymal stem cells, both embryonic stem cells and induced pluripotent stem cells are possibilities. There are currently unresolved ethical issues with embryonic stem cells and safety concerns with induced pluripotent stem cells. As well as the source of the stem cells involved and the method of delivery, the ideal culture conditions and the value of coculture with mature cells have still not been determined.

45.4.5 Scaffolds/Implants/ Hydrogels

Numerous implants have been used including metal, biosynthetic scaffolds, and hydrogels. The structural scaffolds are used by excising an osteochondral plug and then press fitting it into the remaining defect. The hydrogels can be injected or moulded into the defect. Titanium implants have also been used as a carrier for mesenchymal stem cells. While some of the scaffolds and hydrogels have been used on their own as an inductive material for bone marrow blood, and therefore stem cells, they are increasingly being used as carriers for autologous cells, inductive factors, and cultured stem cells.

45.4.6 Tissue Engineering

Tissue engineering involves ex vivo tissue expansion to create cartilaginous material, which is then re-implanted. These can be created from relatively few cells to create pieces of cartilage up to 3 cm in diameter. Commonly, stem cells are used for this and the process is termed regenerative medicine.

45.5 Transgenic Models

Gene therapies have been investigated in animal models for articular cartilage. Genes are either upregulated or downregulated to either improve the ability of cartilage or to decrease cartilage degradation. This has been done in both small (rat) and large (porcine and equine) models. The porcine work used liposomal and viral mediated gene transfer to deliver bone morphogenetic protein-2 complementary deoxyribonucleic acid ex vivo to periosteal cells prior to seeding the cells in a polyglycolic acid matrix to be implanted into the joint.

45.6 Outcome Measures

There are numerous outcome measures that can be used, and the most appropriate for your research question should be used.

45.6.1 Clinical/Lameness

Measures of lameness are increasingly developed and used as valid measures of symptoms. Pressure pads can also be used to determine changes in the ability of the animal to weight bear evenly or to avoid weight bearing through the affected limb.

45.6.2 Macroscopic Appearance

The visual appearance of the joint should be recorded using photographs and a description kept. Goebel et al suggested a new visual scoring system and compared it to the existing scores.[12] It was found to correlate with the magnetic resonance observation of cartilage repair tissue score.

45.6.3 Histology and Immunohistochemistry

Depending upon the size of the joint being examined and the techniques being used to analyze the histology, specimens need to either be processed expediently or fixed and therefore preserved for later analysis using standard techniques (snap freezing can be useful to ensure antigens are not masked but can be hard to perform in larger blocks of tissue where formalin fixation can allow longer processing times without tissue degradation).

Samples are best stained as a batch with hematoxylin and eosin for standard light microscopy and histological scoring. While grading systems have been suggested for individual animals for arthritis, these scores are less relevant for discreet cartilage defects. Researchers have used the International Cartilage Repair Society I and II visual histological assessment scores, which combines six different components. There is now a trend to add these scores together to get an overall score, but the weighting of the individual components has not been validated and therefore researchers should be aware of the limitation of a combined score. Polarized light allows a clear identification of areas of hyaline cartilage as these appear "glassy" (the original definition of hyaline) where collagen fibers are well aligned.

Histological identification of glycosaminoglycans (Alcian blue) and collagens (Picrosirius red) will assist in determining whether the tissue is predominantly hyaline or fibrocartilage-like.[13]

Semiquantitative analysis of matrix constituents can be performed using immunohistochemistry to help determine the similarity to hyaline cartilage. Use fluorophore-assisted carbohydrate electrophoresis to both quantitatively and qualitatively analyze the glycosaminoglycan.

Collagen II is the most abundant in adult hyaline cartilage, whereas type I is found in fibrocartilage. In fibrocartilage, staining for collagen types III and VI is weak and relatively homogeneous, whereas in hyaline cartilage it is strongly associated with chondrocytes and the pericellular matrix, but is not present in the interterritorial matrix. Tissues can be treated with hyaluronidase (with or without trypsin) to help unmask the collagens.

Sections will then be incubated with primary mono- or polyclonal antibodies against collagen types I, II, III, and VI, followed by fluorescently labeled secondary antibodies and visualized by fluorescence microscopy. Monoclonal antibodies against specific glycosaminoglycans can also be performed.

45.6.4 Confocal Microscopy

Confocal microscopy has been widely used to examine cartilage explants. It collects only the in-focus light allowing clear definition at higher magnifications. Laser scanning confocal arthroscopy has been used to assess cartilage in situ in matrix-induced autologous chondrocyte implantation repairs in sheep. This technology is currently unavailable for use in human clinical practice.

45.6.5 Biochemical

Following digestion of the extracellular matrix and ribonucleic acid extraction, genetic expression can be analyzed using standard polymerase chain reaction or quantitatively using real-time quantitative reverse transcription–polymerase chain reaction. Genes typically examined include *Col I, Col II, Col X, Aggrecan,* and *sox-9.* Some investigators use the ratio of *Col II: Col I* as a marker of hyaline rather than fibrocartilage.

The cartilage content can also be determined by testing for protein and antibody expression using Western blot or enzyme-linked immunosorbent assays, respectively.

45.6.6 Mechanical

This involves the use of mechanical forces to determine the physical properties of the cartilage. Researchers need to be aware that this testing can damage the cartilage being tested and might compromise subsequent cell viability and therefore histology. As with most other factors in selecting an animal, there are significant interspecies differences in the mechanical properties of the distal femoral cartilage.

Samples are usually examined ex vivo. Macroscopic samples can be mechanically tested using confined compression, and the bulk modulus and sheer modulus can be calculated. Apparatus is designed to restrict radial expansion of the specimen to assess uniaxial deformation. This will also allow testing of creep and stress relaxation of samples. A number of researchers used an in vivo arthroscopic indentation probe, but this is not commercially available any longer. An alternative of using ultrasound water jet indentation has been described but ex vivo methods are more commonly used.

45.6.7 Imaging

While plain radiographs and computed tomography are of little use for cartilage assessment, magnetic resonance imaging can be used. Dual gadolinium-enhanced magnetic resonance imaging for cartilage scanning is increasingly popular as a method for diagnosis and treatment in both humans and animals, but this requires injection of gadolinium. Current consensus is in favor of T2 mapping to obtain localized quantitation of magnetic resonance imaging signal.

45.7 Time Points

Another critical area is the length of time to run the experiment. As well as the obvious time delay, there are considerable cost implications, particularly when large animal housing is involved. While short time points are acceptable to look at the effects in heterotopic models, this should not be the case for articular cartilage defects of arthritis models. It is known that cartilage repair strategies in humans can take up to 2 to 3 years to mature fully. This is often considered impractical in large animals, and there is also some question of the validity of results past the 1-year point. While having time points earlier than 1 year are interesting to see how the repair is evolving, researchers should be wary of using these as an end point. The repair could either look as though it has not worked, but is just immature, or could looked healed, but has not had time to fail under physiological loading. In either circumstance, the work could be considered invalid due to an inappropriate time point being used. Appropriate planning is important to ensure your results can sufficiently test your hypothesis.

45.8 Practical Recommendations

45.8.1 Screening

Animals come in varying states of health and are prone to disease just like humans. Careful screening needs to occur to ensure that animals start and remain as healthy as possible throughout the experiments. Knowledge of naturally occurring cartilage defects and their natural history in the varying species needs to be taken into account.

> **Practical Tips**
>
> - Thorough review of the literature.
> - Get to know your veterinary staff and department.
> - Plan early: Licenses and ethical approvals can take much longer than you anticipate.
> - Be aware that things may not necessarily work the way you expect.

45.8.2 Limitations

As with all experiments, carefully considered controls are necessary to ensure that results are valid. Untreated controls as well as the effects of any carriers need to be determined to elucidate the effects of specific interventions. One of the benefits of a unilateral model is that cartilage from the contralateral limb can be harvested as an internal control of normal cartilage.

References

[1] Chu CR, Szczodry M, Bruno S. Animal models for cartilage regeneration and repair. Tissue Eng Part B Rev 2010; 16: 105–115

[2] Ahern BJ, Parvizi J, Boston R, Schaer TP. Preclinical animal models in single site cartilage defect testing: a systematic review. Osteoarthritis Cartilage 2009; 17: 705–713

[3] Sah RL, Ratcliffe A. Translational models for musculoskeletal tissue engineering and regenerative medicine. Tissue Eng Part B Rev 2010; 16: 1–3

[4] Hurtig MB, Buschmann MD, Fortier LA et al. Preclinical studies for cartilage repair: recommendations from the International Cartilage Repair Society. Cartilage 2011; 2: 137–152

[5] Simon TM, Aberman HM. Cartilage regeneration and repair testing in a surrogate large animal model. Tissue Eng Part B Rev 2010; 16: 65–79

[6] Mika J, Clanton TO, Pretzel D, Schneider G, Ambrose CG, Kinne RW. Surgical preparation for articular cartilage regeneration without penetration of the subchondral bone plate: in vitro and in vivo studies in humans and sheep. Am J Sports Med 2011; 39: 624–631

[7] Malda J, Benders KE, Klein TJ et al. Comparative study of depth-dependent characteristics of equine and human osteochondral tissue from the medial and lateral femoral condyles. Osteoarthritis Cartilage 2012; 20: 1147–1151

[8] Simon WH. Scale effects in animal joints. I. Articular cartilage thickness and compressive stress. Arthritis Rheum 1970; 13: 244–256

[9] Simon WH. Scale effects in animal joints. II. Thickness and elasticity in the deformability of articular cartilage. Arthritis Rheum 1971; 14: 493–502

[10] Frisbie DD, Cross MW, McIlwraith CW. A comparative study of articular cartilage thickness in the stifle of animal species used in human pre-clinical studies compared to articular cartilage thickness in the human knee. Vet Comp Orthop Traumatol 2006; 19: 142–146

[11] Proffen BL, McElfresh M, Fleming BC, Murray MM. A comparative anatomical study of the human knee and six animal species. Knee 2011; 19: 493–499

[12] Goebel L, Orth P, Muller A, Zurakowski D, Bucker a, Cucchiarini M, Madry H. Experimental scoring systems for macroscopic articular cartilage repair correlate with the MOCART score assessed by a high-field MRI at 9.4 T–comparative evaluation of five macroscopic scoring systems in a large animal cartilage defect model Osteoarthr Cartil 2012; 20: 1046–1055

[13] Roberts S, Menage J, Sandell LJ, Evans EH, Richardson JB. Immunohistochemical study of collagen types I and II and procollagen IIA in human cartilage repair tissue following autologous chondrocyte implantation. Knee 2009; 16: 398–404

Further Reading

An YH, Friedman RJ. Animal models in orthopaedic research. Boca Raton, FL: CRC Press; 1998

46 In Vivo Soft Tissue Models

Melanie Jean Coathup, Catherine Jane Pendegrass, Allen Edward Goodship, and Gordon William Blunn

This chapter describes the use of a plethora of different animal models for the investigation of meniscal, ligament, and tendon repair and regeneration. The purpose of this review is to inform the reader of the work that has been done, how it has been done, and where appropriate, how to improve on it. We believe that the advent of international standards, which define the requirements, specifications, and guidelines needed to optimally and consistently ensure the animal model systems investigated generate results that are repeatable, reliable, and of good quality, would be extremely advantageous and would minimize the numbers of animals used in this research. International standards would allow greater and more effective comparisons between studies, thereby maximizing good-quality scientific output through fewer animals. Animal models are needed for pretreatment evaluation prior to assessment in humans; however, where possible, investigators must always endeavor to reduce, refine, and replace animal use. A power analysis should always be carried out prior to commencing an investigation. Where possible, nonexperimental models should always be used, such as naturally occurring models and preclinical animals attending veterinary clinics. This chapter is also intended to assist investigators in fulfilling their obligation to plan and conduct animal experiments in accordance with the highest scientific, humane, and ethical principles.

This chapter is written with several goals: (1) to provide a foundation of generalized principles that will guide researchers in choosing optimal animal model systems and in the design of new model systems; (2) to review the current animal models available for advancing therapeutic options for meniscal, tendon, and ligament repair, regeneration, replacement, and attachment; and (3) to describe any shortcomings within these current models in order to highlight the need for further innovation and the development of more effective clinical therapies and patient care.

A single ideal animal model in which meniscal, tendon, or ligament tissue regeneration can or should be assessed is currently not available. In vivo models form part of a range of research methods that are used to test a specific biological hypothesis. The most effective model systems should meet several research criteria.[1] While animal models do not replicate the human scenario, they should provide an environment that matches, to the greatest extent possible, the appropriate physiological environment.[2] They should provide objective and quantifiable parameters to assess the success (quantity and quality) and functional performance of the repaired, reattached, or regenerated tissue.[3] They should detect and predict clinically relevant differences in biological performance between the parameters investigated.

46.1 The Meniscus

Many in vivo animal models have been developed to investigate the injury, repair, and replacement of knee menisci. These models are reported to have menisci that are structurally and anatomically similar to humans with comparable physiological responses (injury, healing, and remodeling). However, no one animal model has established itself as the most appropriate to be used when investigating all aspects of meniscal research, and many species are currently being used to successfully test specific hypotheses related to focused areas of meniscal investigation. In general, small animal models have been used to provide an assessment of the biological healing response to new materials implanted in the knee joint. Whether damage to the meniscus occurs at the time of trauma or sometime after is not clear, and therefore the mechanics of knee joint loading are imperative to understand treatment and recovery after injury. Therefore, the main disadvantage in the use of small animal models is that the implants are not subjected to the high loads that would occur during human knee motion. In addition, the accurate placement of defects and tears in the meniscus of small animals is very challenging due to its small size, and this aspect can play a great role in determining the repair outcome. Large animal models such as pigs, goats, and sheep offer the opportunity to investigate the meniscal healing response to new materials that are subject to immediate substantial loads. However, these models are often costly and time-consuming to conduct. The use of sheep models are reported to be advantageous because they are representative of humans in terms of structural properties, vascularization patterns, cell density, the presence of an articulating lamellar collagen structure, and in terms of cross-sectional size. These factors influence meniscal repair. Canine models offer additional advantageous postoperative management options. For example, after meniscal surgery, dogs can readily be managed with slings to keep them nonweight bearing or with bandages for support and to limit range of motion. In addition, controlled physical rehabilitation regimens using underwater treadmills, range of motion exercises, and other such activities can be utilized. Prior to beginning an experimental study, it is essential that a comprehensive review of the various animal models be performed in order to ensure the use of the most appropriate species relevant to your hypothesis.

The ability of meniscal tissue to heal is closely related to its blood supply, and meniscal tears are often classified according to the location of the defect relative to the blood supply. At birth, the whole meniscus is vascularized. However, an avascular area soon develops in the inner circumference of the meniscus, and in the second decade blood vessels are seen only in the outer third. This progressive loss of vascularization within the inner two-thirds of the meniscus may be due to weight bearing and knee movement. Tears that occur within the outer vascularized region of the menisci show good healing capabilities; however, tears within the inner avascular region have a diminished natural ability to heal. The vascular anatomy of the menisci can differ among animal species. Although the vascular supply of both the medial and lateral menisci originate in the peripheral capsular attachment in both humans and animals, the extent of vascular penetration into the meniscus can vary significantly. This is one of the most critical factors to recognize and account for when studying meniscal biology, response to injury, treatment, and healing. Investigators must be careful to confirm the location of the meniscal lesion they create and whether it is in the avascular or vascular portion.

46.1.1 Meniscal Tear Models

As discussed, tears in the avascular zone of the meniscus cannot heal entirely and spontaneously. Animal models that focus on attempts to induce healing in the avascular zone have had some success. In 1983, a canine meniscal model was the first to demonstrate that rasping of the damaged meniscus in the vascularized area promoted an injury response in the avascular region. A small transverse incision was introduced that produced a bridging vascular channel that redirected blood flow from the vascular zone into a longitudinal tear in the avascular zone. Rasping increases the production of interleukin-1-alpha, transforming growth factor-beta, platelet-derived growth factor, and proliferating cell nuclear antigen. This protein network has been demonstrated to improve vascular induction and meniscal healing. Further studies have also reported a significant increase in the healing of menisci within avascular zones when treated with a form of abrasion therapy when compared with control groups. The most common abrasion therapy techniques used are rasping or trephination, in which radially orientated channels are introduced to encourage vascular and cellular migration from the peripheral vascular portion to the tear site. A study by Klompmaker et al[1] used a canine vascular channel access model to investigate the use of a porous polyurethane implant in meniscal healing by creating lesions within the avascular region. In this study, the right or left lateral meniscus was approached using a lateral incision to the knee joint capsule without detachment of any ligaments. A wedge-shaped defect was created with its base at the periphery and with the top of the defect reaching inwards to at least half of the width of the meniscal body. A longitudinal lesion was created well within the avascular midsubstance and which extended into both anterior and posterior meniscal horns. The porous polyurethane implant was sutured into the defect and partial and complete healing was reported in the experimental group where both type I and type II collagen, the two major collagen types of normal meniscal fibrocartilage, could be detected in this newly formed fibrocartilage. After the fibrocartilage had formed, vascularity was seen to decrease and was reported to be completely absent in the mature tissue. Within all empty, control lesions, no regeneration of fibrocartilage was seen. This study concluded that the implant guided vascular tissue from the periphery toward the lesion, resulting in healing of the tear. Over recent years, similar tear models have been developed in rabbits, dogs, sheep, and goats, and include procedures such as a synovial flap sewn into the tear, the application of a fibrin clot attached to the exposed collagen within the tear site, the use of small intestine mucosa, and trephination. Although success has been reported, each of these procedures has disadvantages when performed clinically. For example, a concern with the vascular channel access model is that it destroys healthy meniscal tissue resulting in poor meniscal function when bearing a load, even if the tear is repaired. The trephination models also have the same disadvantages, and it is technically very difficult to raise a pedicle of synovium and suture it into the meniscal tear. Although the application of fibrin glue has been shown to induce the proliferation of fibrous connective tissue that later develops into cartilaginous tissue 12 to 24 weeks postapplication, the disadvantage with this technique is the difficulty of keeping fibrin clots on the tear without immobilization of the operated leg.

More recently, studies have focused on the use of growth factors, gene therapy, and the application of mesenchymal stem cells (MSCs) on the repair and regeneration of meniscal tissue. The use of platelet-rich plasma in a rabbit meniscal model demonstrated increased histological fibrocartilage tissue scoring 12 weeks postsurgery in defects containing platelet-rich plasma when compared with control. Vascular endothelial growth factor (VEGF)-coated sutures have been investigated in the repair of sheep menisci. Following a 6-week follow-up period, results showed that none in the VEGF-coated suture group demonstrated healing, whereas defect healing was identified in half of those in the control group. These results were in agreement with another study where VEGF coated sutures (compared with Ethibond sutures; Ethicon, Somerville, NJ) were investigated at 8 weeks follow-up, and no significant increase in angiogenesis or meniscal healing was found in the VEGF-given groups. Transplanted autologous chondrocytes harvested from articular cartilage and placed within the avascular portions of a meniscal defect in a porcine model reported the ability of seeded chondrocytes to heal the tear. The avascular meniscal tear model has also been used in rabbits, and the effect of transplanted bone marrow cells within a fibrin glue carrier investigated. Earlier histological maturation and more rapid healing was seen in the cell given group when compared to defects containing fibrin glue only. Adaptations to this model have been also been used. In 2003, Murphy et al[2] resected the medial meniscus and anterior cruciate ligament (ACL) in order to investigate the effect of bone marrow–derived MSCs injected intra-articularly on the regeneration of meniscal tissue. This study identified implanted cells within the regenerated meniscus and stated that the cells stimulated meniscal regeneration. These meniscal lesions have also been created in a porcine model and results showed that both autologous and allogeneic chondrocytes delivered in a biodegradable Vicryl mesh (Ethicon) enhanced healing of the avascular lesions.

46.1.2 Meniscal Injury and Osteoarthritis

Several animal models have been employed to demonstrate the direct relationship between meniscal injury and the development of osteoarthritis. While not described in detail in this chapter, these models include the rabbit ACL tear, menisectomy models, the canine Pond-Nuki model, canine meniscectomy or meniscal release models, and sheep and monkey models. Novel and more complex models are also being developed. For example, Killian et al[3] have developed a model that attempts to reproduce acute, high-impact injury patterns within the meniscus and ACL following trauma in a rabbit model. This study showed that unconstrained high-intensity impacts on the tibiofemoral joint led to meniscal damage in conjunction with rupture of the ACL. Both acute and chronic changes to the menisci were identified, and the authors proposed this model to be more realistic in the progression of osteoarthritis compared with surgically transected models. Future work is needed to investigate the meniscal healing response in this model. Despite recent advances in the materials and methods used, a large proportion of meniscal tears in patients remain irreparable, and partial or total meniscectomy is often necessary regardless of the recognized consequences of cartilage degeneration and osteoarthrosis. In these cases, there is a need to protect the articular cartilage by replacing the meniscus.

46.1.3 Partial and Total Replacement Meniscal Models

Meniscal replacement presents a useful reconstructive option for patients with loss of the meniscus due to previous meniscectomy or an irreparable meniscus tear. The possibility to entirely reproduce the meniscus structure and function either through allograft transplantation or synthetic scaffold implantation is highly attractive. In the case of extensive destruction or a complete loss of the meniscus, partial and total meniscal replacement animal models have been developed to investigate restoring knee biomechanics in order to prevent the development of early osteoarthritis. Ideally, a meniscal replacement should mimic the shape and biomechanical properties of the meniscus. An ideal scaffold should have the basic structure of the meniscus and be biodegradable and bioabsorbable in the long term. The structure should also be strong enough to withstand the load in the joint and maintain its structural integrity without damaging articular cartilage. The basic biology of allograft meniscal transplantation has been studied in various animal models, and the results have been dependent on the conservation methods: fresh tissue, cryopreserved, fresh frozen, lyophilized, and glutaraldehyde-preserved allografts. While meniscal allografts have been shown to heal the capsule and relieve pain, their use is limited due to problems with availability, size matching, cost and risk of disease transmission, as well as graft remodeling and shrinkage after implantation. Incomplete cellular repopulation of deep frozen meniscal allografts after total meniscectomy and allograft transplantation in a rabbit model has been reported. Results showed the central core of the allograft remained acellular 12 and 26 weeks postsurgery; however, those cells that did repopulate the graft demonstrated active collagen remodeling. Synthetic scaffold materials have also been investigated as meniscal alternatives. Large wedge-shaped lesions have been created in the menisci of dogs. Lesions were repaired with a meniscal replacement manufactured from carbon fiber and an organic polymer, prepared from physical mixtures of poly(L-lactide) and a segmented polyurethane. Results at 4 and 8 weeks postoperation were unconvincing and showed the reconstructed area was invaded almost completely by fibrous tissue. A large meniscal defect created in the canine model has also been used to investigate the healing capacity of small intestine submucosa, and results demonstrated success in the repair of posterior vascular defects but not for complete meniscal substitution. A polyvinyl alcohol-hydrogel meniscus composed of porous 50/50 copoly(L-lactide/epsilon-caprolactone) was shown to be chondroprotective when investigated in a rabbit model. However, problems were reported with the durability of the polymer, the fixation method, and lack of tissue adherence. The polyvinyl alcohol hydrogel implant of Kobayashi et al[4] was one of the first nonporous permanent replacement approaches to be investigated. In this study, an implant with a compressive strength and viscoelastic properties similar to the human meniscus, was investigated following a 2-year in vivo period in a rabbit model. The implant proved to be chondroprotective; however, no sham-operated controls were included to evaluate the influence of replacement surgery on the cartilage condition. A 2-year canine model was used to investigate porous polyurethane scaffolds as total meniscal substitutes. Compressive properties of the implant increased at evaluation up to 2-years postimplantation,

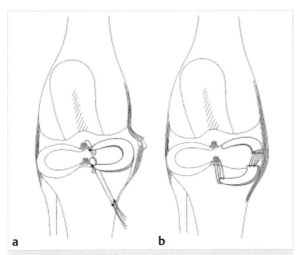

Fig. 46.1 **(a)** The total replacement model: total medial meniscectomy; the medial cruciate ligament (MCL) is cut, the implant fixed to the capsule with suture via two transosseous drill holes, and the MCL is reconstructed. **(b)** Partial replacement model: partial medial meniscectomy of the anterior part. The MCL is intact, and the implant is sutured to the anterior cruciate ligament, the remnant of the original meniscus, and the capsule.[5]

and results showed no difference when compared with the properties of native menisci. However, the material used was not strong enough to resist shear forces within the knee joint, and the collagen type and orientation were reported to be nonmeniscus-like.

Chiari and coworkers[5] developed an ovine model of total and partial meniscus replacement. The sheep model has been used in many studies because the mechanical properties of the meniscus are similar to the human menisci, and the contact stresses transmitted to the tibial plateau are within the range of that of human knees. In the total meniscus replacement animal group, surgery involved cutting the medial collateral ligament (MCL) slightly above the joint line (▶ Fig. 46.1). This was described as necessary in order to achieve good exposure of the posterior aspect of the joint. The meniscus was circumferentially dissected from the capsule; the posterior horn of the meniscus was exposed by flexion, external rotation, and valgus stress of the joint, and the meniscus was detached at its posterior and anterior horns. Two 3 mm tunnels were drilled using a guidewire from the medial tibial condyle to the footprints of the anterior and posterior meniscal horns. The implant was then fixed with two nonresorbable anchoring sutures inserted through the implant at its horns. The sutures were pulled through the bone tunnels and tied to each other in a knot on the tibial surface. Two silk threads were tied to the polylactic acid fibers protruding from the implant at its horns and pulled into the bone tunnels. The capsule was closed. Simultaneously, several additional sutures were

made between the implant and the capsule. The anterior and posterior horns of the implant were fixed to the meniscal ligaments. The MCL was reconstructed with four sutures, using resorbable sutures. In the partial replacement group, the anterior portion of the meniscus was exposed by detaching the capsule at the periphery, while the MCL was left intact. The anterior portion of the meniscus was cut out radially at the level of the MCL. The size of the implant was adjusted using a scalpel so that it corresponded to the resected portion of the meniscus. The implant was then sutured to the remaining portion of the meniscus and to the remnants of the anterior horn fixation near the ACL. The capsule was closed. Simultaneously, several additional sutures were made between the implant and the capsule.

Surgeons are often confronted with loss of the inner portions of the meniscus in partial meniscus defects and only a peripheral rim remains. The ovine model developed by Chiari et al[5] created a different type of defect (anterior partial resection with the MCL left untouched), and a limitation of this model is that the defect does not reflect the clinical situation. However, this type of partial resection was used to successfully study the integration of an implant to the residual meniscus throughout its radial diameter. Blunn et al also developed a similar ovine partial meniscectomy model to investigate the use of xenograft (▶ Fig. 46.2).

Tissue engineering has recently been proposed as a possible solution for meniscal regeneration. This model has been used further to investigate the use of a porous scaffold based on a hyaluronic acid and polycaprolactone matrix augmented with circumferential lactic acid fibers. Cultured autologous chondrocytes were seeded onto the scaffold and results demonstrated improved fibrocartilaginous tissue deposition compared with cell-free constructs; however, the cell-seeded scaffolds did not show better cartilage conditions compared with control. Kang et al[6] demonstrated the feasibility of regenerating whole-meniscal cartilage in a rabbit total meniscectomy model using allogeneic meniscal cells seeded onto a mechanically stabilized polymer (polygylcolic-polylactic acid) scaffold. Neomenisci engineered without cell seeding showed significant failure of maintenance of the original scaffold shape and size. When total meniscal substitution was investigated in the ovine model at 4 months postoperation, stem cells seeded into a resorbable scaffold also showed promising results. A collagenous sponge loaded with MSCs and placed within a partial meniscus defect in rabbits also reported stem cells to augment the repair process.

In terms of microstructure, physiology, and material properties, there is no evidence to suggest that one animal model is best for the study of meniscal biology. No matter the animal model used, it is the responsibility of the investigators to carefully define the valid levels of comparison for each model and to interpret the results within these established confines.

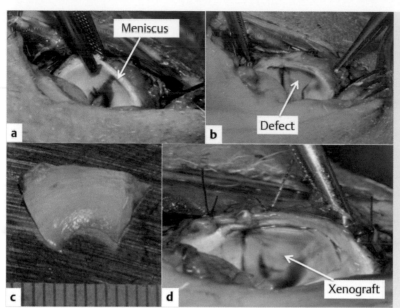

Fig. 46.2 (a) The ovine meniscus was exposed and a 10 mm segment of meniscus removed. (b, c) Xenograft was implanted within the defect and (d) in vivo regeneration observed 12 weeks postoperatively. (Pictures are provided courtesy of Professor Gordon Blunn.)

46.2 Ligaments

Ligaments are soft connective tissues composed of closely packed collagen fiber bundles orientated in a parallel fashion to provide for the articulation and stability of joints in the musculoskeletal system. Their main function is to transmit tensile loads. Tendons and ligaments may share many characteristics; however, there are distinct differences between the two. While tendons have one bony and one muscular attachment point and produce motion across the joints, ligaments are attached to bone at both ends and act to limit motion at the joint to the appropriate planes. The structures should be further subdivided into intrasynovial and extrasynovial tendons and intra-articular and extra-articular ligaments. Synovial fluid is the lubricating fluid found in most mobile joints as well as around certain specialized tendons. This fluid is contained by a joint capsule or around some tendons by a tendon sheath lubricating these structures. Therefore, the blood supply to these intrasynovial structures is more limited, and their response to injury is different to that of tendons and ligaments that are not surrounded by fluid. Therefore, tendons are modeled as either intrasynovial tendons, such as flexor tendons in the hand, or extrasynovial tendons, such as the supraspinatous tendon in the shoulder or the Achilles tendon at the ankle. Similarly, ligaments are modeled as intrasynovial (or intra-articular) ligaments such as the ACL or extrasynovial (or extra-articular) such as the lateral cruciate ligament and MCL at the knee. It is therefore appropriate to model these types of tissues differently. Correctly matching the type of tissue and injury is important in the animal model that has been chosen in order to optimally test a hypothesis.

Animal models proposed for the study of ligament injuries include the rat, rabbit, dog, goat, and sheep. In general and because of surgical accessibility, smaller animal models have been satisfactory for modeling extra-articular ligaments, whereas larger animals have been used mainly for modeling ACL injuries. The majority of models used have examined the healing response of ligaments to injury or their response to a change in activity level (especially immobilization). Ligament injury models include (1) complete tears with a defect or gap between the torn ends, (2) complete ligament division without gap formation, (3) partial ligament disruption, either through partial transection or through the creation of a window defect, and (4) ligament reconstruction or (5) replacement.

46.2.1 Extra-articular Injury Models

Extra-articular ligaments such as the MCL of the knee have a high propensity for healing without surgical management, and the ability of the MCL to heal offers an opportunity for the examination of the mechanism of healing. Because of its accessibility, size, and bony attachments, the MCL has been one of the most commonly used models for studying extra-articular ligament healing. The rat model has been used to model the MCL; however, its small size makes manipulation of the tissues more difficult and the experimental injuries may be less repeatable. The rabbit model has been the most widely used model to study extra-articular ligaments. Frank et al[7] developed a complete MCL tear model by pulling a 3–0 braided steel suture transversely through the MCL substance to rupture and damage the length of the ligament. This technique was developed in the rabbit model and gave similar results to the scalpel cut technique. To create more clinically realistic midsubstance "mop-end" tears with simultaneous damage to the insertion sites, studies have ruptured rabbit MCLs by pulling a 2.5 mm diameter stainless steel rod medially when placed beneath the MCL. Injuries were treated either nonoperatively (with no immobilization) or by surgical repair, and results demonstrated no statistical difference in the mechanical properties between groups at 6 and 12 weeks postinjury. Several subfailure injury models have also been successfully developed. Subfailure models are created by partial laceration (simple side cut with repair or center straight cut) as opposed to complete laceration (straight cut with repair or Z step cut with repair). A surgical injury model with a partial laceration in the midsubstance (approximately 60% of the width) of the rabbit MCL and ACL leaving intact fibers either side has been commonly used. However, the creation of a cleanly severed ligament injury is not a true replication of the condition seen in human patients and is therefore considered a limitation in the use of this model. A sheep model of subfailure MCL injury was therefore developed by manually flexing the knee joint until ligament damage occurred. Extensive injury was seen throughout the length of the ligament, and the strength of the MCL was reported to reduce to 13% of normal. However, MCL strength and compliance returned to normal 6 weeks postinjury. The animal models mentioned previously are poorly controlled and do not consistently recreate the cellular and matrix damage induced by a grade I, II, or III MCL sprain injury. However, results from many of these animal models are in agreement with clinical reports where positive outcomes have been reported. For the clinical treatment of isolated extra-articular ligament injury, it is generally considered that a nonoperative approach followed by early motion and functional rehabilitation is the preferred method of treatment.

Despite the obvious functional improvements following MCL healing, many animal studies have shown that the mechanical properties, histomorphological appearance, and biochemical composition of the healed MCL remain poor when compared to those of the normal MCL. Ligament healing involves a complex, coordinated series of events that result in the formation of a neoligament that is more scar-like than the native tissue. Therefore, animal models have been used to further investigate methods to improve the quality and increase the rate of healing. High doses of platelet-derived growth factor when applied in a fibrin sealant caused a significant increase in the structural properties of the femur-MCL-tibia complex in a rabbit model. A study has also shown that MSCs implanted into an injured rat MCL differentiated into fibroblasts. Bioscaffolds derived from porcine small intestine submucosa have demonstrated a significant increase in the quality of healing tissue when applied to a 6 mm gap injury in the rabbit MCL. However, collectively, results from animal studies have shown that the healing response varies and appears to be species, dosage, and treatment specific. In addition, the method and timing of the treatment is also known to cause differences in tissue response.

46.2.2 Intra-articular Injury Models

The success reported in the healing of extra-articular ligaments has not been achieved with intra-articular ligaments, and surgical repair of the midsubstance and/or immobilization has been inadequate with failure of the repairing ligament over time. Because the cruciate ligaments have a limited capacity to heal, the results of nonsurgical management of a midsubstance rupture have been very poor. As a result, direct repair is generally not performed clinically, and ligament reconstruction is the preferred treatment for most cruciate injuries. Presently, arthroscopic reconstruction using autograft remains the gold standard for the management of ACL tears. Autograft gives high mechanical strength and compatibility with high revascularization and remodeling capacities. Surgical reconstruction of the cruciate ligaments has been investigated using tissue autograft and allograft. Bone-patellar, tendon-bone, or hamstrings tendon and soft tissue allografts are regularly performed to gain knee stability. Complications associated with these reconstruction surgeries include donor site morbidity, allergic reactions and disease transmission, extensor deficit of the knee, degeneration of tissue replacement graft, hamstring muscle weakness, and bone tunnel enlargement. There has been recent interest in discovering methods to stimulate repair and/or regeneration of the ACL rather than replacing it. Successful ACL repair has the theoretical advantages of preserving the broad insertion sites and the proprioceptive nerve fibers of the native ACL, as well as being a less invasive procedure compared to ACL reconstruction.

Animal models used have included the dog, rat, and rabbit, and primarily have evaluated the effects of ligament transection with or without repair. These models are attractive because of their size, cost, and ease of care. In canines, untreated ACL transections showed no evidence of healing, with incomplete healing observed even in partial tears. A canine ACL central defect model was used to investigate the effect of basic fibroblast growth factor pallets on the healing response. In this study, the ACL was exposed through a medial peripatellar arthrotomy and a central wound made in the ACL and paratenon using a specially designed 3.5-mm blade. The resulting wound was 3.5 mm in width and 100 microns in height. In this model, all wounds were made through the vascularized tissue covering the ligaments of the paratenon or the epiligament (MCL and ACL wounds). No significant differences were found when groups were compared; however, results showed increased healing of the ligament with increased vascularity. Little or no new tissue formation was seen in the control specimens. Inherent limitations of animal models include anatomy, biomechanics, and uncontrolled postoperative rehabilitation programs. The porcine model has been commonly used because of its size, its dependence on the ACL for function, its similarity with human gait biomechanics, and the similarity of the baseline coagulation values and platelet sedimentation characteristics to human blood. Central ACL defects in the rabbit and rat model have been used to successfully compare hyaluronic acid as well as stem cells in ACL repair; however, direct application of these results to human cases must be considered with caution.

In the human model of ACL injury, we can assess healing by measuring gait and activity level, identify reoperation for the meniscus, and evaluate the articular cartilage. In relation to this and in some animal models, we can measure lameness, evaluate a re-tear of the meniscus, and observe articular cartilage. However, animal models are extremely ACL dependent in contrast to human, where normal gait is not an ACL-dependent function. In animal models, postmortem laxity measurements reveal significant increases as opposed to normal, which appear greater in laxity than that seen in the human condition. The biomechanical properties of an ACL construct in animal models can be measured postmortem; however, direct measurement of the yield, energy, and material properties of a human graft are not completely understood. Therefore, there is no single direct measure in an animal model that will directly correlate with a condition in the human, and the best expected outcome of a translational animal model is in the biosafety of the material used and in the comparison of treatment groups.

From this review of ligament repair and replacement models, it is clear that the choice of laboratory animal is critical. This review is written to guide investigators to carefully consider their choice of animal model and to ensure it reflects the requirements of the hypothesis and outcome measures, while taking into account the need for replacement, refinement, and reduction in the use of animals.

46.3 Tendons

Because tendinopathy typically occurs in athletes and active individuals, it is widely believed to occur from overuse. Tendon overuse injuries account for 30 to 50% of all sports-related injuries. In order to gain a more complete understanding of tendinopathy, researchers have developed a variety of methods for inducing tendon conditions in animal models, including chemical and mechanical interference. There are no animals that have the same tendon characteristics as humans, and therefore a variety of animal models are necessary because each represents only certain aspects of the pathogenesis and features of tendinopathy.

46.3.1 Naturally Occurring Tendinopathy Models

Horses and dogs naturally develop tendinopathy when trained and raced. There are many anatomical and biomechanical differences between quadrupeds and bipeds during activity; however, naturally occurring strain-induced injuries of specific tendons do occur. There are similarities to specific human tendinopathy, such as superficial digital flexor tendon injury in the horse and Achilles tendinopathy in man. However, these animals are not practical models to use given limited access and high costs.

46.3.2 Induced Tendinopathy Models

Induced animal models fall into two categories: (1) mechanical loading and (2) the introduction of chemicals. Mechanical loading is the most popular method to induce tendinopathy in animals and three methods are commonly used: (1) forced treadmill running, (2) tendon loading by artificial muscle stimulation, and (3) direct repetitive stretching by an external loading device.

Animals are forced to run on a treadmill in order to mimic tendon overuse in humans. While mechanical methods cause chronic tendinopathy rather than acute tendinopathy, they do require more time and effort for producing tendon changes. This method has been used to produce tendinopathy in the supraspinatus tendon and Achilles tendon of rats. Increased cellularity, collagen disorganization, changes in cell morphology, and larger cross-section area similar to tendinopathy were observed. Some studies have reported a lack of inflammation within tendons after treadmill exercising. While forced treadmill running uses naturally generated cyclical loading, which is believed to be the major extrinsic risk factor for tendinopathy, it shows variable success in producing the pathological features of tendinopathy because it can be difficult to force all rodents to run sufficiently fast or intensely to reach the level necessary for overuse. One study reported no changes in the Achilles tendons of rats based on gross observation, geometric measurements, and mechanical testing analyses using the same exercise protocol that produced injuries in the supraspinatus tendon. In addition, it was reported that tendons heal with rest within as short as 2 weeks after running. It was concluded that the model may not be reproducible of the healing response observed clinically.

As tendons transmit the contractile forces of the muscle to the skeleton for motion or stabilization, muscle stimulation has been used to induce tendinopathy in the flexor digitorium profundus and Achilles tendon by electrical stimulation of muscles by surface electrodes, mainly in rat and rabbit models. Increases in tear size, tear area, and tear density compared with control unloaded tendons was reported; however, no tenderness, lameness, nodules, swelling, or reduction in the range of motion and gross claw flexion strength were noted. However, tendon degradation and the development of tendinopathic changes were reported in a rabbit Achilles tendon model following combined treatment of active muscle stimulation and passive ankle joint movements. Another method to induce direct tendon overload is by stretching the tendon repetitively and directly using a single application of subcyclic load using an external device. Histology showed no inflammation up to 3 days poststretching; however, there was fiber space widening and severe matrix disruption with major fiber angulations, thinning, and discontinuities. However, because the follow-up time was so short, further work is required to investigate whether these changes would be repaired. Unlike treadmill running, where the induced loading likely varies among animals, both the artificial muscle stimulation and direct repetitive tendon stretching methods have the advantage of applying a direct controlled load to the tendon. Variations introduced from animal compliance, muscle fatigue, and stress of animal during running are eliminated, theoretically producing more consistent results.

Intratendinous injection of chemicals that are associated with clinical samples of tendinopathy has been used in the development of tendinopathy in animal models. The chemicals investigated include collagenase, cytokines, prostaglandin 1, prostaglandin 2, and fluoroquinolone. These models produce more consistent tendon damage compared with treadmill running; however, an acute tendon injury is induced and these models cannot mimic the entire tendinopathy process.

46.3.3 The Tendon Enthesis

Musculoskeletal disorders are frequently related to tendon and tendon-bone interface damage and degeneration, which are predominately age, disease, or activity induced. The attachment of a tendon or ligament to a bone, termed an enthesis, is divided according to morphology into indirect (also known as fibrous or periosteal) and direct (also known as fibrocartilaginous or chondral). Indirect attachments occur where the superficial layer of the tendon blends with the periosteum, and the deep layers are comprised of perforating Sharpey's fibers that enter the bone. Epiphyseal tendon attachments, such as the patellar tendon insertion, are typically of the direct type, where there is a zonal transition from dense connective tissue in the tendon, through fibrocartilage and mineralized fibrocartilage, to subchondral bone. The dynamic nature of the normal enthesis has been highlighted in studies comparing the morphological changes associated with immobilization or physical activity, with mechanical usage being necessary to maintain normal structure and composition.

46.3.4 Enthesis Reconstruction and Experimental Animal Models

Irrespective of anatomical location, once a tendon has torn, repair of the enthesis is the only treatment to restore function. Reattachment of tendons to bone is clinically challenging because of the vastly different biomechanical properties of each tissue type. Following damage, the interface is never fully, functionally or morphologically, restored. Furthermore, the underlying factors that govern repair of these stages, whether biological or mechanical factors, or a combination of both, are unknown. Interestingly in the rat, unlike other species, successful functional and morphological restoration of the tendon-bone enthesis, in the absence of intervention, is observed following surgical detachment.

In order to advance treatments using new materials and techniques for reattachment of the tendon to bone, clinically relevant animal models are required. Several animal models have been used, both in vivo and in vitro, for tendon research. In vitro models, using cadaveric specimens, are useful for biomechanical experiments and provide basic understanding of shoulder and knee function. In vivo models enable assessment of living processes, including tendon healing, tendinopathy, instability, and biological responses to surgery. However, intrinsic differences between test species make translation to human pathologies difficult. Most experimental animals are quadrupeds, which use their forelimbs for weight bearing during locomotion, with little or no overhead activity. A number of animal models are currently used to study tendon pathologies; however, there is a lack of validation for these animal models. In a quadruped, paralysis of the supraspinatus muscle results in loss of range of abduction and strength, but subsidiary muscles around the shoulder can compensate for this. As a result, recovery of the supraspinatus enthesis cannot be assessed functionally. Despite this, the canine supraspinatus model has been used to assess enthesis reconstruction in a number of studies. In a quadruped, the extensor mechanism of the hind limb relies solely on the patellar tendon enthesis, which is histologically comparable to the human rotator cuff insertion, and its function is easily assessed. Pendegrass et al[8] have developed an ovine model to investigate tendon bone healing. The patellar tendon was surgically dissected from its insertion at the tibial tuberosity and immediately reattached using suture anchors (▶ Fig. 46.3 and ▶ Fig. 46.4).

Rat models have been developed to study enthesis regeneration. For example, degeneration of the rotator cuff has been modeled using specific exercise regimes to induce chronic changes in the supraspinatus tendon. However, these models fail to address the degenerative changes that occur at the enthesis following rotator cuff tears. During the period of time following rotator cuff tears, and prior to surgical repair, disuse will cause degenerative changes in the enthesis and the tendon. The dynamic nature of the enthesis has been highlighted in studies comparing morphological changes associated with immobilization and physical activity. Immobilization reduces the amount of fibrocartilage and mineralized fibrocartilage present at the enthesis, hence reduces the gradation of the interface and its ability to reduce stress concentrations. Off-loading the enthesis would result in reproduction of the clinical situation; morphological, cellular, and biochemical changes that are seen with disuse; and following rotator cuff tear, the subsequent period of disuse before surgical repair. In addition, studies that have successfully induced chronic tears in rats acknowledge that their rapid self-healing potential and the lack of fatty infiltration of the muscle make the model difficult to reconcile with human rotator cuff disease. Ovine models are not limited in the same way because sheep do not demonstrate the same rapid self-healing potential. Sheep and goats provide convenient models for tendon repair due to availability, ease of animal handling, housing, cost, and society acceptance as research animals. Sheep infraspinatus has been shown to be similar to human supraspinatus; however, the sheep infraspinatus is not intra-articular, hence there is a bursa under the tendon so the repair has some contact with synovial fluid that lubricates the bursa. The bursa is unlikely to have a similar volume of synovial fluid that is contained in the human shoulder joint, so although the repair site has some similar characteristics to the human condition, it is not precisely representative. Tenotomy of the infraspinatus tendon and reattachment to the proximal humerus is successful in terms of addressing the histological and biochemical processes of healing; however, biomechanical studies can only be performed by pull-out tests because gait analysis does not provide adequate data for restoration of function. Rumian et al[9] previously developed an ovine tendon disuse model. They have shown that off-loading the patella tendon using an external fixator caused a significant reduction in the structural and material properties of stiffness (79%), ultimate load (69%), energy absorbed (61%), elastic modulus (76%), and ultimate stress (72%) of the tendon compared with controls. This research, however, did not investigate the enthesis junction or osteopenia in the underlying bone. Pendegrass et al[8] aim to develop this in an in vivo ovine model by off-loading the patella tendon to induce disuse in the tendon and in the bone underlying its attachment. This would be more representative of the clinical scenario that surgeons are frequently faced with when repairing rotator cuffs.

Embryological enthesis development has been shown to occur through a process similar to endochondral ossification (EO). Bone morphogenetic proteins are known to lead to EO, hence white New Zealand rabbit models looking at bone morphogenetic protein-2 EO in the flexor digitorum communis tendon midsubstance have been used. However, enthesis formation induced in the tendon midsubstance encounters a very different mechanical environment to the natural enthesis, even if the interface is off-loaded during healing. This should be taken into

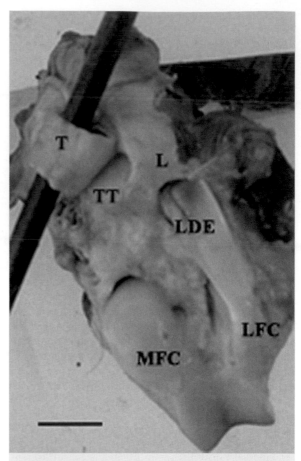

Fig. 46.3 Deep dissection of the ovine stifle joint showing central patellar tendon (*T*) insertion into tibial tuberosity (*TT*). Discrete proximal-lateral band (*L*) forming tunnel containing the long digital extensor tendon (*LDE*). Medial and Lateral femoral condyles are displayed (*MFC* and *LFC*).

consideration when using animal models for EO-induced formation of entheses.

Detaching tendons and immediate reattachment does not represent clinical situations; however, it can be a valuable tool to evaluate suture anchors, suture techniques and patterns, scaffolds, growth factors, and other types of biological augmentation strategies to enhance healing. Goats have been used to evaluate histological and biomechanical tendon healing to cortical bone compared with a cancellous trough and found it to be akin to healing in the human. Acute studies of suture anchors, suture patterns, low intensity pulse ultrasound, bone morphogenetic proteins, and swine small intestinal submucosa. To minimize spontaneous healing, a period of detachment can be enforced prior to reattaching the tendon, or the end of the tendon can be trimmed back to remove any femoral condyle or medial femoral condyle at the margins; however, neither represent the chronic condition observed clinically or overuse injury observed in sports-related injuries.

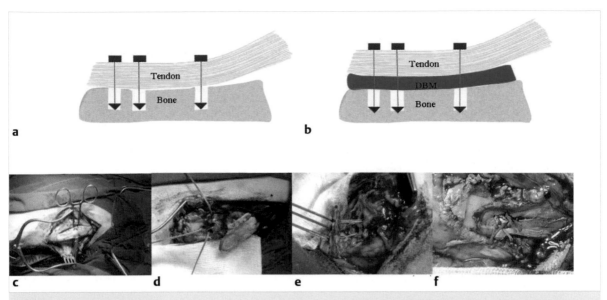

Fig. 46.4 A study[8] using an ovine model to assess enthesis reconstruction following tendon reattachment with demineralized bone matrix augmentation versus unaugmented controls. (**a**) Summary schematic of control group surgery. (**b**) Summary schematic of demineralized bone matrix group surgery. Photographs showing isolation of the patellar tendon (**c**), the sharp dissection of the patellar tendon from the tibial tuberosity, and insertion of suture anchors during surgery (**d**). Also shown are positioning of demineralized bone matrix in the demineralized bone matrix group (**e**) and the suture anchors knotted and tied down during surgery (**f**).

46.4 Conclusion

Animal models for research into tendon and ligament (and their respective entheses) injuries must enable hypotheses associated with disease mechanisms and treatments to be tested. These models must be suitable for the specific condition being investigated, and as such no single model would be appropriate for all studies. A number of factors should be considered prior to commencing research to ensure that a minimal number of animals are used and that all surgical procedures are as consistent with clinical standards as possible. In addition, investigators should consider whether they are investigating tendons or ligaments, and whether they are intra- or extrasynovial, or intra- or extra-articular, respectively. Other factors to consider should include the size of the animal and whether its anatomical features are in keeping with those of the human condition, and the techniques and outcome measure assessments that are available.

Where function is not an outcome measure and integration into a specific tissue is not critical (e.g., for studies in basic biocompatibility), larger animal models provide more implantation sites compared with smaller animals. When considering the need to reduce the number of animals used, fewer large animals could be used as opposed to a large cohort of smaller animals and investigators should consider this when planning their study.

References

[1] Klompmaker J, Veth RP, Jansen HW et al. Meniscal repair by fibrocartilage in the dog: characterization of the repair tissue and the role of vascularity. Biomaterials 1996; 17: 1685–1691

[2] Murphy JM, Fink DJ, Hunziker EB, Barry FP. Stem cell therapy in a caprine model of osteoarthritis. Arthritis Rheum 2003; 48: 3464–3474

[3] Killian ML, Isaac DI, Haut RC, Déjardin LM, Leetun D, Donahue TL. Traumatic anterior cruciate ligament tear and its implications on meniscal degradation: a preliminary novel lapine osteoarthritis model. J Surg Res 2010; 164: 234–241

[4] Kobayashi M, Toguchida J, Oka M. Preliminary study of polyvinyl alcohol-hydrogel (PVA-H) artificial meniscus. Biomaterials 2003; 24: 639–647

[5] Chiari C, Koller U, Dorotka R et al. A tissue engineering approach to meniscus regeneration in a sheep model. Osteoarthritis Cartilage 2006; 14: 1056–1065

[6] Kang SW, Son SM, Lee JS et al. Regeneration of whole meniscus using meniscal cells and polymer scaffolds in a rabbit total meniscectomy model. J Biomed Mater Res A 2006; 78: 659–671

[7] Frank C, Woo SL-Y, Amiel D, Harwood F, Gomez M, Akeson W. Medial collateral ligament healing. A multidisciplinary assessment in rabbits. Am J Sports Med 1983; 11: 379–389

[8] Sundar S, Pendegrass CJ, Oddy MJ, Blunn GW. Tendon re-attachment to metal prostheses in an in vivo animal model using demineralised bone matrix. J Bone Joint Surg Br 2009; 91: 1257–1262

[9] Rumian AP, Draper ER, Wallace AL, Goodship AE. The influence of the mechanical environment on remodelling of the patellar tendon. J Bone Joint Surg Br 2009; 91: 557–564

Part 9

Tissue Engineering

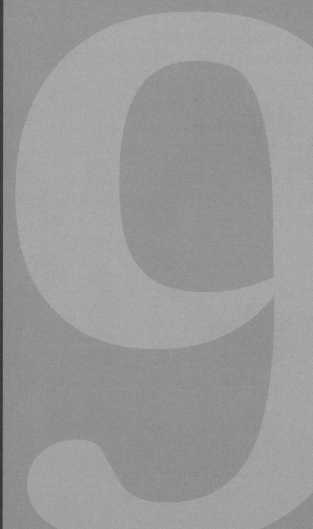

47 Scaffolds for Tissue Engineering and Materials for Repair

Christopher C. West

The use of synthetic materials for orthopedic applications is well established and has significantly improved the quality of life in patients suffering from tissue loss and degeneration. To date, the majority of these implants have been metals and ceramics. However, as the global population demographics change and people live longer, patients are now outliving their implants and require successive and often more complex operations to replace them; therefore, alternative materials are required to meet these challenges.

Initial biomaterial and implant research focused on finding inert substrates that could replace lost or damaged tissue, but evoke minimal effects on the native tissue. Coupled with advances in cell-based therapies and the emergence of regenerative medicine, there has been a significant shift in focus from looking at the application of inert materials that replace lost and damaged tissue, to trying to identify biocompatible and bioactive materials that can stimulate and coordinate the replacement and regeneration of tissue.

This chapter focuses on the theory behind the identification of materials that can be used to stimulate growth and differentiation of cells for the purposes of repair and regeneration of orthopedic tissues.

47.1 Identifying the Problem

The first stage is to identify the specific problem you are trying to address and therefore the best possible combination of cells, scaffolds, and growth factors to address this. The potential application for scaffolds and biomaterials in orthopedic tissue engineering is huge, and so are the number of different biomaterials and fabrication methods available (▶ Fig. 47.1).

Therefore, identifying the most appropriate material to the specific need is fundamental because no single biomaterial can satisfy all problems. For example, in addressing massive bone loss, a scaffold may be required to act as a structural replacement to the bone while the cellular component replaces the lost tissue. Here, the scaffold is required to have mechanical strength as well as the bioactive properties necessary to stimulate regeneration. If the scaffold is designed to be biodegradable, it must be

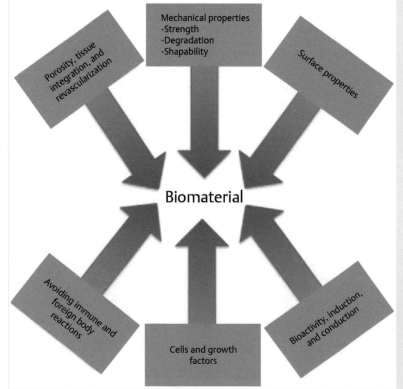

Fig. 47.1 Factors to consider when designing a new biomaterial.

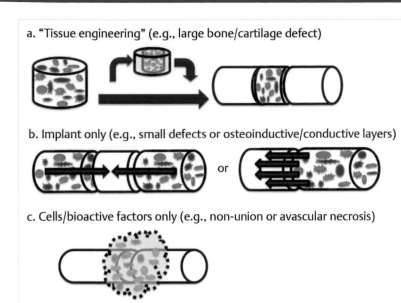

a. "Tissue engineering" (e.g., large bone/cartilage defect)

b. Implant only (e.g., small defects or osteoinductive/conductive layers)

or

c. Cells/bioactive factors only (e.g., non-union or avascular necrosis)

Fig. 47.2 Different approaches to the use of biomaterials, cells, and bioactive factors in orthopaedic repair and regeneration.

designed with a resorption rate that allows the mechanical strength of the scaffold to remain until the cellular component has remodeled and can resume its natural role. In addition, the potential implications of this type of construct are the need for significant periods of in vitro cell culture in a suitable bioreactor to attain the required number of cells prior to differentiation (▶ Fig. 47.2a). However, there are other scenarios where the aim of the scaffold is to allow the ingress of native stem cells, progenitors cells, and blood vessels to repopulate the graft. Hence, the role of the scaffold is to promote ingress and facilitate differentiation of the native cells (e.g., small bone defects, coating of orthopedic implants; ▶ Fig. 47.2b). Thirdly, in some situations, the aim might simply be to deliver factors or cells directly to the site of injury to either stimulate, supplement, or replace existing stem cell populations (e.g., nonunions, avascular necrosis; ▶ Fig. 47.2c).

47.2 Biomaterials and the Stem Cell Niche

The stem cell niche refers to the immediate environment that surrounds a stem cell and comprises a complex number of factors that provide signals and stimuli to the cell. The sum effects of these signals can maintain the cell in a quiescent state, or at appropriate times cause the cell to proliferate and differentiate depending on the need. Interactions between the cell, its neighbors, the basement membrane, soluble factors, and the extracellular matrix (ECM) are all fundamental in this process. Therefore, it is crucial that we understand these processes and aim to mimic them when considering designing scaffolds and biomaterials. Factors as simple as the shape that the cell is maintained in can have a significant impact on its

capacity to differentiate. Maintaining a spherical morphology has been shown to be important in chondrogenesis of mesenchymal stem cells (MSCs), and therefore substrates that maintain cells in a more spherical shape have shown good potential compared to substrates that cause the spreading out of cells into a flattened fibroblastic type morphology.[1] Further studies have demonstrated that the hardness of the substrate on which a stem cell attaches is able to predict the behavior of the cells, with cells preferentially differentiating toward a tissue that mimics the hardness of the substrate on which they are grown.

47.2.1 Example from the Literature: Nanoscale Effects on Cellular Differentiation

An elegant example of the importance of cells and the surface with which they directly interact was shown by the work of Dalby et al.[2] In their study, they used electron beam lithography, a technology used in the manufacture of Blu-Ray disks, to fabricate ultraprecise nanotopographies. The polymethylmethacrylate culture surface was embossed with nanopits of 120 nm diameter and 100 nm depth, and the arrangement of these pits was varied to form five distinct patterns of varying symmetry and disorder (▶ Fig. 47.3).

They demonstrated that variations in the nanotopography had significant effects on MSC attachment, morphology, gene regulation, and protein and mineral production. They observed that using disordered patterns, they were able to stimulate osteogenesis as observed by the increased production of osteopontin, osteocalcin, upregulation of genes specific to osteogenesis, and production of mineralized bone matrix when compared to the ordered

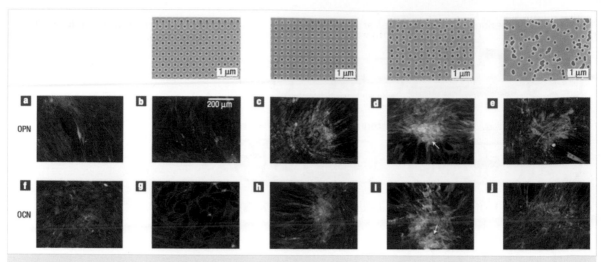

Fig. 47.3 Osteopontin (OPN) and osteocalcin (OCN) staining of osteoprogenitors after 21 days of culture.

and symmetrical patterns. The effects seen by the change in nanopatterning were in the absence of any other inducing agents such as growth factors; however, the distinct differentiation profile that was observed had a similar efficiency to those cultured in osteogenic media. In a similar series of experiments, the same group also identified nanopatterned surfaces that could maintain MSC phenotype and growth over prolonged periods of culture.[3]

47.3 Metals as Biomaterials

Metals form the majority of orthopedic implantable materials that are in current clinical use and are the material that is most routinely used in load-bearing implants and internal fixation devices. However, their design and function has undergone significant change and advancements. When manufactured appropriately, they display high-tensile, high-fatigue, and high-yield strengths with low reactivity of the native tissues. However, these same features that are seen as advantageous are responsible for the ultimate failure of many of these devices.

The high strength of the implant can shield the surrounding tissue from its normal stress and strains. This results in an associated atrophy and weakening of the bone resulting in bone degeneration. Furthermore, due to the inert nature of many metals, there is no osseointegration at the interface between the metal and the host tissue. This results in a layer of connective tissue developing between the implant and the prosthesis, causing a natural weakness. Therefore, much attention has been placed on developing osteoconductive and osteoinductive surfaces that will cause seamless integration of the implant and the host tissue through their influence on native or implanted tissue stem cells (► Fig. 47.2b).

Porosity in orthopedic implants is advantageous because it can facilitate tissue adhesion, growth, and if appropriate vascularization, thus turning an inert structure into a bioactive scaffold that integrates with the host. In addition, varying the degree of porosity of an implant will also have effects on the elastic modulus and can be tailored to that of the tissue to prevent issues such as stress shielding.

While most metals are relatively inert and are not biologically active, many of their oxides and alloys show excellent osteoinductive and -conductive properties. There have been many techniques described to increase the bioactivity and osteoconductivity of metallic implants and biomaterials including mechanical methods, plasma sprays, chemical treatments, and surface treatments, all of which aim to create a more bioactive interface.

This would have many significant advantages including rapid tissue integration, enhanced differentiation of stem cell populations, and increased bonding at the tissue-implant interface.

47.3.1 Example from the Literature: Coating of Titanium Implants with Collagen, RGD Peptide, and Chondroitin Sulfate

In an attempt to enhance osteogenesis and improve integration of the implant, the researchers hypothesized that using components of the bone ECM may enhance bone healing and osteogenesis around implants. Using a tibial titanium nail model in rats, they coated the surfaces of the titanium nails with different components of the ECM including type I collagen, chondroitin sulphate, and the RGD peptide sequence (Arg-Gly-Asp). Each of these components is known to be important in osteogenesis and has been previously shown to enhance bone growth and repair when used as a scaffold. Here, the authors chose to coat the surface of the titanium to create an osteoinductice and osteoconductive interface to enhance bone repair and integration.

They demonstrated that the addition of ECM proteins significantly enhanced bone remodeling in the early stages (days 7 and 14), which led to increased new bone formation in the later stages (day 28).

47.4 Glass as Biomaterials

Bioactive glasses have demonstrated excellent characteristics for potential applications in tissue engineering. They have high levels of bioactivity when compared to metals and ceramics, and also the ability to alter their biomechanics and degradation kinetics. This enhanced bioactivity is through the ability of bioactive glasses to form a tight bond with tissues through the formation of hydroxycarbonate apatite layer on their surface. A significant drawback of bioactive glass when used alone is its low strength and high stiffness resulting in low fracture toughness. Therefore, although bioactive glass has shown wide-ranging ability to induce osteogenesis, this function has largely been exploited in nonweight-bearing applications such as powders and bone cements to enhance bone healing. When used as a porous scaffold, their mechanical properties are even worse. As with polymers, bioactive glasses have been successfully combined with other biomaterials to enhance their overall effect. When combined with polymers and ceramics, they can impart enhanced bioactivity and degradation kinetics, and benefit from the superior mechanical properties of the other biomaterials.

47.5 Polymers as Biomaterials

Polymers are the most widely used biomaterials and have been utilized in a diverse range of applications including sutures, heart valves, surgical mesh, and screws.

They are excellent candidates for biomaterials because they are easy to manufacture and produce in a cost-efficient manner with highly reproducible characteristics. Polymers are incredibly versatile and can be manipulated to have the desired physical and mechanical properties for their intended application. They can be manufactured in many different forms including solids, gels, liquids, and fibers. In addition, they can be used directly, in combination with other materials, or coated onto surfaces. They can be both biodegradable and bioactive, with many examples of polymers supporting and enhancing differentiation of skeletal progenitor cells. ▶ Table 47.1 summarizes some of the most common classes of polymers in use in musculoskeletal therapies.[4,5]

47.5.1 Example from the Literature: High-Throughput Approaches to Identify Synthetic Polymers as Novel Biomaterials

Previous attempts to identify novel biomaterials have been hampered by the slow process of screening and identification that would only permit a small number of materials to be tested at any one time. High-throughput strategies have revolutionized this process, and the use of this technology allows thousands of biomaterials to be tested for their performance over a range of properties simultaneously and in parallel.

The Bradley Group (www.combichem.co.uk) has pioneered the use of microarrays for the identification of novel biomaterials that have been applied to a number of clinical uses including bone,[6] cartilage,[7] hepatic,[8] and vascular prostheses.[9] Polymer microarrays are fabricated using contact printing of polymers onto a standard microscope slide. This allows microscopic spots of thousands of individual polymers to be printed and screened on a single microscope slide (▶ Fig. 47.4).

In this example, a microarray was fabricated to screen, analyze, and compare 135 binary polymer blends that were generated by combining seven individual polymers in different combinations and ratios. Bone marrow–derived STRO-1+ skeletal stem cells were used and allowed the investigators to rapidly identify polymers that could act as noncytotoxic scaffolds for the attachment and proliferation of these musculoskeletal progenitor cells. Candidate polymers were rapidly identified and scaled up to produce matrices for in vitro and in vivo models. Through this platform, the researchers identified and produced three-dimensional polymer scaffolds that supported STRO-1+ stem cell attachment, proliferation, and differentiation that could be used in bone repair.

47.6 Hydrogels as Biomaterials

Hydrogels are three-dimensional structures formed by the crosslinking of either natural or synthetic homopolymers, copolymers, or macromers. Hydrogels have been extensively employed in tissue engineering and regenerative strategies due to their ability to imitate the native ECM and the stem cell niche. The high water content of hydrogels results in excellent biocompatibilty and biodegradability and the mechanical properties can be easily manipulated. This makes hydrogels an ideal candidate for tissue regeneration and cellular support.

Natural hydrogels include proteins found in the ECM of human tissues such as collagen and hyaluronic acid (HA), proteins derived from plants and algae such as cellulose and alginate, and those derived from animal cell lines such as Matrigel (Corning Life Sciences, Harrodsburg, KY), which contains ECM proteins produced from a

Table 47.1 Classes of Polymers Used in Musculoskeletal Therapies

Polymer	Musculoskeletal applications	Features/Outcomes
Polyphosphazene	Bone cements, tissue engineering	Biodegradable and highly tunable with changes in side groups. Comparable effect to poly(lactic-co-glycolic acid) when tested in vivo. Able to neutralize acidic degradation products of other materials. Promotes attachment and proliferation of osteoblasts.
Poly(α-hydroxyacids) [polylactide, poly-l-lactide acid, poly(lactic-co-glycolic acid), polyglycolic acid]	Tissue engineering, drug delivery (also used as sutures, stents, dressings)	Most widely used and investigated biomaterials. Highly tunable and easy to combine with other materials. Acidic degradation products cause strong inflammatory response. Random degradation can lead to premature failure of scaffolds. Hydrophobic and therefore needs modification to support cellular adhesion. Supports attachment, proliferation, and differentiation of osteoblasts and stem cells.
Poly(L-lactide-co-e-caprolactone)	Multiple uses including intramedullary fracture pins, craniofacial repair, bone and cartilage regeneration, tissue engineering	Biodegradable polymer with U.S. Food and Drug Administration approval as medical device. Many uses on own or often in combination with other materials such as ceramics (added strength and mineralization). Has shown to promote attachment and proliferation of osteoblasts.
Poly(propylene fumarate)	Tissue engineering	Biodegradable; however, acidic degradation products can cause inflammatory reaction. Highly tunable with variable crosslinking. Liquid before crosslinking; therefore, easy to fabricate into custom-made shapes or directly inject. Good biomechanical strength. Enhance osteoconductivity when combined with ceramics. Able to support cell attachment and proliferation.
Poly(vinyl alcohol)	Joint resurfacing—cartilage replacement	Nondegradable. Minimal immune response.
Poly(1,4-butylene succinate)	Tissue engineering	Biodegradable with harmless degradation products. Able to support attachment, proliferation, and phenotype of osteoblasts when manufactured appropriately.
Poly(acrylate)s	Bone replacement, tissue engineering	Nondegradable. Many individual polyacrylates can be prepared from a huge range of monomers. Excellent tunability. Favorable biomechanical properties. Able to support stem and progenitor cell attachment, proliferation, and differentiation.

Puppi D, Chiellini F, Piras AM, Chiellini E. Polymeric materials for bone and cartilage repair. Prog Polym Sci 2010;35:403–440; and Seal BL, Otero TC, Panitch A. Polymeric biomaterials for tissue and organ regeneration. Mater Sci Eng Rep 2001;34:147–230.

mouse sarcoma cell line. While these hydrogels have been used extensively, the use of natural products should be avoided where possible, especially in clinical application. Products derived from natural sources show significant batch-to-batch variation due to inherent biodiversity and as such are poorly defined. In addition to this, those derived from animal products can induce immune responses and risk contamination with pathogens.

Synthetic hydrogels offer significant advantages over natural alternatives by eliminating batch-to-batch variability and any risk of infection or immunogenicity. In addition to this, they offer much greater tunability such as molecular weight, crosslinking, chemical composition, addition of growth factors, mechanical strength, and degradability. The ability to consistently predict, control, and reproduce these factors offers significant advantages

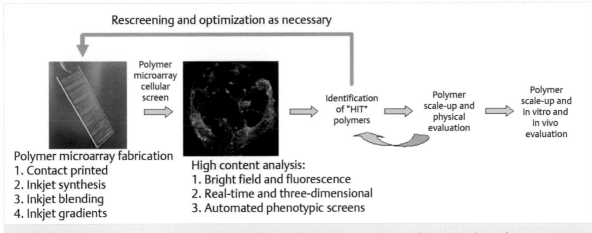

Fig. 47.4 Work flow developed by the Bradley Group showing high-throughput screening, analysis, and scale up of an extensive polymer library.

Table 47.2 A summary of the practical differences between natural and synthetic biomaterials.

	Advantages	Disadvantages
Natural	• Full, rapid, and natural degradation (this is not always beneficial when long-term support is needed [e.g., bone]) • Can function at a molecular level not just macroscopic	• Immunogenicity • Potential for transmission of pathogens • Lot-to-lot variability • Poor biomechanical properties • Limited tunability
Synthetic	• Minimal lot-to-lot variation • Mechanical and chemical properties easily altered • Cheap and easily scalable • Many currently in clinical use with approval from the U. S. Food and Drug Administration • Easy to combine and blend with other materials	• Toxicity • Chronic inflammation • Biocompatibility hard to predict and must be tested • Incomplete degradation with harmful degradation products

for synthetic hydrogels as a construct for tissue engineering (▶ Table 47.2).

The potential role of hydrogels extends beyond their function as a scaffold for tissue engineering, and their role as a potential delivery vehicle for drugs, cells, and other bioactive factors has also been widely investigated. The hydrophilic and biocompatible profile of hydrogels makes them ideal candidates for drug delivery vehicles. By controlling the intrinsic factors of the hydrogel such as crosslinking density and degradation rates, the delivery kinetics of the drug can be engineered to meet the specific needs of the intended application.

While most interest in the application of stem cells in regenerative medicine has focused on the potential to generate new tissue, recent interest has also focused on the paracrine and trophic effects of stem cells and their indirect ability to stimulate regeneration. Many in vivo studies that have implanted stem cells have shown significant regeneration; however, cell tracking studies have shown that the proportion of transplanted cells in the regenerated tissue is very small compared to the proportion of native cells. This suggests that one of the roles that

these transplanted cells potentiate is paracrine stimulation of host cells to enhance regeneration. Therefore, their role as biological drug stores is an expanding area of interest.[10] Hydrogels may have significant roles in this capacity because they can support the cell or cell aggregates during in vivo implantation. They will allow the diffusion of nutrients in and out, but also provide a physical barrier between the transplanted cells and the cells of the host providing immune isolation of the transplant.

47.6.1 Example: In Vivo Chondrogenesis of Mesenchymal Stem Cells Encapsulated in a Hydrogel

Differentiation of stem cells in vitro is relatively easy to control due to the ability to precisely control the media in which they are contained and the specific type, concentration, and duration of the growth factors the cells are exposed to. In vivo, this degree of control is much harder to achieve, and it is made more complicated by the immune response generated by the host and the diffusion of factors through a scaffold. Bian et al used two different hydrogels to address the problems faced by in vivo implantation of MSCs in a subcutaneous implantation model in nude mice.[11] They created alginate microspheres that were loaded with transforming growth factor-β3, a growth factor known to be critical in chondrogenesis of MSCs, which were suspended in an HA-based hydrogel along with the MSCs. They were able to show a sustained and controlled release of transforming growth factor-β3 from alginate microspheres when compared to direct encapsulation within the HA. A major complication of cartilage engineering is the hypertrophy of cartilage resulting in excessive type I and X and collagen compared to type II. In an attempt to prevent this, the authors used parathyroid hormone loaded microspheres within the same HA hydrogel, and demonstrated a reduction in the amount of type X collagen and calcification within the constructs. This example demonstrates the ability to tailor hydrogels to deliver cells and biofactors with high degrees of temporal and spatial organization.

47.7 Conclusion

The challenges that face scientists and clinicians in delivering clinically applicable, durable biomaterials and tissue-engineered grafts remain significant. The solution will rely on the successful marriage between cells, scaffolds, and bioactive factors to achieve the desired outcome.[12]

Jargon Simplified

- Biomaterial: Any substance, either natural or synthetic, that interacts with biological tissues.
- Biocompatible: A material that is compatible with living cells, tissues, organs, or systems, and posing no risk of injury, toxicity, or rejection by the immune system.
- Biodegradable: A material that is degraded; however, the degradation products of these materials may persist in vivo.
- Bioresorbable: A material that degrades and is subsequently eliminated from the host.
- Biomechanics: Mechanical laws as applied to living structure and biomaterials. Often used to measure strength, elasticit,y and compressive forces in scaffold and biomaterials.
- Osteoinductive: A material that promotes osteogenesis and new bone formation.
- Osteoconductive: A material that allows bone growth to occur on it.

Understanding the specific problem and the potential tools available is fundamental to achieving these goals. This chapter has given an introduction and examples of these technologies with the aim to empower researchers to make effective decisions about the most appropriate research strategy.

References

[1] Gao L, McBeath R, Chen CS. Stem cell shape regulates a chondrogenic versus myogenic fate through Rac1 and N-cadherin. Stem Cells 2010;28(3):564–572

[2] Dalby MJ, Gadegaard N, Tare R et al. The control of human mesenchymal cell differentiation using nanoscale symmetry and disorder. Nat Mater 2007; 6: 997–1003

[3] McMurray RJ, Gadegaard N, Tsimbouri PM et al. Nanoscale surfaces for the long-term maintenance of mesenchymal stem cell phenotype and multipotency. Nat Mater 2011; 10: 637–644

[4] Puppi D, Chiellini F, Piras AM, Chiellini E. Polymeric materials for bone and cartilage repair. Prog Polym Sci 2010; 35: 403–440

[5] Seal BL, Otero TC, Panitch A. Polymeric biomaterials for tissue and organ regeneration. Mater Sci Eng Rep 2001; 34: 147–230

[6] Khan F, Tare RS, Kanczler JM, Oreffo ROC, Bradley M. Strategies for cell manipulation and skeletal tissue engineering using high-throughput polymer blend formulation and microarray techniques. Biomaterials 2010; 31: 2216–2228

[7] Khan F, Tare RS, Oreffo ROC, Bradley M. Versatile biocompatible polymer hydrogels: scaffolds for cell growth. Angew Chem Int Ed Engl 2009; 48: 978–982

[8] Hay DC, Pernagallo S, Diaz-Mochon JJ et al. Unbiased screening of polymer libraries to define novel substrates for functional hepatocytes with inducible drug metabolism. Stem Cell Res (Amst) 2011; 6: 92–102

[9] Pernagallo S, Tura O, Wu M, et al. Novel biopolymers to enhance endothelialisation of intra-vascular devices. Adv Healthc Mater 2012;1(5):646–656

[10] Caplan AI, Correa D. The MSC: an injury drugstore. Cell Stem Cell 2011; 9: 11–15

[11] Bian L, Zhai DY, Tous E, Rai R, Mauck RL, Burdick JA. Enhanced MSC chondrogenesis following delivery of TGF-β3 from alginate microspheres within hyaluronic acid hydrogels in vitro and in vivo. Biomaterials 2011; 27: 6425-6434

[12] Ramalingam M, Ramakrishna P, Best P, Biomaterials and stem cells in regenerative medicine. Boca Raton, FL: CRC Press LLC; 2012

48 Use of Growth Factors in Musculoskeletal Research

Iain R. Murray

Growth factors (GFs) are naturally occurring substances that bind to receptors on the cell surface and are capable of stimulating diverse cellular processes including proliferation and differentiation. GFs are usually a protein or hormone and most are pleiotropic, causing multiple biological effects with some stimulating changes in numerous cell types whereas others are specific to a particular cell type. Individual GFs tend to occur as members of larger families of structurally and evolutionarily related proteins. Although the term cytokine is sometimes used interchangeably with GF, cytokines are a unique family of GFs secreted primarily from leukocytes that stimulate both the humeral and immune responses, as well as activation of phagocytes.

GFs are known to play an important role in both normal and abnormal skeletal growth and development. Indeed, some of the most dramatic successes in pediatric orthopedics have resulted from the identification of deficiencies in cell signaling molecules that are crucial to skeletal development, such as vitamin D in rickets, thyroid hormone in cretinism, and growth hormone in hypopituitarism. The importance of GFs in skeletal development has been emphasized by the recent discoveries that the skeletal deformities of achondroplasia, Apert syndrome, Crouzon syndrome, Pfeiffer syndrome, and Jackson-Weiss syndrome are all caused by mutations for the fibroblast GF (FGF) family of signaling molecules. However, the systemic roles of GFs in development are beyond the scope of the current chapter, which will focus on applications involving the local delivery of GFs in isolation or in combinations with mesenchymal stem cells (MSCs) for tissue regeneration and healing.

48.1 Mechanism by Which Growth Factors Regulate Cell Behavior

Although GFs differ in their specific mechanisms of action on the basis of their structure and target cells, the mechanisms by which these proteins modify gene expression and ultimately promote gene translation into the proteins of interest can be generalized (▶ Fig. 48.1). GFs bind

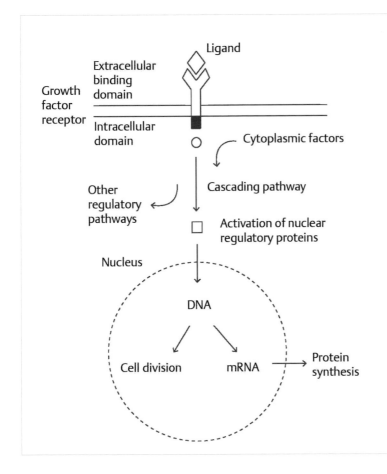

Fig. 48.1 Overview of the mechanisms by which growth factors (GFs) influence cell behavior. A specific cell surface receptor "recognizes" each GF ligand in the extracellular environment, its shape fitting that growth factor precisely. Binding of a GF activates the intracellular domain of the receptor and sets in motion a cascading signaling pathway, usually involving phosphorylation of proteins that ultimately activate nuclear regulatory proteins that trigger cell division or transcription of deoxyribonucleic acid (DNA) sequences to messenger ribonucleic acid (mRNA) and subsequent production of proteins.

with large, specific transmembrane receptor molecules present on the surface of target cells. These receptors convert information carried by GFs into a form usable by the cell. As such, the presence or absence of specific functional receptors defines a cell's ability to respond to signals in the extracellular environment. Receptors may also add to the information carried by the signaling molecule, thereby integrating intracellular information to the delivered message. GF receptors are linked to various genes in the nucleus by a cascade of reactions in the cytoplasm, resulting in cell division or transcription of deoxyribonucleic acid sequences to messenger ribonucleic acid and protein production. Stimulation of this cascade often activates several genes and may therefore generate multiple effects. Each family of GF has a corresponding family of receptors. Although there are marked structural differences among receptor families, many of the links in the gene-activating cascade are shared between families. Therefore, binding of different GFs to their respective receptors may result in the same cellular effect. GFs may act through endocrine, paracrine, and autocrine regulation. In the endocrine pathway, cell-signaling molecules are released by the secreting cell into the circulation to act on distant target cells. In the paracrine pathway, the cell-signaling molecules are secreted locally to act on neighboring cells. The autocrine pathway is characterized by cellular self-activation.

48.2 Actions of Growth Factors

In contributing to tissue healing and regeneration, GFs may exert effects in five broad categories. The majority of GFs contribute to regeneration through several of these actions.

1. **Cellular proliferation:** At the site of injury, GFs may stimulate proliferation of progenitors to ensure that the pool of progenitors lost through differentiation is replenished.
2. **Cell migration:** Tissue formation during healing requires the orchestrated movement of cells in particular directions to specific locations. Cells often migrate in response to and toward specific signals including GFs in a process known as chemotaxis.
3. **Cell survival at the site of injury:** Injured tissue represents a harsh microenvironment where inflammation, low oxygen concentration, and loss of trophic factors may contribute to poor survival of host and transplanted MSCs. GFs contribute to the suppression of harmful inflammation and revival of endogenous tissues.[1]
4. **Differentiation of progenitors:** GFs are key regulators of lineage fate and its progression.[2]
5. **Angiogenesis:** Tissue regeneration is dependent on angiogenesis. GFs promote new blood vessel formation essential for the delivery of oxygen, nutrients, and progenitors to the site of injury.

48.3 Growth Factors in Mesenchymal Stem Cell Transplantation

Individual or synergistic combinations of GFs can be delivered directly to sites of injury where they act directly on host cells to bring about their therapeutic effect. However, GFs are increasingly being used in combination with MSCs, whose ability to differentiate into bone, fat, muscle, and cartilage while beneficially modifying local immune environments and creating a regenerative microenvironment has made them a promising substrate for musculoskeletal regeneration.[1,2] Concomitant delivery of GFs may augment both the regenerative potential of transplanted MSCs while optimizing a regenerative microenvironment through actions on cells within target tissues.

In addition, GFs are playing an increasing role in the preparation and preconditioning of MSCs prior to delivery. Although MSCs are easy to isolate, relatively safe, and do not require immunosuppression, there currently exists a gap between the number of MSCs that can be obtained from the donor site and the number required for implantation to regenerate tissue. Standard methods of MSC expansion are not fully suitable due to time- and age-related constraints for autologous therapies. Furthermore, experiments in small animals have shown that MSCs do not persist well in the graft environment. Either the cells do not incorporate into the host tissue, or if there is incorporation, the cells are rapidly lost. This is likely to reflect the various threats that MSCs face at the site of delivery leading to loss of cells (▶ Fig. 48.2). Through their effects on proliferation, survival, and differentiation of MSCs, pretreatment with GFs may prove helpful in addressing these issues prior to delivery.

48.4 Selected Growth Factors and Their Actions

Growth factors with potential clinical applications in the augmentation of healing of musculoskeletal and connective tissues can be categorized on the basis of their biological activities and clinical use. They include the transforming growth factor beta (TGFβ) superfamily (includes the TGFβ$_{1-3}$ and the bone morphogenetic proteins [BMPs] among others), Wnt, FGFs, and epidermal GFs, vascular endothelial GFs, insulinlike GF, and platelet-derived growth factor beta (PDGFβ) (▶ Table 48.1).

48.4.1 Transforming Growth Factor Beta

The TGFβs form part of the wider TGFβ superfamily, which consists of many GFs and morphogens that have roles in skeletogenesis and skeletal homeostasis. This

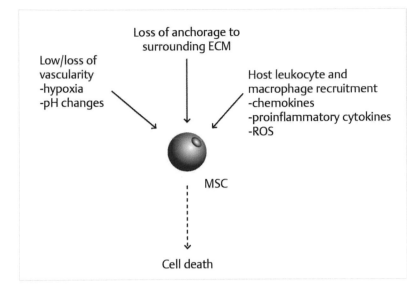

Fig. 48.2 Mesenchymal stem cells (MSC) face various threats at sites of delivery. Low vascularity results in hypoxia and pH changes, whereas host leukocytes and macrophages both release chemokines and proinflammatory cytokines while generating reactive oxygen species (ROS) that may activate apoptotic cascades. Loss of attachment to extracellular matrix (ECM) of these anchorage dependent cells may also result in apoptosis. (Modified from Rodrigues M, Griffith LG, Wells A. Growth factor regulation of proliferation and survival of multipotential stromal cells. Stem Cell Res Thera 2010;1:32.)

Table 48.1 Selected Growth Factors and Their Effects on the Regulation of Skeletal Tissue

Growth Factor	Biological activity on target progenitors and tissue (author, year)
TGFβ • TGFβ$_1$ • TGFβ$_2$ • TGFβ$_3$	MSC proliferation (Ogawa, 2010), chondrogenic differentiation (Noth, 2002), osteogenic differentiation (Joyce, 1990) MSC proliferation (Ogawa, 2010), chondrogenic differentiation (Noth, 2002), osteogenic differentiation (Joyce, 1990) MSC proliferation (Ogawa, 2010), chondrogenic differentiation (Noth, 2002), osteogenic differentiation (Joyce, 1990)
BMP • BMP$_2$ • BMP$_4$ • BMP$_6$ • BMP$_7$	MSC proliferation (Chang, 2010), osteogenic differentiation (Luu, 2007), chondrogenic differentiation (Sekiya, 2001) Osteogenic differentiation (Kann, 2010) Osteogenic differentiation (Luu, 2007) Osteogenic differentiation (Luu, 2007)
Wnt • Wnt$_{3a}$ • Wnt$_{5a}$	Modulates MSC proliferation (Baksh, 2007; Qiu, 2007), MSC survival (Boland, 2004), modulates osteogenic differentiation of MSCs (Cho, 2006), modulates chondrogenic differentiation of MSCs (Day, 2005) Modulates osteogenic differentiation of MSCs (Cho, 2006), modulates chondrogenic differentiation of MSCs (Day, 2005)
FGFs • FGF$_1$ • FGF$_2$ • FGF$_6$ • FGF$_7$ • FGF$_{10}$	Fibroblast proliferation (Hutley, 2004), promotes angiogenesis (Javerzat, 2002) Fibroblast proliferation (Hutley, 2004), myogenic and fibroblast migration (Tanaka, 1998), promotes angiogenesis (Javerzat, 2002) Myogenic differentiation (Lefaucheur, 1995) Keratinocyte proliferation (Tagashira, 1997), keratinocyte migration (Tsuboi,1993), keratinocyte differentiation (Werner, 1993) Keratinocyte proliferation (Tagashira, 1997)
EGF	MSC proliferation (Tamama, 2006), modulates osteogenic differentiation of MSCs (Sibilia, 2003), modulates chondrogenic differentiation of MSCs (Sibilia, 2003)
VEGF	Promotes angiogenesis (D'Amore, 1999)
IGFs • IGF$_1$	MSC proliferation (Haider, 2008), MSC survival (Haider, 2008), modulates chondrogenesis (Longobardi, 2006)
PDGF	MSC proliferation (Tokunaga, 2008), modulates osteogenic differentiation (Kratchmarova, 2005; Ng 2008)

Abbreviations: BMP, bone morphogenetic protein; EGF, epidermal growth factor; FGF, fibroblast growth factor; IGF, insulinlike growth factor; MSC, mesenchymal stem cell; PDGF, platelet-derived growth factor; TGF, transforming growth factor; VEGF, vascular endothelial growth factor.

family also includes the BMPs (considered separately subsequently), growth and differentiation factors, anti-Mullerian hormone, and activin.

Although also capable of stimulating osteogenesis, TGFβs (of which there are three isoforms, $TGFβ_{1-3}$) are best known for their effects on the chondrogenic differentiation of MSCs.[3] TGFβ stimulates cell replication and extracellular matrix formation while inhibiting the alloreactive immune response. In vitro, MSCs exposed to TGFβ show increased proliferation and a bias toward the chondrogenic lineage. While all three isoforms induce proliferation of MSCs and chondrocyte formation, $TGFβ_3$ has the most pronounced effect on chondrogenesis and consistently increases proliferation of MSCs.[4] Cartilage-specific gene expression occurs through intracellular signaling cascades involving SMAD proteins, the mitogen activated protein kinases, p38, extracellular-signal regulated kinase-1, and c-Jun N-terminal kinase.[5]

Animal studies have evaluated the influence of TGFβ on the healing of cartilage defects and fractures. Several studies have demonstrated that the effects of TGFβ are highly dose dependent, with high levels favoring chondrogenesis, while low doses favor osteogenic differentiation. Guo et al[6] investigated whether $TGFβ_1$-modified MSCs to enhance the repair of full thickness articular cartilage damage in a rabbit model. The MSCs transfected with $TGFβ_1$ were seeded onto a biomimetic scaffold in vitro and allografted into cartilage defects. The proliferation and generation of cartilaginous matrix by $TGFβ_1$-transfected MSCs was substantially greater than in MSCs without $TGFβ_1$ with evidence of surface hyaline cartilage-specific extracellular matrix synthesis and reconstruction of the subchondral bone at 24 weeks. Park et al[7] described an enhanced neocartilage formation by rabbit MSCs using a hydrogel plus $TGFβ_1$.

Studies have also demonstrated stimulation of bone regeneration by two- to four-fold a following local application of exogenous TGFβ in animal models of implant fixation.[8] These studies demonstrate that the effect of $TGFβ_1$ is highly dose dependent such that intermediate doses cause more bone to form than low or high doses. Using a knockout mouse model, absence of $TGFβ_1$ has also been shown to be detrimental to bone mineralization.[9]

TGFβs have yet to be evaluated in clinical settings in orthopedics.

48.4.2 Bone Morphogenetic Proteins

Over 20 different BMPs have been isolated that primarily influence cellular proliferation and osteogenic differentiation.[10] BMP_3 has been shown to increase MSC proliferation three-fold. While BMP_2, BMP_4, BMP_6, and BMP_7 all promote the osteogenic differentiation of MSCs, BMP_2 has the greatest impact. The effect of BMP_2 on proliferation and osteogenic differentiation of MSCs is thought to occur

via sustained signaling of mitogen activated protein kinases Frk, whereas the mitogenic effect of BMP_3 has been found to be mediated by TGFβ/activin signaling.

BMP_2 and BMP_7 are now available clinically and have been used successfully in fracture acceleration studies, distraction osteogenesis studies, and nonunion studies. Importantly, the beneficial effect of these factors on the healing of fractures and nonunions has now been evaluated in randomized controlled trials. McKee et al[11] studied the effect of $rhBMP_7$ applied without a collagen carrier in fresh open fractures of the tibia that were all managed with intramedullary nailing. At 6 months, the treatment group had an improved functional outcome as assessed by weight-bearing status and pain. Friedlaender et al[12] compared the addition of fresh autograft or $rhBMP_7$ in a type I collagen carrier to management with intramedullary nailing in 124 tibial nonunions. At 2 years, there was no statistical difference between the control and treatment groups. The authors concluded that $rhBMP_7$ was equivalent to autograft in the management of nonunion, but noted that pain at the donor site was reported in 20% of the autograft group. Treatment with BMP_2 has also been evaluated in large prospective studies. A total of 450 patients were stratified for grade of open fracture before being randomized to a control group and two further groups in which patients received a BMP_2 impregnated sponge at different doses (0.75 mg/mL and 1.5 mg/mL).[13] At 12 months, those treated with the higher dose of BMP_2 had a statistically significant ($p < 0.003$) accelerated healing, fewer invasive secondary interventions, and a lower rate of nonunion than the control group.

As the TGFβ and BMP family of GFs all affect bone formation at different rates and some have a greater effect on proliferation, synergistic pairs of these GFs can be used at optimal does and at specific points during the bone regeneration process. As such, the combined treatment of $TGFβ_3$ with BMP_2 on MSCs has been shown to enhance chondrogenic differentiation in vivo.

48.4.3 Wnt

The Wnt family of 19 genes produces secreted proteins that modulate cell proliferation, differentiation, and apoptosis. They are crucial to normal embryonic tissue development and the regeneration of adult tissues, including bone.[14] There are conflicting reports on the effect of Wnt signaling on the proliferation on MSCs. One set of studies suggests that canonical Wnt signaling maintains progenitors in an undifferentiated but self-renewing state. By activating the canonical Wnt pathway through frizzled 1 and 4, Wnt_{3a} increases both proliferation and survival while preventing osteogenic differentiation in MSCs from multiple sources. Other studies conclude that canonical signaling initiated by Wnt_{3a} inhibits human MSC proliferation. These contrasting findings may reflect the findings of a third group of studies that suggest that Wnt_{3a} signaling at low levels promotes proliferation whereas at higher levels inhibits MSC proliferation.

Wnt_{5a}, a noncanonical Wnt, competes for Wnt_{3a} binding to the frizzled receptor and negates the positive effect of Wnt_{3a} on MSC proliferation. Conversely, Wnt_4, also a noncanonical Wnt, does not influence MSC proliferation. Part of the controversy surrounding Wnt signaling may result from the extensive crosstalk between Wnts and other signaling pathways influencing the fate of progenitors in particular the integrated pathways of TGFβ and Wnt.

In addition to effects being dose dependent, Quarto and colleagues[15] reported that the effects of Wnt_{3a} were dependent on the differentiation state, the cell type, and the age of recipient using in vitro and in vivo models of bone regeneration. When added to undifferentiated MSCs, Wnt_{3a} inhibited osteogenic differentiation. By contrast, when added to calvarial osteoblasts, Wnt_{3a} had an inhibitory effect in cells from juvenile mice but induced bone production in cells from adult animals. These results were in accordance with previous investigations.

48.4.4 Fibroblast Growth Factors

FGF was originally identified as a protein capable of promoting fibroblast proliferation and is now known to represent a group with at least 22 members. FGFs exert multiple functions through the binding into and activation of FGF receptors, with main signaling occurring through the RAS/mitogen activated protein kinase pathway. FGFs function both in vivo and in vitro to influence cellular proliferation, migration, differentiation, angiogenesis, and wound healing.

The biological activity of FGFs in the proliferation of fibroblasts and stimulation of angiogenesis facilitate their potential use in wound healing. Both FGF_1 and FGF_2 are known to be released by damaged endothelial cells and macrophages at wound sites, and if FGF_2 is blocked, wound angiogenesis is almost completely impaired. FGF is also known to induce scar-free healing. FGF_7 and FGF_{10} play a role in the stimulation of the migration and proliferation of keratinocytes. Among the FGFs, studies of wound healing and skin regeneration have primarily been conducted on FGF_2.

Muscle regeneration has also been shown to be controlled by the FGFs, which are abundant in regenerating areas of muscle. FGF_6 is of particular interest because of its specificity to muscle and its characteristic upregulation during muscle regeneration. FGF_2 has been shown to promote recruitment of skeletal muscle satellite cells using a single myofiber culture model.

Following injury of tendons and ligaments, the level of FGF_2 and its receptors has been shown to increase in vivo, with FGF_2 playing a significant role in the recruitment and differentiation of progenitors. The effect of FGF_2 on bone marrow MSCs were investigated for applications in the repair of tendons and ligaments. At low concentrations (3 ng/mL), FGF_2 triggered both cell proliferation and genes related to tendon and ligament tissue. However, treatment with a high dose (30 ng/mL) did not result in beneficial effects. Chan et al[16] demonstrated that collagen type III expression and cellular proliferation increased after 7 days with increasing dosage of FGF_2 injected into a defect at the midpart of the patellar tendon. Using a rabbit model of anterior cruciate ligament repair, FGF_2 incorporated into a gelatin hydrogel and combined with a polylactic acid woven fabric resulted in regeneration of anterior cruciate ligament and bone with enhanced mechanical strength.

The FGF receptors are also widely expressed in developing bone and several common autosomal dominant disorders of bone growth including achondroplasia have been shown to result from mutations of the FGFR genes. Possible effects of FGF_2 on osteogenesis and bone regeneration have also been reported. Tabata et al[17] studied the role of FGF_2 in a rabbit skull defect model—the implants showed dramatic improvement in defect closure, bone mineral density, and bone regeneration in groups treated with varying doses (2 to 200 μg) when compared to an untreated group.

Clinical trials are now under way evaluating a potential therapeutic role of FGFs in wound healing.

48.5 Platelet-Rich Plasma

The escalating interest in GFs for the treatment of musculoskeletal disorders is exemplified by the popularity of platelet-rich plasma (PRP), particularly for soft tissue injuries. PRP can be defined as the volume of the plasma fraction of autologous blood having a platelet concentration above baseline. The α granules within platelets are bound by a membrane and contain more than 30 bioactive proteins, many of which have a fundamental role in hemostasis or tissue healing. The properties of PRP are based on the production and release of multiple growth and differentiation factors from α granules within activated platelets. Platelets actively secrete these proteins within 10 minutes of clotting, with 95% of presynthesized GFs secreted within 1 hour. After the initial burst of GFs, the platelets synthesize and secrete additional such factors for the remaining days of their lifespan. The granular proteins include PDGFs, TGFβs, platelet factor 4, interleukin-1, platelet-derived angiogenesis factor, vascular endothelial GF, epidermal GF, insulinlike GF, osteocalcin, osteonectin, fibrinogen, vitronectin, fibronectin, and thrombospondin-1. PRP also contains proteins such as fibrin, fibronectin, vitronectin, and thrombospondin, which act as cell adhesion molecules, important for the migration of osteoblasts, fibroblasts, and epithelial cells.

Adult MSCs, osteoblasts, fibroblasts, endothelial cells, and epidermal cells express receptors specific to the PRP-derived GFs.

PRP is harvested from a patient's own peripheral blood, centrifuged to obtain a concentrated amount of platelets, placed in a small volume of plasma, and readministered at the site of injury. Prior to delivery, it must be activated (typically using bovine thrombin) to stimulate release of the granular contents, with the forming clot providing a vehicle for delivery and containment of the secreted proteins.

Several animal studies have provided encouraging results supporting the beneficial effect of PRPs on bone healing. The use of PRP has been observed to improve bone healing in defects in the rabbit calvaria and to facilitate the incorporation of particulate cancellous bone grafts in mandibular reconstructions in goats. The effect of PRP on tendon healing in animal studies has been mixed.

In clinical studies, details of the quantity of PRP used and the methods of application are procedure specific. However, the current literature is complicated by a lack of standardization of study protocols, platelet-separation techniques, and outcome measures. As a result, there is uncertainty about the evidence to support the increasing clinical use of PRP and autologous blood concentrates as a treatment modality for orthopedic bone and soft tissue injuries. Published randomized controlled trials evaluating PRP for clinical orthopedic applications are summarized in ▶ Table 48.2.

48.6 Growth Factors as an Alternative to Serum for In Vitro Culture

Current limitations to the use of MSCs for regeneration include providing sufficient numbers of these stromal cells in a timely manner. To bring about MSC expansion, fetal bovine serum (FBS) is currently employed because human serum does not fully support growth of MSCs in vitro. However, complications arise in the use of FBS for MSC transplants in vivo as FBS contains undefined elements that can vary in inducing proliferation. Contaminants in FBS can cause infections, and components of nonhuman origin can trigger host immune reactions.[18] Commercially developed serum-free and animal supplement–free media have been produced using synthetic supplements. However, the proprietary composition of these products remains a barrier to clinical use. The use of GFs as culture supplements instead of FBS offers a promising alternative. Combination treatments with PDGF-BB, FGF_2, and $TGF\beta_1$ show the most encouraging results in serum-free expansion of MSCs. This treatment has not only brought about a synergistic effect on MSC proliferation, but has also retained the phenotype, differentiation, and colony forming potential of these cells.

48.7 Clinical Considerations

The diverse actions of GFs, often varying with dose, cell type, and host factors, highlights the importance of tailoring any potential GF-based treatments to an individual patient's injury. Each clinical situation represents a unique microenvironment with different numbers of host progenitors, variations in levels of endogenous GFs, and variable receptor expression. Furthermore, the type of cells present and the number of growth receptors on these cells are also known to vary at different stages of the healing process. This must be considered when extrapolating experimental evidence and clinical studies into clinical practice.

48.8 Challenges to Clinical Translation

Clear challenges to clinical translation still remain. Despite the reputed genetic stability of MSCs, there have been reports of MSCs displaying localized genetic alterations in the presence of GFs. Similarly, there still remains the scare that the increased proliferation of GFs combined with the immunosuppressive effects of MSCs might result in tumor growth. It is therefore important to have proper modes of GF delivery, which is localized, controlled, and of a time-limited nature. Controlled release of GFs or presentation of the GF in bioengineered form are some of the ways in which this can be achieved.

48.9 Conclusion

GFs are key regulators of normal tissue regeneration and healing in response to injury. Harnessing the capacity of GFs to promote cellular proliferation, migration, survival, and differentiation while contributing to angiogenesis will undoubtedly form an integral part of future therapies in orthopedics. We now have agents including BMP_2 and BMP_7 that have been demonstrated to have a beneficial effect on the healing of fractures and nonunions in randomized controlled trials. Other agents such as FGF have shown promise in large animal studies, whereas others including TGFβ have been evaluated in small animals. Combination treatments of GFs are drawing much attention due to their synergistic effects. Caution must be used in extrapolating the findings of the rapidly expanding body of research. However, more studies are required to evaluate the range of agents and combinations available and to determine the optimum methods, dosing, and time of delivery.

Table 48.2 Randomized Controlled Trials Evaluating Platelet-Rich Plasma for Clinical Applications in Orthopedics

Author (Year)	Indication	Study design	Participants	Author's conclusions
Dallari (2007)	Bone healing in HTOs for genu varus	RCT (ABG + PRP; ABG + BMC + PRP)	23	Increased osteoid on biopsy with PRP groups but no clinical difference
Everts (2008)	Subacromial decompression	RCT (PRP; no PRP)	40	Faster recovery, earlier return to ADLs and reduced requirement for pain medication in PRP group
Orrego (2008)	ACL reconstruction	RCT (PRP; PRP + bone plug: bone plug; neither PRP or bone plug)	108	Enhancing effect of PRP on graft maturation
Nin (2010)	ACL reconstruction	RCT (PRP enriched; no PRP)	100	No clinical or biomechanical difference at 2 years
De Vos (2010)	Chronic Achilles tendinopathy	Double blind RCT (PRP; saline)	54	No difference in pain or activity
Peerbooms (2010)	Lateral epicondylitis	Multicenter RCT (PRP; corticosteroid injection)	100	Reduced pain and improved function in PRP group
Vogrin (2010)	ACL reconstruction	RCT (PRP enriched graft; unenriched graft)	50	Improved AP stability with PRP enrichment, improved vascularity of graft at 6 weeks with PRP
Randelli (2011)	Arthroscopic rotator cuff repair	RCT (PRP + autologous thrombin; no PRP)	53	Reduced pain in first postoperative months and improved healing in grade 1 and 2 tiers in PRP group
Sys (2011)	Lumbar fusion	RCT (BG + PRP; BG)	40	No difference overall
Cervillin (2012)	Patellar tendon ACL donor site healing	RCT (PRP; no PRP)	40	No significant improvement in defect filling; improved VISA but not VAS pain scores with PRP
Rodeo (2012)	Arthroscopic RC repair	RCT (arthroscopic RC repair + PRP; arthroscopic RC repair)	79	No beneficial effect of PRP
De Almeida (2012)	Patellar tendon ACL donor site healing	RCT (PRP; no PRP)	27	PRP reduced postoperative pain and improved harvest site healing on MRI at 6 months

Abbreviations: ABG, autologous bone graft; ACL, anterior cruciate ligament; ADL, activities of daily living; AP, anteroposterior; BG, bone graft; BMC, bone marrow cell; HTO, high tibial osteotomy; MRI, magnetic resonance imaging; PRP, platelet-rich plasma; RCT, randomized controlled trial; RC, rotator cuff; VAS, visual analogue score; VISA, Victorian Institute of Sport Assessment.

References

[1] Caplan AI, Correa D. The MSC: an injury drugstore. Cell Stem Cell 2011; 9: 11–15

[2] Pittenger MF, Mackay AM, Beck SC et al. Multilineage potential of adult human mesenchymal stem cells. Science 1999; 284: 143–147

[3] Sekiya I, Vuoristo JT, Larson BL, Prockop DJ. In vitro cartilage formation by human adult stem cells from bone marrow stroma defines the sequence of cellular and molecular events during chondrogenesis. Proc Natl Acad Sci U S A 2002; 99: 4397–4402

[4] Ogawa T, Akazawa T, Tabata Y. In vitro proliferation and chondrogenic differentiation of rat bone marrow stem cells cultured with gelatin hydrogel microspheres for TGF-beta1 release. J Biomater Sci Polym Ed 2010; 21: 609–621

[5] Schmierer B, Hill CS. TGFbeta-SMAD signal transduction: molecular specificity and functional flexibility. Nat Rev Mol Cell Biol 2007; 8: 970–982

[6] Guo X, Zheng Q, Kulbatski I et al. Bone regeneration with active angiogenesis by basic fibroblast growth factor gene transfected mesenchymal stem cells seeded on porous beta-TCP ceramic scaffolds. Biomed Mater 2006; 1: 93–99

[7] Park JS, Yang HJ, Woo DG, Yang HN, Na K, Park KH. Chondrogenic differentiation of mesenchymal stem cells embedded in a scaffold by long-term release of TGF-beta 3 complexed with chondroitin sulfate. J Biomed Mater Res A 2010; 92: 806–816

[8] Sumner DR, Turner TM, Urban RM et al. Locally delivered rhTGF-beta2 enhances bone ingrowth and bone regeneration at local and remote sites of skeletal injury. J Orthop Res 2001; 19: 85–94

[9] Atti E, Gomez S, Wahl SM, Mendelsohn R, Paschalis E, Boskey AL. Effects of transforming growth factor-beta deficiency on bone development: a Fourier transform-infrared imaging analysis. Bone 2002; 31: 675–684

[10] Luu HH, Song WX, Luo X et al. Distinct roles of bone morphogenetic proteins in osteogenic differentiation of mesenchymal stem cells. J Orthop Res 2007; 25: 665–677

[11] McKee MDSE, Waddell JP. The effect of human recombinant bone morphogenetic protein (rhBMP-7) on the healing of open tibial shaft fractures: results of a multi-center, prospective randomized clinical trial (abstract). Procs Orthopaedic Trauma Association 18th Annual Meeting 2002

[12] Friedlaender GE, Perry CR, Cole JD et al. Osteogenic protein-1 (bone morphogenetic protein-7) in the treatment of tibial nonunions. J Bone Joint Surg Am 2001; 83-A Suppl 1: S151–S158

[13] Govender S, Csimma C, Genant HK et al. BMP-2 Evaluation in Surgery for Tibial Trauma (BESTT) Study Group.. Recombinant human bone morphogenetic protein-2 for treatment of open tibial fractures: a prospective, controlled, randomized study of four hundred and fifty patients. J Bone Joint Surg Am 2002; 84-A: 2123–2134

[14] Westendorf JJ, Kahler RA, Schroeder TM. Wnt signaling in osteoblasts and bone diseases. Gene 2004; 341: 19–39

[15] Quarto R, Mastrogiacomo M, Cancedda R et al. Repair of large bone defects with the use of autologous bone marrow stromal cells. N Engl J Med 2001; 344: 385–386

[16] Chan YS, Li Y, Foster W et al. Antifibrotic effects of suramin in injured skeletal muscle after laceration. J Appl Physiol (1985) 2003; 95: 771–780

[17] Tabata Y, Yamada K, Miyamoto S et al. Bone regeneration by basic fibroblast growth factor complexed with biodegradable hydrogels. Biomaterials 1998; 19: 807–815

[18] Müller AM, Mehrkens A, Schäfer DJ et al. Towards an intraoperative engineering of osteogenic and vasculogenic grafts from the stromal vascular fraction of human adipose tissue. Eur Cell Mater 2010; 19: 127–135

49 Stem Cells for Musculoskeletal Repair

Kurt D. Hankenson

Stem cells are precursors that differentiate to become terminally fated functional cells of tissues and organs. They have properties of self-renewal and have the ability to reconstitute the cells of damaged tissue. This chapter will focus on mesenchymal stem cells (MSCs) in bone regeneration. There is a desire to use stem cells in bone repair both to accelerate healing and to enhance the regeneration of hard-to-heal factures. An increase in bone formation could be accomplished by enhancing the direct formation of bone by osteoblasts (intramembranous bone formation) or by increasing the amount of bone formed on a cartilaginous template produced by chondrocytes (endochondral bone formation). The amount of precursor cartilage formed by chondrocytes could be enhanced or the rate of bone formation on the cartilaginous template accelerated. Both osteoblasts and chondrocytes differentiate from MSCs. MSCs are derived from a wide variety of sources, most commonly marrow and adipose; these cells can also be derived from induced pluripotent stem cells or embryonic stem cells. Interestingly, MSCs not only can contribute to the formation of bone and cartilage but also support vascularization, modulate inflammatory responses, secrete cytokines and growth factors, and produce an extracellular matrix conducive to the progression of healing. While MSCs show promise in preclinical models of bone repair and in isolated clinical cases, the promise of MSCs for bone regeneration has not been fully realized. Methods for cultivation, activation, and delivery must be better developed before the utilization of stem cells for tissue engineering of bone achieves robust clinically application. This chapter will consider MSC origin during bone regeneration, sources for and isolation of MSCs, evaluation of MSC proliferation and differentiation, and ultimately the utilization of MSCs to heal bone.

49.1 Introduction to Mesenchymal Stem Cells

Bone healing requires a robust mesenchymal cell response in order to build new bone through either endochondral (cartilage-mediated) or intramembranous (direct appositional) bone formation. Undifferentiated mesenchymal cells give rise to both osteoblasts and chondrocytes, and additionally promote angiogenesis. Thus, stem cell approaches that enhance the mesenchymal phase of bone repair have great potential for promoting bone regeneration.

Stem cells are undifferentiated progenitor cells that have the ability to become differentiated tissue forming cells and that are also capable of self-renewal. Another trait assigned to stem cells is the ability to reconstitute an ablated tissue. Thus hematopoietic stem cells, the classical stem cell, exist in a quiescent state, self-renew, and can reconstitute ablated marrow developing into all of the progenitor cells that give rise to fully differentiated inflammatory cells and blood cells.

Similar to hematopoetic stem cells, bone marrow is also the tissue from which MSCs were first isolated. In the 1960s, Friedenstein described the ability to isolate cells from marrow that had a high proliferation potential and that could form bone.[1] In early years, these cells were referred to as marrow stromal cells (also abbreviated as MSCs), because of their ability to also promote hematopoiesis. The bone-forming ability of these cells was largely ignored until the early 1990s, when the cells were first referred to as "mesenchymal stem cells," which also, coincidentally, used the same abbreviation. A variety of additional nomenclature has been used to refer to the cells over time, but both the "marrow stromal cell" and "mesenchymal stem cell" designations have been most prominently used. Over the past ten years the acronym MSC as mesenchymal stem cell has been used most frequently because of its broader application to cells that are derived from tissues other than marrow.

These MSCs exist in a limited number and have the ability to differentiate to become osteoblasts, adipocytes, and chondrocytes, as well as hematopoietic supportive stroma (▶ Fig. 49.1). In addition, these cells are believed to be capable of self-renewal.[2] With their ability to become both chondrocytes and osteoblasts, investigators began to realize their great potential for regenerating bone. Since these early years, thousands of papers have been published that have focused on a variety of topics related to MSCs, including their isolation, cultivation, delivery approaches, therapeutic potential, and safety. Indeed, a variety of commercial entities have been developed that seek to capitalize on MSCs for healing tissues, most relevant to this chapter, bone.

Whether an absence of stem cells or dysfunction causes poor, delayed, and nonunion bone healing remains a debatable topic. Theoretically, it is conceivable that stem cell dysfunction could be a contributor to poor healing, but this is not fully understood. Stem cell number declines with age, and this is also true with MSCs, but whether a lack of MSCs or poor activation of MSCs during healing is directly associated with age-associated decline in healing has not been definitively established in either animal models or humans. Regardless of whether there is an inherent deficiency in MSCs, it is prudent to be able to capitalize on their unique properties to promote bone regeneration.

It is also notable that MSCs not only differentiate to become bone-forming cells, they also possess unique

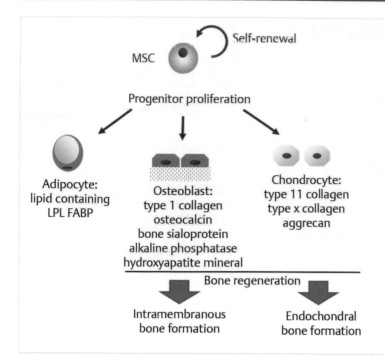

Fig. 49.1 Mesenchymal stem cell (MSC) differentiation. MSCs are capable of self-renewal. These cells can then undergo expansion as progenitors, before achieving terminal differentiation. This schematic emphasizes the primary differentiation fates of adipogenesis, osteoblastogenesis, and chondrogenesis. While MSCs may be come terminal cells of other tissue types, those cell fates have less relevance in bone regeneration. Each terminal fate is associated with distinct functional markers that can be used to assess differentiation capacity in vitro and in vivo, as described in ▶ Fig. 49.5. FABP, fatty acid binding protein; LPL, lipoprotein lipase.

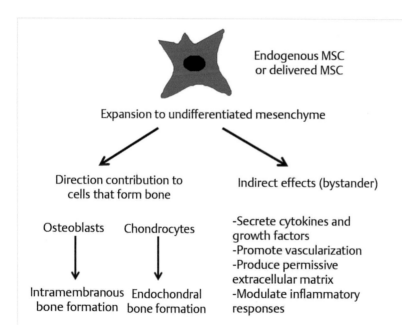

Fig. 49.2 Potential roles of mesenchymal stem cells (MSCs) in bone regeneration. MSCs—whether harvested and cultured or endogenous—may play a variety of roles in bone healing. MSCs can directly differentiate to become bone-forming osteoblasts (intramembranous bone formation) or they can undergo differentiation to become chondrocytes, which then undergo endochondral ossification. Undifferentiated mesenchymal cells can also play indirect roles in bone healing. They produce cytokines and growth factors that drive vascularization and also may recruit other cells involved in later stages of fracture healing. These mesenchymal cells can produce a provisional extracellular matrix that supports healing. Finally, mesenchymal progenitors are immunomodulatory.

properties as "bystander" cells (▶ Fig. 49.2). They produce anti-inflammatory cytokines, are "immunoprivileged," and do not produce a substantial immunological reaction. In addition, they produce additional growth factors that drive the healing cascade, in particular, promoting vascularization. Finally, MSCs also contribute to the production of a provisional matrix that is essential for supporting subsequent phases of the healing cascade. Thus, research has shown the ability of MSCs to modulate healing, repair, and remodeling in tissues such as heart and muscle, even

when not directly contributing to tissue formation. Thus, while MSCs have been a focus for bone tissue engineering because of their ability to form bone and cartilage tissue, the cells could also play additional roles in healing bone.

While stem cells hold great promise for tissue engineering applications to increase bone regeneration, there are a variety of shortcomings that have limited their usefulness. In this chapter, these limitations and methods to address these limitations will be considered. Approaches for isolation, cultivation, differentiation, and delivery will be

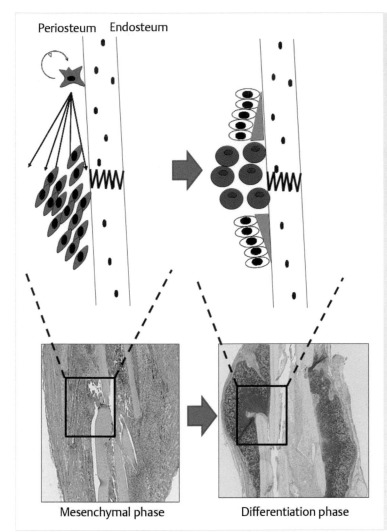

Periosteum Endosteum

Mesenchymal phase   Differentiation phase

Fig. 49.3 Mesenchymal stem cell (MSC) contribution to endochondral and intramembranous bone formation. The illustration demonstrates that MSCs in the periosteum proliferate to form undifferentiated mesenchymal cells (*blue cells*) (mesenchymal phase of healing) that form a soft callus. These MSCs then undergo differentiation to chondrocytes (*red cells*) or osteoblasts that produce osteoid directly (*green*). Histological images demonstrate the appearance of the undifferentiated mesenchyme at the fracture site in the mesenchymal phase. These cells then differentiate to become chondrocytes and bone-forming osteoblasts. Histological images were harvested at day 5 postfracture (mesenchymal phase) or day 10 postfracture (differentiation phase) from mice with closed tibial fractures. Paraffin-embedded decalcified bone sections were stained with safranin-O (red staining).

discussed. Where appropriate, the gaps in our knowledge base and potential strategies for addressing these gaps will be indicated.

49.2 The Physiological Origin of Mesenchymal Stem Cells during Bone Regeneration

Before considering MSCs as a therapeutic to repair bone, it is useful to consider the endogenous origin and function of MSCs during bone regeneration. Bone regeneration is complex, and mesenchymal cells are activated to populate a bone injury site secondary to a poorly described inflammatory response. Interfering with the inflammatory response can decrease mesenchymal influx, but the cytokines that are directly required for inducing mesenchymal influx are not well described. Furthermore, while some literature suggests that both local and distant progenitor cells contribute to repair, must

recent data, using genetic models of cell tracking in mouse models, support the concept that local cells are the primary contributor to healing.

Bone marrow ablation delays fracture repair supporting an essential role for the marrow in bone regeneration; however, whether this is secondary to a loss of MSCs has not been fully established. The strongest evidence of the contribution of MSCs in the marrow to healing bone is developed from studies of mice with genetically engineered, lineage-specific markers that can identify the origin of cells and whether those marked cells develop into osteoblasts or chondrocytes.[3]

Periosteum appears to be the major contributor of MSCs to bone repair (▶ Fig. 49.3). Physical disruption of the periosteum by periosteal stripping delays healing. After injury, periosteal cells proliferate extensively during the mesenchymal phase of healing and then directly develop into both cartilage-forming chondrocytes and bone-forming osteoblasts in the fracture callus. The periosteum is also the primary source of chondrocytes in a gap defect model in a mouse, and this remains true when donor bone is grafted prior to injury so that the periosteum has an endosteal location.[3]

This work was recently extended by another research group working in a mouse model that temporally labels mesenchymal progenitors with a fluorescing protein at the time of fracture. They show definitively that periosteal MSCs have pronounced proliferation and that those cells can become both chondrocytes and osteoblasts. As well, MSCs from the marrow and endosteum also contribute to the healing response, but to a somewhat lesser degree. In this study, the fluorescing protein was expressed based on the expression profile of the alpha smooth muscle actin gene. While this protein is not specific for MSCs, it is a useful marker for cells that show mesenchymal multipotency. In uninjured bone, alpha smooth muscle actin–expressing cells are associated with the vasculature as well localized to the periosteum and are found sporadically in the marrow and endosteum.[4]

Circulating stem cells may also have a minor contribution to endogenous repair; however, there is relatively little evidence of this in experimental models of bone healing. When bone morphogenetic protein (BMP)-containing collagen pellets are implanted in muscle or subcutaneously, this can induce the migration of cells from the marrow to the pellet that can then give rise to both cartilage-forming chondrocytes (which then undergo endochondral ossification) and bone-forming osteoblasts. More definitive proof that endogenous MSCs could migrate from the bone marrow to an injury site was provided with studies of systemic injection of a CXCR4 antagonist, which blocked healing.[5] CXCR4 is an essential receptor involved in cell homing and migration. Similarly, CXCR4 agonists can promote healing. However, presence in low numbers in regenerate tissue is not necessarily indicative of direct contribution to healing, thus whether circulating cells directly contribute to the formation of bone tissue under normal healing situations remains controversial. In most studies of injecting high numbers of MSCs in systemic circulation during the process of bone healing, relatively few cells home to the injury site and those that do likely do not differentiate into osteoblasts or chondrocytes and therefore do not contribute to the callus. However, despite not contributing directly to bone tissue formation, it remains possible that the injection of cells systemically could enhance healing through bystander effects, as previously described (production of proinflammatory cytokines, recruitment of other cell types, etc.).

These studies using lineage-marked mice are extremely valuable in discriminating the origin and fate of cells; however, it is worth considering that at this time the mouse remains the most amenable model for these studies. Studies must be done in larger animal models that more accurately mimic bone healing in humans to best understand the sources of cells into healing bone. This is necessary because if we identify which cell populations give rise to osteoblasts and chondrocytes, and which serve modulatory roles in normal healing bone, we can be guided in a more rational manner as we consider stem cells for therapies.

49.3 Sources of Mesenchymal Stem Cells

While the most relevant sources of MSCs for normal physiological bone repair are the bone and the marrow, MSCs can also be isolated from other tissues. MSCs are present in adipose, muscle, and can systemically circulate. In addition, MSCs can be derived from induced pluripotent cells and from embryonic stem cells. The ideal source of MSCs for bone repair regenerative therapies would be autologous, easily accessible, pain-free, and would result in large amounts of cells that behave in the expected and desired manner.

As previously mentioned, MSCs were first isolated from bone marrow, and bone marrow remains a common source of cells; however, bone marrow–derived MSCs are rare. They occur in every 10,000 to 100,000 nucleated cells, depending on species examined and methodologies utilized for isolation. Therefore, to get a purified population of MSCs requires that they be separated from hematopoietic cells in marrow samples. The first methodology to isolate MSCs involved plating cells on tissue culture plastic and allowing single cells to adhere and to form fibroblastoid colonies. In this case, contaminating hematopoetic cells are removed because they are nonadherent cells, and then the rapidly expanding progenitor populations are able to "out-compete" remaining potential contaminating cells. However, this approach can still result in significant cell heterogeneity (▶ Fig. 49.4).

Bone marrow is readily accessible, and given that surgeons frequently use cancellous autograft for regeneration—which contains marrow in many cases—there is significant orthopedic surgeon comfort in the utilization of marrow as a source of MSCs.[6] Indeed, it is hypothesized that one important positive benefit to healing with autograft material is the potential contribution of transplanted cells; again, it is not well established that the cells from autograft material contribute in any significant manner to healed bone in humans.

An important question to consider regardless of the source of the MSCs is the degree of processing that is required for a viable therapeutic. Specifically, is it necessary to process and isolate the MSCs or is it sufficient to deliver MSCs in admixtures of cells in minimally processed autologous or allogeneic material? These approaches of using minimally processed tissue to deliver "stem cells" have been used clinically, but there is no definitive data in humans to support that these minimally processed samples contribute cells that are involved in bone regeneration.

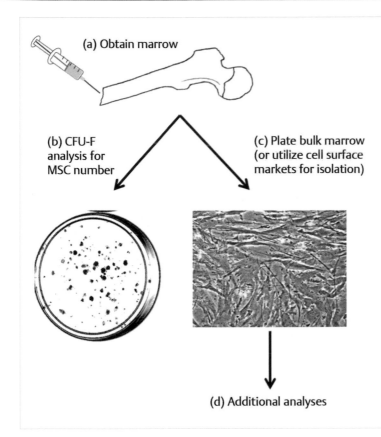

(a) Obtain marrow

(b) CFU-F analysis for MSC number

(c) Plate bulk marrow (or utilize cell surface markets for isolation)

(d) Additional analyses

Fig. 49.4 Mesenchymal stem cell (MSC) harvest and growth. (**a**) MSCs are obtained from a variety of tissues, most commonly marrow. (**b**) Cell suspensions are plated at low density to permit colony formation. Colonies can be stained and enumerated to generate colony forming unit-fibroblast number. (**c**) Bulk marrow can be plated to permit growth of adherent mesenchymal cells. These MSCs can be selected based on cell surface markers using flow-cytometry or magnetic bead separation. (**d**) MSC populations can be assessed for stem cell function and differentiation (▶ Fig. 49.5).

Interestingly, MSCs also exist in solid bone, though there is some controversy about the source of an expanded cell population in these studies. The first studies used bone harvested using curettage or marrow reaming. Marrow is washed from isolated bone and then the bone is treated with collagenase. Bone chips are filtered away, and the cells that remain are plated and proliferate. Cells derived from bone have tridifferentiation potential and are similar to bone marrow–derived MSCs.[7] Despite having fewer total nucleated cells, there are apparently many more MSCs as evaluated using colony forming unit-fibroblast (CFU-F) analysis, suggesting the presence of more MSCs per total nucleated cell. Intriguingly, it is not entirely clear whether the cells that are present in these studies of whole bone are derived from within the bone or whether they exist on bone surfaces, for instance, representing the periosteum or the endosteum. Recent published work using fluorescent labeling shows that cells that can become MSCs may have transdifferentiated from osteocytes that were embedded in bony lacunae.[8]

As previously discussed, periosteum is well recognized both experimentally and clinically as being a primary contributor of cells that form both cartilage and bone at the time of bone injury. It is a well-established standard of care that orthopedic surgeons not disturb or remove periosteum and that indeed when periosteum is removed the ability to heal is decreased. Experimentally, in rodent models, work has clearly shown the essential role of the periosteum in healing, as bone that is stripped of periosteum is incapable of repair. Furthermore, periosteum appears to contribute the bulk of cells to fracture healing in a mouse model.[4] However, although periosteum is plentiful and represents the source of progenitor cells for naturally occurring fracture, it is generally considered a more difficult tissue to harvest compared to bone marrow.[6] In addition, another complicating factor with respect to isolating periosteal cells is that the cellular layer of the periosteum (the cambrium layer) is strongly attached to the bone surface. Thus, developing methodologies that permit the harvest of periosteal donor tissue and cultivation of enough cells could be useful. Alternatively, developing tissue engineering strategies that seek to activate the endogenous periosteal progenitors may hold even greater promise.[3]

Although there is no evidence that adipose tissue is an endogenous source of MSCs for in vivo bone repair, harvesting MSCs from fat presents another possible source for therapeutic use. Adipose-derived MSCs are able to undergo osteogenic, chondrogenic, and adipogenic differentiation similar to MSCs from other tissue types. Adipose is a readily available source of progenitor cells for both autologous and allogeneic applications. Adipose-derived MSCs are present in the stromal vascular fraction of fat and are easily isolated by separating adipose-containing cells from other nucleated cells in fat using density centrifugation. Adipose is easily harvested through lipoaspiration and can then be used to isolate adipose-derived MSCs.[9]

49.4 Mesenchymal Stem Cell Isolation and Enumeration

As previously indicated, initial methods to isolate MSCs utilized their differential adhesion and growth abilities on tissue culture plastic. This is still a method widely used today to isolate MSCs from both humans and animal models (▶ Fig. 49.4). Thus, bulk cell extracts are plated at high density (because of the relative rarity of MSCs in marrow), and the fibroblastoid MSCs will adhere to tissue culture substratum and then proliferate. MSCs can also be identified and isolated using cell-surface markers coupled with either laser-assisted flow cytometry or magnetic bead separation methods.[10] A spectrum of cell surface markers have been shown to be useful for isolating MSCs, although, as opposed to hematopoietic stem cells, a "gold standard" for isolating MSCs does not exist. Further complicating isolating MSCs using cell sorting is that cell surface markers remain poorly described in mouse models. The first antibody shown to isolate human MSC was the antibody Stro1. Stro1-positive cells were shown to have MSC properties. Continued refinements in the identification of markers of human MSCs have identified CD156 as a potential useful, MSC-specific marker. Additional common cell surface markers, albeit, not a complete list, and not specific for MSC, have included CD44, Sca1, Thy1, CD105, and CD106. Most cell surface antibody approaches to identify MSCs use a combination of positive and negative cell surface selection, specifically negatively selecting for hematopoietic origin cells (CD45 negative) such as monocyte cells (CD11b negative).

The gold standard for enumerating the number of isolated MSCs is based on their ability to form fibroblastoid colonies when plated on plastic. Numerous studies have shown that the number of CFU-F is directly correlated with the number of endogenous progenitors (▶ Fig. 49.4). Essentially, MSCs are plated to plastic in limited dilution, and then single cells will form individual colonies derived from a single parent progenitor cell. These colonies show significant heterogeneity in growth based on colony size. These same colonies can also be assessed for multipotency—particularly osteoblastogenesis and chondrogenesis (and adipogenesis)—using protocols that will be described in the next section and in ▶ Fig. 49.5. Comparing MSCs from different sources has consistently shown that bone marrow–derived MSCs form fewer colonies than when derived from adipose or periosteum, respectively. In addition, it is worth noting that CFU-F numbers decrease with age and with unloading of bone, and a variety of genetically modified mouse models have shown

---

Evaluating putative MSC

1. Is a cell an MSC?
   a. Can single cells be massively expanded (clonal expansion) and do those cells show the ability to differentiate to osteoblasts and/or chondrocytes both in vitro and in vivo?
      - Isolate single MSC
   b. Can the cells be passaged and maintain multipotency?
   c. Can the cells replace ablated tissue (bone injury)?
2. What is the functionality of an MSC?
   a. How many MSC in a mixed population of cells?
      - Measure using CRU-F assay
   b. What is the proliferation potential of the MSC?
      - Measure using cell counting; cell cycle analysis; DNA content; 3H incorporation; metabolic activity
   c. What is the differentiation potential of the MSC?
   d. Can the MSC maintain multipotency over passage?
   e. Can the MSC ocontribute to form bone and/or cartilage tissue in vivo or in bone regeneration models?

Evaluating MSC differentiation potential for fracture

3. Evaluating osteoblastogenesis
   a. In vitro
      - Gene expression (bone specific genes such as osteocalcin; bone sialoprotein, alkaline phosphatase)
      - Protein production (alkaline phosphatase activity, osteocalcin production)
      - Mineralization (stain with calcium binding dye)
   b. In vivo
      - Subcutaneous implantation of MSC on ceramic carriers
      - Delivery to a bone injury site
4. Evaluating chondrogenesis
   a. In vitro
      - Various culture methodologies, including Hanging-drop, high-density monolayer culture, Pellet culture
      - Gene expression (aggrecan, type II collagen)
      - Proteoglycan production (GAG content, stain with Alcian blue)
      - Cartilage formation (histology to demonstrate chondrocyte cells in cartilage tissue)
   b. In vivo
      - Can cartilage that is formed in vitro develop into bone when implanted in vivo at ectopic sites or during bone regeneration sites?

Fig. 49.5 Approaches to evaluate mesenchymal stem cells (MSCs). It is essential to validate MSCs prior to potential clinical application. (a) Determining whether a putative MSC is truly a stem cell can be done by demonstrating, expansion, self-renewal, and multipotency, and finally, the contribution of these cells to repopulating injured tissue can be assessed. (b) Numerous differentiation protocols exist for assessing osteoblastogenesis and chondrogenesis, using a battery of cellular and molecular assays.

differences CFU-F depending on whether the gene products have a positive or negative effect on the MSC lineage.

49.5 Mesenchymal Stem Cell Self-Renewal and Proliferation

Gold standards for defining a stem cell include the demonstration of extensive self-renewal and tissue repopulation (reconstitution) (▶ Fig. 49.5a). A self-renewing cell should be capable of long-term cell division in an undifferentiated state to expand the pool of cells that can then undergo differentiation. Self-renewal can occur in a symmetric manner, meaning the two daughters cells are both undifferentiated stem cells, or in an asymmetric manner, where one daughter cell is capable of ongoing proliferation while the other is more differentiated. The process of asymmetric self-renewal has not been definitively demonstrated for MSCs, and in fact, very few studies have demonstrated MSC self-renewal in an in vivo context. In vitro self-renewal can be shown by multiple cell divisions and expansion of the pool of undifferentiated cells. However, expansion must occur in an undifferentiated state, and in many cases, MSCs under in vitro expansion conditions undergo changes consistent with differentiation. Developing enhanced methods for growing and expanding MSCs and maintaining multipotency is essential.

Demonstrating self-renewal in vivo is something that would be done most effectively with murine models by showing that cells can be discretely identified and that daughter cells can be serially transplanted. This has been a technically challenging experiment because of the limited engraftment of MSCs, particularly to bone and cartilage, and then also because issues of poor cell surface markers for isolation of murine MSCs are also complicating factors.

Similar to issues with demonstrating self-renewal, there are significant concerns with demonstrating repopulation/reconstitution of musculoskeletal tissues by putative MSCs. While repopulation ability has been a hallmark of hematopoietic stem cells, as well as cancer stem cells, the ability of isolated MSCs to form a complete bone or cartilage entity in vivo is technically challenging. A few research groups have elegantly demonstrated the ability of a limited numbers of MSCs to form bone-like ossicles when implanted subcutaneously in matrix carriers, and these experiments are surrogates for demonstration of MSC to expand, differentiate, and repopulate.

49.6 Mesenchymal Differentiation and the Ability to Form Bone and Cartilage

The final set of experiments that define a cell as a stem cell is the ability to differentiate to a terminal fated cell type both in vitro and in vivo (in the case of MSCs for the purposes of this chapter, osteoblasts and chondrocytes) (▶ Fig. 49.5b).

Standard protocols for assessing differentiation to osteoblast and chondrocyte lineage exist and are readily available. Many factors are known to influence MSC differentiation to both the chondrocyte and osteoblast lineages. Growth factors that have been used to regulate MSC differentiation include but are not limited to BMP, fibroblast growth factor, Notch, transforming growth factor (TGF)-beta, and Wnt ligands.[11] In addition, other physiologic stimuli, such as hypoxia, cell-to-cell interaction, cell adhesion, and mechanical loading, can influence osteoblastogenesis and chondrogenesis.

Manipulating BMP signaling is undoubtedly the standard approach for inducing osteoblastogenesis and can also induce chondrogenesis in the correct physiological context, whereas induction of MSCs with TGF-beta is appropriate and the gold standard for induction to chondrogenesis.

BMPs were first isolated as proteins capable of inducing both intramembranous and endochondral bone formation. Both BMP and TGF-beta proteins are members of the TGF-beta superfamily and bind to heterodimeric receptor complexes on cell surfaces. Receptor binding leads to phosphorylation of Smad proteins, which enables their activity as transcription factors for many downstream target genes. For osteoblastogenesis, one of the characteristic target genes is *Runx2*. *Runx2* is a master regulator of osteoblastogenesis. Downstream of *Runx2* expression is the expression of the transcription factor Osterix, which has also been shown to be required for mineralization of the skeleton. While BMP2, 4, and 7 have been most highly studied as osteoblast differentiation inducers, a variety of other BMPs also induce MSC osteoblastogenesis.

Downstream of TGF-beta signaling through SMADs for chondrogenesis is the activation of the Sox trio of transcription factors. Sox9 in particular is required for chondrogenesis. While much of the work on MSC differentiation to chondrocytes has been related to the development of articular chondrocytes, in reality maintenance of chondrocytes in an articular chondrocyte state is extremely challenging and in general MSCs that are induced to become chondrocytes invariably will undergo hypertrophy and terminal differentiation to mineralization, and then undergo endochondral ossification.

Wnt/beta-catenin signaling is another growth factor signaling pathway that influences the differentiation of both osteoblasts and chondrocytes. In canonical Wnt signaling, Wnt molecules bind to a frizzled receptor and interact with LRP coreceptors, leading to the accumulation and translocation of beta-catenin to the nucleus where it interacts with T-cell–specific factor and lymphoid enhancer-binding factor 1. Wnts can also signal in a noncanonical manner, and in this case do not increase beta-catenin. In general, canonical Wnt signal stimulates osteoblastogenesis and regulates proper endochondral ossification. However, the effects of Wnt signaling on MSC function are complex and influenced by the cell type, receptors, Wnts that are present, and both the presence and absence of inhibitory and activating cofactors, such as sclerostin (inhibitor) or Rspondins (activators).

Notch signaling is a third prominent growth factor that regulates MSC differentiation. Notch is a transmembrane receptor and interacts with a ligand that is also membrane bound on adjacent cells. Proteolytic cleavage of Notch liberates the Notch intracellular domain, which then translocates to the nucleus where it binds to CSL along with the coactivator Mastermind-like, activating the transcription of a variety of genes, including the canonical Hey and Hes family genes. It is interesting to note that Hey/Hes transcription factors are also activated by BMP signaling. Notch effects on osteoblastogenesis and chondrogenesis are complex. Notch signaling appears to inhibit the initial differentiation phase of bipotent MSCs to enter chondrogenic and osteogenic lineages, and maintain self-renewal and multipotency. Similarly during osteogenesis, enhanced Notch signaling appears to enhance committed preosteoblasts but inhibits terminal differentiation. Finally, Notch signaling appears to be primarily inhibitory to early stages of chondrogenesis but is required for terminal hypertrophic chondrocyte differentiation.

It is interesting to note that differentiation of MSCs to osteoblasts or chondrocytes is also influenced by mechanical cues. MSC that are in high-density nonadherent cultures—either as pellets or using hanging drop methods or sequestered in various nonadhesive biomaterials—are more prone to undergo chondrogenesis, whereas MSCs that adhere to tissue culture plates or mineralized surfaces will undergo differentiation to osteoblasts. Terminal osteoblast differentiation also requires collagen maturation with ascorbic acid and a phosphate donor source to be able to form the calcium phosphate crystal, hydroxyapatite, which is the base mineralized structure of bone.

49.7 Utilizing Mesenchymal Stem Cells Clinically to Heal Bone

Autologous bone grafting remains a gold standard for promoting healing of hard-to-heal long bone fractures, particularly in situations where there is endogenous bone loss. Bone grafting provides both scaffolding as well as endogenous living bone tissue that contains growth factors and endogenous cells. However, autologous bone grafting can result in donor site morbidity and there is a limit to the amount of obtainable tissue. For those clinical scenarios where autologous bone grafting is undesirable, devitalized and sterilized allografts are readily available.

While allograft material can serve as a scaffold and filler, it lacks viable cells, and there is likely a significant limitation to bioactive growth factors that may be present in the processed tissue. Recombinant proteins—specifically BMP2 and BMP7—have been used clinically to promote bone repair; however, there has been a limit to the efficacy of growth factor delivery for bone repair. Therefore, utilizing MSC-based therapies to promote bone regeneration remains a reasonable clinical goal. Unfortunately, to date, the utilization of isolated and grown MSCs, whether autologous or allogeneic, to heal bone has not gained widespread acceptance or regulatory approval. Specifically, additional research must seek to better understand both normal and deficient healing to determine ideal clinical scenarios for MSC-based therapies. Equally important, there must be recognition that not all healing scenarios are the same; thus, designing comparative animal model experiments that mimic specific clinical human scenarios is an absolute necessity. For instance, long bone healing models that utilize both intramembranous and endochondral bone healing are likely very different from highly stabilized gap defect models that heal primarily through intramembranous bone formation. Thus, MSC-based bone regeneration therapeutic approaches could take one of several approaches depending on the clinical scenario of clinical need. Specifically, a number of issues must be better considered to develop the clinical utility of MSCs for bone regeneration:

1. Activation of endogenous MSCs versus delivery of isolated MSCs
2. Autologous versus allogenic cell sources
3. Tissue sources of MSCs
4. MSC pretreatment methodologies
5. Delivery approaches of MSCs

These five considerations will be discussed in the following subsections.

49.7.1 Activating Endogenous Mesenchymal Stem Cells Using Growth Factors

Whether there is a deficiency in MSCs at fracture sites remains controversial. Clearly in some clinical situations, where there is a profound loss of tissue, or in some cases of poor healing, for example, with geriatric fracture healing, there may be a deficiency in endogenous MSCs. However, in many cases, endogenous MSC numbers may be sufficient for proper healing, but a deficiency may exist in MSC activation, thus, a viable clinical approach is that endogenous MSCs can be activated by delivery of osteoinductive factors.

As mentioned, the delivery of purified growth factor to a bone injury site can activate both intramembranous and endochondral bone formation, but clinical results over the past decade with recombinant BMP to promote long bone healing have been less successful than predicted with animal models. Due to their potent osteoinductive effects—even at ectopic sites—BMPs cannot be given systemically, necessitating treatment at the site of fracture. Activating of growth factor pathways other than BMP is possible; however, none of the possible systemic treatments for bone regeneration is currently approved. For instance, the Wnt signaling pathway can be stimulated using systemically administered agents to increase bone formation. There is clinical development of antibodies to block two Wnt signaling inhibitors, Dickkopf 1 (Dkk1) and Sclerostin. Blocking Dkk with a systemically administered antibody in a murine fracture model increased bone healing. Sclerostin binds to Wnt molecules blocking signaling, and antibodies that block scerlostin have been developed clinically to increase bone mass. Sclerostin antibodies could be similarly used to enhance bone regeneration.[12] Therapeutics based on the parathyroid hormone 1–34 amino acid sequences are clinically used to restore lost bone in osteoporosis, and similarly a parathyroid hormone–based therapeutic could be used to activate local bone formation for bone healing. While these systemic agents show significant promise for enhancing bone healing, there is a need to continue to develop both locally and systemically delivered therapeutics to enhance fracture healing by activating endogenous MSCs. However, to achieve this goal will require continued basic science research both of MSCs in vitro as well as an enhanced understanding of signals in vivo that promote MSC activation.

A relatively common readily available source of osteoinductive growth factors that is used in fracture repair is platelet-rich plasma. Platelet-rich plasma contains many growth factors and has been shown to improve fracture repair both in controlled studies and in case studies. Similarly, demineralized bone matrix (DBM) contains osteoinductive growth factors that exist embedded in bone tissue; however, the positive effects of DBM on bone regeneration may have more to do with the scaffold properties of DBM as opposed to the growth factors, which have been shown to be highly variable in concentration and dependent upon processing. Both the utilization of DBM and/or platelet-rich plasma to activate endogenous MSCs requires greater research in animal models. There may be clinical scenarios whereby these cheaper alternatives to purified growth factors could be useful adjuncts to activating MSCs, but controlled studies in animal models assessing the usefulness in conditions where MSC activation is documented to be deficient will be required.

49.7.2 Autologous versus Allogeneic Mesenchymal Stem Cells

Because of their inherent immunomodulatory properties, it is conceivable that allogeneic MSCs can be used therapeutically. Allogeneic MSCs are being pursued as clinical therapeutics for a number of potential therapeutic disease areas. The potential benefit of using allogeneic cells is that "off-the-shelf" MSC-based therapeutics could be developed as opposed to the need to harvest and cultivate autologous MSCs from a patient at the time of surgery. Animal models have used allogeneic MSCs in a variety of species and bone healing models, but relatively few of these studies have directly compared the performance of allogeneic and autologous cells to determine which may perform more optimally. Furthermore, in these comparisons, it will be necessary to evaluate whether any potential positive benefits are based on the implanted cells contributing directly to new tissue formation or whether they play a more important bystander role in recruiting endogenous cells. These types of analyses will be most amenable to animal models, whereby transplanted cells can be tracked both noninvasively and invasively.

49.7.3 Ideal Tissue Source for Isolation of Mesenchymal Stem Cells

MSCs were first isolated from bone marrow, and thus the majority of studies that investigate either in vitro differentiation characteristics or in vivo healing potential have focused on bone marrow–derived cells. Work that directly compares osteoblastogenesis of bone marrow–derived MSCs to adipose-derived MSCa (the next most common MSC source for bone regeneration studies) shows that the bone marrow–derived MSCs have much greater osteoblast potential both in vitro and in vivo relative to the adipose cells. On the other hand, adipose-derived MSCs appear much more likely to differentiate to become adipocytes. Similar to osteoblast differentiation, more research has focused on bone marrow–derived MSC chondrogenesis rather than adipose-derived MSCs, but the adipose-derived MSCs are fully capable of chondrogenic differentiation. Most research on the delivery of MSCs for bone regeneration has similarly focused on bone marrow–derived MSC, relative to adipose-derived MSCs. The direct comparison of delivered cells from various tissue sources in promoting bone regeneration is somewhat limited; however, the few studies that have directly compared in vivo long bone healing capacity of bone marrow–derived MSCs and adipose-derived MSCs suggest that those from bone marrow show enhanced capacity to promote bone healing; however, the results are not entirely definitive, as some studies suggest that adipose-derived cells perform as well as bone marrow.

MSCs from other cell sources have also been studied in bone regeneration, including MSCs from umbilicus, Wharton's jelly, and periosteum, but results to date are not definitive. Regardless of the direct ability of MSCs from any source to become bone-forming osteoblasts or chondrocytes that can go through endochondral ossification, MSCs can of course still play important roles in recruiting of endogenous cell types, immunomodulation, or as vehicles for delivery of bone inducing growth factors, such as BMPs, which can then activate endogenous MSCs to regenerate bone.

49.7.4 Pretreatment Approaches for Isolated Mesenchymal Stem Cells

Two other factors that must be considered with respect to the isolation, cultivation, and delivery of MSCs are determining ideal methods for expansion of cells in an undifferentiated manner, and then determining whether it is advisable to pretreat the cells with differentiation inducers prior to implantation.

Methodologies for expanding MSCs in an undifferentiated state have been described, including using serum-free growth media supplemented with growth factors. Extensive research over the past 15 years has particularly demonstrated that growing MSCs in the presence of fibroblast growth factor-2 (or basic fibroblast growth factor) maintains the cells in an undifferentiated state and permits rapid expansion of the cells. Growth in hypoxic conditions has also been suggested as a mechanism to expand MSCs. However, there are relatively few direct comparisons of different cultivation methods for MSCs that have extended the studies to in vivo bone regeneration models, and this would be a necessary requirement to understanding best growth conditions for MSCs that are used therapeutically.

With respect to the pretreatment of cells to become osteoblasts or chondrocytes prior to therapeutic utilization, a variety of animal studies have shown that osteoblast preinduction can result in more implanted cells becoming osteoblasts. Most of these models have used subcutaneous implantation of cells, but similar results have been obtained using bone regeneration models. Alternatively, inducing chondrogenesis via TGF-beta prior to implanting MSCs on a scaffold allowed for endochondral ossification rather than the intramembranous ossification.[13] Another approach to use implanted MSCs to drive endochondral ossification could be to develop three-dimensional cartilage constructs in vitro using biomaterials and then directly implanting those constructs. Implantation of preformed cartilage in this manner has been used in at least one recently published report, and this approach could hold new promise as a method for utilizing MSCs for bone regeneration.

49.7.5 Delivery Approaches of Mesenchymal Stem Cells to Heal Bone

When we consider delivery of harvested MSCs to bone, there are several strategies that can be evaluated

(▶ Fig. 49.6). MSCs can be locally delivered—the most common approach—or systemically delivered. Direct delivery of MSCs to the fracture site in the simplest manner could include the implantation of autologous bone grafts and/or bone marrow aspirates. These sources contain MSCs that can undergo both chondrogenic and osteoblastogenic differentiation, but MSCs exist in these preparations in very low numbers. The robustness of healing and the timing of healing is directly related to MSC concentration, and thus if the purpose of marrow aspirates or autologous bone treatment is delivery of MSCs, then these cell delivery approaches are not ideal. To optimize these approaches, it would be ideal to be able to concentrate the MSC numbers in the samples. Commercially available products sold as bone-grafting agents that attempt to concentrate cell numbers and perhaps purify MSCs are used clinically. These products attempt to isolate and concentrate autograft or allograft cells before reimplantation—some of which are MSCs; however, few studies have been published that examine the bone regeneration capacities of these concentrated cell products.

The advantage of isolated, purified, and expanded MSCs being delivered directly rather than harvesting mixed cell populations of bone marrow is that it can allow for the profound expansion of stem cells that can then be highly concentrated. It is well described that the extent of bone formation in vivo is directly related to cell number, thus this a potential advantage of isolating and expanding MSCs. Furthermore, separation of MSCs from non-MSCs has advantages in that potentially deleterious or unexpected effects of non-MSCs can be eliminated. However, there are potential concerns with isolating MSCs, cultivating them, and expanding the number of progenitors, namely tissue culture processing of the cells in vitro may alter the behavior and bone healing capacity. Work from a variety of investigators has demonstrated that increased cell passage of MSCs will decrease osteogenic and chondrogenic capacity, thus a need to balance expanding cell numbers with maintenance of ideal differentiation characteristics becomes crucially important.

Mechanisms to directly deliver isolated MSCs could include direct injection or implanting them in a carrier (▶ Fig. 49.6). Most frequently, experimental approaches have used MSCs in combination with an osteoconductive scaffold ("tissue engineering strategy"), whereas fewer experimental studies have attempted direct percutaneous injection of isolated cells.

The benefits of delivering MSCs on a wide variety of mineralized and nonmineralized scaffolds has been validated in many animal models, including mice, rats, rabbits, dogs, sheep, and goats, over the past 20 years since first described in a canine model by Bruder et al in 1998.[14] These studies have used not only simple long bone fracture models, but complete and partial long bone defects, as well as calvarial defects. The results of these

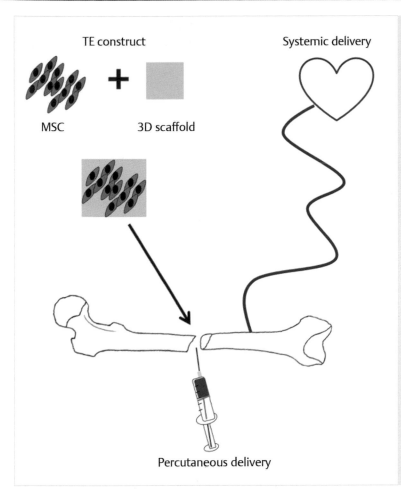

TE construct

MSC   +   3D scaffold

Systemic delivery

Percutaneous delivery

Fig. 49.6 Mesenchymal stem cell (MSC) delivery for bone regeneration. (**a**) The most common approach for delivering MSCs is in combination with a matrix carrier. (**b**) MSCs can also be delivered systemically via venous injection. (**c**) Another approach to deliver MSCs is the direct injection of cells at a site of injury. New biomaterials as well as some naturally occurring biomatrices permit injection and then when in the body the injected solutions can solidify to generate a three-dimensional (3D) structure that maintains cells at an injury site. TE, tissue engineering.

studies have been somewhat variable. While many models do show that MSCs can contribute to increased bone regeneration, whether the MSCs do this via directly forming tissue or directing local cells to form more bone is less clear. Furthermore, variability in responses may be associated with many factors that have already been discussed including cell dose, delivery approaches, ideal cultivation conditions, or the experimental models that are utilized.

Isolated and tissue culture–expanded MSCs can also be directly injected in the systemic circulation. The advantages of systemic, venous delivery of MSCs are obvious, in that an MSC-based therapeutic would be easily administered. Unfortunately, experimental approaches to deliver MSCs systemically for bone healing have been somewhat hampered by early observations that MSCs showed a propensity to be sequestered in either the liver or the lungs. This observation necessitated extensive research that focused on developing better systemic delivery approaches. Those studies that have been successful with systemic delivery of MSCs in animal models show that MSCs will home directly to sites of bone injury preferentially, when administered systemically, but they have not been shown to directly contribute to healing in this context by

becoming bone-forming cells.[15] Whether the systemically delivered MSCs may have indirect effects on healing has not been well established. Thus, more extensive research will need to be completed to determine whether there are potential benefits of systemic delivery and whether the effects are related to direct differentiation of the cells to become bone-forming osteoblasts or chondrocytes or whether the effects are indirect.

49.8 Conclusion

Utilizing MSCs to promote bone regeneration has profound clinical potential. Research must focus on determining whether ideal therapeutic approaches attempt to activate endogenous MSCs, utilize minimally processed samples that contain some MSCs (e.g., marrow or autologous bone), or whether it is better to use harvested MSCs that have been cultivated in vitro. Likely, the ideal therapeutic approach will be highly dependent upon each unique clinical scenario. Some situations may be more amenable to activating endogenous cells, whereas others may require the delivery of expanded and processed cells. Research must focus on better understanding normal fracture biology, as well as understanding the pathogenesis behind deficient healing. Particular emphasis must be placed on an improved understanding that different bones in different clinical situations likely will benefit from differing treatment approaches.

If it is determined that using isolated MSCs is the best therapeutic approach for a given condition, research must continue to focus on developing a more nuanced understanding of normal MSC biology, including how various growth factors and the resultant signaling pathways can activate differentiation or maintain pluripotency and self-renewal. Research must focus on comparing different cell sources, isolation methods, and delivery methods in animal models that are relevant to a wide variety of human bone regeneration conditions (▶ Fig. 49.5).

While this review has focused on MSCs in bone regeneration, it is also notable that investigative groups continue to pursue MSCs for repair of other musculoskeletal tissues, including but not limited to muscle, tendon, ligament, and articular cartilage. Indeed, much work has focused on using MSCs to repair damaged articular cartilage. MSCs readily form chondrocytes, as discussed throughout this chapter, but the two biggest hurdles to clinical translation are the inability to maintain the phenotype of MSC-derived cartilage by preventing cartilage mineralization and the lack of integration of cartilage engineered from MSC with native cartilage. Many of the technical considerations and perspectives on MSCs presented with respect to bone healing are readily transferable to repair of other musculoskeletal tissues, including cartilage. Any MSC-based therapy, whether for bone healing, cartilage healing, or healing of tendon, ligament, meniscus, or muscle, must have a solid foundation in understanding normal and pathological healing as well as a full understanding of the biology of the MSC.

References

[1] Friedenstein AJ. Osteogenic stem cells in the bone marrow. Bone and Min Res 1990; 7: 243–272

[2] Caplan AI. Mesenchymal stem cells. J Orthop Res 1991; 9: 641–650

[3] Colnot C. Skeletal cell fate decisions within periosteum and bone marrow during bone regeneration. J Bone Miner Res 2009; 24: 274–282

[4] Grcevic D, Pejda S, Matthews BG et al. In vivo fate mapping identifies mesenchymal progenitor cells. Stem Cells 2012; 30: 187–196

[5] Pitchford SC, Furze RC, Jones CP, Wengner AM, Rankin SM. Differential mobilization of subsets of progenitor cells from the bone marrow. Cell Stem Cell 2009; 4: 62–72

[6] Colnot C. Cell sources for bone tissue engineering: insights from basic science. Tissue Eng Part B Rev 2011; 17: 449–457

[7] Tuli R, Seghatoleslami MR, Tuli S et al. A simple, high-yield method for obtaining multipotential mesenchymal progenitor cells from trabecular bone. Mol Biotechnol 2003; 23: 37–49

[8] Torreggiani E, Matthews BG, Pejda S et al. Preosteocytes/osteocytes have the potential to dedifferentiate becoming a source of osteoblasts. PLoS ONE 2013; 8: e75204

[9] Levi B, Longaker MT. Concise review: adipose-derived stromal cells for skeletal regenerative medicine. Stem Cells 2011; 29: 576–582

[10] Kode JA, Mukherjee S, Joglekar MV, Hardikar AA. Mesenchymal stem cells: immunobiology and role in immunomodulation and tissue regeneration. Cytotherapy 2009; 11: 377–391

[11] Lin GL, Hankenson KD. Integration of BMP, Wnt, and notch signaling pathways in osteoblast differentiation. J Cell Biochem 2011; 112: 3491–3501

[12] Tian X, Jee WS, Li X, Paszty C, Ke HZ. Sclerostin antibody increases bone mass by stimulating bone formation and inhibiting bone resorption in a hindlimb-immobilization rat model. Bone 2011; 48: 197–201

[13] Janicki P, Kasten P, Kleinschmidt K, Luginbuehl R, Richter W. Chondrogenic pre-induction of human mesenchymal stem cells on beta-TCP: enhanced bone quality by endochondral heterotopic bone formation. Acta Biomater 2010; 6: 3292–3301

[14] Bruder SP, Kraus KH, Goldberg VM, Kadiyala S. The effect of implants loaded with autologous mesenchymal stem cells on the healing of canine segmental bone defects. J Bone Joint Surg Am 1998; 80: 985–996

[15] Ushiku C, Adams DJ, Jiang X, Wang L, Rowe DW. Long bone fracture repair in mice harboring GFP reporters for cells within the osteoblastic lineage. J Orthop Res 2010; 28: 1338–1347

Further Reading

Bianco P, Robey PG, Simmons PJ. Mesenchymal stem cells: revisiting history, concepts, and assays. Cell Stem Cell 2008; 2: 313–319

Colnot C. Cell sources for bone tissue engineering: insights from basic science. Tissue Eng Part B Rev 2011; 17: 449–457

Dimarino AM, Caplan AI, Bonfield TL. Mesenchymal stem cells in tissue repair. Front Immunol 2013; 4: 201

Fleming JE, Jr, Cornell CN, Muschler GF. Bone cells and matrices in orthopedic tissue engineering. Orthop Clin North Am 2000; 31: 357–374

Owen M, Friedenstein AJ. Stromal stem cells: marrow-derived osteogenic precursors. Ciba Found Symp 1988; 136: 42–60

50 Biological Evaluation and Testing of Medical Devices

Dieter R. Dannhorn

In order to exclude potential biological hazards or to control residual risks as much as possible, the consolidated Medical Device Directive 93/42/EEC (MDD)[1] and the Active Implantable Medical Device Directive 90/385/EEC (AIMDD),[2] request that medical device manufacturers establish a risk management process pursuant to European Norm (EN) International Organization for Standardization (ISO) 14971.[3] This risk management process must include, among others, a comprehensive and conclusive biological evaluation. For this purpose, the provisions of EN ISO 10993–1[4] and, as applicable, of the 18 subparts of this basic standard must be observed. For some particular medical devices, even specific product-related international standards have been developed, which must be observed in addition to the aforementioned EN ISO 10993 series of standards. Such product specific "vertical" standards are, for example, EN ISO 11979–5 for intraocular lenses,[5] EN ISO 9394 for contact lenses and contact lens care products,[6] and EN ISO 7405 for medical devices used in dentistry.[7]

With only a few exceptions, all aforementioned international standards have been harmonized under the MDD and the AIMDD. Harmonized standards are European standards that were elaborated at the instigation of the European Commission and that were finally referenced in the *Official Journal of the European Union* (OJEU).

Based upon the regulation of the MDD and the AIMDD, "Member states shall presume compliance with the essential requirements to Article 3 in respect of devices which are in conformity with the relevant national standards adopted pursuant to the harmonized standards the reference of which have been published in the Official Journal of the European Union" (MDD Article 5.1). Consequently, if medical device manufacturers deliver documented evidence that they have complied with harmonized standards, European competent authorities as well as European notified bodies will presume conformity with the applicable essential requirements as mentioned in Article 3 and listed in Annex I of the applicable MDD.

Based upon this regulatory background, harmonized standards are of particular importance and must be observed during the whole life cycle of a medical device.

A complete and updated list of harmonized standards applicable for medical devices is available from the European Commission's homepage (▶ Table 50.1).

Therefore, in order to give documented evidence for the biocompatibility of a medical device, the EN ISO 10993 series of standards provides appropriate and reliable guidance as to which aspects are to be considered for the biological safety assessment and how this assessment is being performed based upon testing and literature research within a risk management process.

It shall be noted that the EN ISO 10993 series of standards still allows room for interpretation, and, therefore, may not fully satisfy non-European regulators. With the aim to provide more precise rules, additional standards and guidelines were developed by certain national organizations which must be observed for medical device registrations in certain countries such the United States and Japan:

- U.S. Food and Drug Administration (FDA) Blue Book Memorandum # G95–1: Use of International Standard ISO 10993, "Biological Evaluation of Medical Devices—Part 1: Evaluation and Testing"[8]
- New U.S. Food and Drug Administration draft guidance: Use of International Standard ISO- 10993, "Biological Evaluation of Medical Devices Part 1: Evaluation and Testing," issued on April 23, 2013[9]
- American Society for Testing of Materials F748–06 (2010) Standard Practice for Selecting Generic Biological Test Methods for Materials and Devices[10]
- Ministry of Health, Labour and Welfare Notification No. 0213001: Basic Principles of Biological Safety Evaluation Required for Application for Approval to manufacture (Import) Medical Devices. February 13, 2003[11]
- Notification Number 36 of the Japanese Pharmaceutical and Food Safety Bureau, Ministry of Health, Labour and Welfare, March 19, 2003: "Test Methods for Biological Safety Evaluation of Medical Devices, Assessment of Medical Devices"[12]

Table 50.1 Harmonized Standards for Medical Devices

Type of device	Applicable directive	Internet link
Active implantable medical devices	AIMDD 90/380/EEC	http://eur-lex.europa.eu/LexUriServ/LexUriServ.do?uri=OJ:C:2013:022:0001:0006:EN:PDF; OJEU 022 dated 24/01/2013
All other medical devices except in vitro diagnostic devices	MDD 93/42/EEC	http://eur-lex.europa.eu/legal-content/EN/TXT/PDF/?uri=uriserv:OJ.C_.2014.149.01.0003.01.ENG; OJEU 149 dated 16/05/2014

These national regulations are intended to be more stringent than the basic EN ISO 10993–1 standard, giving less room for interpretation. For Japanese submissions, medical device manufacturers must be prepared to do some additional testing in compliance with Japanese requirements, as the technical conduct of certain biological tests as well as the respective biological end points differ from the ISO requirements.

Jargon Simplified: Abbreviations

- AIMDD: Active Implantable Medical Device Directive 90/385/EC
- ASTM: American Society for Testing of Materials
- EN: European Norm
- FDA: U.S. Food and Drug Administration
- ISO: International Organization for Standardization
- MDD: Medical Device Directive 93/42/EEC
- OJEU: Official Journal of the European Union
- MHLW: Japanese Ministry of Health, Labour and Welfare

Jargon Simplified: Terms and Definitions (EN ISO 10993–1; EN ISO 14971)

- Final product: Medical device in its "as-used" state, as defined by the manufacturer's specifications or labeling
- Material: Any synthetic or natural polymer, metal, alloy, ceramic, or other nonviable substance ... used as a medical device or any part thereof
- Harm: Physical injury or damage to the health of people, or damage to property or the environment Hazard: Potential source of harm
- Risk: Combination of the probability of occurrence of harm and the severity of that harm

---

50.1 Historical Development of European Norm International Organization for Standardization 10993 Series of Standards

Since 1989, European Committee for Standardization/Technical Committee 206—in liaison with ISO/Technical Committee 194—developed standards to guide the biological safety assessment of medical devices and to propose appropriate test and evaluation procedures. Meanwhile, 18 working groups have become active[13] and developed 25 published ISO standards (number includes updates), with active contribution of 22 countries and 25 additional countries observing the process.[14]

With regard to the EN ISO 10993 series of standards, the standards in ▶ Table 50.2 have been prepared by the various Working Groups of European Committee for Standardization/Technical Committee 206 and ISO/Technical Committee 194.

The standardization work is not completed after publishing a final version or after formal harmonization by referencing the standard in the *Official Journal of the European Union*. Based upon the regulations of the ISO, all standards are being reviewed regularly and, if necessary, revised. Therefore, ▶ Table 50.2 only represents the current status of standardization (November 2012). Furthermore, additional standards will be prepared if needed. Therefore, ISO/TC 194 WG 17 is currently working on biocompatibility issues of nanomaterials.

Jargon Simplified: Abbreviations

- CEN/TC: European Committee for Standardization/Technical Committee working on a particular topic
- ISO/TC: International Standardization Organization/Technical Committee working on a particular topic
- ISO/TS: International Standardization Organization/Technical Specification

---

50.2 Biological Categorization of Medical Devices

Following the categorization rules of EN ISO 10993–1 Chapter 5, the following categorization by nature of body contact must be considered for the purpose of defining an appropriate biological evaluation program:
1. **Surface-contacting devices** with contact to
   - Intact skin surfaces
   - Intact mucosal membranes
   - Breached or compromised body surfaces
2. **External communicating devices** with contact to
   - Blood path, indirect contact to the blood path for entry into the vascular system
   - Tissue, bone, or dentin
   - Circulating blood
3. **Implant devices** with contact to
   - Tissue or bone
   - Blood

Further to this, the following categorization regarding duration of body contact is proposed:
1. **Limited exposure:** Devices whose cumulative single, multiple, or repeated use or contact is up to 24 hours
2. **Prolonged exposure:** Devices whose cumulative single, multiple, or repeated use or contact is likely to exceed 24 hours but not 30 days

Table 50.2 Parts of European Norm International Organization for Standardization 10993 Series of Standards

Part:Year[a]	Title	Working group	Harmonized[a]
-1:2009/AC:2010	Evaluation and testing within a risk management process	WG 1	Yes 02/12/2009 & 18/01/2011
-2:2006	Animal welfare	WG 3	No
-3:2009	Tests for genotoxicity, carcinogenicity, and reproduction toxicity	WG 6	Yes 02/12/2009
-4:2009	Selection of tests for interaction with blood (WG 9)	WG 9	Yes 02/12/2009
-5:2009	Tests for in vitro cytotoxicity	WG 5	Yes 02/12/2009
-6:2009	Tests for local effects after implantation	WG 10	Yes 02/12/2009
-7:2008/AC:2009	Ethylene oxide sterilization residuals	WG 11	Yes 19/02/2009 & 07/07/2010
(-8:2000)	(Guidance on the selection and qualification of reference materials for biological tests. Withdrawn. Integrated in Part 12)	(WG12)	(No)
-9:2009	Framework for identification and quantification of potential degradation products	WG2	Yes 02/12/2009
-10:2010	Test for irritation and skin sensitization (Current version not harmonized)	WG 8	Previous version expired 21/03/2009; current version not harmonized
-11:2009	Tests for systemic toxicity	WG 11	Yes 02/12/2009
-12:2012	Sample preparation and reference materials	WG 12	Yes 24/01/2013
-13:2010	Identification and quantification of degradation products from polymeric medical devices	WG 2	Yes 18/01/2011
-14:2009	Identification and quantification of degradation products from ceramic medical devices	WG 2	Yes 02/12/2009
-15:2009	Identification and quantification of degradation products from metals and alloys	WG 2	Yes 02/12/2009
-16:2010	Toxicokinetic study design for degradation products and leachables	WG 13	Yes 07/07/2010
-17:2009	Establishment of allowable limits for leachable substances	WG 15	Yes 02/12/2009
-18:2009	Characterization of materials	WG 14	Yes 02/12/2009
-19:2006	Physicochemical, mechanical, and morphological characterization	WG 14; ISO/TS	No
-20:2006	Principles and methods for immunotoxicological testing of medical devices	WG 15 ISO/TS	No

[a] Status per February 2015

3. **Permanent contact:** Devices whose cumulative single, multiple, or repeated use or contact exceeds 30 days.

If a medical device has neither direct nor indirect contact to the human body or a patient, no biocompatibility assessment needs to be performed. However, based upon the provisions of EN ISO 14971 (risk management), biocompatibility testing may additionally be necessary to not expose other persons to biological hazards (e.g., doctors, nurses, or nonpatient operators).

50.2.1 Examples from the Market

- Contact lens: Surface device with permanent contact to mucosal membrane
- Wound dressing: Surface device with permanent contact to breached surfaces
- Laparoscope: External communicating device with limited exposure to tissue
- Blood administration set: External communicating device with prolonged exposure to blood path

- Vascular stent: Implant device with permanent contact to blood
- Bone cement: Implant device with permanent contact to tissue or bone

50.3 General Principles to be Applied

Clause 4 ("General principles applying to biological evaluation of medical devices") and Clause 6 ("Biological evaluation process") of EN ISO 10993–1 describe both general and specific provisions that must be followed in order to attain a reliable biological assessment for a medical device. In addition to that, ANSI/AAMI/ISO TIR15499:2012,[15] which is a "technical information report" prepared by a group of authors responsible for the preparation of the EN ISO 10993 series of standards, gives further guidance and interpretation support regarding EN ISO 10993-1. In an attempt to summarize, the following principles were found to be of particular importance:

1. The process of biological evaluation must be based upon a well-structured biological evaluation program, which is in accordance with a risk management system following EN ISO 14971.[3] This program "shall be planned, carried out and documented by knowledgeable and experienced professionals" (Clause 4.1), who will assess any relevant "advantages and disadvantages" of a material or final product under consideration, and who draw "informed decisions" (Clause 4.1) relative to the intended use of a given medical device.
2. The biological evaluation process should follow the flowchart provided in EN ISO 10993–1, Chapter 4, Figure 1. This chart gives a compulsory route to follow and assists to select appropriate chemical and biological test procedures as well as to appropriately include existing chemical, toxicological, and human exposure data from literature before a final biological assessment report can be issued.
3. The biological evaluation must consider potential risks relating to final products as well as to raw materials, breakdown products, leachables, extractables, and metabolites. Therefore, degradable devices must be evaluated extensively following the requirements of EN ISO 10993–9,[16] -13,[17] -14,[18] and -15.[19] Further to this, the biological evaluation must also evaluate the influence of intended additives (e.g., colors or plasticizers), process contaminants (e.g., oil or lubricants), and residues (e.g., detergents after cleaning the final product).
4. The biological evaluation must also investigate the potential influence of other products or components or treatments that may interact with the device under consideration. This could be, for example, the packaging materials, permitted accessories to be used in combination with the product, pharmaceutical products being in contact or medical treatments (e.g., X-ray) to potentially interact with the device, or its primary packaging.
5. Because biocompatibility of a final product is not only based upon its particular chemistry, physical and morphological properties of the device or material under consideration must also be evaluated and tested. This may require testing of certain mechanical properties as well as surface properties such as porosity, surface morphology, or surface charging. For this purpose, the provisions of EN ISO 10993–18 ("Chemical characterization of materials"[20]) and ISO/TS 10993–19 ("Physico-chemical, morphological and topographical characterization of materials"[21]) apply.
6. In order to avoid unnecessary animal testing, EN ISO 10993–1 requests to start the biological evaluation process always with a physical and chemical material characterization (Clause 4.3) and also to use in vitro test procedures before in vivo tests are initiated (Clause 4.6). Further to this, EN ISO 10993–1 Clause 6.2.1 describes particular conditions where animal experimental studies are not justifiable in terms of EN ISO 10993–2.[22] Such conditions occur if previous study results and/or conclusive toxicological data are available for chemically identical products or materials, or if preclinical and clinical data (including a human history of safe use) exists for a chemically identical material or final product.
7. Another important general requirement of EN ISO 10993–1 is found in Clause 4.6. According to this, "all tests shall be conducted according to recognized current/valid best laboratory/quality practices, for example Good Laboratory Practice (GLP) or ISO/IEC 17025." Therefore, any subject matter expert preparing a written biological assessment report must check the available documents whether the reported study results were obtained under such a quality management system. The guidelines for Good Laboratory Practice[23] are available free of charge from public sources, whereas the ISO/IEC 17025 standard,[24] like any other official standard, must be purchased from one of the national standardization organizations.
8. Following the general principles of risk management, the biocompatibility files must be kept updated by the responsible manufacturer during the entire life cycle of a medical device or material under consideration. Therefore, EN ISO 10993–1 specifies five conditions in Clause 4.7 where a biological re-evaluation must be performed:
   a) If a material's specifications or its supplier changes
   b) If the manufacturing formulation, processing, primary packaging, or sterilization changes
   c) If shelf life and/or transportation routines are changed
   d) If the intended use of a product (i.e., its nature and/or duration of body contact) is changed

e) If any evidence becomes available that a product may cause unexpected adverse effects in humans

Considering these points, a medical device manufacturer must also re-evaluate biological hazards if changes occur to parts of the manufacturing equipment, to manufacturing aids (e.g., lubricants, grease, cooling agents), or to manufacturing processes (e.g., temperature profiles during manufacturing or introduction of product surface modifications).

In the case of "minor" changes (e.g., new supplier, changes to manufacturing equipment or manufacturing conditions), the medical device manufacturer may initiate some limited comparative physicochemical and biological tests to investigate whether the aforementioned changes are likely to have a relevant impact on the biocompatibility of the modified material.

50.3.1 Example from Laboratory Practice

If a medical device manufacturer wants to change his supplier of an implantable grade polypropylene, how could he practically approach the required biological safety re-evaluation?

In a first step, the specifications of the polypropylene raw material of the old supplier must be compared to the specifications of the material provided from the potentially new supplier. There should be no critical differences between the materials.

In a second step, the two polypropylene materials should undergo comparative physicochemical material characterizations. A quick and easy test for organic leachables/extractables would be to perform gas chromatographic fingerprint investigations, coupled with a mass spectrophotometer using both polar and nonpolar extraction vehicles. The respective chromatograms should show no relevant differences between the two materials.

In order to exclude potential biological hazards from inorganic substances, the two polypropylene materials could be subjected to comparative infrared spectroscopy and inductively coupled plasma analyses. Again, both materials should provide essentially identical test results. At least, the "new" material should not present with additional peaks or impurities as compared to the "old" material.

After successfully completing this chemical material characterization work, some in vitro testing should be performed in order to exclude potentially low-concentration toxic substances that may be responsible for a potential toxic reaction. Therefore, a comparative cytotoxicity test pursuant to EN ISO 10993–5[25] is proposed as a biological end point. Growth inhibition levels of the "new" material should not be higher than the "old" material and —following the requirements of the standards—should be below 30% for the undiluted extract.

If the polypropylene raw material is finally intended to be used as an implantable material, a bacterial in vitro genotoxicity test (Ames test) pursuant to EN ISO 10993–3[26] is recommended as a second biological end point. Genotoxicity may be caused by very low concentrations of genotoxic substances. Therefore, this test may be advisable even if chemical material characterization did not reveal obvious differences between the "old" and the "new" materials.

In summary, if this series of chemical testing and in vitro biological testing was completed successfully, no further biocompatibility tests need to be repeated for the "new" material. All tests previously performed with the "old" material are fully applicable for the "new" material, and duplicative testing can be avoided.

This approach, which we would call a "bridging approach," was initially suggested by NAMSA Inc. in 1996[27] and further detailed in 2007,[28] in order to avoid multiple testing of identical materials. This strategy, systematically applied, can widely be applied in order to justify minor changes to medical device materials, manufacturing processes, cleaning procedures, or even to reprocessing and sterilization of final product, without a need to repeat the whole animal experimental biocompatibility testing that was previously performed for the initial material or final product.

50.4 Requirements for Sample Preparation

An appropriate sample preparation and selection of reference materials, comparative devices, as well as positive and negative controls are crucial for obtaining meaningful experimental results. Therefore, EN ISO 10993–12[29] addresses the following topics:
- Test sample selection
- Selection of representative portions from a device
- Test sample preparation
- Experimental controls
- Selection of and requirements for reference materials
- Preparation of extracts

An appropriate test sample may be the final product, a representative sample from the final product, or a particularly manufactured test item that has been processed in the same manner as intended for the final product. If applicable, this must also include cleaning and sterilization processes, aging or reprocessing processes, or intended or unintended degradation processes (e.g., through aging during shelf life).

If the final product or material cannot be tested directly, exaggerated extraction is performed with both polar and nonpolar extraction media in order to identify potential chemical hazards relating to leachable or extractable substances and manufacturing residues.

Extractions must be performed in clean, chemically inert, and closed containers that are gently agitated during extraction. Extraction vehicles as well as extraction temperatures may vary for different materials, test procedures, and medical purposes, and must be justified appropriately. Extraction vehicles must be appropriate to the nature and use of the final product, and must be compatible with the intended test procedure (e.g., not dissolve or etch the product or material).

Because extraction is a complex process, standardized procedures are requested with defined temperature conditions and defined extraction periods using appropriate polar and nonpolar extraction vehicles at defined surface-area-to-volume ratios. Based upon the provisions of Clause 10.3.1, the following extraction temperatures and periods shall be applied, as appropriate:

- 37 ± 1°C for 72 ± 2 hours
- 50 ± 2°C for 72 ± 2 hours
- 70 ± 2°C for 24 ± 2 hours
- 121 ± 2°C for 1 ± 0.1 hours

Clause 10.3.5 proposes the following extraction vehicles:
- Polar extraction vehicles: water, physiological saline solution, cell culture medium without serum
- Nonpolar extraction vehicles: freshly refined vegetable oil (e.g., cottonseed or sesame oil)
- Additional extraction vehicles: ethanol/water mixtures, ethanol/saline mixtures, physiologically diluted polyethylene glycol 400, dimethyl-sulfoxide, and culture media with serum

The latter is preferred for devices or material extractions that are to be tested for cytotoxicity or in vitro genotoxicity. A cell culture medium containing serum is considered to represent both polar and nonpolar extraction conditions.

Regularly formed test samples where a surface area can clearly be determined must be extracted based upon the surface-area-to-volume ratios as provided in Clause 10.3.3 Table 1 of the standard. For thin materials (< 0.5 mm thickness), 6 cm^2/mL extraction vehicle must be used. For materials > 0.5 mm thickness, 3 cm^2/mL extraction vehicle is required. For irregularly shaped materials, a gravimetric approach is to be used. Depending on the nature of the investigational material, 0.1 mg/mL (membranes, textiles) or 0.2 mg/mL extraction vehicle (powders, pellets, foam, nonabsorbent molded items) is required. For the extraction of absorbent materials and hydrocolloids, a saturation step with extraction vehicle is proposed before an additional volume representing 0.1 g or 1.0 cm^2 test material per mL extraction vehicle is achieved.

50.5 Biological Evaluation Tests

In addition to the aforementioned general principles, EN ISO 10993–1 refers to a series of specific biological test models that must be considered when planning the biological part of a biocompatibility assessment program. The biological evaluation tests applicable for a given medical device or material are listed in relation to the intended nature and duration of body contact (Clause 5, see previous discussion) in Annex A. This table "Evaluation tests for consideration" is not intended to serve as a "checklist," but it provides a "framework for the development of an assessment program," allowing for product-specific adjustments based on a risk management output. Such adjustments may be due to the particular short-term or long-term hazards relating to a device under normal conditions of use. Therefore, EN ISO 10993–1 principally allows for a strategy of reduced experimental testing provided that this strategy is appropriately justified in the final biological assessment report. It shall be noted that this approach is well supported by ANSI/AAMI/ISO TR15499.[15]

Even though EN ISO 10993–1 is a harmonized international standard, the FDA issued a guideline that amends the Table A.1 of EN ISO 10993–1 for some medical device categories. According to this "Blue Book Memorandum G95–1,"[8] for example, the hazard of acute toxicity must be evaluated for all categories except skin contact and limited mucosal membrane contact.

Furthermore, both EN ISO 10993–1 and Blue Book Memorandum #G95–1 declare that serious biological hazards such as chronic toxicity, carcinogenicity, reproductive and developmental toxicity, biodegradation, and immunotoxicity must be addressed for any medical device or material if applicable from a risk management point of view.

It shall be noted that the FDA just recently published a new draft guideline document that is intended to later replace the aforementioned Blue Book Memorandum #G95–1. This document, which was published on April 23, 2013, "for comment purposes only," gives extensive guidance on the issue of biocompatibility assessment of medical devices and provides helpful additional information and recommendations from an FDA perspective.

▶ Table 50.3 and ▶ Table 50.4 summarize the "evaluation tests for consideration" as of EN ISO 10993–1 Annex A and Blue Book Memorandum G95–1 and the new draft FDA guidance as of April 23, 2013.

50.6 Description of Biological Evaluation Test Models

In order to provide reliable and validated biological test procedures, the EN ISO 10993 series of standards provides numerous subparts describing the applicable test

Table 50.3 Evaluation Tests for Consideration, European Norm International Organization for Standardization 10993–1 Table A.1 and U. S. Food and Drug Administration Blue Book Memorandum G95–1/Draft U.S. Food and Drug Administration Guideline, April 23, 2013

Device categorization by			Biologic effect							
Nature of body contact		Contact duration								
Category	Contact	A - limited (≤ 24 h) B - prolonged (≥ 24 h to 30 d) C - permanent (> 30 d)	Cytotoxicity	Sensitization	Irritation or intracutaneous reactivity	Systemic toxicity (acute)	Subchronic toxicity (subacute toxicity)	Genotoxicity	Implantation	Hemocompatibility
Surface device	Intact skin	A	X	X	X					
		B	X	X	X					
		C	X	X	X					
	Mucosal membrane	A	X	X	X					
		B	X	X	X	O	O		O	
		C	X	X	X	O	X	X	O	
	Breached or compromised surface	A	X	X	X	O				
		B	X	X	X	O	O		O	
		C	X	X	X	O	X	X	O	
External communicating device	Blood path, indirect	A	X	X	X	X				X
		B	X	X	X	X	O			X
		C	X	X	O	X	X	X	O	X
	Tissue/bone/dentin	A	X	X	X	O				
		B	X	X	X	X	X	X	X	
		C	X	X	X	X	X	X	X	
	Circulating blood	A	X	X	X	X		O		X
		B	X	X	X	X	X	X	X	X
		C	X	X	X	X	X	X	X	X
Implant device	Tissue/bone	A	X	X	X	O				
		B	X	X	X	X	X	X	X	
		C	X	X	X	X	X	X	X	
	Blood	A	X	X	X	X	X		X	X
		B	X	X	X	X	X	X	X	X
		C	X	X	X	X	X	X	X	X

"X" marks the biological evaluation tests as proposed by EN ISO 10993–1 Annex A, and "o" marks additional evaluation tests as mentioned in the Blue Book Memorandum G95–1 and the draft U.S. Food and Drug Administration guidance dated April 23, 2013. According to this guidance, these tests "should be addressed in the submission, either by inclusion of the testing or a rational for its omission."

Table 50.4 Supplementary Evaluation Tests for Consideration, U.S. Food and Drug Administration Blue Book Memorandum G95–1/Draft U.S. Food and Drug Administration Guideline April 23, 2013

Device categorization by			Biologic effect			
Nature of body contact		Contact duration				
Category	Contact	A - limited (≤ 24 h) B - prolonged (> 24 h to 30 d) C - permanent (> 30 d)	Chronic toxicity	Carcinogenicity	Reproductive/ developmental toxicity	Biodegradable
Surface device	Intact skin	A				
		B				
		C				
	Mucosal membrane	A				
		B				
		C	O			
	Breached or compro-mised surface	A				
		B				
		C	O			
External communicating device	Blood path, indirect	A				
		B				
		C	O	O		
	Tissue/bone/dentin	A				
		B				
		C	O	O		
	Circulating blood	A				
		B				
		C	O	O		
Implant device	Tissue/bone	A				
		B				
		C	O	O		
	Blood	A				
		B				
		C	O	O		

"X" marks the biological evaluation tests as proposed by EN ISO 10993–1 Annex A, and "o" marks additional evaluation tests as mentioned in the Blue Book Memorandum G95–1 and the draft U.S. Food and Drug Administration guidance, dated April 23, 2013. According to this guidance, these tests "should be addressed in the submission, either by inclusion of the testing or a rational for its omission."

procedures for all of those biological hazards addressed in EN ISO 10993–1. The following paragraphs are intended to briefly describe these test procedures without describing the technical details of the tests.

50.6.1 Chemical Characterization of Materials (EN ISO 10993–18)[20]

As requested by EN ISO 10993–1, the chemical characterization of the materials used for medical devices as well as the chemical nature of the final medical device must always be investigated before animal experimental tests are initiated. This includes both identification and quantification of the chemical constituents of a medical device and potential leachable and/or extractable substances, considering the intended nature and duration of contact to the human body (see previous discussion).

Due to the fact that medical devices may be manufactured from thousands of polymeric, metallic, ceramic, or even from natural macromolecules, EN ISO 10993–18 only provides general principles to apply and gives a list of chemical/physicochemical methods that may be applied in order to analyze polymeric materials (Clause 7.2), metals and alloys (Clause 7.3), ceramics (Clause 7.4), and natural macromolecules (Clause 7.5).

In general, EN ISO 10993–18 proposes a "stepwise process linked to risk assessment." This implies that chemical characterization requires a series of tests that finally allow a conclusion on the identity and quantity of leaching/extractable substances, followed by a toxicological risk assessment of those substances.

Regarding the test procedures, validated analytical methods must be used (i.e., methods that are accurate, precise, and specific). Furthermore, the methods must be robust, reasonably sensitive, and must allow for repeatable analytical results. In addition to the respective quantitative analytical results, the laboratory must also provide applicable limits of detection and limits of quantification.

Based upon both qualitative and quantitative data, a toxicological risk analysis must be performed following the principles of EN ISO 10993–17.[30]

Jargon Simplified: Determination of Leachables and Extractables

- Exhaustive extraction: Extraction conducted until the amount of extractable material in a subsequent extraction is less than 10% by gravimetric analysis of that detected in the initial extraction.
- Exaggerated extraction: Extraction that is intended to result in a greater amount of a chemical constituent being released as compared to the amount generated under the simulated conditions of use.

Key Concepts: Typical Analytical Methods

- DMTA: Dynamic mechanical thermal analysis
- DSC: Differential scanning calorimetry
- EDX-SEM: Electron dispersal X-ray analysis—scanning electron microscopy
- FTIR: Fourier transform infrared spectroscopy
- GC: Gas chromatography
- LC: Liquid chromatography
- MS: Mass spectroscopy (often in combination with GC and LC)
- GPC: Gel permeation chromatography
- HPLC: High-performance liquid chromatography
- ICP: Inductively coupled plasma
- IR: Infrared spectroscopy
- NMR: Nuclear magnetic resonance spectroscopy
- UV/VIS: Ultraviolet/visual light spectroscopy
- SPX: X-ray photoelectron spectroscopy
- SRF: X-ray fluorescence
- 2D PAGE: Two-dimensional polyacrylamide gel electrophoresis

---

50.6.2 Tests for in Vitro Cytotoxicity (EN ISO 10993–5)[25]

Cytotoxicity testing is considered to be one of the most elementary and widespread in vitro test systems to be used for medical devices. Depending on the particular type of medical device, the standard proposes to perform an extract test, a direct test, or an indirect contact test.

The extract test provides both qualitative and quantitative results and can be applied to any solid medical device that allows direct extraction with a polar or nonpolar extraction vehicle. It is well established to use a "complete" culture medium (e.g., Dulbecco's Modified Eagle's medium containing 10% fetal calf serum) in order to apply both polar (aqueous culture medium) and nonpolar (fetal calf serum) extraction conditions in one and the same test. After extraction, the test cells (e.g., L929 mouse fibroblasts) are exposed to the extracted culture medium as to determine cell damage, cell growth, growth inhibition, and/or specific aspects of cellular metabolism. From our experience as an accredited test laboratory, this extraction test represents the most common form of in vitro cytotoxicity testing.

The direct contact test also provides both qualitative and quantitative results, and is applicable for both liquid and solid products. The test cells, suspended in an appropriate culture medium, are allowed to be in direct contact with the test material whereby cell damage, cell growth, growth inhibition, and/or specific aspects of cellular metabolism are determined in relation to the investigated product.

The indirect contact test can only provide qualitative results and may be justified only for certain medical devices, such as dental impression materials or other in situ polymerizing materials, where other procedures for cytotoxicity testing are considered inappropriate. The main disadvantages of the indirect tests, such as the agar diffusion test and the filter diffusion test, are that they only provide a limited sensitivity as compared to the extract test. Furthermore, the agar diffusion test will only detect leachable substances that can diffuse through the hydrophilic agar layer. Cytotoxicity (zone of inhibition) is then determined by use of a vital stain that allows distinguishing viable from nonviable test cells available in the exposed agar gel.

With regard to the qualitative and quantitative determination of cytotoxic effects, EN ISO 10993–5 proposes five reactivity grades: "none" (0), "slight" (1), "mild" (2), "moderate" (3), and "severe" (4). Numerical grades of cytotoxic reactions greater than 2 are considered a "cytotoxic effect." If photometric determinations identify a reduction of cell viability by more than 30% as compared to nonexposed control samples, this is also considered a "cytotoxic effect."

50.6.3 Tests for Delayed Type Hypersensitivity (EN ISO 10993–10)[31]

Sensitization testing is particularly important for medical devices that are intended to come into contact with skin and mucosal membranes. Sensitization testing is, however, also requested for all other types of body contact listed in EN ISO 10993–1 (see ▸ Table 50.3 and ▸ Table 50.4). It shall be noted that the risk of sensitization—and likewise the risk of genotoxicity—represents a biological reactivity that may also occur with extremely low concentrations of the respective sensitizing substance. Allergic reactions are independent of dose. They become visible only after repeated exposure to the sensitizer (delayed reaction), and allergic skin reaction (e.g., erythema) is not localized. Therefore, sensitization testing may not be waived even if physicochemical analyses did not reveal quantifiable amounts of potentially toxic leachable/extractable substances.[9]

There are three major models for testing the sensitizing capacity of a medical device or material:
1. Guinea pig maximization test according to Magnusson and Kligman
2. Guinea pig closed patch test according to Buehler
3. Murine local lymph node assay (LLNA)

Among these three, the guinea pig maximization test can be assumed to be the most frequently applied and most accepted test model. Typically, polar (saline solution) and nonpolar (cotton seed oil) extracts of the test article are prepared and injected intradermally together with Freund's Complete Adjuvant (intradermal induction phase). Seven days later, the test article extracts are exposed to the induction area for another 48 hours (topical induction phase). Another 7 days later (i.e., 14 days after completion of the intradermal induction phase), the test animals are challenged with a topical dose of the test extracts for 24 hours (challenge phase). For that, the extracts are placed on a previously untreated skin area. Final reading of the study results is performed 24 and 48 hours after completion of the challenge phase. If the test animals show no visible skin reaction (score 0), the test material is considered nonsensitizing.

The closed patch test is a direct exposure test where the material under evaluation is typically applied directly to the shaved skin of guinea pigs. The test item or extract is exposed to the animal skin as closed patches repeatedly. During induction phase, the test animals receive nine exposures for 6 hours each during 3 weeks. Fourteen days after the last induction treatment, animals are challenged for 6 hours with a single topical dose of the test item or extract. The final reading of the study results is performed 24 hours after completion of the challenge exposure. If the test animals show no visible skin reaction (score 0), the test material is considered nonsensitizing.

The murine LLNA makes use of murine lymph nodes of mice and determines a potential increase of lymphocyte proliferation in the investigational lymph node. The test has been validated to provide an alternative to the aforementioned guinea pig assays and was just recently introduced to EN ISO 10993–10. However, it shall be noted that the LLNA has initially been validated for sensitization testing of a single chemical substance. Therefore, if complex medical devices are tested (applying more than one material), or if medical devices are made from metal alloys, non-European health authorities may not accept study results based upon the LLNA alone. Therefore, this LLNA test model can be used to screen for allergic contact sensitization, but the guinea pig sensitization models should be preferred for regulatory purposes of complex medical devices.

Jargon Simplified: Terms and Definitions

- **Allergen:** Substance or material capable to induce an allergic reaction. Synonymous to "sensitizer."
- **Skin sensitization:** T-cell–mediated delayed-type hypersensitization. The allergen induces an immunological memory in these cells, which results in an allergic reaction after secondary contact with the respective allergen.
- **Immunotoxicity:** Toxic reaction of a chemical substance, affecting the normal functioning of the human immune system. An impaired immune system and a modified immune function may result in autoimmune diseases, elevated rates of infectious diseases, or even cancer. For testing of immunotoxicity, ISO/TS 10993–20 is applicable.[32]

50.6.4 Tests for Irritation (EN ISO 10993–10)[31]

Depending on the intended nature and duration of body contact, EN ISO 10993–10 describes a variety of irritation tests, all based upon animal models.

The test material or final medical device may be applied directly to the skin in the form of a polar and nonpolar extract. The treatment may include a single exposure only or a repeated dosing, depending on the intended use of the material or medical device under consideration. Reading of the biological reactivity is performed 1, 24, 48, and 72 hours after removal of the test material using a scoring system for erythema and eschar formation as well as for edema formation. In addition, the observed irritation scores may further be substantiated by histopathological evaluations of the contact sites with the human body.

EN ISO 10993–10 describes the following irritation test models:

1. Dermal skin irritation test in albino rabbits of either sex
2. Ocular irritation test in albino rabbits of either sex
3. Oral mucosa irritation test in Syrian hamsters of either sex
4. Penile irritation test in male albino rabbits or guinea pigs
5. Rectal irritation test in albino rabbits of either sex
6. Vaginal irritation test in female albino rabbits
7. Intracutaneous reactivity test in albino rabbits of either sex

---

Jargon Simplified: Terms and Definitions

- Erythema: Reddening of the skin or mucous membrane due to increased peripheral blood flow
- Eschar formation: Dry scab or slough formed on the skin or mucous membrane
- Edema formation: Swelling of skin or mucous membrane due to an abnormal serous fluid accumulation in the tissue

---

The irritation tests listed under points one to six allow investigation of a material or final device and their polar and nonpolar extracts directly on the intended target tissue. The intracutaneous reactivity test (model seven) has a different approach. Both polar and nonpolar extracts of a device or material are prepared and injected intracutaneously (five injections per extract and solvent controls) to the shaved skin of the rabbit back. At 24, 48, and 72 hours after injection, erythema and eschar formation and edema is documented. Finally, the irritation response is calculated to be "negligible," "slight," "moderate," or "severe." Due to the invasiveness of this test, the intracutaneous reactivity test can be regarded as sensitive and predicting test model for both skin and mucous membrane applications. Therefore, this test model is widely accepted by European notified bodies and international health authorities.

50.6.5 Tests for Systemic Toxicity (EN ISO 10993–11)[33]

EN ISO 10993–11 defines systemic toxicity as "a potential adverse effect of the use of medical devices. Generalized effects, as well as organ and organ system effects can result from absorption, distribution and metabolism of leachates from the device or its materials to parts of the body with which they are not in direct contact." Therefore, tests for systemic toxicity are designed to investigate these "generalized" effects, whereas irritation studies and implantation studies primarily focus on the local effects to adjacent tissues that may be caused by an investigational device or material. In the case of implant devices, a combined systemic toxicity and implantation study can investigate both generalized systemic effects and local tolerability aspects, in one animal experimental study.

The standard differentiates the following types of systemic toxicity studies:

1. Test for acute systemic toxicity: ≥ 5 rodent animals (or ≥ 3 nonrodent animals) are exposed to a single, multiple, or continuous dose of a test sample or extract for ≤ 24 hours.
2. Test for subacute systemic toxicity: ≥ 10 rodent animals (or ≥ 6 nonrodent animals), equal numbers per sex, are exposed to multiple or continuous doses of the test sample or extract between 24 hours and 28 days.
3. Test for subchronic systemic toxicity: ≥ 20 rodent animals (or ≥ 8 nonrodent animals), equal numbers per sex, are exposed to multiple or continuous doses of the test sample or extract for less than 10% of the lifespan of the respective test animal. For rodent species, this is typically 90 days or 14 to 28 days for subchronic intravenous studies.
4. Test for chronic systemic toxicity: ≥ 40 rodent animals, equal numbers per sex, are exposed to multiple or continuous doses of the test sample or extract for more than 10% of the lifespan of the respective rodent species. Chronic toxicity studies usually have duration of 6 to 12 months.

For systemic toxicity studies, the route of exposure (medical devices, materials, or their leachable substances) "shall be the most clinically relevant to the use of the device" (Clause 4.6). Typical routes of application are, in alphabetical order, dermal, implantation, inhalation, intradermal, intramuscular, intraperitoneal, intravenous, oral, or subcutaneous (Annex A). The standard also provides recommendations to the dosage volumes that may be applied to various animal species and routes of administration (Annex B).

Depending on the particular medical device, material, or extract investigated, clinical signs and observations are documented during the treatment phase. Such signs can be respiratory effects, motor activities, convulsion, reflexes, ocular signs, cardiovascular signs, or any other relevant observations (Annex C). If appropriate, particularly in subacute, subchronic, and chronic toxicity studies, hematological investigations, clinical chemistry, and urinalyses are performed before, during, and after dosing (Annex D). After completion of the treatment phase, all animals are euthanized and histopathological evaluations are performed on all relevant organs and tissues. Selected organs are weighed in addition (Annex E). Finally, all study results are compared to the results of negative control animals and/or to historical controls.

It shall be noted that the aspect of immunotoxicity pursuant to ISO/TS 10993–20[32] can be combined with long-term systemic toxicity and also with implantation studies. According to this Technical Specification, indications for inflammation, immunosuppression, immunostimulation, hypersensitivity, and autoimmunity are searched, using various in vivo and in vitro assays. Examples of such assays are listed in Table 2 of the standard.

50.6.6 Tests for Genotoxicity (EN ISO 10993–3)[26]

Genetic toxicity must be regarded a major hazard to be excluded for any medical device because genetic damage to chromosomes and/or to the genome may result in heritable diseases or cancer in exposed human subjects.

Therefore, EN ISO 10993–3 requests a series of in vitro and in vivo tests and describes strategies for the selection of an appropriate sequence of testing. If a medical device manufacturer follows these rules, potential hazards of genotoxicity can be excluded as much as possible.

As mentioned before, the genotoxicity may be caused by very low concentrations of hazardous substances released from a medical device or material. Therefore, genotoxicity must be tested and scientifically excluded even if physicochemical material characterization does not exhibit relevant concentrations of potentially hazardous substances.

For testing, the standard describes two optional strategies:

Option 1: Testing for gene mutations in bacteria according to Organisation for Economic Co-operation and Development (OECD) guideline 471 (Bacterial Reverse Mutation Test, "Ames" Test[34]) and testing for gene mutations in mammalian cells according to OECD Guideline 476 (In Vitro Mammalian Cell Gene Mutation Test[35]) and test for clastogenicity in mammalian cells according to OECD 473 (In Vitro Mammalian Chromosome Aberration Test[36]).

Option 2: Testing for gene mutations in bacteria according to OECD guideline 471 (Bacterial Reverse Mutation Test, "Ames" Test[34]) and testing for gene mutations in mammalian cells according to OECD Guideline 476 (In Vitro Mammalian Cell Gene Mutation Test[35]), specifically a mouse lymphoma test covering both end points of clastogenicity and gene mutations.

From our experience as a test laboratory, it seems that international competent authorities such as the FDA for the United States of America and the Ministry of Health, Labour and Welfare for Japan expect applicants to follow Option 1, thus providing test results for the said three independent test models.

In the following, the three most common in vitro tests are described.

Bacterial reverse mutation test (Ames test): For the purpose of this test, five genetically deficient strains of *Salmonella typhimurium* are exposed with and without metabolic activation to polar and nonpolar extracts of the medical device or material under investigation. If reverse mutations occur in their tryptophan and histidine gene, the test will be considered positive.

In vitro mammalian cell gene mutation test: For the purpose of identifying mutagenic potential in mammalian cells, a mouse lymphoma forward mutation test is performed. Mouse L5178Y lymphoma cells are tested with and without metabolic activation regarding the ability of polar and nonpolar product extracts to induce homozygous thymidine kinase mutants. If such mutations occur, the test is considered positive.

Chromosome aberration test: The hazard of medical devices or materials to cause chromosomal aberrations can be investigated in cultures of Chinese hamster cells or in human lymphocytes. The cells are exposed to product or material extracts in the presence and absence of metabolic activation, and metaphase plates are then checked for chromosomal aberrations. If increased chromosomal aberrations are observed in the investigational probes, the test is considered positive.

In case the aforementioned tests of Option 1 and Option 2 provided negative results (i.e., no indication of genotoxicity), further animal experimental genotoxicity testing is normally not required. If any of the in vitro tests provided positive results, either in vivo mutagenicity testing shall be followed or, preferably, the respective critical material should be categorized as mutagenic and not be used for the purpose of a medical device.

Jargon Simplified: Terms and Definitions

- OECD: Organisation for Economic Co-operation and Development
- Gene mutation: Genetic toxicity resulting in changes to the DNA or genes of the genome
- Clastogenicity: Genetic toxicity resulting in changes in the chromosome structure like disruptions or breakage of chromosomes

50.6.7 Tests for Local Effects after Implantation (EN ISO 10993–6)[37]

According to EN ISO 10993–1 Table A.1 (see previous discussion), all implantable medical devices must prove that they do not cause local pathological effects in relevant animal tissues that appropriately stand for those tissues where the final devices are intended to be used in humans. Therefore, implantation studies are typically performed in small animals like mice, rats, guinea pigs, or rabbits, using particularly manufactured test specimens or the appropriate size and shape. Only for particular scientific or medical reasons, the use of large animals such as dogs, sheep, goats, or pigs may be justified.

Implantation studies are indicated for solid nonbiodegradable devices and materials, degradable and/or resorbable materials, as well as nonsolid devices or materials such as liquids, pastes, porous materials, and particulates. Relative to the intended implantation sites in humans, the test animals receive study materials implanted into muscle tissue, subcutis or bone. However, other implantation sites like brain tissue, peritoneum, blood vessels or even heart tissue may be required in order to prove local tolerability in the intended target organ.

Depending on the intended purpose of the investigational product or material in humans, EN ISO 10993–6 recommends implantation periods of 1 to 4 weeks for implants with limited or prolonged exposure, and 12, 26, 52, 78, or in exceptionally cases even 104 weeks for permanent implants. A minimum of three animals, allowing for a minimum of 10 test specimens and 10 control specimens, must be used per investigated implantation period. At the end of the respective implantation period, the test animals are euthanized in line with EN ISO 10993–2, and relevant tissues are analyzed macroscopically and microscopically for biological responses. Histopathological findings are to be documented by photomicrographs.

If degradable or resorbable materials are tested, an implantation period must be selected that shows a nearly completed degradation or resorption, with some residual material remaining in the implanted tissue. Therefore, in vitro degradation data are always required to appropriately plan an implantation study for such materials.

In the case of bone implants, the interface between the bone tissue and the implant material must be particularly documented in order to evaluate biological tissue reactions such as bone degeneration or osseointegration in the vicinity of the implant.

It shall be noted that EN ISO 10993–6 is not focusing on functional implantation studies, where implantable medical devices are investigated regarding their mechanical and/or biological functionality and safety. Such studies may, however, be necessary for innovative medical implant devices before clinical studies in humans can be initiated (e.g., ISO 11979–5 for intraocular lenses[5]).

50.6.8 Tests for Interaction with Blood (EN ISO 10993–4)[38]

Hemocompatibility must be evaluated and tested for all medical devices that are intended to be in direct or indirect contact with blood. This may be an external communicating device such as a blood bag (indirect contact to the blood path) or a central venous catheter (direct contact to circulating blood), or an implant device with direct contact to blood (e.g., a coronary stent).

For the evaluation of hemocompatibility, potential adverse effects of the device geometry, surface properties, contact conditions, and resulting dynamic effects on the blood flow are investigated. Such adverse effects may relate to cellular blood components as well as to plasma proteins or enzymes. Therefore, the standard requests to consider the following categories for testing, as appropriate, for a given medical device: thrombosis, coagulation, platelets, hematology, and complement system. In two tables, the standard provides a list of exemplary blood-contacting medical devices and indicates which of the aforementioned categories should be investigated in particular. In addition, the standard gives an overview of applicable in vitro, ex vivo, and in vivo evaluation methods for the aforementioned five categories (▶ Table 50.3 and ▶ Table 50.4 and Annex of the Standard B).

Among these tests, both static (batch tests) and dynamic (blood is kept moving) testing conditions are included. Frequently used routine procedures are, among others, tests for hemolysis, complement activation, prothrombin time, partial thromboplastin time, blood clotting time, platelet aggregation, complete blood count, hematocrit, and hemoglobin content of erythrocytes.

50.6.9 Tests for Carcinogenicity, Reproduction, and Developmental Toxicity (EN ISO 10993–3)[26]

According to EN ISO 10993–1 carcinogenicity testing (Clause 6.2.2.11), reproduction, and developmental toxicity (Clause 6.2.2.12) of a medical device should only be considered "if there are suggestive data from other sources." Therefore, animal experimental testing of these serious hazards is only indicated if the chemical composition of a final device or materials used for manufacturing suggests that such hazards may exist. Furthermore, during the design phase and manufacturing of a medical device, special care must be taken to select materials and processes that are known not to cause a risk of carcinogenicity, reproduction, or developmental toxicity.

Based upon these requirements, the potential of carcinogenicity, reproductive, and developmental toxicity is typically evaluated on the basis of genotoxicity test results (EN ISO 10993–3), physicochemical materials characterization (EN ISO 10993–18), and toxicological literature data for the chemical ingredients and manufacturing aids used.

For a quick toxicological survey, the following toxicological fact databases may be particularly helpful:

- RTECS Search database: http://ccinfoweb.ccohs.ca/rtecs/search.html
- TOXNET Toxicology Data Network: http://toxnet.nlm.nih.gov/

Within TOXNET, 14 subdatabases are provided that focus on particular biological hazards such as genotoxicity (GENETOX database), carcinogenicity (CCRIS database), or developmental and reproductive toxicity (DART database).

50.6.10 Evaluation of Intended and Nonintended Degradation (EN ISO 10993–9)[16]

Poly(glycolic acid), poly(lactic acid), and their copolymers were the first synthetic biodegradable materials used in the medical device industry for the purpose of surgical suture materials, back in the early 1970s.[39] Since then, numerous other degradable materials and medical applications have been developed.

Based upon the provisions set out in EN ISO 10993–1 Clauses 5.3 and 6.2.2.13, biodegradation and related biocompatibility aspects must be experimentally investigated (1) for the starting components of manufacture, (2) for intermediate reaction products, and (3) for the fully polymerized material. This particularly applies to medical devices that are designed to be biodegradable, intended to be implanted for longer than 30 days, or which may release potentially toxic substances during the intended body contact. Further to that, the presence and nature of degradation products must also be investigated and toxicologically evaluated if the conditions of manufacture, sterilization, transport, storage, and clinical use of a material or device may provoke degradation processes.

For further guidance, ISO TC 194 WG 2 developed four standards that are intended to provide general (Part 9) and particular strategies (Parts 13, 14, and 15) for the investigation and risk assessment of such materials:

- EN ISO 10993–9: Framework for identification and quantification of potential degradation products[16]
- EN ISO 10993–13: Identification and quantification of degradation products from polymeric medical devices[17]
- EN ISO 10993–14: Identification and quantification of degradation products from ceramics[18]
- EN ISO 10993–15: Identification and quantification of degradation products from metals and alloys[19]

In addition to synthetic degradable materials, numerous degradable materials from materials of animal origin have been developed. For such materials, ISO TC194 SC1 developed another three harmonized standards and a technical report to give particular guidance for the development, manufacturing, and testing of such materials, particularly addressing biological risks such as transmissible diseases:

- EN ISO 22442–1: Medical devices utilizing animal tissues and their derivatives–Part 1: Application of risk management[40]
- EN ISO 22442–2: Medical devices utilizing animal tissues and their derivatives–Part 2: Controls on sourcing, collection, and handling[41]
- EN ISO 22442–3: Medical devices utilizing animal tissues and their derivatives–Part 3: Validation of the elimination and/or inactivation of viruses and transmissible spongiform encephalopathy agents[42]
- ISO/TR 22442–4: Medical devices utilizing animal tissues and their derivatives–Part 4: Principles for elimination and/or inactivation of transmissible spongiform encephalopathy agents and validation assays for those processes.[43]

The ISO standards 10993–9, –13, –14, and –15 require in vitro and in vivo degradation studies to identify the mechanism of degradation, determine the rates and chemical identities of degradation products, and analyze the interaction and potential toxicity of degradation products in relation to the surrounding tissues (local tolerability) and the rest of the body (systemic effects). For that a combination of physicochemical investigations, histopathological assessments and toxicological literature research in appropriate databases is necessary.

In cases of well-known, clinically accepted degradable implant materials and degradation products, animal experimental investigations may not be required. For innovative biodegradable materials, where the mechanisms of absorption, distribution, metabolism, and excretion of the degradation products are unknown or nonpredictable, toxicokinetic studies according to EN ISO 10993–16[44] are required. For that, radiolabeled materials and degradation products are applied to investigational organisms, and the disposition and fate of these substances (i.e., their time-course of movement through the body) is analyzed.

50.7 Preparation of a Summarizing Expert Testimony

After successfully going through the biological testing, literature search, and risk evaluation process, European notified bodies and international competent authorities will request a summarizing "overall biological safety assessment" or expert testimony according to EN ISO 10993–1 Clause 7, which confirms that a medical device or material under consideration is biocompatible in terms of the EN ISO 10993–1 standard or other applicable product-specific vertical standard[5,6,7] and, in case of non-European registrations, with other particular national regulations.[8,10,11,12]

This summarizing document, which we typically call "Declaration of Compliance with EN ISO 10993–1," has the form from an expert assessment that contains the following elements:

- Regulatory background to the applicable MDD and/or other applicable regulations
- Confirmation that the biological evaluation process was performed within a risk management system of EN ISO 14971
- Technical description, intended purpose and medical indications/contraindications of the medical device or material under consideration
- Legal identification of manufacturer by name and location
- Classification of the device following the applicable MDD and/or other applicable regulations
- Classification of the device regarding its nature and duration of body contact (EN ISO 10993–1)
- Identification of all applicable biological risk categories in terms of EN ISO 10993–1, potentially applicable vertical product standards, and/or other applicable regulatory guidelines
- Compilation of any relevant test reports (biological evaluation tests, material characterization, other tests) dealing with the investigational device or material and critical evaluation of the study design, conduct, and results in view of the provisions and specifications set out in the respective EN ISO 10993 standard or other applicable regulation
- Rationale for the selection of particular tests; rationale and justification for the waiving of tests
- Compilation of relevant scientific and toxicological literature allowing for a biological risk assessment of the medical device or material under consideration as well as of potential leachable and extractable substances and degradation products
- Compilation of potentially available medical literature and postmarket surveillance data of the medical device or material under consideration allowing for a critical assessment of a possibly existing human use history and practical experience
- Signed and dated concluding statement of the expert that the device or material under consideration can be considered biocompatible in terms of the applicable standards and guidelines and considering the intended use as specified in the manufacturer's instructions for use
- Signed and dated curriculum vitae of the biological expert confirming his/her scientific expertise and practical as well as medical device regulatory experience

It shall be noted that each of the evaluable biological risk categories, such as cytotoxicity, irritation, sensitization, etc., must be addressed and evaluated individually for the medical device or material under consideration. General statements like "titanium is known to be biocompatible for implantable medical devices," even if appropriate literate has been quoted, are not adequate for the purpose of a "Declaration of Compliance with EN ISO 10993–1" and will typically not be accepted by European notified bodies or by non-European competent authorities. As a minimum, final medical devices made from "standardized" materials—i.e., materials documented for the respective intended purpose in national or international norms/standards—must experimentally prove their identity with the specifications of the "standardized" materials regarding their chemical nature and surface cleanliness before omission of animal experimental testing can be duly justified.

Therefore, in case tests required by EN ISO 10993–1 or other applicable standards have not been experimentally executed, or any modifications to the test design and conduct occurred or if the EN ISO 10993–12 requirements for sample preparation were not followed, appropriate justification must be provided for each waiving of a test as well as for each procedural deviation from the applicable standard.

With regard to toxicological and medical literature data, the expert must investigate whether the literature data can be expected to be applicable and representative for the medical device or material under consideration. Literature data can only be expected to represent a particular medical device if the materials of manufacture, the manufacturing processes, the manufacturing and environmental conditions, as well as other impacting treatments (e.g., cleaning, reprocessing, sterilization, and packaging) are identical or comparable to the device or material under consideration. Such similar products are be classified as "substantially equivalent" or as a "predicate device," and study results obtained and documented for such devices or materials can be utilized for the device or material under evaluation.

A valuable guidance as to how to predicate devices may be used in the biological risk assessment of a particular medical device is provided in the FDA guideline document "The 510(k) Program: Evaluating Substantially Equivalence in Premarket Notifications [510(k)]."[45] Even if there is no such 510(k) registration analogue in Europe, this guideline helps explain the technical, chemical, mechanical, and clinical criteria that qualify other medical devices as "substantially equivalent."

References

[1] Council Directive 93/42/EEC of 14 June 1993 concerning medical devices. (OJ L 169, 12.7.1993, p. 1) latest amended by Directive 2007/47/EC of the European Parliament and of the Council of 5 September 2007. http://eur-lex.europa.eu/LexUriServ/LexUriServ.do?uri=CONSLEG:1993L0042:20071011:en:PDF

[2] Council Directive 90/385/EEC of 20 June 1990 on the approximation of the laws of the Member States relating to active implantable medical devices (OJ L 189, 20.7.1990, p.17). http://eur-lex.europa.eu/LexUriServ/LexUriServ.do?uri=CONSLEG:1990L0385:20071011:EN:PDF

[3] European Norm International Organization for Standardization 14971:2012 Medical devices - Application of risk management to medical devices (ISO 14971:2007, Corrected version 2007–10–01

[4] European Norm International Organization for Standardization 10993–1:2009 Biological evaluation of medical devices - Part 1: Evaluation and testing within a risk management process

[5] European Norm International Organization for Standardization 11979–5:2006 Ophthalmic implants - Intraocular lenses - Part 5: Biocompatibility

[6] European Norm International Organization for Standardization 9394:2012 Ophthalmic optics - Contact lenses and contact lens care products - Determination of biocompatibility by ocular study with rabbit eyes

[7] European Norm International Organization for Standardization 7405:2008 Dentistry - Evaluation of biocompatibility of medical devices used in dentistry (Amendment A1:2013)

[8] Blue Book Memorandum U.S. Food and Drug Administration. (1995) Use of International Standard ISO 10993, "Biological Evaluation of Medical Devices – Part 1: Evaluation and Testing." General Program Memorandum - # G95–1. FDA, Department of Health and Human Services, last updated 05/03/2009. http://www.fda.gov/MedicalDevices/DeviceRegulationandGuidance/GuidanceDocuments/ucm080735.htm

[9] U.S. Food and Drug Administration. (2013) Draft Guidance for Industry and Food and Drug Administration Staff: Use of International Standard ISO 10993, "Biological Evaluation of Medical Devices Part 1: Evaluation and Testing." Document issued on 23 April 2013 for comment purposes only

[10] American Society for Testing of Materials F748–06(2010) Standard Practice for Selecting Generic Biological Test Methods for Materials and Devices

[11] Notification No. 0213001: Basic Principles of Biological Safety Evaluation. Required for Application for Approval to manufacture (Import) Medical Devices. Pharmaceutical and Food Safety Bureau, Ministry of Health, Labour and Welfare February 13, 2003. http://www.pmda.go.jp/english/service/pdf/notifications/0213001.pdf

[12] Notice from the Office Medical Devices Evaluation Number 36 of the Japanese Pharmaceutical and Food Safety Bureau, Ministry of Health, Labour and Welfare, March 19, 2003: "Testing Methods to Evaluate Biological Safety of Medical Devices, Notice from the Office Medical Devices Evaluation Number 36." http://dmd.nihs.go.jp/iso-tc194/guide_sankou.pdf

[13] International Organization for Standardization. TC 194 Biological evaluation of medical devices. Subcommittees/Working Groups. http://www.iso.org/iso/home/standards_development/list_of_iso_-technical_committees/iso_technical_committee.htm?commid=54508

[14] International Organization for Standardization. TC 194 Biological evaluation of medical devices. http://www.iso.org/iso/home/standards_development/list_of_iso_technical_committees/iso_technical_-committee.htm?commid=54508

[15] ANSI/AAMI/ISO TIR15499:2012 Biological evaluation of medical devices - Guidance on the conduct of biological evaluation within a risk management process.

[16] European Norm International Organization for Standardization 10993–9:2009 Biological evaluation of medical devices – Part 9 Framework for identification and quantification of potential degradation products

[17] European Norm International Organization for Standardization 10993–13:2010 Biological evaluation of medical devices – Part 13 Identification and quantification of degradation products from polymeric medical devices

[18] European Norm International Organization for Standardization 10993–14:2009 Biological evaluation of medical devices – Part 14 Identification and quantification of degradation products from ceramic medical devices

[19] European Norm International Organization for Standardization 10993–15:2009 Biological evaluation of medical devices – Part 15 Identification and quantification of degradation products from metals and alloys

[20] European Norm International Organization for Standardization 10993–18:2009 Biological evaluation of medical devices – Part 18 Characterization of materials

[21] International Organization for Standardization/Technical Specification 10993–19:2006 Biological evaluation of medical devices – Part 19 Physico-chemical, mechanical and morphological characterization

[22] European Norm International Organization for Standardization 10993–2:2006 Biological evaluation of medical devices – Part 2 Animal welfare

[23] Organisation for Economic Co-operative and Development. (1998) OECD Series on Principles of Good Laboratory Practice and Compliance Monitoring. OECD Principles on Good Laboratory Practice (as revised in 1997). Organisation for Economic Co-operation and Development ENV/MC/CHEM(98)17. http://www.oecd-ilibrary.org/docserver/download/fulltext/9760011e.pdf?expires-1352222617&id=id&accname=guest&checksum=1A4DC32FBBD6352A3-F1ED47F893C9D6B

[24] DIN European Norm International Organization for Standardization/IEC 17025:2007 General requirements for the competence of testing and calibration laboratories (ISO/IEC 17025:2005); German and English version EN ISO/IEC 17025:2005, Corrigenda to DIN EN ISO/IEC 17025:2005–08; German and English version EN ISO/IEC 17025:2005/AC:2006

[25] European Norm International Organization for Standardization 10993–5:2009 Biological evaluation of medical devices – Part 5 Tests for in vitro cytotoxicity

[26] European Norm International Organization for Standardization 10993–3:2009 Biological evaluation of medical devices – Part 3 Tests for genotoxicity, carcinogenicity and reproduction toxicity

[27] Upman PJ, Charton R. 1996. Satisfying medical device biocompatibility requirements: what's a supplier to do? http://www.namsa.com/Portals/0/Documents/Biocomp-WhatsaSupplierToDo-W6–95.pdf

[28] Albert D, Hoffmann A. 2007. Using chemical characterization to show equivalency. MDDI Medical Device and Diagnostic Industry News Products and Suppliers. Publication date: May 1, 2007. http://www.mddionline.com/print/1793

[29] European Norm International Organization for Standardization 10993–12:2012 Biological evaluation of medical devices – Part 12 Sample preparation and reference materials

[30] European Norm International Organization for Standardization 10993–17:2009 Biological evaluation of medical devices - Part 17: Establishment of allowable limits for leachable substances

[31] European Norm International Organization for Standardization 10993–10:2010 Biological evaluation of medical devices - Part 10: Test for irritation and skin sensitization

[32] International Organization for Standardization/Technical Specification 10993–20:2006 Biological evaluation of medical devices - Part 20: Principles and methods for immunotoxicological testing of medical devices

[33] European Norm International Organization for Standardization 10993–11:2009 Biological evaluation of medical devices - Part 11: Test for systemic toxicity

[34] Guideline Organisation for Economic Co-operative and Development. 471:1997, Bacterial Reverse Mutation Test. http://www.oecd-ilibrary.org/docserver/download/9747101e.pdf?expires-1355473191&id=id&accname=guest&checksum=921F6E23A6F858916457-CEE8D83112DC

[35] Guideline Organisation for Economic Co-operative and Development. 476:1997, In Vitro Mammalian Cell Gene Mutation Test. http://www.oecd-ilibrary.org/docserver/download/9747601e.pdf?expires-1355473259&id=id&accname=guest&checksum=B3C24AC8C24-B0A6BAF0942CEC2FAC929

[36] Guideline Organisation for Economic Co-operative and Development. 473:1997, In Vitro Mammalian Chromosome Aberration Test. http://www.oecd-ilibrary.org/docserver/download/9747301e.pdf?expires-1355473312&id=id&accname=guest&checksum=3626035677DC8C248010CC9D8CE8B230

[37] European Norm International Organization for Standardization 10993–6:2009 Biological evaluation of medical devices - Part 6: Tests for local effects after implantation

[38] European Norm International Organization for Standardization 10993–4:2009 Biological evaluation of medical devices - Part 6: Selection of tests for interaction with blood

[39] Teiser M, Abramson S, Langer R, Kohn J. Degradable and resorbable biomaterials. In: Ratner BD, Hoffman AS, Schoen FJ, Lemons JE (eds.) Biomaterials science: an introduction to materials in medicine. 3 e. Bridgewater, NJ: Elsevier Academic Press; 2012

[40] European Norm International Organization for Standardization 22442–1:2007 Medical devices utilizing animal tissues and their derivatives–Part 1: Application of risk management

[41] European Norm International Organization for Standardization 22442–2:2007 Medical devices utilizing animal tissues and their derivatives–Part 2: Controls on sourcing, collection and handling

[42] European Norm International Organization for Standardization 22442–3:2007 Medical devices utilizing animal tissues and their derivatives–Part 3: Validation of the elimination and/or inactivation of viruses and transmissible spongiform encephalopathy (TSE) agents

[43] International Organization for Standardization/Technical Report 22442–4:2010 Medical devices utilizing animal tissues and their derivatives–Part 4: Principles for elimination and/or inactivation of transmissible spongiform encephalopathy (TSE) agents and validation assays for those processes

[44] European Norm International Organization for Standardization 10993–16:2010 Biological evaluation of medical devices - Part 16: Toxicokinetic study design for degradation products and leachables

[45] U.S. Department of Health and Human Services. FDA CDRH (2011) Draft Guidance for Industry and Food and Drug Administration Staff. The 510(k) Program: Evaluating Substantial Equivalence in Premarket Notifications [(510(k)]. Date of issue: December 27, 2011. http://www.fda.gov/downloads/MedicalDevices/DeviceRegulationandGuidance/GuidanceDocuments/UCM284443.pdf

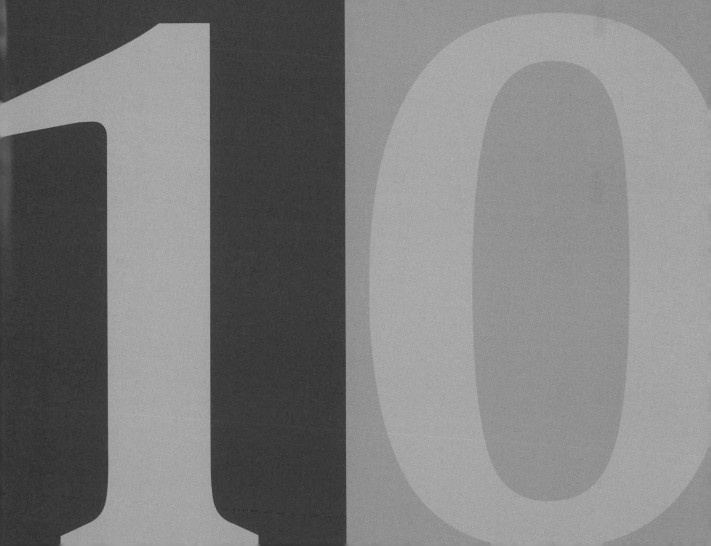

Part 10
Statistics for Experimental Research

51 Study Design

Taco Johan Blokhuis

Study design in experimental research is fundamentally different from study design in clinical research for several reasons. First, the question to be answered in a clinical trial usually comes from well-documented effects of, for example, a new treatment method. After finishing the preclinical studies, and possibly even a phase 1, phase 2, or phase 3 clinical trial, a randomized controlled trial is designed and conducted. Most of the prerequisites for the design of a randomized controlled trial are lacking in experimental research, and this will have direct consequences for the study design in experimental work. Second, the aim of experimental studies is to detect the mechanism behind an effect, or understand a causal relationship, rather than to investigate the effect itself as in clinical studies.

For these reasons, designing and conducting experimental studies can be perceived as difficult, or convincing the animal ethics committee can be seen as impossible. This section on statistics aims to suggest improvements in the study design, helping you to increase the scientific level of your work. This first chapter will discuss some of the specific aspects of study design in experimental studies, and the rest of this section will go into more detail concerning the statistical aspects of experimental research.

51.1 Hypothesis

The study you are about to start will usually begin with a question. This question has arisen from either literature, previous work you and your colleagues performed, or has come up during a discussion. A question, however, is not the best starting point for the design of a proper study, as it will leave too many open ends in the design. Instead of starting with a question, starting with a hypothesis will create a solid basis for your design. Formulation of a hypothesis helps the scientist to think about aspects of the issue at hand and avoids performing unnecessary studies that have to be repeated afterwards in a different manner. The hypothesis actually consists of two parts: the null hypothesis and the alternative hypothesis. The null hypothesis is the default hypothesis, assuming a steady state or no relationship between two variables. The alternative hypothesis states that there is an effect of treatment or a relation between two variables. In a specific experiment, the null hypothesis is tested against the alternative hypothesis. Formulation of a good hypothesis reflects the thought given to a study design, but will also determine specific aspects of the design and analysis. For example, when the hypothesis states that the effect of treatment A will be greater than the effect of treatment B,

one-sided testing can be performed in the analysis, thus increasing the value of a specific experiment.

However, in experimental research, hypotheses are not always available due to a lack of data. Starting from a thought or a question rather than from proper data from previous experiments, studies are sometimes necessary to create a solid and well-defined hypothesis. In such cases, results from literature, preliminary work, and thorough knowledge of pathophysiology are the starting points for the design of a hypothesis-finding study.

51.2 Research Question

The key issue in study design is the research question. The research question has to be clear and unambiguous, although this is not as simple as it may seem. The question has to be based upon a hypothesis that has to be tested in the study, and the study therefore has to be designed in such a manner that the research question can be answered by the study without leaving any answers open. Especially in animal studies, from an ethical perspective, the study has to be designed using as few animals as possible, yet enough to answer the question(s) appropriately; otherwise, the study result will be useless altogether. It is therefore important for the scientist to appreciate the importance of the research question and not to embark upon a study that may seem interesting at the start, but at the end only results in more questions. Apart from clear and unambiguous, the question has to be precise. Compare, for example, the following two questions: (1) What is the effect of my new intervention on the survival of septic rats? and (2) Can my new intervention, applied within 12 hours after intraperitoneal injection of 5 mg/kg lipopolysaccharide, decrease the 48-hour mortality in adult male wistar rats by 25%? In the first question, methods and end points are unclear, and as a consequence the study design will be unclear. The second question describes the study design in great detail, and although some aspects are left open such as weight of the animals, the question is clear, unambiguous, and precise. The question already contains key aspects of the study design and is likely to be answered by the suggested design.

51.3 End Points

Measuring what you want is the only way to answer the research question that was formulated so precisely. Choosing the correct end points is therefore important. For example, the alkaline phosphatase (ALP)/deoxyribonucleic acid (DNA) ratio in an in vitro study on osteogenic capacity of specific cell types appears to give an exact measurement of the outcome. However, looking closer at the data the increase in ALP/DNA ratio does not say whether all cells express some ALP or some cells express a lot of ALP. In the first case, you may want to continue the same model, whereas in the second case you may want to select the few positive cells and work with those. In experimental research, the material is often unique and limited. You only have funding for a group of 20 animals or the cells you work with come from a unique source. It is therefore crucial to think about the end points you want to use before starting your experimental study. Do you end points answer your question? Are your end points relevant? Is the expertise and experience available in your center? Do you have enough funding for the end points you have in mind, or are alternative end points available? Is the timing of your end point correct? These are questions you have to answer while designing an experimental study because they have important consequences for the execution of the study, and often cannot be changed once the study has started.

Before you start your study, one specific end point has to be chosen as the primary outcome measure. This is important in calculating the sample size, as discussed elsewhere in this section. Ideally, choosing the primary outcome measure should be done regarding the clinical relevance of the end point, the effect size you want to determine in your study, and the known variation in size of the end point. In experimental research, this is not always possible, for example because the normal variation in the population you want to study is not known. It may therefore be necessary to perform a pilot study to determine the normal variation of the end point of interest before you start the final study.

51.4 Outcome and Analysis

You have designed and executed an experimental study with correct end points and a sufficient sample size. Analyzing the data will then be the next step, and this requires some consideration as well. Choosing the correct statistical test (e.g., parametric versus nonparametric) will be described elsewhere in this section, and other precautions such as limiting bias are described elsewhere in this book. These are key issues and should be considered before the start of the experimental study. For example, randomization of the animals has to be planned and done at the start of the study. Once the study is running, there is often no way to correct for omitting vital measures like this, and the quality of your study will be at risk. For these reasons, early consultation of a statistician should be done, preferably before the start of the study.

51.5 Conclusion

Experimental studies differ from clinical studies, both in aim and in design. Statistics are a vital part of the study design. Several key issues have to be addressed in designing an experimental study, and by taking these issues into account the quality of your scientific work can be maintained at the highest level. This section on statistics is written to aid you in these aspects of experimental studies.

Further Reading

Altman DG. Practical statistics for medical research. London: Chapman & Hall; 1990

Petrie A. Statistics in orthopaedic papers. J Bone Joint Surg Br 2006; 88: 1121–1136

52 Power and Sample Size Calculation

Nan van Geloven, Rob de Haan, Marcel Dijkgraaf, Michael Tanck, Johannes B. Reitsma

52.1 Why Perform a Sample Size Calculation Prior to a Study?

Why do we want to determine the sample size before a study starts? The importance of a sample size calculation is based on ethical grounds. If the number of subjects tested in a study is too small to pick up a possible effect in the population, study subjects are tested in vain. The study will easily result in a false-negative conclusion. On the other hand, testing too many subjects may also lead to undesirable situations. If an intervention turns out to be effective, too many subjects have missed out on this intervention. If the intervention is not effective, too many have been exposed to this ineffective intervention. For these reasons, a trial should always consider what number of subjects would be appropriate to answer the study question. Sample size calculations prior to a study can help focus on the number of subjects that is needed and sufficient for a study. Moreover, a sample size calculation helps one to focus on a clinically relevant effect, instead of the erroneous strategy of testing as many subjects as needed to reach statistical difference of an irrelevant effect.

For clinical studies, several regulatory authorities demand a sample size calculation before the start of inclusion of subjects. The CONSORT statement (guideline for reporting clinical trials) states that a researcher should calculate study size beforehand and should report this calculation in the methods section of the resulting scientific paper. For experimental research, the guidelines are less strict, although all animal ethics committees will require a detailed sample size calculation before approving a research protocol. Finally, the logistic planning of a study benefits from a sample size calculation and helps you as a researcher to perform your studies in a more controlled manner.

52.2 What is Power and Statistical Significance?

The term "power" pops up everywhere in medical research, certainly in sample size calculations. Often, the term power is interpreted as a synonym for the number of patients tested in a study. "Our study did not have enough power to control for possible confounders" is understood as "you didn't test enough patients to account for several effects." "Our study had 80% power to detect an odds ratio of 1.1 at a significance level of 5%" is understood as "you have tested enough patients to pick up a possible effect."

Although these interpretations are not (absolutely) wrong, in order to use the concept of power in a sample size calculation, we need to understand its exact meaning. Formally: *the power of a study testing the null hypothesis H_0 against the alternative hypothesis H_1 is the probability that the test (based on a sample from this population) rejects H_0, given H_0 is false (in the whole population).*

So the power is the chance of correctly rejecting a null hypothesis (rejecting a null hypothesis given it should be rejected). Because in most tests, H_0 is stated as "no difference between groups or no effect of intervention" (e.g., H_0 = "no difference in survival between treated and control group"), rejecting H_0 means you have reason to believe there is a difference. In other words, the power reflects the ability to pick up an effect that is present in a population using a test based on a sample from that population (true positive).

The power of a study is closely related to the so called type II error (β), the probability of falsely accepting H_0. The power of a study is $1 - \beta$, so it is the probability of rightfully rejecting H_0 (▶ Table 52.1).

The significance level α is stated in ▶ Table 52.1. Alpha is the probability of falsely rejecting H_0 (i.e., falsely picking up an effect [false-positive]). Note that α only concerns situations in which no true effect exists in the population.

In a sample size calculation, one determines the number of patients needed to test the hypothesis with large enough power and small enough significance level. In this way, one protects oneself against false-negative and false-positive conclusions.

Table 52.1 Possible Conclusions and Errors of a Study in Relation to the Truth

		Whole population	
		Effect exists H_1 is true	No effect exists H_0 is true
Study conclusion	Effect observed H_1 appears true	True positive Power $(1 - \beta)$	False-positive Type I error (α)
	No effect observed H_0 appears true	False-negative Type II error (β)	True negative $(1 - \alpha)$

52.3 What Information is Needed to Calculate a Sample Size?

To make a sample size calculation, one will need information about each of the following values:

a) *Desired power of the study 1-β.* How much power do you want in the study? Or, stated differently, how certain do you want to be of preventing a type II error?

b) *Desired significance level α.* How certain do you want to be of preventing a type I error?

c) *Desired test direction.* One- or two-sided test?

d) *Clinically relevant (or expected) difference.* Which difference or which effect are you trying to find?

e) *Expected variance/standard deviation.* How much variation is expected in subjects belonging to the same study group?

f) *Test to be used in statistical analysis.* How will the hypothesis test be performed in the analysis phase of the study?

g) *Attrition rate.* Anticipate on the number of included subjects who will not be available for the study analysis.

52.4 Where to Find the Information Needed for a Sample Size Calculation

In this section, we advise on how to determine or choose the necessary input values for a sample size calculation.

- *Desired power of the study.* 80% is a common power level used in sample size calculations. It means you accept a chance of 20% (one in five) of failing to detect an effect in your study sample that is indeed present in the population (false-negative). If you want to reduce the change to miss out a certain effect, you should increase the power level, for instance to 90%. Increasing the power level will increase the sample size.

- *Desired significance level α.* Five percent is a common significance level used in hypothesis testing. This means you accept a chance of 0.05 to detect an effect in your study that is not present in the whole population (false-positive). A reason to lower the significance level might be that multiple tests are done and you do not want to detect an effect just by increasing the odds of finding a false-positive. Lowering the significance level will increase sample size.

- *Desired test direction.* A two-sided test is standard. It means that you test the possibility that treatment A is better than treatment B and the other option (treatment B better than treatment A) simultaneously. A one-sided test can only be considered when a clear rationale is provided about why only one direction of

the alternative hypothesis is tested (ethical committees and journals are quite strict on this point, some even reject all one-sided tests). See, for example, Knottnerus and Bouter[1] or Peace[2] for considerations about using a one-sided test for sample size calculation.

- *Clinically relevant (or expected) difference.* Here you have to define the difference that you would like to detect with your study. It can be the effect that has been found in previous studies and that you would like to reproduce. Or in situations where there are no previous studies, you can define a difference that you consider clinically relevant. Information can be found in previous studies found in literature or can be based on expectation from clinical practice. Because a small effect is more difficult to pick up than a large effect, decreasing the difference (~effect) will increase sample size. Note: Frequently, available time and resources do not allow the conduct of a clinical trial large enough to reliably detect the smallest clinically relevant effect. In these cases, one may choose a larger difference, with the realization that should the trial result be negative, it will not reliably exclude the possibility of a smaller but clinically important treatment difference.[3] In general, you have to find a balance between defining a large(r) effect that is easier to pick up (i.e., requiring fewer subjects) and running the risk of obtaining a nonsignificant result if the difference turns out smaller.

- *Expected variance/standard deviation.* This should be based on pilot data or previous projects in your institute or comparable studies found in literature. If high variation exists between subjects, a difference between groups or an effect of intervention will be harder to pick up, so more spread in the data will increase sample size.

- *Test to be used in the statistical analysis.* A power calculation will always be based on one particular statistical analysis. Therefore, the sample size calculation forces you to think about the planned data analysis in a very early phase of the study.

- *Attrition rate.* Previous studies in the same population will give an estimate of the expected number of included subjects who will not be available for analysis. This may be caused by dropout or withdrawal from the study. Study burden, follow-up length, and age, for example, will influence the attrition rate. The simplest form of attrition (i.e., attrition not related to the intervention or the outcome) can be easily corrected for in the sample size calculation. After calculation of sample size, adjust so that the number needed remains after expected loss of study subjects. For example, if an attrition rate of 10% is expected, divide the number needed by 0.9 (1 − attrition rate).

Because one never knows the exact difference, spread, or dropout of a study beforehand, a sample size calculation remains a difficult exercise. Repeat the calculation using slightly different input values and check the consequences of these modifications. If absolutely no information is available for the estimation or the necessary input values, one may consider doing a pilot study first.

52.5 Which Software Can be Used for Sample Size Calculations?

Several computer programs exist for performing sample size calculations. On the Internet, several free power programs exist. Reliability of these free programs is not always ensured. We advise you to use a reliable registered program available in your institution for your power calculations and contact your local statistician at an early stage.

52.6 How to Write Down a Sample Size Calculation

Writing down your sample size calculation will aid the local (animal or clinical) ethics committee in understanding your calculations and in interpreting your data. It is advisable to carefully consider writing down your calculation, and to include all steps and considerations as described in this chapter. For example, you are designing a study in which you want to investigate the symptoms of patients undergoing surgery for a chronic inflammatory disease (CID), especially fever. Suppose, you want to compare the temperature in the CID group with a healthy control group undergoing cosmetic surgery, and a clinically relevant difference is determined to be 0.5°C. Previous studies have shown the temperature of healthy individuals (controls) to be 37°C, with a standard deviation of 0.4°C. We assume a normal distribution and that the spread of the temperature is equal in both groups. Using the appropriate software, the sample size is calculated at 12 per arm. The full description of your calculation can be described as follows:

A sample size of 12 in each group (or 24 in total) will have 80% power to detect a difference in means of at least 0.5°C using a two group t-test with a 0.05 two-sided significance level. In this calculation we used the following assumptions: We expect the healthy patients undergoing a cosmetic surgery have a mean temperature of 37°C. We assume that both groups show equal variability in temperature and that the common standard deviation is 0.4° C. A mean temperature of 37.5°C or higher in the CRS patients is considered a relevant sign of fever. We anticipate that only 85% of included patients will have valid measurements. We therefore plan to include 28 patients in total, 14 in the CID group and 14 in the healthy control group.

When asked to report a sample size calculation, this statement is a good starting point. You should customize this statement and complete it with references on which you based the assumptions. A paragraph on a sample size calculation is very explicit; a reader has to be able to reproduce your calculations.

52.7 Advanced Topics

Several situations exist that call for more advanced sample size calculations. Here, we point out some of these situations to make you aware of the need for extra effort when the situation occurs.

- *Equivalence design.* In an equivalence design, you do not want to test for differences; instead, you want to show equivalence. In such a design, you will need to specify your interpretation of equivalent. Perfect equivalence can never be demonstrated. A limit has to be determined of which small difference between groups will be considered not meaningful and lead to the conclusion of equivalence; this is called the equivalence limit difference. Also, the expected difference between groups has to be given. A special type of equivalence designs is a noninferiority design. In this design, one is interested in equivalence in only one test direction. For instance, when a new, less invasive diagnostic procedure is compared to the current invasive one, the new procedure does not have to prove better than the current one. If it has at least similar diagnostic strength as the invasive one, it would be preferred.
- *Clustered design.* When randomization of patients is not done individually but in clusters (e.g., per treating physician or per department), it is expected that the outcome of patients within a cluster are not independent of each other. In the sample size calculation, the correlation between patients needs to be accounted for. Also when multiple observations per patient are obtained, the power calculation has to be suited to take along the correlation between measurements in the same patient.
- *Advanced analyses.* Planned statistical analyses such as survival analysis, regression analysis, and reliability analysis call for their own specific sample size calculation.

References

[1] Knottnerus JA, Bouter LM. The ethics of sample size: two-sided testing and one-sided thinking. J Clin Epidemiol 2001; 54: 109–110
[2] Peace KE. The alternative hypothesis: one-sided or two-sided? J Clin Epidemiol 1989; 42: 473–476
[3] Lewis RJ. Power analysis and sample size determination: concepts and software tools. Presented at the 2000 Annual Meeting of the Society for Academic Emergency Medicine in San Francisco, California

Further Reading

Carley S, Dosman S, Jones SR, Harrison M. Simple nomograms to calculate sample size in diagnostic studies. Emerg Med J 2005; 22: 180–181

Donner A. Sample size requirements for the comparison of two or more coefficients of inter-observer agreement. Stat Med 1998; 17: 1157–1168

Garson GD. 2009. Chi-square significance tests. Statnotes: topics in multivariate analysis. November 6, 2009. http://faculty.chass.ncsu.edu/garson/pa765/statnote.htm

Jones SR, Carley S, Harrison M. An introduction to power and sample size estimation. Emerg Med J 2003; 20: 453–458

Kerry SM, Bland JM. Sample size in cluster randomisation. BMJ 1998; 316: 549

Li J, Fine J. On sample size for sensitivity and specificity in prospective diagnostic accuracy studies. Stat Med 2004; 23: 2537–2550

Walter SD, Eliasziw M, Donner A. Sample size and optimal designs for reliability studies. Stat Med 1998; 17: 101–110

53 Nonparametric versus Parametric Tests

Nicholas Clement

The terms "nonparametric" and "parametric" are used as broad classifications of statistical procedures used to analyze and determine the significance of data between groups.[1] A basic fundamental knowledge of statistical concepts is needed to understand these two terms. These statistical fundamentals include random variables, probability distributions, parameters, population, sample, sampling distributions, and the central limit theorem. These will be covered in this chapter at a superficial level to enable a basic understanding of statistics to be achieved.

The field of statistics exists because it is generally impossible to gather data from all individuals of interest (i.e., the whole population at risk). Hence, the only alternative is to study a smaller subset (sample) of the population at risk, with the ultimate aim being to know the outcome for the whole population.[1] "Parameters" are used to describe the study population; these include quantities such as means, standard deviations, and proportions. Logistically, it is normally not possible to obtain data for the whole population, and hence we cannot determine the parameters of the population. Using a subset (sample) of the population, we can calculate estimates of the parameters for the whole population. When parameters are calculated from the sample data, they are called "statistics"; hence, a statistic estimates a parameter.

There is no exact definition of what constitutes parametric or nonparametric data. However, for practical purposes, parametric statistical procedures rely on assumptions about the shape of the distribution (assumed to have a normal distribution) in the underlying population and about the form or parameters (means and standard deviations) of the assumed distribution.[1] Nonparametric statistical procedures rely on no or few assumptions about the shape or parameters of the population distribution from which the sample was drawn. Hence, before either a parametric or a nonparametric test can be used to analyze the sample data, descriptive statistics must be performed. This chapter will cover how to perform statistical analysis of quantitative and qualitative data, covering data cleaning, descriptive statistics, and parametric and nonparametric statistical tests.

53.1 Data Types

To enable descriptive statistics to be performed, a knowledge of the data type is essential. There are two data types: quantitative and qualitative data (▸ Fig. 53.1).[2]

53.1.1 Cleaning the Data

Data cleaning is an important step that must be performed; do not overlook this step with a view to trying to analyze data quickly, because doing so will result in erroneous conclusions. This process basically entails assessing the sample data to identify "out of range" numbers that need to be amended before statistical analysis takes place.[3] Qualitative variables are best recorded into numerical codes (e.g., male gender = 1 and female gender = 2). Relying upon a string/text variable may result in three groups for gender. For example, male, MALE, and female, due to capitals being used for some males and not

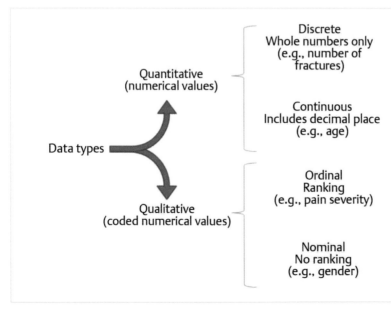

Fig. 53.1 A flow diagram demonstrating the different types of data.

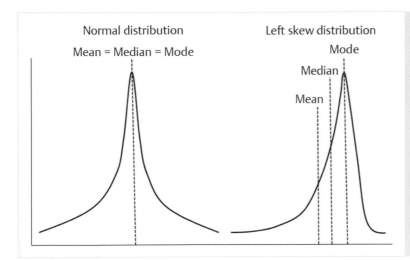

Fig. 53.2 Distribution of two different quantitative data distributions (normal and a left skewed population).

for others. It is also important to record each variable in separate columns (e.g., a blood pressure measurement of 140/80 should be recorded as separate variables in different columns). This will allow systolic and diastolic pressures to be analyzed independently. Frequency tables are useful to identify out-of-range figures; this will highlight variables that are simply not possible (e.g., age 205 years, which has probably had a decimal place missing and is more likely to be 20.5 years old).

53.1.2 Descriptive Statistics

Basic descriptive statistical analysis enables the sample population to be described in relation to a normal population.[2] Quantitative and qualitative variables are described differently. Quantitative variables are described according to their central tendency, normality, spread, and confidence intervals. Qualitative variables, however, do not have these properties and are generally described as frequencies or percentages.

53.1.3 Quantitative Variables

Central Tendency

There are three measures of central tendency: mean, median, and mode (▶ Fig. 53.2).[2] The sample mean is the average value of the data collected (total of all variables/n). An alternative measure is the sample median, which is the ranked value that is in the middle of the dataset (e.g., ages 24, 28, 34, 45, and 58 will result in a median age of 34). Hence it is the value that divides the distribution of the scores into two equal halves. The mode is the most frequently occurring value in the sample data, which is normally quoted with a percentage of the sample population that falls within that value. The mean and the median are the most commonly used measure of central tendency in medical research: The distribution of the data dictates which measure should be used.[4] If the data

is normally distributed, all measures (mean, median, and mode) should be equal, and the mean is generally quoted. However, if the data is skewed, which may be to the right or left, the median is a more appropriate measure (▶ Fig. 53.2).

Normality

It is essential to check the normality of the sample population to allow the appropriate descriptive and correct statistical tests to be performed. There are three methods of doing this: by using graphs, descriptive statistics (skewness and kurtosis), or by statistical tests.

A histogram is the simplest way to observe whether the sample data is distributed normally or skewed (▶ Fig. 53.3).[3] Alternatively, Q-Q plots can be used to help decide the normality of the data. This plot compares the quantiles (Q) of data distribution with the quantiles (Q) of a standardized theoretical distribution (i.e., normal distribution). If the distributions match, the points will demonstrate a straight line (▶ Fig. 53.3a), signifying a normally distributed population. In contrast, if the plots illustrate a curve (▶ Fig. 53.3b), this indicates different patterns of distribution representative of a skewed population.[3] Deviations at the ends of plot indicate outliers within the population.

The value derived from the skewness indicates whether the data is skewed to the right (>0), normal (~ 0), or to left (<0).[2] The skewness ranges from −3 to 3, with an acceptable range for normally distributed data lying between −1 to 1. Skewness should not be used in isolation; kurtosis measures the relative peakness of the bell shaped curve (▶ Fig. 53.4). A range between −1 and 1 indicates a normal distribution of the population (▶ Fig. 53.3).

Komolgorov-Smirnov and Shapiro-Wilk are formal statistical tests that can be performed where significant differences are observed for data that is skewed.[3] Reliance upon these tests is dependent upon the sample size,

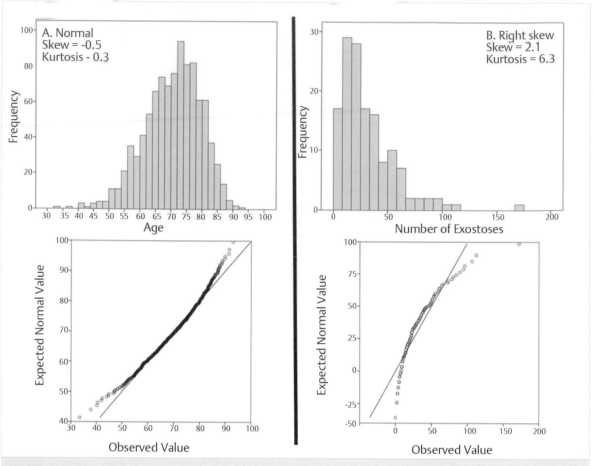

Fig. 53.3 Histogram and Q-Q plots for a normally distributed population (**a**) and a skewed population (**b**).

where the likelihood of obtaining a significant result (skewed) from a small sample ($n < 30$) is low. In contrast, for larger sample sizes ($n > 100$), a minor deviation from normal may produce a significant result but demonstrate a relatively normally distribution. So how do we know what is normal and what is not? A general rule is that for small samples ($n < 30$), a skewed distribution should be assumed for the population. Moderate samples ($n = 30$ to 100) that are statistically significant (skewed) are accepted, but if a nonsignificant result is obtained, double check using graphs, skewness, and kurtosis to affirm normality. In contrast, nonsignificant results (normal distribution) for large samples ($n > 100$) are accepted, but if significance is demonstrated this should be checked using graphs, skewness, and kurtosis to affirm a skewed population.[2]

Measures of Spread

An important descriptor to be presented with quantitative data is the variability or the spread of the data points.[4] A simple method of presenting this is the range of scores, being the minimum and maximum scores within the dataset. However, this does not give an indication of how the data is distributed between these points for the study sample (▶ Fig. 53.4). Standard deviation of the data is used to demonstrate how the data is distributed around the mean. The standard deviation is calculated from the square root of the variance, which is measure of spread (corrected sum of the squares about the mean). One standard deviation includes 68%, two standard deviations include 95%, and three standard deviations include 99% of the sample population.[2] The smaller the standard deviation, the more the data is centered around the mean score, whereas the greater the standard deviation the greater to spread of the data around the mean (▶ Fig. 53.4). When quoting a mean, it is convention to accompany this with a standard deviation, often in brackets subsequent to the mean. A small standard deviation is not always a good thing; for example, if the standard deviation for the sample population was small, this would suggest that the intervention may only be applicable to a specific age group. Alternatively, a small standard deviation in an outcome score demonstrates consistency of the intervention.

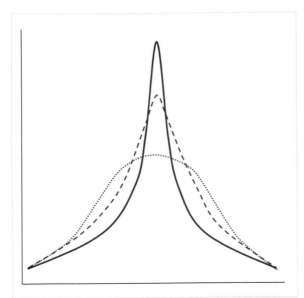

Fig. 53.4 Three normally distributed populations with differing kurtosis, where the *solid line* has a kurtosis > 0, the *dashed line* has a kurtosis ~ 0, and the *dotted line* has a kurtosis of < 0. The standard deviation also varies, with the *solid line* having a standard distribution of 1, whereas the *dotted line* has a standard deviation of 2.

Data that demonstrates a skewed distribution the interquartile range is used instead of the standard deviation. This range excludes values at the extremes of the sample population, giving an indication of how the data is centered around the median. Using 3, 4, **4**, 6, 8, **8**, 10, 10, **11**, 12, 31 as a sample population, the median is 8 with the lower quartile being 4 and the upper quartile being 11. The interquartile range is the difference between the upper quartile and the lower quartile (e.g., the interquartile range for the example is 11 − 4 = 7).

Confidence Intervals

Due to the use of a sample population, if a study was repeated multiple times, the mean and standard deviation would vary. Using the theory of "sampling distribution of the mean," the mean of all means obtained from repeated samples would give a more specific estimate for the population. However, due to finite budgets and ethical constraints, repeated studies are not feasible. Using the central limit theorem with a large enough sample, an interval estimate can be calculated between which we are confident the true mean lies.[2] This is normally quoted as the 95% confidence interval, whereby we can be 95% sure that the true mean lies between these two values. The confidence limits are calculated using the standard error of the mean, which is defined as the standard deviation divided by the square root of the sample size. The standard error of the mean is then multiplied by 1.96 to give 95% confidence intervals (e.g., sample mean ±

[standard error of the mean × 1.96]). This confidence interval indicates the quality of the result; for example, if the difference in an outcome score was 6 with 95%, confidence intervals of ± 5 (2.55 × 1.96) may be due to a small sample size or a wide variation in the difference between the groups. Confidence intervals are generally used when illustrating a difference after an intervention; for example, a change in an outcome score before and after total knee replacement.

53.1.4 Qualitative Variables

Descriptive statistics of categorical variables is limited; frequency tables are probably adequate.[2] Ordinal variables may benefit from visual presentation using a bar or pie chart (e.g., very satisfied, satisfied, neutral, unsatisfied, and very unsatisfied).

53.2 Data Interpretation

The null hypothesis is the key concept to statistical analysis, where the assumption is made that any observed difference is a chance occurrence. The collected data is then used to disprove the null hypothesis, and if a statistically significant result is obtained then the null hypothesis is rejected. The observed difference must therefore be real and not have occurred by chance. Most researchers are willing to accept a 5% probability that the difference occurred by chance, hence the commonly quoted p value of 0.05 is equal to that 5% probability that the result is due to chance.[4]

Errors can arise when accepting or rejecting the null hypothesis.[5] A type I error occurs when a significant difference is found but in reality no difference exists. The null hypothesis is wrongly rejected (i.e., one of the 5% of results that occur by chance). A type II error occurs when no significant difference is identified but in reality a difference does exist. This may be due to a small sample size, hence the importance of a power calculation before undertaking a study (see Chapter 52). These two errors are inversely related, decreasing the accepted p value reduces type I error but increases type II error and vice versa.[5]

53.2.1 Statistical Tests

There are multiple statistical tests available, but the specific test used is dependent upon the type of analysis being performed and whether the data demonstrates a parametric or nonparametric characteristics.[3] ► Table 53.1 illustrates which statistical test is most appropriate according to these criteria.

The first part of the following section deals with which statistical test should be used according to the data analysis required and data parameters; both quantitative and qualitative data will be discussed.

Table 53.1 Statistical Tests That are Appropriate for a Given Sample Distribution or Data Type According to the Required Analysis

Type of analysis	Parametric	Nonparametric	
	Normal distribution	Skewed distribution	Nominal data
Two groups	Unpaired t-test	Mann-Whitney U test	Chi-square test or Fisher's exact ($n < 5$)
Intervention in the same group	Paired t-test	Wilcoxon signed rank test	McNemar's test
More than two groups	Analysis of one-way variance	Kruskal Wallis test	Chi-square test
Association between two variables	Pearson correlation	Spearman correlation	Contingency coefficients

Table 53.2 Unpaired t-test for the Improvement in Oxford Knee Score before and after a Total Knee Replacement According to Gender

Independent samples test							
	Levene's test for equality of variances		t-test for equality of means				
	F	Significance	Significance	Mean difference	Standard error difference	95% confidence interval of the difference	
			(Two-tailed)			Lower	Upper
Equal variances assumed	1.865	0.172	0.023	1.44127	0.63368	0.19772	2.68482
Equal variances not assumed			0.024	1.44127	0.63811	0.18887	2.69368

Qualitative Data

Parametric tests will be applied when assumptions of normality are satisfied; if this is not the case, the equivalent nonparametric test will then be discussed.

- Unpaired data: For example, comparison of two different groups after an intervention.

An example of this would be to compare the improvement in the Oxford knee score after a total knee replacement between male and female genders. A power analysis should be performed before the commencement of such a comparative study is undertaken (see Chapter 52). There are three assumptions[5] that must be fulfilled before an unpaired t-test can be performed:
1. Normal distribution for both populations
2. Both groups are random samples
3. Homogeneity of variance (population variances are the same)

The first two assumptions can be checked as described previously for normality and by the study design (see Chapter 51). The third assumption is normally given as part of the output of the statistical package used. Levene's test for equality of variances checks that the population variances are the same.[3] ▶ Table 53.2 demonstrates a typical output from a statistically package for an unpaired t-test, in this case Statistical Package for Social Sciences version 17.0 (SPSS Inc., Chicago, IL). The nonsignificant difference between variances of 0.17 in the third column for Levene's test of equal variances means that the values on the first row ("Equal variances assumed") can be used. This illustrates that there is a 1.4 point difference, with a 95% confidence interval of 0.20 to 2.68 and a p value of 0.023. However, if the p value for Levene's test was significant (< 0.05), the second row would be used ("Equal variances not assumed") because the distribution of the groups is significantly different. SPSS adjusts for this different and returns differing 95% confidence intervals and p values.

When the normality assumptions are not satisfied, a Mann–Whitney U test can be performed. There is, however, a difference in the statistical output from this test, returning a z score and a p value only.[3]

Table 53.3 Paired t-test for the Oxford Knee Score before and after a Total Knee Replacement

	Paired differences					Significance (two-tailed)
	Mean	Standard deviation	Standard error mean	95% confidence interval of the difference		
				Lower	Upper	
Pair 1	15.680	9.787	0.315	15.062	16.298	0.000

- Paired data: For example, before and after an intervention within the same sample population.

An example of this would be the improvement in the Oxford knee score before and after a total knee replacement. Simple descriptive statistics should be performed first, such as the mean or median for pre- and postintervention scores with their respective standard deviation or interquartile range. The difference between these two samples should then be computed as a new variable and checked for normality.[5] ▶ Table 53.3 demonstrates a typical output from a statistical package for a paired t-test (SPSS Inc.).[3] This illustrates that there was a 15.7 point increase in the Oxford knee score after a total knee replacement, and we can be 95% sure that the true value lies between 15.1 and 16.3 points, which is statistically significant. This is also likely to be clinically significant. A minimal clinically important difference is defined as the smallest change of a score to be of importance, which is generally defined as half the standard deviation of the variable.[6,7] Standard deviation for this sample population was 9.8; hence the minimal clinically important difference is 4.9, which has been surpassed by the mean difference and the lower 95% confidence interval limit.

If the normality assumptions were not satisfied, a Wilcoxon signed rank test is performed. In this case, medians of the variables are analyzed rather than the mean. The Wilcoxon signed rank test uses the magnitude of positives and negative as ranks to calculate significance.[3]
- Multiple groups: For example, comparison of three or more different groups after an intervention.

An example of this would be to compare the improvement in the Oxford knee score after a total knee replacement between social quintiles (five ordinal groups, where 1 is the most deprived and 5 is the least deprived). Analysis of one-way variance is an extension of the t-test. The aforementioned three assumptions, for the unpaired t-test, also apply to the sample populations for the analysis of one-way variance. Again, the same principles apply to satisfy these assumptions. The homogeneity of variance test in SPSS for preoperative Oxford knee scores according to social quintile produces ▶ Table 53.4, which indicates no significant difference ($p = 0.377$), and we can assume equal variance for population samples.[3] ▶ Table 53.5 demonstrates that there is a significant difference between groups with a p value of < 0.0001; post

Table 53.4 Homogeneity of Variance Test between Multiple Groups

Test of homogeneity of variances

Difference in Oxford knee score

Levene statistic	df1	df2	Significance
1.057	4	957	0.377

Table 53.5 Analysis of One-Way Variance Results for Difference in Oxford Knee Score According to Social Quintile

	Sum of squares	df	Mean square	F	Significance
Between groups	1639.822	4	409.955	7.664	0.000
Within groups	51192.952	957	53.493		
Total	52832.773	961			

hoc testing needs to be carried out to determine between which groups these differences occur. Bonferroni corrected post hoc analysis is a commonly used technique, which multiples the p value by the number of comparisons performed to adjust the type 1 error (in this case 10).[5] ▶ Table 53.6 demonstrates that on post hoc analysis, with Bonferroni correction, there were only statistically significant differences between social quintiles 1 with 4 ($p = 0.047$) and 5 ($p < 0.001$), and social quintile 2 with 5 ($p < 0.001$). To illustrate the effect of the Bonferroni correction, if a t-test is performed comparing social quintile 1 with 4, the p value is 0.0047 (i.e., 10 times greater to correct for the number of comparisons made).

When assumptions of normality and homogeneity are not satisfied for the sample groups, a Kruskal Wallis test is used.[5] This will return a p value without an option of post hoc analysis, which will need to be performed using multiple Mann–Whitney U tests for each of the comparative groups.[3] The p value would then need to be adjusted according to the number of comparisons made (multiple the p value by number of comparisons made).
- Correlation between two continuous variables: For examples, relationship between two linear variables.

An example of this would be the relationship between preoperative knee function according to the Oxford knee

Table 53.6 Analysis of One-Way Variance with Bonferroni Correction for Post Hoc Analysis

(I) Quintile	(J) Quintile	Mean difference (I-J)	Standard error	Significance	95% confidence interval	
					Lower bound	Upper bound
1	2	0.670	0.861	1.000	−1.75	3.09
	3	1.900	0.880	0.311	−0.58	4.38
	4	2.499[a]	0.882	0.047	0.02	4.98
	5	3.673[a]	0.820	0.000	1.37	5.98
2	1	−0.670	0.861	1.000	−3.09	1.75
	3	1.230	0.743	0.982	-0.86	3.32
	4	1.829	0.745	0.143	−0.27	3.93
	5	3.003[a]	0.671	0.000	1.12	4.89
3	1	−1.900	0.880	0.311	−4.38	0.58
	2	−1.230	0.743	0.982	−3.32	0.86
	4	0.599	0.767	1.000	−1.56	2.76
	5	1.774	0.695	0.108	−0.18	3.73
4	1	−2.499[a]	0.882	0.047	−4.98	−0.02
	2	−1.829	0.745	0.143	−3.93	0.27
	3	−0.599	0.767	1.000	−2.76	1.56
	5	1.175	0.697	0.923	−0.79	3.14
5	1	−3.673[a]	0.820	0.000	−5.98	−1.37
	2	−3.003[a]	0.671	0.000	−4.89	−1.12
	3	−1.774	0.695	0.108	−3.73	0.18
	4	−1.175	0.697	0.923	−3.14	0.79

[a]The mean difference is significant at the 0.05 level.

score and improvement in the score postoperatively. The relationship between these two variables is shown in ▶ Fig. 53.5. This plot demonstrates that with increasing preoperative Oxford knee score, signifying more severe symptoms, the greater the improvement in the postoperative score (reduction of symptoms). To demonstrate the degree of the linear relationship between the two variables, a correlation coefficient is generated.[8] If both variables are normally distributed, a Pearson's correlation is preformed, otherwise a Spearman's correlation is performed.[3] A Spearman's correlation can also be used for categorical ordinal variables such as satisfaction (e.g., very satisfied, satisfied, neutral, unsatisfied, very unsatisfied). ▶ Table 53.7 demonstrates the Pearson's correlation coefficient ($r = 0.335$) generated by SPSS for the plot in ▶ Fig. 53.5, which illustrates the correlation to be significant ($p < 0.001$). The value of r, the correlation coefficient, can be negative or positive.[8] A negative r simply means that there is an inverse relationship between the variables, and as one increases the other decreases, whereas a

positive r means as one variable increases so does the other. The value of r indicates the strength of the correlation, where a value of 0 equates to no correlation and + or −1 equates to a strong correlation (▶ Table 53.8).[9] Using the example in ▶ Table 53.7, there is a "fair" correlation but the p value is small, which is due to the large size of the cohort ($n = 966$). It is important to acknowledge this difference between correlation and significance. A small cohort may result in failure to demonstrate a statistical significance despite a strong correlation, though a larger cohort may produce statistical significance but the correlation may be poor.

The r squared gives the coefficient of determination that indicates the proportion of variance the two variables have in common.[9] Using the example from ▶ Table 53.7, the r squared is 0.112, which means that 11.2% of the change postoperative score is explained by the preoperative score. However, this also means that 88.8% of the change is related to other factors. Precautions must be made to ensure subgroup populations are

Table 53.7 Correlation Coefficient for Preoperative Oxford Knee Score and Improvement Postoperatively

		Preoperative Oxford knee score	Change in Oxford knee score postoperatively
Preoperative Oxford knee score	Pearson correlation	1	0.335[a]
	Significance (two-tailed)		0.000
	N	966	966
Change in Oxford knee score postoperatively	Pearson correlation	0.335[a]	1
	Significance (two-tailed)	0.000	
	N	966	966

[a]Correlation is significant at the 0.01 level (two-tailed).

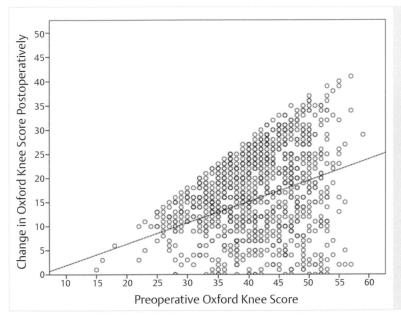

Fig. 53.5 A scattered plot demonstrating correlation between preoperative Oxford knee score with change in the score postoperatively.

Table 53.8 Strength of the Linear Relationship According to the Correlation Coefficient

Correlation coefficient	Strength of linear relationship
1 to 0.8	Very strong
0.6 to < 0.8	Moderately strong
0.3 to < 0.6	Fair
< 0.3	Poor

not different (e.g., gender), where one may be significant and the other is not. Also, outliers can affect the correlation: for example, a 40 entered in place of 4.0 due to failure to acknowledge the decimal point (▶ Fig. 53.6). These two potential errors can be avoided by performing analysis using graphs that will illustrate subgroup differences and outliers (▶ Fig. 53.6).

A potential difficulty when analyzing correlations is the interaction of a third variable. Using the example in ▶ Table 53.7 again, age may also influence postoperative change in the Oxford knee score. The effect of age can be controlled for by using partial correlation.[3] ▶ Table 53.9 illustrates that age has no effect upon change in the Oxford knee score, due to the fact the correlation coefficient has not changed to any great extent ($r = 0.334$).

Chi-square, Fisher's exact, and McNemar tests are all methods of determining statistical significance between groups for categorical variables.[10] Such an example would be using a Chi-square test to reject the null hypothesis that there is no difference in the rate of satisfaction after total knee replacement between male and female genders. A cross-tabulation table can be constructed, according to the counts in each category. ▶ Table 53.10 demonstrates a typical 2 × 2 cross-tabulation table; however, this can vary according to the number of categorical

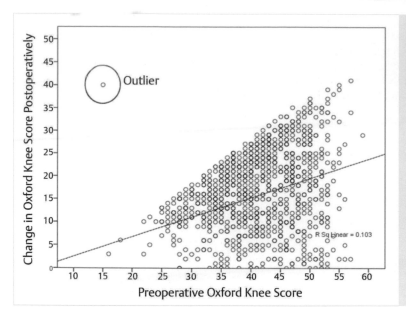

Fig. 53.6 Same scatter plot as ▶ Fig. 53.5, but there is an obvious outlier (*circled*) that needs to be investigated and amended accordingly before further analysis takes place.

Table 53.9 Partial Correlation between Preoperative Oxford Knee Score and Improvement Postoperatively Controlling for Age

Control variables			Preoperative Oxford knee score	Change in Oxford knee score postoperatively
Age	Preoperative Oxford knee score	Correlation	1.000	0.334
		Significance (two-tailed)		0.000
		df	0	963
	Change in Oxford knee score postoperatively	Correlation	0.334	1.000
		Significance (two-tailed)	0.000	
		df	963	0

Table 53.10 A 2 × 2 Cross-Tabulation Table for Satisfaction after a Total Knee Replacement According to Gender

		Satisfied		Total
		Yes	No	
Gender	Male	351	70	421
	Female	468	77	545
Total		819	147	966

Table 53.11 A 2 × 2 Cross-Tabulation Table for the Presence of a Disease According to Groups

		Disease	
		Yes	No
Group	1	a	b
	2	c	d

variables (e.g., 2 × 4 or 3 × 4, etc.). From this table, a Chi-square test can be performed, and for the example in ▶ Table 53.10 the *p* value was 0.28, so we cannot reject the null hypothesis. If there was a significant association observed, the *p* value does not indicate what the association is or the strength of this association. Observing ▶ Table 53.10, the relationship is not clear; however, by calculating the satisfaction rate by gender reveals that males (351/421 = 83.4%) are not as satisfied as females (468/545 = 85.9%). The strength of the association can be calculated using an odds ratio or by the relative risk; however, these can only be calculated for 2 × 2 cross-tabulation table (▶ Table 53.11). The odds ratio is the ratio of the odds of having the disease in group 1 compared to the ratio of the odds of having the disease in group 2 [odds ratio = (a × d) / (b × c)].[10] For the example in ▶ Table 53.10, the odds ratio is 0.83 [(351 × 77) /

(468 × 70)]. This value (< 1) indicates group 1 (males) are less likely to be satisfied, whereas if this value was greater than 1 it would indicate that they would be more likely to satisfied with their knee replacement relative to females. The relative risk is the ratio between having the disease in group 1 compared with having the disease in group 2 [relative risk = (a × (c + d)) / (c × (a + b))]. For the example in ▶ Table 53.10, the relative risk is 0.97 [(351 × 545) / (468 × 421)].

The validity of the Chi-square test is violated when there are small frequencies in the cells within the cross-tabulation table. When the expected count is less than five, a Fisher's exact test is used.[10] Furthermore, if the number of subjects is small ($n < 30$), a Yates' continuity correction has to be made in order to avoid individual values having an overly significant influence on the calculation.

A McNemar test is used when there is matched categorical data that has been gathered from a case control study (i.e., paired nominal data). The McNemar test compares the observations of the discordant pairs in a 2 × 2 table similar to a Chi-square test.[9] An example of this is patients who had pain (yes or no) prior to a surgery compared to the same patients who did not have pain after a total knee replacement.

53.3 Conclusion

It is crucial to clean the collected data before any statistical analysis is performed. The data can then be classified according to their type. Simple descriptive statistics can then be applied to define the sample population and to be categorized as nonparametric or parametric. Interpretation of the data can then performed using the correct nonparametric or parametric statistical test(s) and the type of analysis required. However, the obtained p value needs to be taken into context with the said difference—is it clinically relevant and how strong is the relationship? Statistical analysis is useful, but this needs to be used in conjunction with critical clinical analysis also.

References

[1] Bhandari M, Joensson A. Review of basic statistical principles. In: Clinical research for surgeons. Stuttgart: Thieme; 2009:269–278
[2] Chan YH. Biostatistics 101: data presentation. Singapore Med J 2003; 44: 280–285
[3] Pallant J. SPSS survival manual. 3 e. Maidenhead: Open University Press; 2007
[4] Bhandari M, Joensson A. Statistical means and proportions. In: Clinical research for surgeons. Stuttgart: Thieme; 2009:279–287
[5] Chan YH. Biostatistics 102: quantitative data—parametric & nonparametric tests. Singapore Med J 2003; 44: 391–396
[6] Norman GR, Sloan JA, Wyrwich KW. Interpretation of changes in health-related quality of life: the remarkable universality of half a standard deviation. Med Care 2003; 41: 582–592
[7] Schmitt JS, Di Fabio RP. Reliable change and minimum important difference (MID) proportions facilitated group responsiveness comparisons using individual threshold criteria. J Clin Epidemiol 2004; 57: 1008–1018
[8] Bhandari M, Joensson A. Correlation defined. In: Clinical research for surgeons. Stuttgart: Thieme; 2009:301–8
[9] Chan YH. Biostatistics 104: correlational analysis. Singapore Med J 2003; 44: 614–619
[10] Chan YH. Biostatistics 103: qualitative data - tests of independence. Singapore Med J 2003; 44: 498–503

Further Reading

Kocher MS, Zurakowski D. Clinical epidemiology and biostatistics: a primer for orthopaedic surgeons. J Bone Joint Surg Am 2004; 86-A: 607–620

54 How to Limit Bias in Experimental Research

Paul J. Jenkins

All scientific studies are subject to experimental error, and it is the duty of the investigator to eliminate it where possible, or reduce its impact if it cannot be completely removed. Error may jeopardize the validity of research findings, which may result in useless or harmful treatments being recommended, a waste of limited research resources. Bias is a specific type of error that results in a consistently false result through a systemic flaw in the experiment's methodology. It has been increasingly recognized that clinical and basic scientific research may be subject to significant biases that jeopardize their findings.[1,2]

In order to understand and reduce potential sources of error, an investigator requires a sound understanding of the experimental process (▶ Fig. 54.1). Some study types are inherently more at risk of error than others. Inclusion and exclusion criteria are selected, or a suitable animal model, organ, tissue, cell line, or other biological material is chosen. An outcome measure is selected, and comparison of this outcome measure is made between study groups. The methodology of group allocation is critical to performing a sound experiment. The study results are analyzed, written up, and reported via posters, conference presentations, and papers. These are then disseminated to other researchers via journals and research databases. These results may then be further assimilated by meta-analysis.

54.1 New Techniques in Musculoskeletal Research

Jargon Simplified: Finite Element Analysis

Finite element analysis is a technique that is used to examine the internal stresses, strains, and deformation of materials under loads. It can be applied to simple homogenous materials, or complex heterogeneous biological tissues. Each structure is composed of a multitude of smaller elements that may be rectangles, cubes, or tetrahedrons. They are linked by "nodes" at their edges. The properties of each element and their influence on their neighbor is calculated for the overall structure. This requires intensive computational power for complex materials. Specific biological tissues can be modeled through the creation of a "mesh" from three-dimensional imaging such as computed tomography. The results predicted by the models can be compared to in vitro testing of the tissue under controlled conditions as part of the validation process.

Musculoskeletal research has been enhanced by the development of new techniques to explore biochemical processes, genes, and proteins. New imaging techniques have allowed more detailed structure of cellular and extracellular structure. These new techniques are subject to experimental error, and the investigator should recognize the potential sources of error. Biomechanical research also regularly investigates the material properties of tissues and implants. Design and testing of novel implants requires techniques to evaluate strength, fatigability, and wear in both in vitro and in vivo scenarios. Finite element analysis, while offering myriad new possibilities to understand loading and stress distribution in biological tissues and implants, has specific sources of error and bias that must be recognized.

Techniques in molecular biology and biomechanics are constantly evolving, and it is impossible to provide complete coverage of each of them, along with specific biases. The aim of this chapter is to discuss the types of bias that may occur in research, with particular reference to musculoskeletal research. It will also discuss techniques to reduce these through study design and risk assessment. Using this knowledge, researchers will be able to reduce the influence of bias through careful planning of their research and experiments. They will also be able to analyze new techniques for potential sources of bias.

54.1.1 Key Concepts: Types of Experimental Error

Random error occurs when there is chance variation between individuals or specimens. Biological processes may be influenced by myriad factors, and no two specimens or sets of environmental conditions are identical. These errors can only be reduced by the ubiquitous techniques of increasing repetition, multiple samples, and averaging of results. Statistical techniques exist that may be used to decide whether a difference between groups is a result of chance or represents a real effect. Random errors are generally reduced by increasing the sample size. Sample sizes are limited, however, by experimental design, technical, time, and funding considerations. A researcher can predict the sample size required by performing a power calculation. A power calculation generally requires an estimate of the dispersion of the characteristic in the sample (such as standard deviation) and the minimal detectable difference expected to be measured. In situations where these are not able to established from existing research, a pilot study may be required.

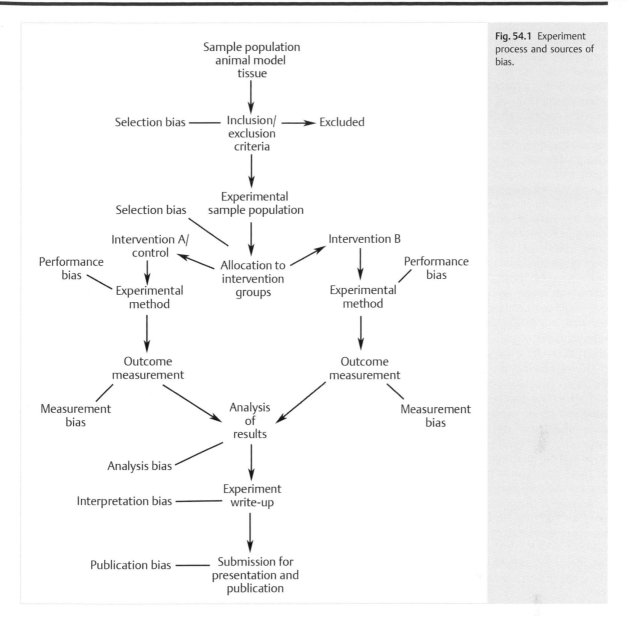

Fig. 54.1 Experiment process and sources of bias.

Systematic error is otherwise known as bias.[3] While random errors can be reduced by repeated experiments, biased studies can never be improved by repetition or sample size. Bias is the tendency of an experiment to produce a finding that is not consistent with the actual situation, through the methodology of performing the experiment. There are five main types of bias and they are influential at different stages of the research path.

54.1.2 Key Concepts: Main Types of Bias

- **Selection bias:** Systematic error introduced in choosing the experimental population and dividing it into groups

- **Performance bias:** Systematic error introduced carrying out the experiment
- **Measurement bias:** Systematic error introduced assessing outcome
- **Analytical and interpretation bias:** Systematic error introduced during the analysis of data and interpretation of results
- **Publication bias:** Systematic error introduced during the submission and presentation of the findings

54.2 Types of Bias

54.2.1 Selection Bias

Selection bias occurs where experimental subjects or specimens are divided into different intervention groups.

The optimum situation would for each group to be completely identical apart from the characteristic of being *deliberately* altered between groups. This could refer to animal model age and gender or cell line characteristics. Confounding is a particular result of selection bias, where a second, unmeasured characteristic is linked with group selection and may also influence a group to have an association with the outcome measure. In animal models that require the induction of a disease state or performance of a surgical procedure, knowledge of the subsequent study group may influence the researcher performing this step, thereby introducing bias.[3]

An experiment may also be planned on tissue obtained from live patients (such as ligament, tendon, cartilage, or bone). In such cases, other forms of selection bias may occur, similar to other clinical studies. Sample bias is a form of selection bias that results from the sample population having different characteristics from a target population such as age, gender, or comorbidity. Sample bias is one of the most common biases present in basic science research, where the tissue or model is not adequately representative of the in vivo process and the generalizability of results is limited.

Referral bias may occur if only a proportion of those in the target population, meeting the inclusion criteria, are considered for the research study. Certain groups of patients may be more likely to participate in research than others, and this may introduce participant bias where the results will have a tendency to reflect the situation in those more likely to participate in research. Some of these effects may be negligible, but often they are unknown and inestimable.

Selection bias can also result from loss to follow-up or post hoc exclusion of subjects. In basic science research, this may occur where a technique does not work as planned in a particular group. If these results are not included, the results may be biased toward or away from the group in which the technique worked.

Reducing Selection Bias

Control of selection bias is easier in prospective experiments where the target population or specimen specification can be tightly controlled to ensure uniformity between group. In retrospective studies, or studies where experimentation is planned on tissue obtained from patients during a study, selection bias is primarily controlled through rigorous study design and participant selection. In animal studies, the specimens should be of the same age and gender at the time of the study. If the disease process is to be induced prior to intervention, this should be performed without knowledge of the subsequent intervention group.

Randomization is one of the most powerful methods of reducing selection bias. It can reduce the effect of unequal distribution of known and unknown characteristics between groups. As such, it is also effective in reducing random error. Practically, this can be performed using many techniques that include sealed envelopes and computerized randomization services. The researcher should be unaware of the randomization sequence. Randomization should occur at the time of intervention. The use of quasirandomization techniques based on study sequence or day of week (among others) offer less protection against bias. Block randomization can be used to ensure that groups remain balanced at the end of a predetermined number of participants (i.e., six or eight) to assist in resource utilization. This may be important if a procedure- or time-intensive assay was required by the protocol. Stratification and minimization are techniques used in the randomization procedure to account for known confounding characteristics, where it is extremely desirable to ensure equal distribution between groups. Decisions regarding stratification and minimization should be taken during the development of the protocol if particularly powerful confounders are recognized. The advice of biostatistician is recommended for these more advanced techniques of randomization because they can have significant implications on power calculations (as studies require to be powered to demonstrate differences between subgroups).

Jargon Simplified: Allocation Concealment

Allocation concealment is the practice of protecting the randomization sequence from prior knowledge to the participants or researchers. This could result from knowledge of random number tables used to generate the sealed envelopes. For this reason, the use of external randomization techniques (which are more accessible in days of Internet access) or sequential numbering of sealed envelopes to prevent tampering with the sequence are used to prevent selection bias.

54.2.2 Performance (Intervention) Bias

If the researcher is aware of what experimental group each specimen is in during the intervention phase, or if a treatment, test, or assay is performed differently in each group performance bias may occur. This varies from bias introduced during the creation of the sample, model, or cell line. It is sometimes also referred to as intervention bias. The most common type of performance bias is ascertainment bias where knowledge of treatment group may alter the researcher's or assessor's performance of the experiment.

Reducing Performance Bias

Animals participating in animal studies should be housed in identical conditions. Cells in cultures should be incubated in the same environmental conditions of temperature, nutrition, and handling. Similarly, experiments on tissue should occur under identical atmospheric (temperature and humidity) conditions and similar times of the day, using the same equipment. The same investigator should perform all interventions, or if this is not possible, investigators should be mixed randomly between groups. If one investigator performed one intervention and another investigator performed another intervention, there may a difference in technique, rather than the intervention itself.

Example of Performance Bias

It was hypothesized that extracorporeal irradiation may be beneficial in the treatment of chondrosarcoma, a tumor that is not normally sensitive to radiation delivered with the tumor in situ. A study was planned to assess the efficacy of radiation in killing chondrosarcoma cells under laboratory conditions. A specimen of chondrosarcoma was removed from a patient. The tumor was split, and half was subjected to irradiation. Cells from this specimen were stored overnight in a fridge at 0°C. In the interim, cells from the other half of the specimen were taken and incubated for cell culture. The following morning, the irradiated cells were also placed in cell culture. After 48 hours, a live:dead assay was performed, and it was found that there were no surviving cells in the half that had been irradiated.

This case is subject to performance bias in that the cells that were irradiated were stored in different conditions and for a different time period prior to culture. This may also have affected the results of the culture; the observed effect could not be solely attributed to irradiation.

The use of placebo interventions is important. The very act of performing the intervention may also affect the outcome. This is especially important in animal studies involving surgical procedures. Placebo surgery is rare in clinical studies in human subjects for ethical reasons. In animal models, the use of placebo surgery allows for the creation of similar surgical trauma and local inflammation, with the only difference being the intervention in question.

Studies of pharmacological agents should use similar volumes of biologically inert substances introduced into the control groups at the same time and under the same conditions.

54.2.3 Measurement Bias

Measurement bias is an extremely important source of bias in basic science research. The preselected outcome requires measurement using instruments and a scale. The instrument may not be properly calibrated (a set of scales not "zeroed") or the scale may lack the precision to identify the change occurring (i.e., the use of a ruler to detect a change on the micrometer scale).

> ### Jargon Simplified: Calibration
>
> Calibration is the adjusting of a measuring instrument to check its accuracy by comparing the results obtained by it to a known standard. A researcher should be fully aware of the calibration process for any instrument being used. The calibration process should be reported in any write-up of the experiment or publication.
>
> Ascertainment bias also affects measurement: If a researcher is aware of the experimental allocation, this may affect knowingly or unknowingly their application of a measure.

Example of Measurement Bias

As part of a study, a researcher had to examine histological slides of ligament tissue and quantify the degree of staining for elastin. The specimens came from two groups of patients: those with generalized ligamentous laxity and those without. The researcher had to grade the specimens on a scale from 0 to 5 based on the degree of staining.

If the researcher knew which patients had generalized ligamentous laxity, their quantification of staining may have introduced a measurement bias. This could have been reduced by concealing the allocation from the researcher or by having the slides assessed by an independent researcher. The process could also have been repeated and averaged to assess reliability and reproducibility.

A specific form of measurement bias may arise from the instrument (instrument bias) or the scale used for measurement (insensitive measure bias). A researcher will use a variety of instruments, and all of these require correct calibration and maintenance.

Reducing Measurement Bias

Blinding is an important technique in the reduction of performance bias.[4] Blinding is the prevention of the trial participant, investigator, and assessor from knowing which group the participant is in. This definition highlights the importance of having the performance of the intervention independent from the assessment of outcome. In basic research, where the subject may be an animal, tissue, or cell line, the blinding of the participant is less relevant. Participant blinding may, however, be important in studies where tissue has been obtained from human patients, because knowledge of study group allocation may result in unrecognized differences in treatment prior to tissue harvest.

Blinding may be impossible in some studies such as investigations requiring surgical procedures. In the use of biological material and pharmacological agents, the substances can be identified by means of codes so the investigator is unaware of which substance is being used until the code is broken at the end of the study. Such substances can be obtained from manufacturers in special masked containers, or could be made within the laboratory by an independent technician, without knowledge of allocation.

Blinding is commonly referred to a single-blind, double-blind, or triple-blind. Single-blind studies are more common in clinical settings where the participant is unaware of which group they are in or whether they are receiving an active treatment or placebo. Double-blind studies refer to those where the investigator is also unaware what intervention each subject is receiving treatment. Triple-blind studies refer to those where the outcome assessment is made independently from the intervention, without knowledge of the experimental group. The blinded, independent assessment of outcomes is the most common method by which researchers in basic science experiments can reduce performance and measurement bias. In common discussions, double-blind means that both participant and researcher are unaware of treatment group.

Calibration involves the comparison of the results obtained by the testing machine when testing a known reference standard under controlled conditions. Temperature and humidity may also affect the calibration and performance of a measuring device such as a strain gauge, thermometer, or mechanical testing machine. Repeatability must also be established by repeated calibration by different individuals. Some machines may include automatic calibration techniques to reduce such errors.

Example: Mechanical Testing of Bone

Standard mechanical testing of whole cadaveric bone specimens and small animal bones, along with other tissue, is well established. These tests require pretest preparation and storage that may affect material properties. Investigators should be aware of the effect of different storage (i.e., formaldehyde versus saline versus buffered phosphate) and the effect of different freezing techniques and how these may bias the results. Mechanical properties may also change over time and with refreezing. Standardization of tests such as three-point and four-point bending will allow comparison of experimental findings with other research groups and previous studies. More recently, synthetic bones have been introduced with properties that aim to simulate their biological counterparts. These have the advantage of availability and ease of storage and handling, but researchers should be aware that selection bias may occur through imperfect simulation of biological materials.

54.2.4 Analytical and Interpretation Bias

Once an experiment has been performed, the data is collected, assimilated, checked for errors and omissions, and finally analyzed. There may be cases where it is judged that an experiment has not worked or produced an outlier. These require careful handling as post hoc exclusion may introduce analytical bias.

Reducing Analytical and Interpretation Bias

It is extremely important that the statistical methods and analysis are agreed during the design of the experiment. Rules should be developed to handle outliers and potential loss to follow-up. Ideally, an independent biostatistician should be involved in the analysis of the data. Care should be taken in particular with the use of complex multivariable modeling techniques and post hoc subgroup analysis. A researcher who has been involved with a study from its inception may not be able to dispassionately evaluate his or her findings.

When the results are written up for publication, interpretation is required. This interpretation encompasses acceptance or rejection of the null hypothesis, along with treatment effect. It is quite common to see statements such as "there was a difference, which was not statistically significant" and "there was a trend toward statistical significance." Both of these statements are often made by researchers who have not adequately defined the hypothesis under test and the conditions under which they will accept or reject the hypothesis.

Jargon Defined: Publication Bias

Publication bias occurs when studies that reject the null hypothesis (positive outcome) have a greater tendency to achieve publication than those who report no difference between groups.

Individual researchers can guard against publication bias by actively seeking to publish papers that do not show differences within groups, or that produce findings at odds with what was expected. The registration of trials with national and international registries can ensure that proper assessment can be made of the extent of publication bias in a particular area. Publication bias can influence the results of subsequent meta-analysis, with results skewed toward positive findings. Journal editors and reviewers also have a duty to consider these studies for publication, particularly if the studies are methodologically sound and all steps possible have been taken to reduce bias.

54.2.5 Reducing Bias through Guidelines

The reporting of animal and basic science research in the biomedical literature is recognized as being inadequate.

This situation has been compounded by the vast expansion in the number of papers published per year and an increase in the number of available techniques, with less recognition and reporting of the potential pitfalls. Serious omissions are regularly noted in the reporting of trial methodology and results.[1,2] A large number of trials failed to adequately describe randomization, blinding, or statistical analysis techniques, and should therefore be assumed to be subject to bias. The Animals in Research: Reporting In Vivo Experiments (ARRIVE) guidelines have been designed to provide guidance on what information to report when describing animal research.[5] This was based on the CONSORT statement. They include number, species, strain, gender, genetic background, housing and husbandry, and experimental, statistical, and analytical methods (including blinding and randomization).

54.3 Conclusion

Bias is highly prevalent throughout scientific research. Biomedical researchers require an awareness of all the potential sources of bias when they are designing, performing, analyzing, writing up, and submitting their experiments. The best guards against bias are the performance of prospective experiments, under controlled conditions, with adequate allocation concealment. Independent researchers may be required for protocol development, experimental techniques, and data analysis. The development of guidelines such as the ARRIVE guidelines will assist researchers in the planning and reporting of studies.

References

[1] Kilkenny C, Parsons N, Kadyszewski E et al. Survey of the quality of experimental design, statistical analysis and reporting of research using animals. PLoS ONE 2009; 4: e7824

[2] Watters MP, Goodman NW. Comparison of basic methods in clinical studies and in vitro tissue and cell culture studies reported in three anaesthesia journals. Br J Anaesth 1999; 82: 295–298

[3] Agabegi SS, Stern PJ. Bias in research. Am J Orthop (Belle Mead NJ) 2008;37–5:242–248

[4] Schulz KF, Grimes DA. Blinding in randomised trials: hiding who got what. Lancet 2002; 359: 696–700

[5] Kilkenny C, Browne WJ, Cuthill IC, Emerson M, Altman DG. Improving bioscience research reporting: the ARRIVE guidelines for reporting animal research. PLoS Biol 2010; 8: e1000412

Index

– glycosaminoglycan (GAG) content 221
– image acquisition 219, 221, *221*
– imaging coils 218, *219*, **219**, *220*
– magnetic field strengths **220**, *221*
– magnetic relaxation times **219**
– magnetic resonance spectroscopy (MRS) 220, *220*, 221, *221*
– multinuclear coils *220*, **220**
– phase coherence loss 219
– principles 218, *218*
– proton (spin) density weighting 219
– quality assurance 223, *223*
– quantitative 225
– signal to noise ratio (SNR) 220–221, *221*
– spin-lattice (longitudinal) relaxation time (T1) 219
– spin-spin (transverse) relaxation time (T2) 219
– T1 mapping **222**
– T1ρ imaging **224**
– T2 mapping, *see* T2 mapping
– ultra-small superparamagnetic particles of iron oxide (USPIO) **223**
multiplex ligation-dependent probe amplification 314
multiplex PCR 314
murine LLNA test 404
Murphy, J. M. 358
muscle regeneration 10
muscle stem cells *272*, **278**
muscle testing
– clinical relevance **114**
– musculoskeletal dynamics **113**, *114*
– strength clinical assessment **123**
musculoskeletal dynamics
– active angle reproduction test 114, *115*
– closed kinetic chain lower limb tasks **110**
– Codman's paradox **112**
– gait (walking) **110**
–– See also gait analysis
– gait (walking), clinical relevance **111**
– inverse dynamics, *see* inverse dynamics
– kinematics **110**
– kinetic chains **110**
– kinetics **110**
– motor unit action potential (electromyography) 110
– muscle testing 113, *114*
– muscle testing clinical relevance **114**
– open kinetic chain upper limb tasks **112**
– passive angle reproduction test 114
– passive movement threshold to detection 115
– proprioception assessment **114**
– proprioception assessment clinical relevance **115**

– shoulder joint 112–113, *113*
– single limb squats 112, *112*
– squats, dips 111, *112*
– stairs, step down *111*, **111**
–– See also stair climbing
– stairs, step down clinical relevance **111**
– tendinopathy 111
mutant proteins 252

N

nanoindentation 66
nanopores 247
nested PCR 314
New Ulm Differentiation Function 183, *184*, 187
Newton's second law 136
Newton-Euler equations 136
next-generation sequencing
– applications **247**
– by ligation **247**
– ion semiconductor 247
– nanopores 247
– overview **247**
– pyrosequencing 247
– reversible terminator 247
– single molecule real-time 247
Niemeyer, F. 187
Notch signaling 390
Nottingham Leg Extensor Power Rig 124, *125*
nucleic acid hybridization, *see* in situ hybridization

O

OAI database 227
OmniViz 317
one-way variance analysis 425, *425–426*
open reading frame 254
organ culture models
– definitions **288**
– dynamic 288, *289*
– joint harvesting *286*, 289
– overview **282**, **288**
– static 288, *289*
orthopedic biomechanics laboratory
– collaborations, partnerships 15
– finite element method 14
– functional tissue engineering 13
– imaging applications 13
– implant subsidence monitoring *14*
– in vitro biomechanical analysis 13, *14*
– in vivo biomechanical analysis 13
– infrastructure, equipment 15, *16*
– kinematics applications 13
– medical devices evaluation 13
– modeling and simulation computation analysis 13, *14*
– motion measurement 13, *14*
– optical systems applications 13
– research directions **12**

– robotics applications 13
– simulation software 15
osteoarthritis 225, *226*
osteomyelitis 343, **345**
osteopenia
– BMD values 205
– imaging 206
osteoporosis
– BMD values 205
– bone healing, animal models **337**
– imaging 206
Oxford Medical Research Council scale 124, *124*

P

parallel-plate fluid flow chamber studies *292*, **292**, 298
partial correlations 427, *428*
passive angle reproduction test 114
patellofemoral joint force magnitude *32*
Pauwels, F. 183
PCR
– allele-specific 313
– assembly 313
– hot-start 313
– methylation-specific 314
– multiplex 314
– nested 314
– overview *312*, **312**
– pulsatile fluid flow **295**
– quantitative **314**, *315*
– RT-PCR 314
– single-target single nucleotide polymorphism *318*, **318**
– step-down (touchdown) 314
Pearson's correlation coefficient 425, *427*
PECAM-1 immunohistochemistry *265*, **265**
pedobarography **118**, *119*
Pérez, M. 185
Perkin Elmer Life Sciences 317
Perlau, R. 114
phage hybrid vectors **249**
Photoshop technique *266*, *267*
PICO framework 2
pigs
– in animal research generally *329*, **330**, 331
– soft tissue models 356
pin-on-disk tribometer 89, *89*
pin-on-plate tribometer 89, *89*, 90, *90*
Pittenger, M. F. 274
plasmids **248**, 249
plate fixation 74
platelet-rich plasma (PRP) **379**, *381*, 391
plexus brachialis lesions 140, *142–143*
Poisson's ratio 170, *170*
poly (α-hydroxyacids) *372*
poly(1,4-butylene succinate) *372*
poly(acrylate)s *372*

poly(L-lactide-co-e-caprolactone) *372*
poly(propylene fumarate) *372*
poly(vinyl alcohol) *372*
polyetheretherketone, static testing 44
polymerase chain reaction, *see* PCR
polyphosphazene *372*
power output clinical assessment **124**, *125*
preclinical research, *see* evidence-based research
Prendergast, P. J. 183, 185
proprioception assessment **114**
proprioception assessment clinical relevance **115**
prostheses, implants
– articular cartilage repair models **353**
– implant-associated infections 347
– load profile development 39
– medical device validation case study *21*, **21**, *22*
– medical devices evaluation 13
– polymer scaffolds *372*
– prosthetic joint infections 347
– scaffolds 370
–– See also scaffolds
– soft tissue models 357–358
– subsidence monitoring *14*
– titanium implant coatings **370**
prostheses, implants biological evaluation
– abbreviations **396**, **403**
– animal testing 398
– animal tissues, derivatives testing 408
– bacterial reverse mutation test (Ames test) 406
– biocompatibility testing 397–398
– biological categorization **396**
– blood interactions testing (EN ISO 10993-4) **407**
– Blue Book Memorandum #G95-1 395, 400, *402*
– bridging approach 399
– carcinogenicity testing (EN ISO 10993-3) **407**
– chemical characterization of materials (EN ISO 10993-18) **403**
– chromosome aberration test 406
– closed patch test 404
– compliance 395
– cytotoxicity testing (EN ISO 10993-5) **403**
– developmental toxicity testing (EN ISO 10993-3) **407**
– EN ISO 10993 395, **396**, *397*
– EN ISO 10993-1 398, 400, *402*
– EN ISO 10993-2 409
– EN ISO 10993-12 399
– EN ISO 14971 397–398
– EN ISO 22442-1 408
– expert testimony summarization **408**